Cognitive Changes and the Aging Brain

Cognitive Changes and the Aging Brain

Edited by

Kenneth M. Heilman
Department of Neurology, University of Florida College of Medicine

Stephen E. Nadeau
Department of Neurology, University of Florida College of Medicine

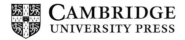

CAMBRIDGE
UNIVERSITY PRESS

University Printing House, Cambridge CB2 8BS, United Kingdom

One Liberty Plaza, 20th Floor, New York, NY 10006, USA

477 Williamstown Road, Port Melbourne, VIC 3207, Australia

314–321, 3rd Floor, Plot 3, Splendor Forum, Jasola District Centre, New Delhi – 110025, India

79 Anson Road, #06–04/06, Singapore 079906

Cambridge University Press is part of the University of Cambridge.

It furthers the University's mission by disseminating knowledge in the pursuit of education, learning, and research at the highest international levels of excellence.

www.cambridge.org
Information on this title: www.cambridge.org/9781108453608
DOI: 10.1017/9781108554350

First published 2020

Printed in the United Kingdom by TJ International Ltd. Padstow Cornwall

A catalogue record for this publication is available from the British Library.

Library of Congress Cataloging-in-Publication Data
Names: Heilman, Kenneth M., 1938– editor. | Nadeau, Stephen E., editor.
Title: Cognitive changes and the aging brain / edited by Kenneth M. Heilman, Stephen E. Nadeau.
Description: Cambridge, United Kingdom ; New York, NY : Cambridge University Press, 2020. | Includes bibliographical references and index.
Identifiers: LCCN 2019036972 (print) | LCCN 2019036973 (ebook) | ISBN 9781108453608 (paperback) | ISBN 9781108554350 (epub)
Subjects: MESH: Brain–physiology | Cognitive Aging | Cognitive Dysfunction | Neurodegenerative Diseases
Classification: LCC QP376 (print) | LCC QP376 (ebook) | NLM WL 300 | DDC 612.8/2–dc23
LC record available at https://lccn.loc.gov/2019036972
LC ebook record available at https://lccn.loc.gov/2019036973

ISBN 978-1-108-45360-8 Paperback

. . . .

This book is dedicated to Donald T. Stuss.

On September 3, 2019, Don died. He was 77. Only now have we learned that he wrote his wonderful chapter while he was terribly ill. This was vintage Don: brilliant and passionate scientist, dedicated educator, and the kindest of men to the very end.

Don's scientific work is legion: Over 200 peer-reviewed publications, over 50 book chapters, two editions of his landmark book, *Principles of Frontal Lobe Function*, two editions of *Cognitive Rehabilitation*, coedited with Gordon Winocur and Ian Robertson, and more than 300 presentations. His publications have been cited over 33,000 times. Early in his career, he worked with two of the founders of American neuropsychology, Frank Benson and Edith Kaplan. His major interest was always in the frontal lobes and executive functions. His creativity and scientific discipline made him a leader in this field for much of his life. One of his earliest papers, "Long-term effects of prefrontal leucotomy – an overview of neuropsychologic residuals," published in 1981, introduced the world to Don and signaled the new and highly productive approaches he was going to take. He also wrote papers about the neuropsychological effects of many different diseases that cause frontal lobe dysfunction, including head trauma, stroke, degenerative diseases, and aging. His curiosity led to studies of humor, memory, word finding, and emotions.

In addition to his creativity and scientific productivity, Don was an extraordinary teacher and mentor. He helped to train many notable neuropsychologists and neurologists.

A list of all Don's accomplishments as an administrator and leader would require several pages; however, most significantly, he was the founding Director of the Rotman Research Institute (1989–2008) and founding President and Scientific Director of the Ontario Brain Institute (2011–2015). His list of honors would also take more pages. Most notably, he was a Fellow of the Royal Society of Canada and received lifetime achievement awards from both the National Academy of Neuropsychology (2011) and the International Neuropsychological Society (2013).

Don was a kind man of gentle humor. The editors of this book and many other neuropsychologists and neurologists will miss our dear friend. His presence was a blessing and he left us with a treasure of knowledge. We feel particularly privileged to be able to include his chapter in this book.

Contents

Contributors

Nicole D. Anderson
Departments of Psychology & Psychiatry, University of Toronto and Rotman Research Institute, Baycrest Health Sciences, Toronto, Canada

Jolie D. Barter
Department of Neuroscience and McKnight Brain Institute, University of Florida, FL, USA

Russell M. Bauer
Brain Rehabilitation Research Center, Malcom Randall VA Medical Center, Departments of Clinical & Health Psychology and Neurology, University of Florida, FL, USA

Anjan Chatterjee
Department of Neurology, Perelman School of Medicine, University of Pennsylvania, PA, USA

Ronald A. Cohen
Center for Cognitive Aging and Memory, Evelyn F. McKnight Brain Institute and Department of Clinical and Health Psychology, University of Florida, FL, USA

Erin C. Conrad
Department of Neurology, Perelman School of Medicine, University of Pennsylvania, PA, USA

Fergus I. M. Craik
University of Toronto, Rotman Research Institute of Baycrest Centre, Toronto, Canada

Steven T. DeKosky
Department of Neurology and McKnight Brain Institute, University of Florida, FL, USA

Paul M. Dockree
School of Psychology and Institute of Neuroscience, Trinity College Dublin, University of Dublin, Dublin, Ireland

Kirk I. Erickson
Department of Psychology and Center for the Neural Basis of Cognition, University of Pittsburgh, PA, USA

Ira S. Fischler
Department of Psychology and Office of Research, University of Florida, FL, USA

Thomas C. Foster
Department of Neuroscience and Genetics and Genomics Program and McKnight Brain Institute, University of Florida, FL, USA

Joseph M. Gullett
Center for Cognitive Aging and Memory, Evelyn F. McKnight Brain Institute and Department of Clinical and Health Psychology, University of Florida, FL, USA

Kenneth M. Heilman
Geriatric Research, Education and Clinical Center at the Malcom Randal Veterans Affairs Medical Center Departments of Neurology and Clinical and Health Psychology, University of Florida, FL, USA

Gabrielle A. Hromas
Departments of Clinical & Health Psychology and Neurology, University of Florida, FL, USA

Glenn J. Larrabee
Independent Practice in Forensic Neuropsychology, Sarasota, FL, USA

Stephen E. Nadeau
Research Service and the Brain Rehabilitation Research Center, Malcom Randall VA Medical Center Department of Neurology, University of Florida College of Medicine, FL, USA

Jamie C. Peven
Department of Psychology and Center for the
Neural Basis of Cognition, University of Pittsburgh,
PA, USA

Eric Porges
Center for Cognitive Aging and Memory
Evelyn F. McKnight Brain Institute and Department
of Clinical and Health Psychology, University of
Florida, FL, USA

Ian H. Robertson
Global Brain Health Institute, Institute of
Neuroscience, Trinity College Dublin, University of
Dublin, Dublin, Ireland

Edmund T. Rolls
Oxford Centre for Computational Neuroscience,
Oxford, UK

Yat-Fung Shea
Department of Medicine, LKS Faculty of Medicine
Queen Mary Hospital, University of Hong Kong,
Hong Kong

Jennifer J. Stamps
Trait Biosciences, Los Alamos, NM, USA

Chelsea M. Stillman
Department of Psychology and Center for the Neural
Basis of Cognition, University of Pittsburgh, PA, USA

Donald T. Stuss
University of Toronto, Rotman Research Institute of
Baycrest Centre, Toronto, Canada

Erin Trifilio
Department of Clinical and Health Psychology,
University of Florida, FL, USA

John B. Williamson
Department of Psychiatry, University of Florida,
FL, USA

Gordon Winocur
Rotman Research Institute, Baycrest Health Sciences,
Toronto, Canada
Department of Psychology, Trent University, Ontario,
Canada
Departments of Psychology & Psychiatry, University
of Toronto, Toronto, Canada

Anthony T. Yachnis
Department of Pathology, Immunology, and
Laboratory Medicine,
University of Florida College of Medicine, FL, USA

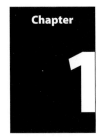

Introduction

Kenneth M. Heilman and Stephen E. Nadeau

In America today, there are 46 million people over the age of 65 and there will be over 98 million by 2060. With aging, there are many neurological diseases that can adversely affect the brain, such as Alzheimer's disease, Lewy body dementia, and Parkinson's disease. These diseases are common and a major cause of disability and suffering. Although, in a small percentage of patients, these diseases can be related to a genetic defect, for the most part we do not fully understand their causes. Perhaps that is why they are called "degenerative diseases." Several decades ago, the diagnosis of Alzheimer's disease was made only in those who were below the age of 65 and had signs of progressive dementia. If a person had cognitive deterioration and was above the age of 65, their disorder was called "senile dementia." One of the reasons this term was used is that many clinicians thought memory loss and cognitive decline were part of normal aging. Fortunately, we have learned that disorders such as Alzheimer's disease are associated with specific pathological changes in the brain, such as neurofibrillary tangles, and that normal aging does not cause this disease. Although the origins of these degenerative brain diseases are still unclear, much progress has been made in understanding their pathophysiology, thereby helping to pave the way for preventative, ameliorative, and curative treatments.

In the absence of any brain disease, from the time we are born until the time we die, our brains are continuously changing. These changes alter many brain functions such that with maturation there is growth and with aging deterioration. Neuroscientists and clinicians who treat brain disorders have three interrogative pronouns they often use in approaching such matters: how, why, and what? How does the brain change with aging and how do these changes affect us? Why does it change? What can be done about these changes? The goal of this book is to try to address these how, why, and what questions.

The word "cognition" comes from the Latin verb *cognosco*, which is a cognate of the Greek verb γι(γ)νώσκω, gi(g)nósko, meaning, "I know." This book is about the effects of aging on cognition, but it is not limited to our ability to know and learn. It also about the influence of aging on sensory perception, creativity, emotions and moods, action programming, and executive functions such as planning, initiating, monitoring, controlling, and completing.

There are many different organizing principles of cognitive function, and in the last two centuries we have learned much about them. One of the most basic principles is that brain processes are organized in a modular fashion. The concept of modularity or localization of specialized functions dates back to the early part of the nineteenth century. Franz Joseph Gall, the founder of phrenology, proposed that different regions of the brain are important for mediating different cognitive functions. Gall also proposed that the larger and more developed a module, the better the performance. Although Gall's postulates generated the pseudoscience of phrenology, in which the shape and size of the skull, quantified through caliper measurements, were thought to indicate an individual's personality and mental abilities, his postulates of modularity and size have received scientific support.

Support for the modularity hypothesis first came from Paul Broca, a French physician and anthropologist, who was strongly influenced by a lecture given by Ernest Aubertin. Aubertin and his father-in-law, Jean-Baptiste Bouillard, were students of Gall. Aubertin believed that speech is mediated by the frontal lobes. After hearing that lecture, Paul Broca reported the case of Louis Victor Leborgne, a patient who had a history of speech loss and a right hemiplegia [1]. Broca noted that, although Leborgne was unable to speak or write, he was able to understand spoken language, a dissociation of two language–speech functions. Leborgne died and a postmortem examination revealed that he had a discrete lesion localized in his left hemisphere, primarily in the inferior portion of the frontal lobe, but also extending to the anterior temporal lobe and deep into the cerebral white matter. The inability of this patient to speak was, according to Broca, caused by a disorder of the special faculty of articulated language [1]. In a subsequent paper published in 1865, Broca described several other patients who had an aphasia associated with a right hemiplegia [2]. Based on these observations of laterality, Broca concluded that in humans, the left hemisphere primarily mediates speech. These observations provided additional evidence of brain modularity.

Double dissociations provide even greater evidence of modularity. In 1864, Carl Wernicke wrote "Der Aphasische Symptomencomplex," describing patients who, unlike the nonfluent patients Broca described, were fluent. In addition, unlike patients with Broca's aphasia, those that Wernicke described exhibited a severe comprehension disorder [3]. Furthermore, whereas patients with Broca's aphasia have anterior perisylvian lesions maximally involving the frontal lobe, patients with Wernicke's aphasia have posterior perisylvian lesions that extensively involve the superior temporal lobe. In Wernicke's important paper, in addition to describing a form of aphasia and its localization, he also introduced the concept of an information-processing network. He suggested that the area that contains the memories of how words sound, located in the left posterior temporal lobe (now called Wernicke's area), is connected to and provides information to the area where the articulation of words is programmed (now called Broca's area).

The second part of Gall's hypothesis, bigger is better, was supported by a study by Geschwind and Levitsky [4]. They reported that the posterior superior temporal lobe, which includes Wernicke's area, is often larger in the left than in the right hemisphere. In addition, Foundas et al. [5] reported that right-handed people with left hemisphere dominance for speech also have a larger left pars triangularis, which is part of Broca's area.

The reasons why certain areas of the cerebral cortex store different forms of information and perform different mental operations are now fairly well understood. By far the most important reason is patterns of connectivity. This can be illustrated with some examples. The daily business of neurons in auditory association cortices is the processing of acoustic input. In the left hemisphere, to a greater extent than in the right, the daily business of neurons in Broca's area is to translate input into spoken words. The network of connections between auditory association cortex and Broca's area, including Wernicke's area and the supramarginal gyrus, in the course of language learning, acquires knowledge of the orderly relationships between acoustic phonological sequences and spoken articulatory sequences. Unimodal and polymodal association cortices acquire knowledge of the world and the objects within it through the repeated sensory input that underlies perception. Connectivity between both unimodal and polymodal association cortices and the perisylvian phonological cortex entrains phonological processing to semantic knowledge. Analogous principles of cortical connectivity apply to all components of language function, including syntax and grammatical morphology. The connectivity principle extends to other regions of the brain. The major inputs to the frontal lobes are sensory (relayed from postcentral association cortices to dorsolateral frontal cortex) and limbic (relayed from limbic structures to the orbitofrontal cortex). The major output of the frontal lobes is to the motor cortex. Thus, prefrontal cortex is predestined by its connectivity patterns to acquire knowledge that enables the translation of sensory and limbic input into orderly plans for action. The fact that frontal-postcentral connectivity is bidirectional conveys additional capacities for working memory and volitional attention that are essential to optimization of information processing and to thinking.

In the preceding paragraph, we spoke of the daily business of neurons in auditory association cortex being the processing of acoustic input. This leads us to another way of understanding regional cortical function – in terms of the position of a region in a trajectory of sensory or motor projections. Thus, primary auditory cortex (Heschl's gyrus) projects to primary and secondary auditory association cortices (superior temporal gyrus and the planum temporale); primary visual cortex (calcarine cortex) projects to primary (occipital and posterior temporal lobes) and secondary visual association cortices (lateral and ventral temporal lobes and parietal lobes); and primary somatosensory cortex (postcentral gyrus) projects to primary and secondary somatosensory association areas (parietal lobes). Sensory association cortices project to polymodal/supramodal cortical regions (angular and supramarginal gyri, Brodmann's area 7 in the superior parietal lobes, the cingulate gyrus, the temporal poles, prefrontal cortex, and the hippocampal system). In the frontal lobes, premotor cortex can usefully be thought of as an association area for motor cortex. These association cortices serve simultaneously as data repositories (long-term memories – knowledge and skills) and data processors. While the idea of projection trajectories is a useful one, it must be borne in mind that within the cortex, connections are reciprocal (two-way). Thus, one cortical region does not send information to another cortical region – it elicits a pattern of neural activity in the connected region, and, through rapid back-and-forth exchange, the two regions (and other connected regions) settle into optimal or quasi-optimal patterns of activity corresponding to attractor states (a recurring theme in this book).

The concept of neural networks, first articulated by Wernicke, is implicit in connectivity principles. Modern imaging techniques seek evidence of anatomic connectivity by measuring functional connectivity – to which there are innumerable references in this book. This is a worthy enterprise provided that one bears in mind that functional connectivity may be state-dependent (e.g., motor cortex supports the representation of movements but also of a component of movement verbs), and that covariance in the activity of neurons in different regions of the brain may be produced not just by their connectivity but also by slowly recurring changes in the electrocortical rhythms in which they are simultaneously engaged.

Although the modularity of cortical function is defined by connectivity patterns, we have only incipient knowledge of the hows and whys of neuronal processing in any given region and essentially no knowledge of the basis for individual differences. Two questions may be asked: (1) What is the fundamental nature of the computational processing that takes place? and (2) How does the cytoarchitecture of a given cortical region endow it with certain, presumably optimal, processing capabilities given its particular functional specialty? Edmund Rolls (Chapter 14) provides some insight into the current state of the science bearing on question one. We have long had tantalizing clues on how to address question two but so far have not been able to make much sense of them.

At the beginning of the twentieth century, Brodmann discovered that the human cerebral cortex has six layers. He also found enormous variation in the thickness and cellular organization of different regions of the cortex. From analysis of microscopic and macroscopic features, Brodmann divided the cortex into a total of 52 areas [6]. Brodmann postulated that the structural differences between cortical regions had to do with differences in their functions. Undoubtedly this is true but, so far, the relationship between structure and function remains largely opaque with limited exceptions, e.g., the extraordinary thickness of layer 4 in calcarine cortex, reflecting the enormous afferent input from the lateral geniculate nuclei conveying visual input.

To perform their functions, neurons have to communicate – entraining each other in patterns of activity. The means of communication is primarily chemical and is achieved through the release of neurotransmitters. Some neurotransmitters provide the basis for data processing, e.g., glutamate (excitatory) and γ-aminobutyric acid (GABA, inhibitory). Others are best regarded as regulatory (acetylcholine, dopamine, norepinephrine, epinephrine, serotonin, and histamine) or modulatory (e.g., endorphins, somatostatin, neuropeptide-Y, and substance P). The brain also contains glia. These are cells that are not neurons but have many important functions in the brain, including providing physical support of neuronal structures, cleaning up after neurons through uptake of potentially toxic materials (e.g., glutamate), maintaining the blood-brain barrier, and forming myelin (the critical insulation around the axons of neurons).

With healthy aging, many changes take place in the brain. These may affect neurons, neural connectivity, neurotransmitter systems, and glia. They may affect some brain regions more than others. For example, the frontal lobes are heavily dependent on connectivity with posterior association areas, the medial dorsal thalamus, the basal ganglia, and limbic structures (e.g., the amygdala, lateral septal nuclei, the insula, the periaqueductal gray, and the nucleus solitarius). Thus, when there is degradation of white matter, frontal lobe functions may be differentially impaired.

This book begins with reviews of aging-related changes in anatomy and physiology. Chapter 4 reviews aging-related changes revealed by imaging studies and, thereby, starts the bridge linking anatomic alterations associated with aging to changes in cognitive functions. Subsequent chapters review aging-related alterations in cognitive functions, including memory, language, motor planning, attention, executive functions, emotions, and creativity. Chapter 5 includes some review of changes in vision that may contribute to disorders of visual perception. Chapter 8 provides references to the large literature on aging-related changes in auditory function. Olfaction is reviewed in Chapter 6. There are certainly aging-related changes in somatosensory functions, but our limited knowledge of their relevance to cognitive functions did not seem to justify a separate chapter.

From the outset of this project, we encouraged authors to think strongly about potential mechanisms. Of course, because of the limitations of existing science, many of the mechanisms elucidated are at best tentative hypotheses. A startling number of mechanisms emerged, as well as a number of recurring mechanistic themes.

There are many means by which aging-related changes can be studied. The vast majority of the studies discussed are cross-sectional, which means that attribution of the differences they reveal to a process that extends across the life span requires an inference that the differences observed do not reflect an incipient degenerative process. Cross-sectional studies that involve more than two age groups can help to confirm such an inference. Longitudinal studies, in principle, can provide the most definitive evidence of changes associated with an aging process, as opposed to incipient dementia, but these studies also have problems, including duration, expense, practice effects, and population attrition. In this book, we encouraged use of the term "aging-related" when we

believed that the preponderance of evidence suggested that the primary mechanism inducing a change was related to aging. Readers should be aware, however, that this is not necessarily a correct conclusion, particularly as it is a challenge to completely rule out the effects of an incipient disease process.

The final chapters discuss what can potentially be done to slow or reverse aging-related decline of cognitive functions, including the role of exercise, cognitive rehabilitation, and the use of pharmacological agents. We now have overwhelming evidence of the protective effect of cognitive reserve in delaying and even preventing dementia. The elucidation of specific mechanisms associated with aging-related cognitive decline, many potentially amenable to treatment (reviewed in Chapter 15), coupled with existing evidence of the value of some interventions (reviewed in Chapters 16–19), may provide pathways to increasing cognitive reserve. Hence, the last chapter of this book: "Preventing Cognitive Decline and Dementia."

We hope that the knowledge gained from reading this book about brain aging may help to differentiate normal aging from brain diseases, reduce the adverse effects of brain aging, provide some assurance to those of us approaching late life that declining episodic memory and anomia are not necessarily symptoms of incipient dementia, and, optimistically, lead to further research on how the adverse effects of brain aging can be reversed, stopped, modified, or best managed.

References

1. Broca P. Remarques sur le siege de la faculte du language articule, suivies d'une observation d'aphemie. *Bulletin de la Societe d'Anthropologie.* 1861;2:330–57.

2. Broca P. Sur le siege de la faculte du langage articule. *Bulletin de la Societe d'Anthropologie.* 1865;6:337–93.

3. Wernicke C. Der Aphasische Symptomenkomplex (Trans.). *Boston Stud Phil Sci.* 1874;4:34–97.

4. Geschwind N, Levitsky W. Human brain: left-right asymmetries in temporal speech region. *Science.* 1968;161:186–7.

5. Foundas AL, Leonard CM, Gilmore RL, Fennell EB, Heilman KM. Pars triangularis asymmetry and language dominance. *Proceedings of the National Academy of Sciences USA.* 1996;93:719–22.

6. Brodmann K. *Vergleichende Lokalisationslehre der Grosshirnrinde in ihren Prinzipien dargestellt auf Grund des Zellenbaues.* Leipzig: Barth; 1909.

Anatomic and Histological Changes of the Aging Brain

Anthony T. Yachnis

1 Introduction

The purpose of this chapter is to describe gross (macroscopic) and microscopic changes that occur in the aging brain. An expert in neurodegenerative disease once said: "Aging is a terminal illness." This leads to a philosophical question: Is there "normal" aging? One might ask if aging is a pathological process that involves changes resulting from less effective genetic regulation of critical brain functions that leads to reduced or less effective protein synthesis, processing, and catabolism. If such changes are mild or limited, the patient may experience "age-related" memory impairment, mild cognitive issues, or could have normal neurologic function. More severe changes may result in the more debilitating signs and symptoms of a neurodegenerative disease. Just as neurodegenerative diseases are now considered "proteinopathies," characterized by dysregulation of Aβ-amyloid, hyperphosphorylation of tau, or nuclear to cytoplasmic translocation of TDP-43, one might consider, to some extent, reduced metabolic function over a person's lifetime as a "proteinopathy of aging." As such, in this chapter no attempt at a rigid definition will be made nor will the term "normal aging" be used since neuropathological changes such cerebral atrophy, neuritic plaques, and neurofibrillary tangles can be found in the brains of elderly individuals who are not cognitively impaired or demented [1–5]. On the other hand, recent studies have suggested that patients may live to advanced age without accumulation of Aβ-amyloid-containing neuritic plaques or only low Braak stages of neuritic plaques [6].

The chapter begins with a brief overview of gross changes seen in association with human aging and then will consider general histological changes seen in neurons and glia. Aging-related white matter changes are commonly observed on neuroimaging studies, and histopathological correlates, including small vessel cerebrovascular changes, will be considered.

Brain arteriolosclerosis and its relationship to "hippocampal sclerosis of aging" – now called "cerebral age-related TDP43 and sclerosis" (CARTS) – will be covered. The accumulation of brain amyloid without tau or other neuropathologies, called "pathological aging," will be discussed along with a review of more recently described conditions that occur during aging such as "primary age-related tauopathy" and "aging-related tau astrogliopathy."

2 Brain Weight and Patterns of Atrophy in Aging

The weight and volume of the brain change throughout life. A peak of brain weight is reached during the third and fourth decades of life, after which a slow decline occurs [7]. It has been estimated that the brain undergoes a 0.1–0.2% per year reduction in volume between the ages of 30 and 50 years, and after age 70, brain volume decreases by 0.3–0.5% per year [8]. These volume reductions involve both gray and white matter. Some studies suggest that cerebral cortical volume is reduced by 9% between the years of 30 and 70 [9]. More recent MRI data confirm CNS volume reductions with a corresponding increase in ventricular volume with normal aging, with the biggest changes observed in the frontal and temporal cortex, putamen, thalamus, and nucleus accumbens [10]. White matter volume steadily increases into the 50s but by age 70, it has declined by 6%, and by age 80, by about 40% relative to age 20 volumes [11].

Aging-related changes observed on gross examination of postmortem brains include mild sulcal widening, gyral narrowing, and mild blunting of the lateral ventricular angles (Figure 2.1). Brain weights are quite variable in the aging population with a normal range of about 1150–1450 g. While brains weighing less than 1100 g often have histological changes associated with neurodegenerative disease,

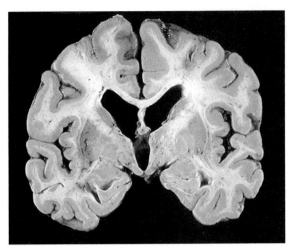

Figure 2.1 Gross coronal section at a mammillary body level showing symmetrical ventriculomegaly with blunting of the lateral ventricular angles. There is mild widening of the sulci, especially in insular regions.

there are many individuals with brain weights that fall within the "normal" range who also have evidence of significant neurodegenerative disease. Significant atrophy of the frontal and temporal lobes and atrophy of the hippocampus with corresponding widening of the temporal horns tend to correlate with a neurodegenerative process.

These gross changes have for many years been assumed to correlate with age-related neuronal loss. Studies attempting to quantitate cell loss during aging are difficult and inherently biased because of the need to define precise anatomical boundaries for counting and the confounding effects of multiple co-morbidities. However, the use of stereologic methods has enabled accurate estimates of neuronal loss. Stereologic studies in humans have estimated that about 10% of cortical neurons are lost throughout the entire life span [7]. However, other studies suggest that neuronal loss or lack thereof may be region specific. For example, there is little to no detectable neuronal loss in the normal aging brain in certain areas such as the superior temporal gyrus, entorhinal cortex, and the putamen [12]. Areas showing subtle age-related neuronal loss may include the hippocampal CA1, subiculum, and substantia nigra [13–15]. Adult neurogenesis, known to occur in locations such as the fascia dentata of the hippocampus, may to some extent offset age-related neuronal loss [16]. Although pathobiologic mechanisms of neuronal loss in aging are still poorly understood, one recent study using single cell whole genome sequencing identified an increase in somatic mutations in individual neurons [17]. Aging-related somatic mutations of individual neurons in the human prefrontal cortex and hippocampus increase roughly linearly with age, especially in the hippocampus [17].

Changes in neurocognitive functions with aging may relate to alterations in the prefrontal cortex [18]. The cytoarchitecture of the prefrontal cortex features mini-columns of neurons (radial arrays of pyramidal neurons traversing laminae II–VI) that have connections with many cortical regions, including the posterior parietal cortex, as well as the striatum and thalamus [19]. These interconnected pathways, in addition to connections with the cingulate gyrus, may serve to mediate executive functions, such as coordination of thought and behavioral goals. Disruptions of mini-columnar processing are implicated in a number of disorders including autism, depression, schizophrenia, drug addiction, and dementia [18]. With aging and in neurodegenerative diseases, the width of mini-columns in the dorsolateral prefrontal cortex is reduced ("mini-column thinning") and one morphometric study showed a relationship between mini-columnar width and IQ decline [20]. An emerging model of Alzheimer's disease pathophysiology suggests that aging-related mini-columnar thinning in the prefrontal and temporal lobe neocortices precedes the mini-columnar degeneration that occurs with onset of dementia [21, 22].

3 General Histological Changes in Neurons and Glia Associated with Aging

The most common age-related neuronal change is the accumulation of lipochrome pigment (lipofuscin) [23–26]. Lipofuscin represents long-term storage of neuronal lysosomal degradation products from the cytoskeleton, cell membrane, mitochondria, and other cellular material. The yellow-brown granular pigment accumulates in the neuronal cytoplasm, often displacing the Nissl substance and other cytoplasmic constituents (Figure 2.2). While many neuronal types accumulate lipofuscin, large neurons of the cerebellar dentate nuclei, globus pallidus, inferior olivary nuclei, anterior horns of the spinal cord, and the brainstem are most prominently affected [27]. Although lipofuscin accumulation is most commonly encountered as a nonspecific reactive change associated with aging, widespread accumulation of

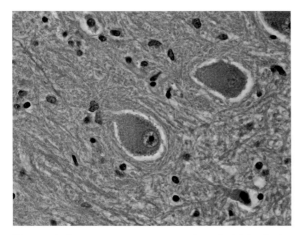

Figure 2.2 Two neurons containing granular yellowish lipofuscin pigment (dentate nucleus of cerebellum). A black and white version of this figure will appear in some formats. For the color version, please refer to the plate section.

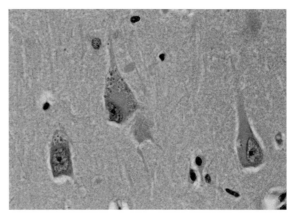

Figure 2.3 Three CA1 neurons showing granulovacuolar degeneration (H&E stain). A black and white version of this figure will appear in some formats. For the color version, please refer to the plate section.

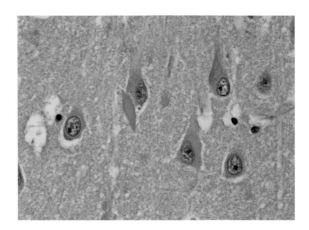

Figure 2.4 Hirano body: eosinophilic rod-shaped structure in close proximity to a hippocampal pyramidal neuron (H&E stain). A black and white version of this figure will appear in some formats. For the color version, please refer to the plate section.

lipochrome pigment occurs in the familial and metabolic cerebral lipofuscinoses, a group of neurodegenerative, lysosomal storage disorders that often induce motor and cognitive disabilities.

Neurons containing tau-positive neurofibrillary tangles (NFT) may be found in the locus coeruleus in patients as young as the teenage years [28, 29]. Widespread NFTs are typical of Alzheimer's disease and the tauopathies, including progressive supranuclear palsy, corticobasal degeneration, and some of the frontotemporal dementias, as well as chronic traumatic encephalopathy. However, a subset of elderly individuals, usually 85 years or older, have NFTs in the mesial temporal region with little or no associated amyloid plaques and yet are cognitively normal or have only mild cognitive changes. This condition is called "primary age-related tauopathy" (PART) [30]. It remains controversial whether this alteration represents a common feature of advanced age or an early stage of Alzheimer-like neuropathology. PART will be discussed further in this chapter under its own topic heading.

Granulovacuolar degeneration and Hirano bodies are two other neuronal changes that increase with aging and are more prominent in neurodegenerative diseases [7, 27]. Granulovacuolar degeneration (of Simchowicz, granulovacuolar bodies) occurs most commonly in hippocampal pyramidal cell neurons of CA1 and in the subiculum (Figure 2.3). Granulovacuolar bodies are cytoplasmic (autophagosomal) vacuoles that measure about 3–5 microns. Each of

these vacuoles contains a 1–2 micron dense core that is composed of tubulin, neurofilament proteins, and tau. They are strongly immunoreactive for TDP-43. Granulovacuolar degeneration is especially striking in Alzheimer's disease and in the frontotemporal dementias, in which it can affect other brain regions, including the amygdala and the nucleus basalis of Meynert [27]. Hirano bodies are eosinophilic rod-like structures seen on routine hematoxylin and eosin stains (Figure 2.4) and, like granulovacuolar degeneration, occur in hippocampal sector CA1 and the subiculum. They have a paracrystalline lattice-like "herringbone" structure when viewed by electron microscopy and are composed of actin and alpha-actinin [27]. Hirano bodies lie within the neuron cell body or its processes. They may develop with normal aging but are increased in people with Alzheimer's disease, frontotemporal dementias like Pick's disease, and prion diseases.

Marinesco bodies are eosinophilic intranuclear inclusions that arise in pigmented neurons of the substantia nigra and locus coeruleus. They are between 2 and 10 microns in diameter. While Marinesco bodies are of little clinical significance in aging, some have noted a similarity of these proteinaceous inclusions to those found in neuronal intranuclear inclusion disease of childhood.

A variety of nonspecific, reactive-like changes occur in astrocytes with aging. The astrocytic cytoskeletal intermediate filament protein glial fibrillary acidic protein (GFAP) has been shown to increase with aging [31]. Increased GFAP may be part of what has been termed a "senescence-associated secretory phenotype" that refers to elevated expression of various brain-related cytokines and the accumulation of proteotoxic aggregates during aging-related senescence of astrocytes [32]. Thorn-shaped astrocytes containing hyperphosporylated forms of tau accumulate with aging with about 50% of individuals having this change by the eighth decade [33]. In fact, a range of tau-related astrocytic changes has been recently grouped under the term "aging-related tau astrogliopathy" (ARTAG) [34]. This will also be discussed below under a separate heading.

Corpora amylacea are probably the most common aging-related change of astrocytes. They are spherical intracytoplasmic bodies [27] that have no pathological significance. They are rare in children under age 10 years but increase with age and are invariably found in individuals over age 40. These 5–20 micron diameter basophilic structures have a concentric lamellated appearance (Figure 2.5) and are located in subpial, perivascular, and subependymal regions. Corpora amylacea are frequent at the base of the brain, including the olfactory tracts, and are common in the medial region of the lentiform nuclei, posterior columns of the spinal cord, and in the white matter adjacent to the caudal extent of the occipital horns of the lateral ventricles. They are strongly PAS-positive amorphous structures that are composed of glycogen-polymers ("polyglucosan bodies"). Although these structures are considered a nonspecific reactive change of astrocytes, patients with mutations of the *GNE1* gene lose a critical glycogen debranching

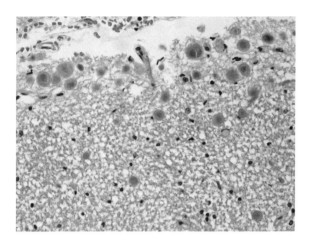

Figure 2.5 Corpora amylacea: 5–20 micron in diameter basophilic entities that are concentric lamellated structures commonly located in subpial, perivascular, and subependymal regions (H&E stain). A black and white version of this figure will appear in some formats. For the color version, please refer to the plate section.

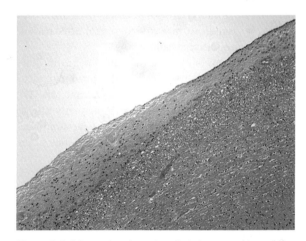

Figure 2.6 Subependymal reactive gliosis (center and lower left of image) that occurred in an area of ependymal denudation (H&E stain). A black and white version of this figure will appear in some formats. For the color version, please refer to the plate section.

enzyme that results in widespread accumulation of corpora amylacea in the central and peripheral nervous systems [35].

The ependymal lining of the ventricular system undergoes focal denudation during aging and this lining is not capable of regeneration. Since ependymal cells are not replaced, a subependymal glial nodule or scar forms at the site of their loss (Figure 2.6). In some areas of cell loss, residual ependymal cells can form reactive rosette-like structures.

Oligodendrocytes generate and maintain myelin sheaths on larger diameter axons, thereby enabling rapid neurotransmission. Degeneration or dysfunction results in local interruption in formation and maintenance of myelin (demyelination), resulting in impaired or blocked impulse conduction along these axons. Neuropathological data on oligodendrocyte changes with aging are limited. However, ultrastructural studies in nonhuman primates reveal degenerative changes, such as localized splitting of the major dense line of myelin and ballooning and reduplication of myelin sheaths [36]. Such changes could affect conduction velocities and may play a role in cognitive decline with aging. Several studies suggest that myelin production by oligodendrocytes may be less efficient with aging, resulting in thinner myelin sheaths and shorter internodes [11, 37].

Microglia are resident histiocytes of the central nervous system that interface with the immune system. Activation results in morphologic transformation to so-called pleomorphic microglia (or "rod-cell" microglia), which respond to low-grade, incomplete necrosis, and chronic infections. Pleomorphic microglia are capable of ingesting destroyed nerve cell fragments ("neuronophagia") and myelin. Transformation into fully developed macrophages occurs with acute, severe tissue destruction, and with active demyelination. Reactive macrophages in the brain arise not only from tissue microglia but also from circulating monocytes.

During aging, microglia display evidence of activation, especially in the white matter. Animal models and postmortem studies in humans show increased expression of class II histocompatibility antigens [38]. It is possible that changes in the microglia with aging may lead to "immune senescence" that increases susceptibility to neurodegeneration, much as decreased immune function in older individuals increases susceptibility to certain forms of neoplasia. This concept has been extensively reviewed elsewhere [39, 40].

4 Mitochondria in CNS Aging

Despite accounting for but 2% of total body weight, the human brain is highly energy consuming and requires 20% of the body's oxygen supply for normal function. Oxygen is utilized to produce ATP during the last step of oxidative phosphorylation in the mitochondria. On one hand, mitochondria provide energy for all fundamental CNS functions, including maintenance of cellular homeostasis and ion balances,

propagation of action potentials, neurotransmitter synthesis, neurotransmitter release (the most energy-consuming activity of all and the chief source of signal in fMRI and fluoro-deoxyglucose PET studies), synaptic plasticity, and cell survival. On the other hand, mitochondria are a source for reactive oxygen species (ROS) that can be harmful when produced in excess or when inadequately counteracted by cellular defenses provided by the superoxide dismutase (SOD) and glutathione systems [41] (see Chapter 3). There is evidence that the balance between energy production and the removal of potentially harmful ROS is altered with brain aging. For example, postmortem studies reveal that there is a progressive increase in protein nitration and oxidation by ROS with increasing age, especially in the hippocampus and frontal cortex [42]. This observation is supported by investigations in living patients showing a gradual decline in glutathione with aging [43]. Regional subcellular susceptibility of mitochondria is suggested by animal studies showing that mitochondria located at synapses are more sensitive to age-related changes in oxygen consumption and calcium metabolism [41]. The ability of mitochondria to proliferate or fuse according to cellular metabolic demands is altered with aging, resulting in the appearance of abnormal interconnected mitochondria in ultrastructural studies [41]. The removal of damaged mitochondria ("mitophagy") may also occur with aging. Although mechanisms of aging-related mitochondrial dysfunction are incompletely understood, the accumulation of mitochondrial DNA mutations may be a contributing factor [41].

5 White Matter Changes with Aging

MRI studies demonstrate "leukoaraiosis" – punctate and, in some cases, confluent areas of increased T2 signal in the deep white matter on T2-weighted MRI scans and diminished signal on CT scans. Leukoaraiosis becomes more prevalent with increasing age. It will be more completely described in Chapter 4. Histological correlates of leukoaraiosis may include pallor of white matter staining on H&E or Luxol fast blue stains, especially in periventricular regions [44]. Fibrous thickening of the walls of small veins in periventricular regions commonly occurs with aging and is referred to as "venous collagenosis" [45]. More widespread aging-related vascular changes, collectively referred to as "small vessel cerebrovascular disease" (discussed below), could degrade the blood–brain barrier [46] by interrupting the articulation between astrocytic end processes and brain capillary endothelial cells [32, 47], thereby degrading the capacity for maintenance of cerebral fluid balance.

Loss or degeneration of axons is another prominent change in the white matter during aging [48, 49]. In a randomly selected group of patients without neurodegenerative disease, it was estimated that a 45% reduction in large myelinated axons occurs between the ages of 20 and 80 years [11]. It is not clear how much of this is due to axonal loss and how much is due to demyelination [37]. Considering estimates of a 10% loss of cortical neurons throughout life [7, 50], it follows that axonal loss during aging results from failure of the neuronal cell body to support and maintain the axon and its functions. Possible reasons for this axonal loss include a decline in axonal protein homeostatic functions ("proteostasis"), which include protein synthesis, folding, transport, secretion, and degradation [49]. These processes are dependent on many different molecular pathways that maintain cellular homeostasis and quality control, including the heat shock response, ubiquitin-proteasome system, autophagy, and the endoplasmic reticulum–associated degradation pathway.

6 Vascular Changes in the Aging Brain

Large vessel atherosclerosis that affects the cerebral basal vasculature occurs with aging and is associated with well-known risk factors, including smoking, hypercholesterolemia, diabetes, hypertension, and inactivity. Small vessel cerebrovascular disease–like changes, characterized by arterial hyalinization and widened perivascular spaces, sometimes containing hemosiderin (Figure 2.7), may occur with aging in the absence of these risk factors. Such changes are typically found in the lenticulostriate branches of the middle cerebral artery, which supply the basal ganglia and the deep white matter. Small vessel changes are usually associated with a clinical history of diabetes or hypertension. However, one large autopsy study found that this association held true only for patients who died before the age of 80 years [51]. Small vessel cerebrovascular disease that affects cerebral arterioles in healthy elderly people, typically 80 years of age or older, has been described under the term "brain arteriolosclerosis" (B-ASC) [52]. Arteriolosclerosis may have a genetic association (*ABCC9*) that links it to "hippocampal sclerosis of

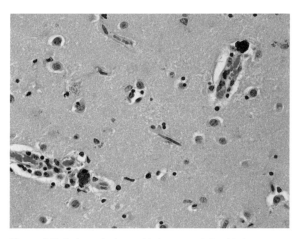

Figure 2.7 Perivascular hemosiderin accumulation (dark concretions – bottom left and top right) seen frequently in the basal ganglia with aging (H&E stain). A black and white version of this figure will appear in some formats. For the color version, please refer to the plate section.

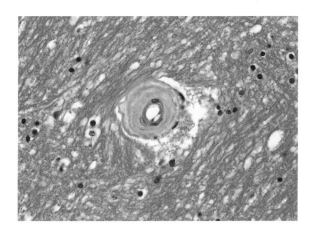

Figure 2.8 Arteriolosclerosis, hyaline type, of a small deep penetrating white matter blood vessel (H&E stain). A black and white version of this figure will appear in some formats. For the color version, please refer to the plate section.

aging" (discussed below) [53]. B-ASC is histologically heterogeneous and may be characterized by intimal fibromuscular proliferation ("hyperplastic type") or by the presence of amorphous, non-amyloid containing material in the arteriolar wall ("hyaline type") (Figure 2.8) [52]. There may be degenerative changes in arteriolar walls, including calcification, and occasionally multiple profiles of arterioles may appear within the same plane of section (Figure 2.9). The latter finding could be due to vascular ectasia with increased tortuosity [52]. Other vascular changes

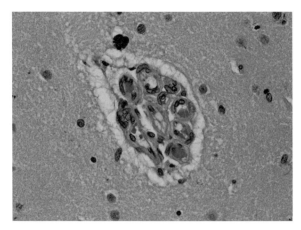

Figure 2.9 Multiple profiles of small blood vessels in the same plane suggesting reduplication (basal ganglia; H&E stain). A black and white version of this figure will appear in some formats. For the color version, please refer to the plate section.

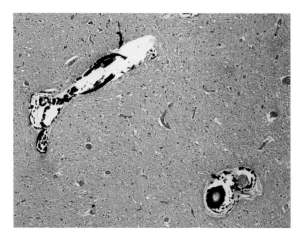

Figure 2.10 Blood vessels of the globus pallidus showing extensive calcification (H&E stain). A black and white version of this figure will appear in some formats. For the color version, please refer to the plate section.

associated with aging include striking concentric calcification of the media of small penetrating arteries of the basal ganglia, which is particularly common in the globus pallidus (Figure 2.10). Calcification of globus pallidus blood vessels is mostly an incidental finding at autopsy and is of uncertain clinical significance. However, it has also been associated with a number of other disorders, especially metabolic abnormalities of calcium and phosphate metabolism, such as hypoparathyroidism.

7 Hippocampal Sclerosis of Aging

Hippocampal sclerosis (HS) of aging is a common aging-related disease in which there is marked neuronal loss and gliosis of the hippocampus and subiculum with minimal or no tau, Aβ or α-synuclein pathology [54, 55]. This disorder should be distinguished from hippocampal sclerosis in young people with intractable temporal lobe epilepsy, who have unilateral disease and neuronal loss in CA1 but not in the subiculum. Patients with HS of aging are typically greater than 85 years of age and usually have a severe episodic memory defect that mimics that of Alzheimer's disease. There is a strong association between HS of aging and brain arteriolosclerosis (B-ASC) [52, 53]. HS and B-ASC have in common a genetic variant of *ABCC9* (rs704180), which suggests a shared pathobiology. B-ASC can exist in the absence of HS [52, 53], but when it is accompanied by HS, there is concomitant TDP-43 pathology that occurs

first in the amygdala, subiculum, and hippocampus and later can be found outside these limbic structures [56, 57]. HS also has been associated with several other genetic changes not found with B-ASC, including GRN/TMEM106B [52]. Because HS commonly affects patients greater than 85 years of age and is associated with TDP-43 pathology, the term "limbic-predominant, age-related TDP-43 encephalopathy" (LATE) was introduced [54]. The frequent association of HS and TDP-43 pathology is reminiscent of pathologic changes observed in a phenotypic spectrum of non-tauopathy frontotemporal lobar degenerations associated with TDP-43 pathology (FTLP-TDP) [52]. In contrast to the FTLD-TDPs, CARTS combines neurodegenerative changes manifest by abnormal TDP-43 accumulation with cerebrovascular dysfunction that may play a role in hippocampal neuronal loss [52].

8 Pathological Aging

Although neuritic and diffuse Aβ-amyloid plaques are associated with dementia and Alzheimer's disease (AD), a subset of older patients have a form of cerebral amyloidosis in which there are neuritic and diffuse amyloid plaques (Figure 2.11) but little or no tau pathology (neurofibrillary tangles). These patients lack the cognitive impairment seen with AD despite having a similar plaque burden [58]. It remains controversial whether this condition, often referred to as "pathological aging," represents a pre-clinical form of

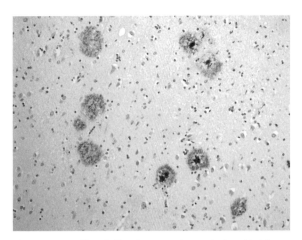

Figure 2.11 Diffuse (left) and neuritic plaques (right, with Aβ-amyloid cores). The patient had no detectable neurofibrillary tangles or Lewy body pathology and was cognitively intact ("pathological aging") (immunohistochemistry for Aβ-amyloid). A black and white version of this figure will appear in some formats. For the color version, please refer to the plate section.

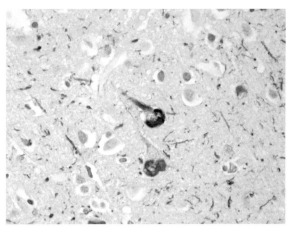

Figure 2.12 Tau-immunoreactive neurofibrillary tangles and neuropil threads in neurons of the transentorhinal cortex. The patient was 88 years old and had no apparent diffuse or neuritic plaques or Lewy body pathology ("primary age-related tauopathy"). A black and white version of this figure will appear in some formats. For the color version, please refer to the plate section.

Alzheimer's disease or a "pathological variant" of normal aging [3, 4, 59]. It has been suggested that cognitively intact patients with amyloid-beta pathology may have protective or resistance factors that reduce or minimize the deleterious effects of such pathology [58].

9 Primary Age-Related Tauopathy (PART)

"Primary age-related tauopathy" (PART) includes a spectrum of low Braak stage neurofibrillary tangle pathologies that occurs commonly in aged individuals and is usually not associated with significant cognitive impairment [30]. It occurs in individuals above age 80, and it is estimated that 20% of patients in their ninth decade are affected by this disorder [30, 52]. The brains of such patients may appear "normal for age" or show mild to moderate cerebral cortical atrophy. Mesial temporal lobe atrophy may be prominent in individuals with dementia. PART is defined by the presence of tau-immunoreactive neurofibrillary tangles in the mesial temporal lobes and typically minimal or no Aβ-amyloid pathology (Figure 2.12). Areas of the brain that can be affected in PART include the transentorhinal cortex, subiculum, hippocampus, and, occasionally, the adjacent temporal lobe neocortex, in aggregate corresponding to lower Braak

stages (I–IV) [60]. Other areas containing tau-positive neurofibrillary tangles include the amygdala, nucleus basalis of Meynert, nucleus accumbens, thalamus, hypothalamus, olfactory bulb and cortex, and the medulla [30]. Cognitive impairment may occur in patients with Braak stages III–IV. Unlike Alzheimer's neuropathology, PART pathology does not progress to the isocortical stages of Braak (V–VI). Also, the *APOE* e4 genotype has not been shown to be a risk factor for this disorder [30].

10 Aging-Related Tau Astrogliopathy (ARTAG)

It has been long recognized that astrocytes in the brains of elderly individuals can contain accumulations of phosphorylated forms of tau and that this accumulation is not associated with better clinicopathologically defined tauopathies in which glial cells are primarily affected, such as progressive supranuclear palsy, multiple systems atrophy, and globular glial tauopathies [34, 61, 62]. In 2016, a multinational and multi-institutional group of neuropathologists put forth a standardized method to evaluate the central nervous system in cases in which there is accumulation of hyperphosporylated tau in astrocytes [34]. "Aging-related tau astrogliopathy" (ARTAG) describes a morphological spectrum of astrocyte pathology that is associated with expression of 4-repeat tau. (Tau is encoded from the *MAPT* gene on chromosome 17. Alternative splicing results in six tau isoforms that may contain either three or four tandem repeats.) Astrocyte morphologies seen in ARTAG include thorn-shaped astrocytes that are similar to those described in progressive supranuclear palsy [63] and are typically located in subpial and subependymal regions. These thorn-shaped astrocytes may be found in the cortex or white matter, as well as in the basal forebrain and brainstem [34, 62]. Another type of astrocyte found in the gray matter in ARTAG shows granular or "fuzzy" immunohistochemical reactivity for tau. Currently, the clinical significance of ARTAG is not well understood.

ARTAG can occur along with other neurodegenerative disorders, including Alzheimer's disease, Lewy body disease, multiple system atrophy, and Creutzfeldt–Jacob disease [62]. Subpial and subependymal clusters of tau-positive astrocytes have also been described in chronic traumatic encephalopathy (CTE); these findings are supportive but not diagnostic of the disorder [64]. According to current consensus criteria, the pathognomonic feature of CTE is the finding of phosphorylated-tau aggregates in neurons, astrocytes, and cell processes at the depths of the sulci around small blood vessels [64]. However, recent work has suggested that ARTAG and CTE may have a common etiologic pathway since both involve the basal forebrain and are more common in men [65].

that occur with aging. Gradual morphologic changes of mild cerebral atrophy with reductions in weight and volume correlate with variable and region-specific neuronal loss in the hippocampus and frontal cortex. Loss of neurons or connections in the prefrontal area may account for thinning of cortical mini-columns of neurons that have extensive connections to other brain regions. Loss of axons in the white matter with reductions in myelin thickness also occur with aging with the latter findings reflecting alterations in oligodendroglial function. Senescence of astrocytes may lead to changes in blood–brain barrier and other functions, while microglial changes could affect CNS immune function. Histological changes that occur with aging are not disease specific but may reflect progressive alterations of basic biochemical functions, including oxidative and protein metabolism, that may lead to pathological accumulations of Aβ-amyloid and hyperphosphorylated forms of tau, α-synuclein, and TDP-43. Neurodegenerative diseases most likely arise within a background of pre-existing aging-related brain changes, including vascular disease, which set the stage for subsequent pathological changes. With more people living to advanced age, we have recognized that non-Alzheimer's disease patterns of brain pathology, including PART, "pathological aging," ARTAG, and CARTS, can often be seen even in the absence of clinical dementia. Further studies are needed to help define the significance of these entities and their role in the spectrum of human brain aging.

11 Conclusions

This chapter has reviewed some of the major central nervous system anatomic and histological changes

References

1. Tomlinson BE, Blessed G, Roth M. Observations on the brains of demented old people. *J Neurol Sci* 1968;7:331–356.

2. Tomlinson BE, Blessed G, Roth M. Observations on the brains of non-demented old people. *J Neurol Sci* 1970;11:205–242.

3. Dickson DW. Senile cerebral amyloidosis (pathological aging) and cognitive status predictions: a neuropathology perspective. *Neurobiol Aging* 1996;17:936–937.

4. Dickson DW, Crystal HA, Mattice LA, et al. Identification of normal and pathological aging in prospectively studied nondemented elderly individuals. *Neurobiol Aging* 1992;13:179–189.

5. Mufson EJ, Malek-Ahmadi M, Perez S, et al. Braak staging, plaque pathology, and APOE status in elderly persons without cognitive impairment. *Neurobiol Aging* 2016;37:147–153.

6. Neltner JH, Abner E, Jicha GA, et al. Brain pathologies in extreme old age. *Neurobiol Aging* 2016;37:1–11.

7. Lowe J. Ageing of the brain. In: Love S, Budka H, Ironside JW, Perry A, eds. *Greenfield's Neuropathology*, 9th edition. CRC Press, Taylor & Francis Group, 2015; 849–857.

8. Esiri MM. Ageing and the brain. *J Pathol* 2007;211:181–187.

9. Allen JS, Bruss J, Brown CK, Damasio H. Normal neuroanatomical variation due to age: the major lobes and a

parcellation of the temporal lobes. *Neurobiol Aging* 2005; **26**:1245–1260.

10. Fjell AM, Walhovd KB. Structural brain changes in aging: courses, causes and cognitive consequences. *Rev Neurosci* 2010;**21**:187–221.

11. Marner L, Nyengaard JR, Tang Y, et al. Marked loss of myelinated nerve fibers in the human brain with age. *J Comp Neurol* 2003;**462**:144–152.

12. Peters A, Morrison JH, Rosene DL, et al. Are neurons lost from the primate cerebral cortex during normal aging? *Cereb Cortex* 1998;**8**:295–300.

13. Simic G, Kostovic I, Winbld B, et al. Volume and number of neurons of the human hippocampal formation in normal aging and Alzheimer's disease. *J Comp Neurol* 1997;**379**:482–494.

14. West MJ, Coleman PD, Flood DG, et al. Differences in the pattern of hippocampal neuronal loss in normal ageing and Alzheimer's disease. *Lancet* 1994;**344**:769–772.

15. Ma SY, Roytt M, Collan Y, et al. Unbiased morphometrical measurements show loss of pigmented nigral neurones with ageing. *Neuropathol Appl Neurobiol* 1999;**25**:394–399.

16. Boldrini M, Fulmore CA, Tartt AN, et al. Human hippocampal neurogenesis persists throughout aging. *Cell Stem Cell* 2018;**22**:589–599.

17. Lodato MA, Rodin RE, Borhson CL, et al. Aging and neurodegeneration are associated with increased mutations in single human neurons. *Science* 2018; **359**:555–559.

18. Opris I, Cassanova MF. Prefrontal cortical minicolumn: from executive control to disrupted cognitive processing. *Brain* 2014;**137**:1863–1875.

19. Opris I. Inter-laminar microcircuits across the neocortex: repair and augmentation. *Front Syst Neurosci* 2013;**7**:80–85.

20. Van Veluw SJ, Sawyer EK, Clover L, et al. Prefrontal cytoarchitecture in normal aging and Alzheimer's disease: relationship with IQ. *Brain Struct Funct* 2012;**217**:797–808.

21. Chance SA. Subtle changes in the aging human brain. *Nutr Health* 2006;**18**;2017–2224.

22. Chance SA, Casanova MF, Switala AE, et al. Minicolumn thinning in the temporal lobe association cortex but not in primary auditory cortex in normal aging. *Acta Neuropathol* 2006;**111**:459–464.

23. Brody H. The deposition of aging pigment in the human cerebral cortex. *J Gerontol* 1960;**15**:258–261.

24. Braak H. Spindle-shaped appendages of IIIab-pyramids filled with lipofuscin: a striking pathological change of the senescent human isocortex. *Acta Neuropathol* (Berl) 1979;**46**:197–202.

25. Keller JN, Dimayuga E, Chen Q, et al. Autophagy, proteasomes, lipofuscin and oxidative stress in the aging brain. *Int J Biochem Cell Biol* 2004;**36**:2376–2391.

26. Gray DA, Woulfe J. Lipofuscin and aging: a matter of toxic waste. *Sci Aging Knowledge Environ* 2005;**5**:re1.

27. Hirano A. Neurons and astrocytes. In: Davis RL, Robertson DM, eds. *Textbook of Neuropathology*, 3rd edition. Williams & Wilkins, 1997; 1–109.

28. Mather M, Harley CW. The locus coeruleus: essential for maintaining cognitive function and the aging brain. *Trends Cogn Sci* 2016;**20**:214–226.

29. Satoh A, Iijima KM. Roles of tau pathology in the locus coeruleus (LC) in age-associated pathophysiology and Alzheimer's disease pathogenesis: potential strategies to protect the LC against aging. *Brain Res.* 2019;**1702**:17–28.

30. Crary JF, Trojanowski JQ, Schneider JA, et al. Primary age-related tauopathy (PART): a common pathology associated with human aging. *Acta Neuropathol* 2014;**128**:755–766.

31. David JP, Ghozali F, Fallet-Bianco C, et al. Glial reaction in the hippocampal formation is highly correlated with aging in the human brain. *Neurosci Lett* 1997;**235**:53–56.

32. Salminen A, Ojala J, Kaarniranta K, et al. Astrocytes in the aging brain express characteristics of senescence-associated secretory phenotype. *Eur J Neurosci* 2011;**34**:3–11.

33. Schultz C, Ghebremedhin E, Del Tredici K, et al. High prevalence of thorn-shaped astrocytes in the aged human medial temporal lobe. *Neurobiol Aging* 2004;**25**:397–405.

34. Kovacs GG, Ferrer I, Grinberg LT, et al. Aging-related tau astrogliopathy (ARTAG): harmonized evaluation strategy. *Acta Neuropathol* 2016;**131**:87–102.

35. Kohler W, Curiel J, Vanderver A. Adult leukodystrophies. *Nat Rev Neurol* 2018;**14**:94–105.

36. Peters A, Sethares C. Aging and the myelinated fibers in the prefrontal cortex and corpus callosum of the monkey. *J Comp Neurol* 2002;**442**:277–291.

37. Nasrabady SE, Rizvi B, Goldman JE, et al. White matter changes in Alzheimer's disease: a focus on myelin and oligodendrocytes. *Acta Neuropathol Commun* 2018;**6**:22–32.

38. Von Bernhardi R, Tichauer JE, Eugenin J. Aging-dependent changes of microglial cells and their relevance for neurodegenerative disorders. *J Neurochem* 2010;**112**:1099–1114.

39. Conde JR, Streit WJ. Microglia in the aging brain. *J Neuropathol Exp Neurol* 2006;**65**:199–203.

40. Streit WJ, Xue QS. Human CNS immune senescence and neurodegeneration. *Curr Opin Neurol* 2014;**29**:93–96.

41. Grimm A, Eckert A. Brain aging and neurodegeneration: from a mitochondrial point of view. *J Neurochem* 2017;**143**:418–431.

42. Venkateshappa C, Harish G, Mahadevan A, et al. Elevated oxidative stress and decreased antioxidant function in the human hippocampus and frontal cortex with increasing age: implications for neurodegeneration in Alzheimer's disease. *Neurochem Res* 2012;**37**:1601–1614.

43. Mandal PK, Tripathy M, Sugunan S. Brain oxidative stress: detection and mapping of anti-oxidant marker "Glutathione" in different brain regions of healthy male/female, MCI and Alzheimer's disease using non-invasive magnetic resonance spectroscopy. *Biochem Biophys Res Commun* 2012;**417**:43–48.

44. Schmidt R, Schmidt H, Haybaeck J, et al. Heterogeneity in age-related white matter changes. *Acta Neuropathol* 2001;**122**:171–185.

45. Moody DM, Brown WR, Challa VR, et al. Periventricular venous collagenosis: association with leukoaraiosis. *Radiology* 1995;**194**:469–476.

46. Popsecu BO, Toescu EC, Popescu LM, et al. Blood–brain barrier alterations in ageing and dementia. *J Neurol Sci* 2009;**283**:99–106.

47. Abbott NJ, Ronnback L, Hansson E. Astrocyte-endothelial interactions at the blood–brain barrier. *Nat Rev Neurosci* 2006;**7**:41–53.

48. Adelbert R, Colman MP. Axon pathology in age-related neurodegenerative disorders. *Neuropathol Appl Neurobiol* 2013;**39**:90–108.

49. Salvadores N, Sanhueza M, Manque P, et al. Axonal degeneration during aging and its functional role in neurodegenerative disorders. *Front Neurosci* 2017;**11**:1–21.

50. Pakkenberg B, Gundersen HJ. Neocortical number in humans: effect of sex and age. *J Comp Neurol* 1997;**384**:312–320.

51. Ighodaro ET, Abner EL, Fardo DW, et al. Risk factors and global cognitive status related to brain arteriolosclerosis in elderly individuals. *J Cereb Blood Flow Metab* 2017;**37**:201–216.

52. Nelson PT, Trojanowski JQ, Abner EL, et al. "New Old Pathologies": AD, PART, and cerebral age-related TDP-43 with sclerosis (CARTS). *J Neuropathol Exp Neurol* 2016;**75**:482–498.

53. Nelson PT, Jicha GA, Wang W-X, et al. ABCC9/SUR2 in the brain: implications for hippocampal sclerosis of aging and a potential therapeutic target. *Ageing Res Rev.* 2015;**24**:111–125.

54. Nelson PT, Dickson DW, Trojanowski JQ, et al. Limbic-predominant age-related TDP-43 encephalopathy (LATE): consensus working group report. *Brain* 2019;**142**:1503–1527.

55. Brenowitz WD, Monsell SE, Schmitt FA, et al. Hippocampal sclerosis of aging is a key Alzheimer's disease mimic: clinical-pathologic correlations and comparisons with both Alzheimer's disease and non-tauopathic frontotemporal lobar degeneration. *J Alzheimers Dis* 2014;**39**:691–702.

56. Cykowski MD, Powell SZ, Schulz PE, et al. Hippocampal sclerosis in older patients: practical examples and guidance with a focus on cerebral age-related TDP-43 with sclerosis. *Arch Pathol Lab Med* 2017;**141**:113–1126.

57. Cykowski MD, Takei H, Van Eldik LJ, et al. Hippocampal sclerosis but not normal aging or Alzheimer disease is associated with TDP-43 pathology in the basal forebrain of aged persons. *J Neuropathol Exp Neurol* 2016;**75**:397–407.

58. Murray ME, Dickson DW. Is pathological aging a successful resistance against amyloid-beta or preclinical Alzheimer's disease? *Alzheimers Res Ther* 2014;**6**:24–28.

59. Morris JC, Storandt M, McKeel DW, et al. Cerebral amyloid deposition and diffuse plaques in "normal aging": evidence for presymptomatic and very mild Alzheimer's disease. *Neurology* 1996;**46**:707–719.

60. Braak H, Alafuzoff I, Arzberger T, et al. Staging of Alzheimer's disease-associated neurofibrillary pathology using paraffin sections and immunohistochemistry. *Acta Neuropathol* 2006;**112**:389–404.

61. Lowe J, Kalaria R. Dementia. In: Love S, Budka H, Ironside JW, Perry A, eds. *Greenfield's Neuropathology*, 9th edition. CRC Press, Taylor & Francis Group, 2015;858–973.

62. Kovacs GG, Robinson JL, Xie SX, et al. Evaluating patterns of aging-related tau astrogliopathy unravels novel insights into brain aging and neurodegenerative disease. *J Neuropathol Exp Neurol* 2017;**76**:270–288.

63. Nishimura M, Namba Y, Ikeda K, et al. Glial fibrillary tangles with straight tubules in the brains of patients with progressive supranuclear palsy. *Neurosci Lett* 1992;**143**:35–38.

64. McKee AC, Cairns NJ, Dickson DW, et al. The first NINDS/NBIB consensus meeting to define neuropathological criteria for the diagnosis of chronic traumatic encephalopathy. *Acta Neuropathol* 2016;**131**:75–86.

65. Liu AK, Goldfinger Questari HE, et al. ARTAG in the basal forebrain: widening the constellation of astrocytic tau pathology. *Acta Neuropathol Comm* 2016;**4**:59.

Chapter 3

Cellular and Molecular Mechanisms for Age-Related Cognitive Decline

Jolie D. Barter and Thomas C. Foster

1 Prefrontal Cortex, Hippocampus, and Animal Models

When attempting to learn the cellular and molecular mechanisms for age-related cognitive decline, one of the first questions is: Where do we look for brain changes associated with aging and cognitive decline? Senescence is associated with selective changes in specific cognitive processes, including a progressive slowing of sensory-motor function, disruption of sleep patterns, difficulties with memory and attention, and increased susceptibility to psychiatric or neurodegenerative disorders. Considerable research has focused on age-related changes in the hippocampus and prefrontal cortex (PFC), since age-related impairments in cognitive processes that depend on these regions appear to emerge early, in middle age. Brain imaging studies confirm that the medial temporal lobe/hippocampus and the PFC are highly vulnerable to age-related changes in structure and activity in humans [1–7]. Moreover, these regions exhibit differences in molecular markers of aging and differential vulnerability to the stressors of aging [8–14]. Even within the hippocampus, there are differences in vulnerability to aging across hippocampal subregions [8, 10, 15]. Importantly, age-related cognitive decline is not uniform or inevitable. There is individual variability in age of onset and the trajectory of decline, emphasizing that chronological age is a poor predictor of functional decline. This variability can be employed to identify mechanisms and biological markers to predict functional decline referred to as biological age.

As with humans, animal models of aging exhibit considerable variability in the onset and progression of cognitive decline, which can be utilized to examine biological variables that may contribute to impairments. Thus, animal models can be employed to identify senescent neurophysiologic and molecular changes that are associated with the onset of cognitive decline. Animal models provide several advantages for examining "normal" cognitive aging. First, it is important to discriminate impairments due to aging from those associated with neurodegenerative diseases [16]. The fact that animal models do not normally develop neurodegenerative diseases, such as Alzheimer's disease, suggests that these animal models may provide a good model of normal brain aging. Indeed, the results from animal studies suggest mechanisms for age-related changes in brain structure and activity in humans, examined with noninvasive techniques [17]. Below, we highlight cognitive processes associated with the PFC and hippocampus and demonstrate similarity in impairments for humans and animal models (i.e., face validity).

1.1 Prefrontal Cortex and Executive Function

The PFC mediates executive functions, a comprehensive term used to describe several cognitive abilities required to accomplish goal-directed behaviors, including motivation, planning, sequencing, set shifting, sustained attention, and working memory. These executive function impairments in humans are the subject of later chapters in this volume (esp. Chapters 7 and 10–12). Deficits in basic cognitive processes that involve increased attentional demand, such as sustained attention, may emerge early and contribute to impairments in executive processes, while other basic cognitive components, such as signal detection or maintenance of information in working memory, remain intact [18, 19]. Animal models support the idea that impaired sustained attention emerges in middle age for a subset of animals, and the propensity for impairment increases with advancing age [19–22].

Simple working memory tasks involve the encoding and short-term maintenance (i.e., seconds or minutes) of stimulus representations, and impairments in working memory are observed as attentional demand is increased (see Chapter 12). For animal models, attentional demand of a working memory task can be increased by increasing the memory load (i.e., working memory capacity). Again, a deficit in working memory capacity emerges in middle age for primates, canines, and rodents [23–28].

Set shifting is a form of cognitive flexibility that requires the ability to shift strategies in response to changes in goals or environmental cues, permitting the rapid adaptation of behavior to a change in contingencies (see Chapter 12). Rhesus monkeys exhibit impaired set shifting starting in middle age, suggesting that impaired cognitive flexibility may occur early in this animal model. In contrast, across a number of species, impairments on set shifting tasks is observed in the oldest group [29–32].

1.2 Hippocampus and Episodic Memory

Memory deficits are a major concern for the elderly. It is estimated that ~40% of people >65 years can be diagnosed with an age-related memory impairment [33]. Episodic memory deficits in humans manifest in middle age [34–36]. Impairment in episodic memory also emerges in middle age in animals models of age-related cognitive decline [37]. The hippocampus is required for encoding episodic memories, linking individual elements to be remembered with the spatial location and time of occurrence of an episode or trial. Episodic memories are rapidly acquired, flexible, and can be updated from trial to trial. Thus, episodic information of what, where, and when is "trial-dependent." Episodic memories are retained over the course of hours or days, months or years, making them distinct from PFC-dependent working memory, which lasts seconds. Episodic memory is also distinct from procedural, semantic, and reference memory, which represent knowledge or facts that are not dependent on a single experience, are acquired with repeated exposures (i.e., trial independent), and remain relatively constant throughout life. Indeed, deficits in semantic, reference, or procedural memory are more common in neurodegenerative diseases.

2 The Ca^{2+} Hypothesis of Aging and the Senescent Synapse

Thirty years ago, observations of age-related changes in Ca^{2+} regulation and alterations in physiological processes that depend on Ca^{2+} led to formulation of the "Ca^{2+} hypothesis of brain aging" [38]. Early studies provided evidence of a small and prolonged increase in intracellular free Ca^{2+} with aging [39]. Physiological studies of hippocampal CA1 pyramidal cells indicated that aging was associated with an increase in the hyperpolarization phase that follows the action potential, reducing cell excitability and burst discharge activity. This after-hyperpolarization depends on cytosolic (intracellular) Ca^{2+} to activate Ca^{2+}-dependent, potassium channels. Thus, the aging-related increase in the after-hyperpolarization provided further evidence of a modest extended rise in the level of intracellular Ca^{2+} [40]. The initial Ca^{2+} hypothesis attempted to link the Ca^{2+} dysregulation to neurodegenerative diseases of aging, suggesting that over time, a small and prolonged increase in Ca^{2+} would have toxic effects, resulting in cell death, similar to that observed following a large increase over a short time period. However, several questions remained. While aging-related impairment in episodic memory function correlates with a decrease in the size of the hippocampus, it is not associated with hippocampal cell loss [41, 42]. Furthermore, cognitive benefits have been observed with acute pharmacological treatments that block voltage-dependent Ca^{2+} channels. More recent research has focused on behavioral changes reflective of senescent physiology related to changes in Ca^{2+}-regulated processes, including cell-to-cell communication.

2.1 The Senescent Synapse

A key to understanding how senescent physiology disrupts cognition has been provided by studies examining the mechanisms of synaptic plasticity, long-term potentiation (LTP), and long-term depression (LTD), underlying episodic memory formation. The expression of LTP is achieved through an increase in synaptic transmission made possible by increases in postsynaptic α-amino-3-hydroxy-5-methyl-4-isoxazolepropionic acid (AMPA) glutamate-sensitive sodium channels. This increase is induced by activation of postsynaptic N-methyl-D-aspartate (NMDA) glutamate receptors. The activation of NMDA receptors produces a large, brief rise in postsynaptic intracellular Ca^{2+}, which activates Ca^{2+} sensitive kinases. This increases the strength of the synaptic response through phosphorylation of AMPA-glutamate channels, which leads to insertion

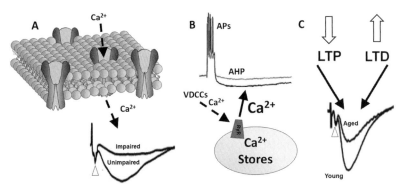

Figure 3.1 Senescent physiology due to a shift in Ca^{2+} regulation. (A) A decrease in Ca^{2+} influx through the NMDA receptor-gated channel of aged cognitively impaired animals is observed as a decrease in the NMDA receptor synaptic response for a given number of afferents activated. (B) During the generation of action potentials (APs), the depolarization activates voltage-dependent Ca^{2+} channels (VDCCs) in the membrane, and the Ca^{2+} influx through VDCCs acts on ryanodine receptors (RyR) on intracellular Ca^{2+} stores to increase Ca^{2+}-induced Ca^{2+} release (CICR). The Ca^{2+} from CICR activates sensitive potassium channels in the membrane to increase the amplitude of the after-hyperpolarization (AHP) in impaired (dark trace) relative to unimpaired (gray trace) animals. The larger after-hyperpolarization reduces cell burst activity and contributes to altered synaptic plasticity. (C) The shift in Ca^{2+} alters the balance of kinase and phosphatase activity, impairing LTP and facilitating induction of LTD. Altered synaptic plasticity promotes a decrease in synaptic transmission through the hippocampus, particularly for aged memory impaired animals. The open arrow heads in panels A and C indicate the fiber potential that precedes the synaptic responses. A black and white version of this figure will appear in some formats. For the color version, please refer to the plate section.

of additional AMPA-glutamate channels into the postsynaptic membrane. Early studies demonstrated that decay of LTP increased in aged animals and correlated with forgetting, suggesting that impaired acquisition and retention of information was related to impairment in the induction and maintenance of LTP [43].

Whereas induction of LTP requires a brief, large increase in intracellular Ca^{2+}, LTD is induced by a modest and prolonged rise in intracellular Ca^{2+}. This activates phosphatases that decrease synaptic transmission through dephosphorylation of AMPA-glutamate channels, resulting in their removal from the postsynaptic membrane. Initial studies of LTD indicated developmental regulation, such that the ability to induce LTD in the hippocampus declined from neonatal to adult periods. Therefore, it was somewhat surprising to discover an increase in susceptibility to induction of LTD with advanced age. The increase in susceptibility to LTD contributes to the increased decay of LTP and correlates with increased forgetting in older animals, suggesting that LTD underlies memory impairment [44, 45]. The shift in synaptic plasticity, favoring LTD over LTP, results in a decrease in synaptic transmission in the hippocampus of older animals [45, 46]. The weakening of synaptic transmission could contribute to the decrease in activation of the hippocampus of

aging-memory impaired humans, recorded as a decrease in the fMRI BOLD signal during learning or recall [17, 47, 48]. Moreover, LTD can reduce dendritic spine number, such that LTD may decrease synaptic connectivity and contribute to the reduction in brain volume [49]. Together, these results point to Ca^{2+} dysregulation as a mechanism for senescent physiology characterized by reduced cell excitability, decreased LTP, increased LTD, and decreased synaptic transmission.

2.2 Mechanism for Ca^{2+} Dysregulation

Altered synaptic plasticity results from dysregulation of extracellular and intracellular Ca^{2+} sources. Starting in middle age, animals with impaired episodic memory exhibit decreased Ca^{2+} influx through NMDA receptor-gated channels at the synapse, which contributes to deficits in the induction of synaptic LTP [37, 46, 50] (Figure 3.1A). In contrast, during an action potential, Ca^{+2} influx through voltage-dependent Ca^{2+} channels (i.e., L-channels) acts on ryanodine receptors to increase Ca^{2+} release from intracellular stores in a process known as Ca^{2+}-induced Ca^{2+} release (CICR) (Figure 3.1B). The increase in CICR activates Ca^{2+}-dependent potassium channels in the membrane, producing a larger after-hyperpolarization. The NMDA receptor is voltage gated as well as ligand gated. Thus, the larger after-hyperpolarization dampens the activation of NMDA channels, further contributing to impaired LTP [37, 51]. Blocking CICR, by blocking ryanodine receptors or depletion of Ca^{2+} from intracellular stores, has a greater effect in reducing the after-hyperpolarization in aged animals [52, 53], indicating an aging-specific mechanism. Moreover, inhibition of CICR promotes LTP and inhibits LTD in aged animals [52, 54]. Thus, the relative shift in Ca^{2+} sources, with reduced extracellular influx of Ca^{2+} from NMDA receptors and increased release of Ca^{2+} from intracellular stores, underlies senescent physiology, which is characterized by a larger after-hyperpolarization, a decrease in NMDA voltage-gated channel activity, decreased synaptic transmission, and reduced synaptic plasticity (Figure 3.1C).

The decrease in NMDA receptor function in the hippocampus is thought to impair synaptic plasticity required for episodic memory [37]. In PFC, a decline in NMDA receptor function on inhibitory interneurons may shift the balance of excitatory/inhibitory activity, decreasing the release of inhibitory transmitter, and increasing neural activity [20, 32, 55, 56]. Pharmacological studies support the idea that a decline in NMDA channel function could contribute to age-related cognitive decline. In humans, the NMDA receptor blockers ketamine and phencyclidine impair episodic memory and the manipulation of information in working memory, leaving the simple, delay-dependent, maintenance of information in working memory intact [57]. There is also some evidence that increased CICR could contribute to cognitive decline as blockade of voltage-dependent Ca^{2+} channels can slow cognitive aging [58–60]. The protective effect appears to be independent of the anti-hypertensive effect of Ca^{2+} channel blockers.

It may be important that brain regions that exhibit Ca^{2+}-dependent plasticity appear to manifest increased vulnerability to the effects of aging and neurodegenerative disease. Synaptic plasticity and changes in cell excitability may compensate for a loss of inputs [47, 48, 61–65]. In addition, neural compensation may include recruitment of more brain regions through network activation [66–68]. However, plasticity mechanisms may also represent a risk factor for the damaging effects of aging [69]. In particular, Ca^{2+}-dependent plasticity generates reactive oxygen species and senescent physiology may represent the co-opting of reduction–oxidation (redox) signaling

pathways, which are normally responsible for feedback regulation of synaptic transmission [70].

3 Redox State versus Oxidative Damage

Several long-standing theories propose that aging is due to endogenous free radicals and the accumulation of damaged lipids, DNA, and proteins [71]. Oxidative damage in the brain increases with age and in neurodegenerative disease. The vulnerability of different cell types, cellular compartments, and brain regions depends on the chemical character of the oxidative moiety, the level of reactive oxidative species production, and the activity of antioxidant enzymes [70]. Research in this area was originally influenced by cell death associated with neurodegenerative disease. More recently, thinking has evolved to consider a continuum of alteration in cellular function short of cell death (Figure 3.2). In this model, redox signaling, involving hydrogen peroxide and nitric oxide, functions to regulate synaptic transmission on a moment-to-moment basis through reversible cysteine nitrosylation and cysteine disulfide bonds.

In middle age, increased or more prolonged activation of redox signaling cascades, sometimes referred to as redox stress, induces the changes in Ca^{2+} regulation that underlie senescent physiology [50, 53]. Oxidizing agents, xanthine/xanthine oxidase or hydrogen peroxide, induce a decrease in the NMDA receptor–mediated synaptic response and increase the after-hyperpolarization in hippocampal slices from young animals. Little or no effect of oxidizing agents was observed for older animals, suggesting that cells were already in an oxidized state. In contrast, bath application of the reducing agent dithiothreitol (DTT) enhanced NMDA receptor-mediated synaptic responses in the PFC and hippocampus of aged animals, and the increase correlated with impaired performance on PFC or hippocampal-dependent tasks, respectively [20, 46]. The redox state influences the formation of cysteine disulfide bonds. The disulfide bonds of ryanodine receptors for intracellular Ca^{2+} stores determine Ca^{2+} release and the after-hyperpolarization amplitude. In the case of NMDA receptors, redox-sensitive disulfide bonds are localized to NMDA receptor subunits and to molecules (e.g., CaMKII) that modify NMDA receptor function. The age-dependent specificity of oxidizing agents and DTT provides strong support for the idea that redox stress mediates senescent physiology.

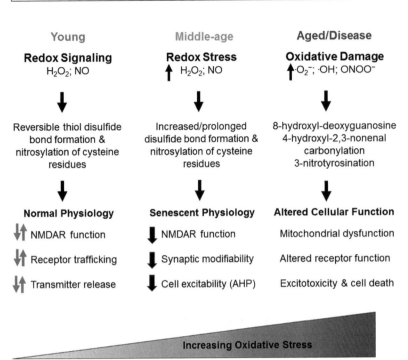

Young	Middle-age	Aged/Disease
Redox Signaling	**Redox Stress**	**Oxidative Damage**
H_2O_2; NO	↑ H_2O_2; NO	↑·O_2^-; ·OH; $ONOO^-$
↓	↓	↓
Reversible thiol disulfide bond formation & nitrosylation of cysteine residues	Increased/prolonged disulfide bond formation & nitrosylation of cysteine residues	8-hydroxyl-deoxyguanosine 4-hydroxyl-2,3-nonenal carbonylation 3-nitrotyrosination
↓	↓	↓
Normal Physiology	**Senescent Physiology**	**Altered Cellular Function**
↓↑ NMDAR function	↓ NMDAR function	Mitochondrial dysfunction
↓↑ Receptor trafficking	↓ Synaptic modifiability	Altered receptor function
↓↑ Transmitter release	↓ Cell excitability (AHP)	Excitotoxicity & cell death

Increasing Oxidative Stress

Figure 3.2 Altered redox homeostasis, from signal transduction to oxidative damage, over the course of aging. In younger individuals, a brief rise in hydrogen peroxide or nitric oxide acts as a signal by forming reversible disulfide bonds or S-nitrosylation to rapidly and reversibly influence synaptic function. With advancing age, increased levels of hydrogen peroxide or nitric oxide will prolong or constitutively activate these signaling processes, resulting in stable physiological changes (senescent physiology). With advanced age or in neurodegenerative disease, increased levels of highly reactive molecules, superoxide, peroxynitrite, and the hydroxyl radical induce the accumulation of irreversible damage, impairment in mitochondrial function, impaired synaptic transmission, and cell death.

The link between redox state and cognition was provided by studies showing that impaired executive function and episodic memory correlated with redox-sensitive NMDA receptor hypofunction in the prefrontal cortex and hippocampus, respectively [20, 46]. A series of studies that employed viral vector-mediated delivery of antioxidant enzymes demonstrated that NMDA receptor hypofunction was due to increased levels of hydrogen peroxide and redox signaling rather than elevated superoxide and oxidative damage [72, 73]. First, overexpression of the antioxidant enzyme superoxide dismutase 1 (SOD1) was associated with decreased oxidative damage. However, SOD1 overexpression impaired memory and synaptic plasticity. This seems counterintuitive, that reduced oxidative damage is associated with impaired cognition and synaptic plasticity. The mechanism involved the SOD1 production of excess hydrogen peroxide from superoxide. Overexpression of catalase, which converts hydrogen peroxide to water, rescued cognition and synaptic plasticity. The results suggest that altered redox signaling and senescent physiology precede oxidative damage. Furthermore, the results link an aging mechanism, increased oxidative stress, to impairment of a mechanism involved in episodic memory function, reduced NMDA receptor function, and altered synaptic plasticity.

4 Interaction of Redox Stress with Other Aging Mechanisms

In addition to redox stress, aging encompasses many other biochemical, physical, and functional changes. Mitochondrial dysfunction, systemic inflammation, and disruption of neuroendocrine regulation are risk factors for neurodegenerative diseases and interact with oxidative stress to contribute to brain aging. For example, microglia are activated during the initiation of neural repair and they normally support neurons under oxidative stress [74]. However, with advancing age, a persistent low-level increase in serum markers of inflammation is observed and is thought to contribute to Alzheimer's disease and age-related memory deficits [75, 76]. In this case, prostaglandins and pro-inflammatory cytokines (IL-1β, IL-6, TNF-α) may cross the blood–brain barrier to activate microglia, increase production of reactive oxygen species, and eliminate synapses through the complement cascade and phagocytosis. Thus, systemic inflammation can enhance redox stress of aging and provide a second hit to the system by eliminating synapses.

The female sex steroid estradiol (E2) is neuroprotective against stressors of aging and neurodegenerative diseases; however, neuroprotection may be lost

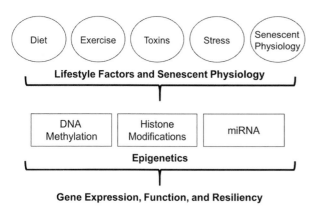

Figure 3.3 Epigenetic mechanisms, including DNA methylation, histone modifications, and miRNA-mediated processes are modified by environment and lifestyle factors (diet, exercise, toxins) and interact with age-related changes in signaling caused by stress (inflammation, oxidative stress) or senescent physiology to determine gene expression. In turn, the ability to express or inhibit gene expression will contribute to variability in resilience and functional decline.

with the decline in E2 levels during reproductive senescence (i.e., menopause) [77]. E2 can have rapid (minutes/hours) and long-term (days) effects on physiology that are diametrically opposite to senescent physiology and involve both membrane and genomic signaling [78]. Anti-aging effects include the ability to increase NMDA receptor function and decrease the amplitude of the after-hyperpolarization [79, 80]. E2 treatment also improves episodic spatial memory that depends on NMDA receptors [37, 79, 81]. The E2-mediated improvement in memory is associated with increased NMDA receptor function [79, 82]. The mechanism for anti-aging effects is unknown but may involve decreased oxidative stress [83, 84].

The therapeutic potential of E2 declines with advanced age or prolonged hormone deprivation. There is now considerable evidence from human and animal models for an E2 "therapeutic window" [77, 79, 85]. For animals in which the therapeutic window is closed (i.e., E2 treatment no longer improves memory), E2 treatment does not increase NMDA receptor function or induce transcription of neuroprotective genes [77, 79, 82, 86]. The mechanism for closing of the therapeutic window is unknown, but likely involves epigenetic regulation of gene expression.

5 Gene Expression and Epigenetic Mechanisms of Brain Aging

5.1 Genes as Markers for Chronological and Biological Aging

Gene expression in the aging brain depends on signals generated by senescent physiology. Thus, there is altered gene expression associated with oxidative stress, Ca^{2+} regulation, and inflammation that begins to emerge by middle age [15, 32, 86–89]. Importantly, variability in cognitive decline is correlated with expression of synaptic and neural activity genes. Moreover, lifestyle factors can affect gene expression through epigenetic modifications, providing a mechanism for environmental influences on cognitive decline.

5.2 Epigenetic Mechanisms

The term "epigenetics" encompasses the processes that induce changes in gene expression that are not due to alterations in the DNA sequence (Figure 3.3). Thus, while all cells have the same DNA, epigenetic mechanisms underlie cell type–specific changes in transcription during differentiation, development, and maturation. Diet, stress, hormone status, and exercise can act through the epigenetic–environmental interface to influence expression of genes involved in resiliency and the progression of cognitive aging. For example, monozygotic twins share the same DNA and epigenetic markers are similar between young twin pairs. However, during aging, differences in environmental and lifestyle factors underlie the emergence of epigenetic differences that correlate with phenotype differences, including cognitive function [90, 91].

Epigenetic mechanisms include post-translational modification on the N-terminal tails of histones (acetylation, methylation, phosphorylation). Signals from the environment induce histone modifications, which in turn alter the DNA structure. Some histone modifications open up the DNA, making it accessible for transcription. However, in the absence of transcription, the increased accessibility also renders the

DNA vulnerable to de novo methylation. DNA methylation represents a relatively stable mechanism for decreasing gene expression, including inhibition of transcription factor binding. For example, the estrogen receptor alpha (ERα) is a transcription factor, activated by E2, which acts on the brain to increase the expression of a multitude of genes that are neuroprotective [77, 86]. The decline in E2 during menopause decreases the transcriptional activity of ERα. In turn, the decline in active transcription is associated with increased DNA methylation and silencing of estrogen-responsive genes, such that the therapeutic benefits of E2 are reduced with long-term E2 deprivation [77, 92, 93].

Animal studies indicate that behavioral and environmental stressors induce epigenetic changes in the PFC and hippocampus [94–96]. For example, DNA methylation associated with early-life events contributes long-term alterations in transcription, decreasing expression of synaptic genes and promoting pathological phenotypes [97]. In older animals that exhibit impairment in behaviors that are PFC-dependent, increased DNA methylation is observed for synaptic genes that exhibit decreased transcription [32, 98]. The mechanisms underlying age-related changes in DNA methylation are unclear. One possibility is that a decline in NMDA receptor function results in decreased activation of cAMP response element-binding protein (CREB), a transcription factor involved in synaptic plasticity [37, 99]. The decreased transcriptional activation of CREB could render synaptic plasticity genes vulnerable to DNA methylation. Interestingly, several genes linked to memory exhibit increased DNA methylation with advancing age; however, environmental stimulation and behavioral training can reverse the methylation state of memory genes [100, 101]. The results are suggestive that the age-related shift in DNA methylation may be reversible through lifestyle and environmental factors. Indeed, mounting evidence supports the idea that the epigenetic–environmental interface contributes to the beneficial effects of diet, exercise, and cognitive stimulation (e.g., environmental enrichment) [102–107].

5.3 MicroRNA

MicroRNA (miRNA) provides another epigenetic process for regulating gene expression, by binding to post-transcriptional target mRNA to inhibit translation. miRNAs are small, phylogenetically conserved, non-coding RNAs. The nucleotide sequence determines the binding of miRNA to target mRNAs. In turn, binding of miRNA removes the mRNA and represses translation. An important aspect of miRNA is that it can be packed into exosomes that are released into the extracellular space. Exosomes are able to cross membranes (e.g., blood–brain barrier). In this way, microvesicles can provide intercellular and inter-organ communication by delivery of miRNAs to influence translation in target recipient cells.

Examination of miRNA from blood or plasma could provide an inexpensive method for obtaining biomarkers of aging and disease. Changes in plasma miRNA levels correlate with cognitive decline in mild cognitive impairment, Alzheimer's disease, and normal aging. Interestingly, cognitive impairment is associated with increased plasma levels of miRNA families, which are typically found enriched in the brain [108]. This suggests that brain-enriched miRNAs found in the plasma may offer insights into brain changes. In addition, it is likely that exosomes from other tissues can enter the brain to deliver miRNA. In particular, miRNAs associated with inflammation and cellular stress are increased in plasma exosomes [108, 109]. In this way, peripheral organs, systemic inflammation, as well as environmental factors, exercise, and nutrition, could act through miRNA to influence translation in the brain.

6 Conclusion

Ideas about the mechanisms for brain aging and cognitive decline have evolved from the original hypotheses that attempted to link altered Ca^{2+} regulation and oxidative stress to neuronal death. Recent work emphasizes that a modest increase in the duration or magnitude of oxidative stress, starting in middle age, acts through redox signaling, inducing senescent physiology through Ca^{2+}-dependent mechanisms for synaptic plasticity and cell excitability involved in memory and executive function. Gene expression in the aging brain has been linked to oxidative stress, Ca^{2+} dysregulation, and inflammation. However, the expression of synaptic and neural activity genes provides a better correlate of variability in cognitive function. In addition to aging physiology, gene expression is influenced by epigenetic changes.

Epigenetic modification may inhibit transcription, rendering cells less responsive to the environment. The epigenetic–environmental interface provides a potential mechanism by which the environment and lifestyle factors can have stable influences on gene expression to impact resiliency and variability in the progression of cognitive aging.

Acknowledgments

Supported by National Institute of Aging grants R37AG036800, RO11049711, and RO1052258 and the Evelyn F. McKnight Brain Research Foundation. This work was partially supported by the University of Florida Claude D. Pepper Older Americans Independence Center (P30-AG028740).

References

1. de Flores R, La Joie R, Chetelat G. Structural imaging of hippocampal subfields in healthy aging and Alzheimer's disease. *Neuroscience*. 2015;**309**:29–50.

2. Kerchner GA, Bernstein JD, Fenesy MC, Deutsch GK, Saranathan M, Zeineh MM, et al. Shared vulnerability of two synaptically-connected medial temporal lobe areas to age and cognitive decline: a seven tesla magnetic resonance imaging study. *J Neurosci*. 2013;**33** (42):16666–72.

3. Kirchhoff BA, Gordon BA, Head D. Prefrontal gray matter volume mediates age effects on memory strategies. *Neuroimage*. 2014;**90**:326–34.

4. Raz N, Gunning FM, Head D, Dupuis JH, McQuain J, Briggs SD, et al. Selective aging of the human cerebral cortex observed in vivo: differential vulnerability of the prefrontal gray matter. *Cereb Cortex*. 1997;**7**(3):268–82.

5. Salat DH, Buckner RL, Snyder AZ, Greve DN, Desikan RS, Busa E, et al. Thinning of the cerebral cortex in aging. *Cereb Cortex*. 2004;**14**(7):721–30.

6. Wolf D, Fischer FU, de Flores R, Chetelat G, Fellgiebel A. Differential associations of age with volume and microstructure of hippocampal subfields in healthy older adults. *Hum Brain Mapp*. 2015;**36**(10):3819–31.

7. Raz N, Ghisletta P, Rodrigue KM, Kennedy KM, Lindenberger U. Trajectories of brain aging in middle-aged and older adults: regional and individual differences. *Neuroimage*. 2010;**51** (2):501–11.

8. Jackson TC, Rani A, Kumar A, Foster TC. Regional hippocampal differences in AKT survival signaling across the lifespan: implications for CA1 vulnerability with aging. *Cell Death Differ*. 2009;**16**(3):439–48.

9. McEwen BS, Morrison JH. The brain on stress: vulnerability and plasticity of the prefrontal cortex over the life course. *Neuron*. 2013;**79**(1):16–29.

10. Wang X, Michaelis EK. Selective neuronal vulnerability to oxidative stress in the brain. *Front Aging Neurosci*. 2010;**2**:12.

11. Abd El Mohsen MM, Iravani MM, Spencer JP, Rose S, Fahim AT, Motawi TM, et al. Age-associated changes in protein oxidation and proteasome activities in rat brain: modulation by antioxidants. *Biochem Biophys Res Commun*. 2005;**336**(2):386–91.

12. Dominguez M, de Oliveira E, Odena MA, Portero M, Pamplona R, Ferrer I. Redox proteomic profiling of neuroketal-adducted proteins in human brain: regional vulnerability at middle age increases in the elderly. *Free Radic Biol Med*. 2016;**95**:1–15.

13. Horvath S, Mah V, Lu AT, Woo JS, Choi OW, Jasinska AJ, et al. The cerebellum ages slowly according to the epigenetic clock. *Aging (Albany NY)*. 2015;**7** (5):294–306.

14. Kumar A, Gibbs JR, Beilina A, Dillman A, Kumaran R, Trabzuni D, et al. Age-associated changes in gene expression in human brain and isolated neurons. *Neurobiol Aging*. 2013;**34**(4):1199–209.

15. Ianov L, De Both M, Chawla MK, Rani A, Kennedy AJ, Piras I, et al. Hippocampal transcriptomic profiles: subfield vulnerability to age and cognitive impairment. *Front Aging Neurosci*. 2017;**9**:383.

16. Foster TC. Biological markers of age-related memory deficits: treatment of senescent physiology. *CNS Drugs*. 2006;**20**(2):153–66.

17. Febo M, Foster TC. Preclinical magnetic resonance imaging and spectroscopy studies of memory, aging, and cognitive decline. *Front Aging Neurosci*. 2016;**8**:158.

18. Goh JO, An Y, Resnick SM. Differential trajectories of age-related changes in components of executive and memory processes. *Psychol Aging*. 2012;**27**(3):707–19.

19. McAvinue LP, Habekost T, Johnson KA, Kyllingsbaek S, Vangkilde S, Bundesen C, et al. Sustained attention, attentional selectivity, and attentional capacity across the lifespan. *Atten Percept Psychophys*. 2012;**74** (8):1570–82.

20. Guidi M, Kumar A, Foster TC. Impaired attention and synaptic senescence of the prefrontal cortex involves redox regulation of NMDA receptors. *J Neurosci*. 2015;**35**(9):3966–77.

21. Jones DN, Barnes JC, Kirkby DL, Higgins GA. Age-associated impairments in a test of attention: evidence for involvement of cholinergic systems. *J Neurosci*. 1995;**15**(11):7282–92.

22. Fortenbaugh FC, DeGutis J, Germine L, Wilmer JB, Grosso M, Russo K, et al. Sustained attention across the life span in a sample of 10,000: dissociating ability and strategy. *Psychol Sci.* 2015;**26**(9):1497–510.

23. Bimonte HA, Nelson ME, Granholm AC. Age-related deficits as working memory load increases: relationships with growth factors. *Neurobiol Aging.* 2003;**24**(1):37–48.

24. Bopp KL, Verhaeghen P. Aging and verbal memory span: a meta-analysis. *J Gerontol B Psychol Sci Soc Sci.* 2005;**60**(5):P223–33.

25. Brockmole JR, Logie RH. Age-related change in visual working memory: a study of 55,753 participants aged 8–75. *Front Psychol.* 2013;**4**:12.

26. Dellu-Hagedorn F, Trunet S, Simon H. Impulsivity in youth predicts early age-related cognitive deficits in rats. *Neurobiol Aging.* 2004;**25** (4):525–37.

27. Moss MB, Killiany RJ, Lai ZC, Rosene DL, Herndon JG. Recognition memory span in rhesus monkeys of advanced age. *Neurobiol Aging.* 1997;**18** (1):13–19.

28. Tapp PD, Siwak CT, Estrada J, Holowachuk D, Milgram NW. Effects of age on measures of complex working memory span in the beagle dog (*Canis familiaris*) using two versions of a spatial list learning paradigm. *Learn Mem.* 2003;**10**(2):148–60.

29. Robbins TW, James M, Owen AM, Sahakian BJ, Lawrence AD, McInnes L, et al. A study of performance on tests from the CANTAB battery sensitive to frontal lobe dysfunction in a large sample of normal volunteers: implications for theories of executive functioning and cognitive aging. Cambridge Neuropsychological Test Automated Battery. *J Int Neuropsychol Soc.* 1998;**4**(5):474–90.

30. Rhodes MG. Age-related differences in performance on the Wisconsin card sorting test: a meta-analytic review. *Psychology Aging.* 2004;**19**(3):482–94.

31. Fisk JE, Sharp CA. Age-related impairment in executive functioning: updating, inhibition, shifting, and access. *J Clin Exp Neuropsychol.* 2004;**26**(7):874–90.

32. Ianov L, Rani A, Beas BS, Kumar A, Foster TC. Transcription profile of aging and cognition-related genes in the medial prefrontal cortex. *Front Aging Neurosci.* 2016;**8**:113.

33. Small GW. What we need to know about age related memory loss. *BMJ.* 2002;**324**(7352):1502–5.

34. Cansino S. Episodic memory decay along the adult lifespan: a review of behavioral and neurophysiological evidence. *Int J Psychophysiol.* 2009;**71**(1):64–9.

35. Uttl B, Graf P. Episodic spatial memory in adulthood. *Psychol Aging.* 1993;**8**(2):257–73.

36. Nyberg L, Lovden M, Riklund K, Lindenberger U, Backman L. Memory aging and brain maintenance. *Trends Cogn Sci.* 2012;**16**(5):292–305.

37. Foster TC. Dissecting the age-related decline on spatial learning and memory tasks in rodent models: N-methyl-D-aspartate receptors and voltage-dependent Ca^{2+} channels in senescent synaptic plasticity. *Prog Neurobiol.* 2012;**96**(3):283–303.

38. Khachaturian ZS. Hypothesis on the regulation of cytosol calcium concentration and the aging brain. *Neurobiol Aging.* 1987;**8**(4):345–6.

39. Michaelis ML, Johe K, Kitos TE. Age-dependent alterations in synaptic membrane systems for Ca^{2+} regulation. *Mech Ageing Dev.* 1984;**25**(1–2):215–25.

40. Landfield PW, Pitler TA. Prolonged Ca^{2+}-dependent afterhyperpolarizations in hippocampal neurons of aged rats. *Science.* 1984;**226**(4678):1089–92.

41. Rapp PR, Gallagher M. Preserved neuron number in the hippocampus of aged rats with spatial learning deficits. *Proc Natl Acad Sci USA.* 1996;**93** (18):9926–30.

42. West MJ, Coleman PD, Flood DG, Troncoso JC. Differences in the pattern of hippocampal neuronal loss in normal ageing and Alzheimer's disease. *Lancet.* 1994;**344**(8925):769–72.

43. Barnes CA, McNaughton BL. An age comparison of the rates of acquisition and forgetting of spatial information in relation to long-term enhancement of hippocampal synapses. *Behav Neurosci.* 1985;**99** (6):1040–8.

44. Foster TC, Kumar A. Susceptibility to induction of long-term depression is associated with impaired memory in aged Fischer 344 rats. *Neurobiol Learn Mem.* 2007;**87**(4):522–35.

45. Norris CM, Korol DL, Foster TC. Increased susceptibility to induction of long-term depression and long-term potentiation reversal during aging. *J Neurosci.* 1996;**16**(17):5382–92.

46. Kumar A, Foster TC. Linking redox regulation of NMDAR synaptic function to cognitive decline during aging. *J Neurosci.* 2013;**33**(40):15710–15.

47. Elman JA, Oh H, Madison CM, Baker SL, Vogel JW, Marks SM, et al. Neural compensation in older people with brain amyloid-beta deposition. *Nat Neurosci.* 2014;**17**(10):1316–18.

48. O'Brien JL, O'Keefe KM, LaViolette PS, DeLuca AN, Blacker D, Dickerson BC, et al. Longitudinal fMRI in elderly reveals loss of hippocampal activation with clinical decline. *Neurology.* 2010;**74** (24):1969–76.

49. Foster TC. Calcium homeostasis and modulation of synaptic plasticity in the aged brain. *Aging Cell*. 2007;**6**(3):319–25.

50. Bodhinathan K, Kumar A, Foster TC. Intracellular redox state alters NMDA receptor response during aging through Ca^{2+}/calmodulin-dependent protein kinase II. *J Neurosci*. 2010;**30**(5):1914–24.

51. Foster TC, Norris CM. Age-associated changes in Ca(2+)-dependent processes: relation to hippocampal synaptic plasticity. *Hippocampus*. 1997;**7**(6):602–12.

52. Kumar A, Foster TC. Enhanced long-term potentiation during aging is masked by processes involving intracellular calcium stores. *J Neurophysiol*. 2004;**91**(6):2437–44.

53. Bodhinathan K, Kumar A, Foster TC. Redox sensitive calcium stores underlie enhanced after hyperpolarization of aged neurons: role for ryanodine receptor mediated calcium signaling. *J Neurophysiol*. 2010;**104**(5):2586–93.

54. Kumar A, Foster TC. Intracellular calcium stores contribute to increased susceptibility to LTD induction during aging. *Brain Res*. 2005;**1031**(1):125–8.

55. Homayoun H, Moghaddam B. NMDA receptor hypofunction produces opposite effects on prefrontal cortex interneurons and pyramidal neurons. *J Neurosci*. 2007;**27**(43):11496–500.

56. Porges EC, Woods AJ, Edden RA, Puts NA, Harris AD, Chen H, et al. Frontal gamma-aminobutyric acid concentrations are associated with cognitive performance in older adults. *Biol Psychiatry Cogn Neurosci Neuroimaging*. 2017;**2**(1):38–44.

57. Morgan CJ, Curran HV. Acute and chronic effects of ketamine upon human memory: a review. *Psychopharmacology (Berl)*. 2006;**188**(4):408–24.

58. Forette F, Seux ML, Staessen JA, Thijs L, Babarskiene MR, Babeanu S, et al. The prevention of dementia with antihypertensive treatment: new evidence from the Systolic Hypertension in Europe (Syst-Eur) study. *Arch Intern Med*. 2002;**162**(18):2046–52.

59. Lovell MA, Abner E, Kryscio R, Xu L, Fister SX, Lynn BC. Calcium channel blockers, progression to dementia, and effects on amyloid beta peptide production. *Oxid Med Cell Longev*. 2015;**2015**:787805.

60. Trompet S, Westendorp RG, Kamper AM, de Craen AJ. Use of calcium antagonists and cognitive decline in old age. The Leiden 85-plus study. *Neurobiol Aging*. 2008;**29**(2):306–8.

61. Barnes CA. Memory deficits associated with senescence: a neurophysiological and behavioral study in the rat. *J Comp Physiol Psychol*. 1979;**93**(1):74–104.

62. Daselaar SM, Iyengar V, Davis SW, Eklund K, Hayes SM, Cabeza RE. Less wiring, more firing: low-performing older adults compensate for impaired white matter with greater neural activity. *Cereb Cortex*. 2015;**25**(4):983–90.

63. Kumar A, Foster TC. Neurophysiology of old neurons and synapses. In: Riddle DR, editor. *Brain Aging: Models, Methods, and Mechanisms*. Frontiers in Neuroscience. Boca Raton, FL, 2007.

64. Neuman KM, Molina-Campos E, Musial TF, Price AL, Oh KJ, Wolke ML, et al. Evidence for Alzheimer's disease-linked synapse loss and compensation in mouse and human hippocampal CA1 pyramidal neurons. *Brain Struct Funct*. 2015;**220**(6):3143–65.

65. Mormino EC, Brandel MG, Madison CM, Marks S, Baker SL, Jagust WJ. Aβ deposition in aging is associated with increases in brain activation during successful memory encoding. *Cereb Cortex*. 2012;**22**(8):1813–23.

66. Kennedy KM, Rodrigue KM, Bischof GN, Hebrank AC, Reuter-Lorenz PA, Park DC. Age trajectories of functional activation under conditions of low and high processing demands: an adult lifespan fMRI study of the aging brain. *Neuroimage*. 2015;**104**:21–34.

67. Reuter-Lorenz PA, Park DC. Human neuroscience and the aging mind: a new look at old problems. *J Gerontol B Psychol Sci Soc Sci*. 2010;**65**(4):405–15.

68. Davis SW, Dennis NA, Daselaar SM, Fleck MS, Cabeza R. Que PASA? The posterior-anterior shift in aging. *Cereb Cortex*. 2008;**18**(5):1201–9.

69. Oberman L, Pascual-Leone A. Changes in plasticity across the lifespan: cause of disease and target for intervention. *Prog Brain Res*. 2013;**207**:91–120.

70. Kumar A, Yegla B, Foster TC. Redox signaling in neurotransmission and cognition during aging. *Antioxid Redox Signal*. 2018;**28**:1724–1745.

71. Harman D. Aging and oxidative stress. *J Int Fed Clin Chem*. 1998;**10**(1):24–7.

72. Lee WH, Kumar A, Rani A, Foster TC. Role of antioxidant enzymes in redox regulation of N-methyl-D-aspartate receptor function and memory in middle-aged rats. *Neurobiol Aging*. 2014;**35**(6):1459–68.

73. Lee WH, Kumar A, Rani A, Herrera J, Xu J, Someya S, et al. Influence of viral vector-mediated delivery of superoxide dismutase and catalase to the hippocampus on spatial learning and memory during aging. *Antioxid Redox Signal*. 2012;**16**(4):339–50.

74. Streit WJ, Xue QS, Tischer J, Bechmann I. Microglial

pathology. *Acta Neuropathol Commun.* 2014;**2**:142.

75. Rafnsson SB, Deary IJ, Smith FB, Whiteman MC, Rumley A, Lowe GD, et al. Cognitive decline and markers of inflammation and hemostasis: the Edinburgh Artery Study. *J Am Geriatr Soc.* 2007;**55**(5):700–7.

76. Scheinert RB, Asokan A, Rani A, Kumar A, Foster TC, Ormerod BK. Some hormone, cytokine and chemokine levels that change across lifespan vary by cognitive status in male Fischer 344 rats. *Brain Behav Immun.* 2015;**49**:216–32.

77. Bean LA, Ianov L, Foster TC. Estrogen receptors, the hippocampus, and memory. *Neuroscientist.* 2014;**20**(5):534–45.

78. Foster TC. Interaction of rapid signal transduction cascades and gene expression in mediating estrogen effects on memory over the life span. *Front Neuroendocrinol.* 2005;**26**(2):51–64.

79. Bean LA, Kumar A, Rani A, Guidi M, Rosario AM, Cruz PE, et al. Re-opening the critical window for estrogen therapy. *J Neurosci.* 2015;**35**(49):16077–93.

80. Kumar A, Foster TC. 17beta-estradiol benzoate decreases the AHP amplitude in CA1 pyramidal neurons. *J Neurophysiol.* 2002;**88**(2):621–6.

81. Foster TC, Sharrow KM, Kumar A, Masse J. Interaction of age and chronic estradiol replacement on memory and markers of brain aging. *Neurobiol Aging.* 2003;**24**(6):839–52.

82. Vedder LC, Bredemann TM, McMahon LL. Estradiol replacement extends the window of opportunity for hippocampal function. *Neurobiol Aging.* 2014;**35**(10):2183–92.

83. Lopez-Grueso R, Gambini J, Abdelaziz KM, Monleon D, Diaz A, El Alami M, et al. Early, but not late onset estrogen replacement

therapy prevents oxidative stress and metabolic alterations caused by ovariectomy. *Antioxid Redox Signal.* 2014;**20**(2):236–46.

84. Moorthy K, Sharma D, Basir SF, Baquer NZ. Administration of estradiol and progesterone modulate the activities of antioxidant enzyme and aminotransferases in naturally menopausal rats. *Exp Gerontol.* 2005;**40**(4):295–302.

85. McCarrey AC, Resnick SM. Postmenopausal hormone therapy and cognition. *Horm Behav.* 2015;**74**:167–72.

86. Aenlle KK, Foster TC. Aging alters the expression of genes for neuroprotection and synaptic function following acute estradiol treatment. *Hippocampus.* 2010;**20**(9):1047–60.

87. Blalock EM, Chen KC, Sharrow K, Herman JP, Porter NM, Foster TC, et al. Gene microarrays in hippocampal aging: statistical profiling identifies novel processes correlated with cognitive impairment. *J Neurosci.* 2003;**23**(9):3807–19.

88. Prolla TA. DNA microarray analysis of the aging brain. *Chem Senses.* 2002;**27**(3):299–306.

89. VanGuilder HD, Bixler GV, Brucklacher RM, Farley JA, Yan H, Warrington JP, et al. Concurrent hippocampal induction of MHC II pathway components and glial activation with advanced aging is not correlated with cognitive impairment. *J Neuroinflammation.* 2011;**8**:138.

90. Fraga MF, Ballestar E, Paz MF, Ropero S, Setien F, Ballestar ML, et al. Epigenetic differences arise during the lifetime of monozygotic twins. *Proc Natl Acad Sci USA.* 2005;**102**(30):10604–9.

91. Starnawska A, Tan Q, McGue M, Mors O, Borglum AD, Christensen K, et al. Epigenome-wide association study of

cognitive functioning in middle-aged monozygotic twins. *Front Aging Neurosci.* 2017;**9**:413.

92. Leu YW, Yan PS, Fan M, Jin VX, Liu JC, Curran EM, et al. Loss of estrogen receptor signaling triggers epigenetic silencing of downstream targets in breast cancer. *Cancer Res.* 2004;**64**(22):8184–92.

93. Moreno-Piovano GS, Varayoud J, Luque EH, Ramos JG. Long-term ovariectomy increases BDNF gene methylation status in mouse hippocampus. *J Steroid Biochem Mol Biol.* 2014;**144 Pt B**:243–52.

94. Carter SD, Mifsud KR, Reul JM. Distinct epigenetic and gene expression changes in rat hippocampal neurons after Morris water maze training. *Front Behav Neurosci.* 2015;**9**:156.

95. Han Y, Han D, Yan Z, Boyd-Kirkup JD, Green CD, Khaitovich P, et al. Stress-associated H3K4 methylation accumulates during postnatal development and aging of rhesus macaque brain. *Aging Cell.* 2012;**11**(6):1055–64.

96. Kenworthy CA, Sengupta A, Luz SM, Ver Hoeve ES, Meda K, Bhatnagar S, et al. Social defeat induces changes in histone acetylation and expression of histone modifying enzymes in the ventral hippocampus, prefrontal cortex, and dorsal raphe nucleus. *Neuroscience.* 2014;**264**:88–98.

97. Oh JE, Chambwe N, Klein S, Gal J, Andrews S, Gleason G, et al. Differential gene body methylation and reduced expression of cell adhesion and neurotransmitter receptor genes in adverse maternal environment. *Transl Psychiatry.* 2013;**3**:e218.

98. Ianov L, Riva A, Kumar A, Foster TC. DNA methylation of synaptic genes in the prefrontal cortex is associated with aging and age-related cognitive impairment. *Front Aging Neurosci.* 2017;**9**:249.

99. Foster TC, Sharrow KM, Masse JR, Norris CM, Kumar A.

Calcineurin links Ca^{2+} dysregulation with brain aging. *J Neurosci*. 2001;**21**(11):4066–73.

100. Penner MR, Parrish RR, Hoang LT, Roth TL, Lubin FD, Barnes CA. Age-related changes in Egr1 transcription and DNA methylation within the hippocampus. *Hippocampus*. 2016;**26**(8):1008–20.

101. Penner MR, Roth TL, Chawla MK, Hoang LT, Roth ED, Lubin FD, et al. Age-related changes in Arc transcription and DNA methylation within the hippocampus. *Neurobiol Aging*. 2011;**32**(12):2198–210.

102. Grinan-Ferre C, Puigoriol-Illamola D, Palomera-Avalos V, Perez-Caceres D, Companys-Alemany J, Camins A, et al. Environmental enrichment modified epigenetic mechanisms in SAMP8 mouse hippocampus by reducing oxidative stress and inflammaging and achieving

neuroprotection. *Front Aging Neurosci*. 2016;**8**:241.

103. Weaver IC, Champagne FA, Brown SE, Dymov S, Sharma S, Meaney MJ, et al. Reversal of maternal programming of stress responses in adult offspring through methyl supplementation: altering epigenetic marking later in life. *J Neurosci*. 2005;**25** (47):11045–54.

104. Zhang TY, Keown CL, Wen X, Li J, Vousden DA, Anacker C, et al. Environmental enrichment increases transcriptional and epigenetic differentiation between mouse dorsal and ventral dentate gyrus. *Nat Commun*. 2018;**9** (1):298.

105. Cechinel LR, Basso CG, Bertoldi K, Schallenberger B, de Meireles LC, Siqueira IR. Treadmill exercise induces age and protocol-dependent epigenetic changes in prefrontal cortex of Wistar rats. *Behav Brain Res*. 2016;**313**:82–7.

106. Cosin-Tomas M, Alvarez-Lopez MJ, Sanchez-Roige S, Lalanza JF, Bayod S, Sanfeliu C, et al. Epigenetic alterations in hippocampus of SAMP8 senescent mice and modulation by voluntary physical exercise. *Front Aging Neurosci*. 2014;**6**:51.

107. Feil R. Environmental and nutritional effects on the epigenetic regulation of genes. *Mutat Res*. 2006;**600** (1–2):46–57.

108. Rani A, O'Shea A, Ianov L, Cohen RA, Woods AJ, Foster TC. miRNA in circulating microvesicles as biomarkers for age-related cognitive decline. *Front Aging Neurosci*. 2017;**9**:323.

109. Freedman JE, Gerstein M, Mick E, Rozowsky J, Levy D, Kitchen R, et al. Diverse human extracellular RNAs are widely detected in human plasma. *Nat Commun*. 2016;**7**:11106.

Chapter 4

Neuroimaging of the Aging Brain

Ronald A. Cohen, Eric Porges, and Joseph M. Gullett

1 Introduction

Aging-associated changes in brain structure and function occur among all humans, though the nature of these changes, their severity, and their functional impact vary. These changes fall into three broad categories: (1) neurodegenerative diseases, (2) other diseases that affect the brain either directly (e.g., stroke) or indirectly (e.g., organ failure), and (3) the effects of normal aging (see Figure 4.1). Since multiple factors, some pathological in nature and others linked to the normal process of aging, can contribute to changes in the brain, there are four things that should be considered when assessing structure and function: (1) the neurodiagnostic assessment of older adults needs to take into consideration the contribution of each of the three categories of change; (2) different cognitive effects may be associated with each of these categories; (3) different structural and functional brain changes may also be associated with each of these categories; and (4) when assessing aging-associated cognitive and functional changes, it is essential to integrate neurodiagnostic data that inform about changes in brain structure and function, as well as underlying neurobiological alterations.

Analyses of human brain and laboratory studies involving animal models have been the source of considerable postmortem data regarding structural and histological changes in the brain that occur with aging. Comparing the brains of older adults without brain disease or injury with those of younger adults provides evidence of aging-associated brain changes not attributable to a specific etiology (Chapter 2). Some of the most common findings from postmortem examination of the brains of aging adults include: (1) cortical atrophy with widening of sulci and volume loss in gyri primarily related to reduced dendritic branching, (2) loss of white matter, and (3) alterations in almost all neurotransmitter systems, including glutamate and GABA systems, which play a major role in synaptic plasticity and learning. Whereas many of the most dramatic changes are found in people with a neurodegenerative disease, some changes also occur among aging adults without significant cognitive or functional decline or a diagnosed neurological disorder. This chapter will focus on the use of neuroimaging approaches to assess the aging brain and current evidence regarding aging-associated changes in brain structure and function.

2 Neuroimaging Approaches

The advent of computed tomography (CT) and, subsequently, magnetic resonance imaging (MRI) and spectroscopy (MRS) during the second half of the twentieth century provided the basis for major advances in the diagnosis of neurological disorders and an understanding of their pathophysiology, as well as changes in the brain associated with aging. It was no longer necessary to rely solely on postmortem analysis to characterize the location, size, and nature of lesions, as neuroimaging enabled the visualization and quantification of brain abnormalities concurrent with the clinical assessment. MRI-based neuroimaging methods offer major advantages in that they are in vivo and generally noninvasive and the acquisition of data reflecting multiple properties of the brain can be achieved within an hour. MRI provides excellent spatial resolution of neuroanatomy and reasonable temporal resolution on functional tasks (though less temporal resolution than can be achieved with electrophysiological methods).

Historically, the majority of clinical neuroimaging research has been directed at brain disorders. However, considerable data were collected from healthy individuals in the context of routine clinical assessment and for purposes of having control groups in research studies. In recent years, there has been growing interest in aging-associated changes in the brain in relation to cognitive changes. We begin by discussing the different neuroimaging modalities and the types of information that these modalities can provide. We then discuss the current neuroimaging literature on changes in brain structure and function associated with aging and include a description of the neuroimaging findings from the "oldest old." Neuroimaging findings among people exhibiting "successful" cognitive and brain aging will be contrasted with neuroimaging findings among people with neurodegenerative diseases and other brain disorders. This discussion, however, is not designed to be a comprehensive review of the entire neuroimaging literature.

MRI approaches fall into three broad categories: structural, functional, and metabolic/physiological. Neuroimaging approaches that provide information about brain structure are the most widely used in routine clinical practice. The largest body of neuroimaging research exists for these approaches, so structural neuroimaging will be considered first.

2.1 Structural Imaging

High-resolution MRI is now the gold standard for noninvasive in vivo assessment of cortical and subcortical structures and is most often used for the detection and measurement of structural brain abnormalities (e.g., lesions). Different types of information about brain structure can be obtained with specific imaging modalities.

2.1.1 Volumetrics and Morphometry

Cerebral cortex, subcortical nuclei (e.g., thalamus and basal ganglia), and cerebral subcortical white matter can now be visualized and quantified using T1 MRI sequences. T1 MRI is the most sensitive to lipid in brain tissue and yields images with excellent spatial resolution, which enables precise visualization of the brain's neuroanatomic features. This can be accomplished with MRI scanners at 1.5 Tesla (T) or less, although the current research standard is 3 T. To adequately characterize smaller units, such as hippocampal subfields, higher resolution scanners (e.g., 7 T) are necessary. Gyri, sulci, and other brain structures can be distinguished based on light–dark contrast. Quantified volumetric and morphometric analyses of brain regions can be accomplished via a variety of methods. Currently, the most common research approaches are voxel-based morphometry

and FreeSurfer. The two methods employ different segmentation and parcellation principles. Using these analytic methods, one can obtain measures of the volume, surface area, thickness, and shape of cortical and subcortical structures. T1 images are also widely used to provide a neuroanatomic framework for co-registration with neuroimaging data collected with other MRI techniques, such as fMRI.

2.1.2 Lesion Analysis

Lesions and other brain abnormalities can also be assessed via T1 imaging, particularly chronic lesions and necrotic brain tissue resulting from injury or infection. However, in the clinical setting, other scan sequences (e.g., T2, proton density, and fluid-attenuated inversion recovery (FLAIR)) are used to characterize brain abnormalities because they are more sensitive than T1 in detecting chronic parenchymal abnormalities. T2 images are sensitive to both lipids and water in brain tissue and therefore highlight areas with high water content, as in stroke and other acute injuries. When quantifying regions of interest, co-registration of these other types of image sequences with T1 images can improve neuroanatomic spatial resolution.

2.1.3 White Matter Lesions

Lesions and other white matter abnormalities can be visualized and quantified using several different MRI modalities. T1 imaging can be used for segmentation and parcellation of white matter via FreeSurfer and other image analysis programs. T2 scans are better for assessing lesions affecting the white matter (see Figure 4.1).

2.1.4 Fluid-Attenuated Inversion Recovery (FLAIR)

FLAIR sequences, which employ specialized T2 sequences, suppress signal from CSF accumulations (e.g., in the ventricles and sulci). FLAIR provides greater contrast of white matter hyperintensities (WMH) occurring in the context of microvascular disease and other brain disorders (e.g., multiple sclerosis). Over the past two decades, many research studies aimed at quantifying WMH associated with vascular cognitive impairment, HIV, and other neurological brain disturbances that affect cognition have employed FLAIR sequences. Figure 4.1 depicts a brain with a large quantity of WMH.

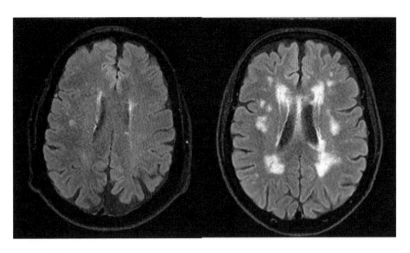

Figure 4.1 White matter hyperintensities (WMHs) exhibited on T2 FLAIR images in two individuals over the age of 85 years, neither with clinical signs of AD, neurodegenerative disease, stroke, or diagnosed cerebrovascular disease. Significant differences in the extent of WMHs are evident, as the right axial slice shows moderate to severe subcortical and periventricular WMHs, whereas minimal WMHs are evident in the scan of the individual on the left. Neither had major cognitive dysfunction, though the individual with extensive WMHs exhibited marked cognitive and psychomotor slowing.

2.1.5 Diffusion Tensor Imaging (DTI)

Diffusion-based MRI, in particular, DTI, is now widely used as a noninvasive method for investigating white matter structure in vivo. Historically, visualization of white matter pathways and their connections to gray matter and subcortical structures was limited to postmortem histological studies. DTI offers the ability to examine the axonal structure of white matter, as well as other characteristics of the axon, such as myelination. Modern DTI techniques provide the ability to examine the microstructural characteristics of white matter and to investigate anatomical changes associated with aging, both in isolation and in association with various clinical disorders and health conditions. DTI is more sensitive than conventional MRI in the detection of subtle white matter changes that might be related to clinically meaningful behavioral or functional changes.

2.2 Functional Imaging

Neuroimaging methods exist that enable the measurement of the functional responses made by the brain. In contrast to structural imaging, which capitalizes on the high spatial resolution provided by MRI, functional neuroimaging is sensitive to both the brain's spatial and temporal characteristics, that is, signal change over time. The two most widely used approaches are fMRI and positron emission tomography (PET). There are advantages and disadvantages to each. The major advantages of PET are: (1) it provides a direct measure of the metabolic activity of the brain during different functional states, and (2)

it utilizes radioactive ligands that can be used to label particular neurotransmitter systems, or as pathological markers (e.g., of amyloid and tau). PET has several disadvantages: (1) it involves the administration of a radioactive substance, which limits how frequently a person can undergo scanning; (2) it is expensive compared with fMRI; and (3) it has less spatial and temporal resolution than fMRI. The most commonly used PET ligand, ^{18}F-fluorodeoxyglucose, accumulates slowly in the brain; thus, long scan times are needed and generally only one task is possible during a scanning session. There exist PET ligands that employ very short-lived isotopes, for example, ^{15}O, but because of their very short half-lives, they cannot be shipped and must be generated on site using a cyclotron.

In contrast to PET, fMRI (1) does not require a radioactive agent; (2) is less expensive; (3) can provide information on brain responses occurring over short blocks of time or, in the case of event-related paradigms, on a trial-by-trial basis; (4) enables performance of multiple tasks in a single scanning session; (5) can be repeated without risk; (6) achieves better spatial resolution; and (7) can be readily co-registered with structural MRI scans. There are some disadvantages: (1) people with metal in their body cannot be scanned without many precautions; (2) it is less amenable to the use of ligands for the study of neurotransmitter systems; and (3) the resulting physiological signal does not provide an absolute or direct measure of metabolic or physiological activity. Activity occurring during a task of interest needs to be compared with a control task or condition. This last issue can be addressed to some extent by employing functional connectivity analysis, which correlates functional activity in different brain regions during a particular state. Because in recent years, fMRI has been employed more extensively than PET for the study of functional brain responses associated with neurological disorders and age-associated cognitive changes, this chapter will primarily focus on fMRI.

The hemodynamic response of the brain naturally varies over time in relation to metabolic demands. fMRI capitalizes on variation in the brain's hemodynamic response over time to changes in physiological state associated with the prevailing task demands. Blood-oxygen-level-dependent (BOLD) signal is evoked based on the required oxygen utilization. It is driven predominantly by synaptic activity. fMRI paradigms fall into two broad categories: task-based fMRI and resting state (rfMRI).

Task-based fMRI has been the dominant approach employed by cognitive neuroscientists. In most fMRI studies, the BOLD response during a cognitive, sensory, motor, or other behavioral task is contrasted with the response occurring during a control task. By subtracting out the areas of brain response that are common to both tasks, it is possible to determine the specific brain areas that are uniquely engaged by the task of interest and the magnitude of the functional response occurring relative to task demands. Early studies employed simple sensory or motor paradigms, such as looking at sequences of two contrasting stimuli or tapping a finger repetitively to elicit activation in the primary brain regions underlying each function (e.g., occipital and primary motor cortex, respectively). There has been rapid proliferation of fMRI paradigms over the past two decades and there are now literally hundreds of paradigms available for studying cognitive, affective, and behavioral processes. This research has provided a wealth of information, but also considerable heterogeneity in findings across studies due to a variety of factors, including the use of different paradigms, task demands, inclusion–exclusion criteria, and participant demographics.

Resting state fMRI does not employ task contrasts. Therefore, during rfMRI, participants lie passively in the scanner in a restful state, which contrasts with task-based fMRI, during which participants engage in specific tasks. The images recorded during the task are compared with control task images, yielding different patterns of activation or deactivation across

brain regions. Network connectivity is the analytic focus of rfMRI. The correlation in activation occurring across brain regions provides the basis for determining the strength of functional connections. During the resting state, greatest activation tends to occur across a set of brain regions that include the anterior and posterior cingulate cortex, pre-cuneus, medial pre-frontal cortex, and the inferior parietal lobe. The consistency of the response of these brain regions during rest led to the concept that they form a "default mode network" (DMN). The primary feature of this network is that it activates when there is not a demand for performance on a specific cognitive task or for the processing of external stimuli. On the other hand, during rest, when a person remains awake, the brain is not dormant nor is cognition absent. Rather, cognition tends to be introspective and less constrained than during task performance. The functional correlations that derive from rfMRI actually reflect the fact that brain activity in the resting state tends to spontaneously oscillate between two different states over many seconds to minutes. One major assumption underlying rfMRI is that functional connectivity observed at rest is an accurate representation of connectivity present during other states. This "state independence" has not been adequately studied and specific instances of state-specific responses have been identified.

2.3 Neuroimaging of Metabolic and Physiological Disturbances

MR-based methods have been developed that provide information about metabolic and pathophysiological changes occurring in the brain. Two methods are particularly relevant to the study of cognition and the aging brain: perfusion imaging with arterial spin labeling (ASL) and magnetic resonance spectroscopy (MRS).

2.3.1 Perfusion MRI

Perfusion-weighted imaging (PWI) enables quantification of blood flow to the brain. It can detect abnormalities in perfusion occurring as a result of a vascular occlusion causing a stroke. PWI usually involves the injection of gadolinium, an MRI contrast agent that enables visualization of blood flow to specific brain regions. It is primarily used during stroke assessment. By contrasting the extent of perfusion abnormalities with the extent of alterations in diffusivity, derived from diffusion-weighted imaging (DWI) and reflecting evolving infarction, it is possible to learn the extent of brain that might be saved if the blockage were rapidly eliminated. PWI, however, has less relevance to the study of normal brain aging.

Alternative MRI-based perfusion-weighted approaches now exist that enable quantification of regional cerebral blood flow and volume without injecting an MRI-contrast agent. While a number of these methods have been developed, arterial spin labeling is the most widely studied approach. ASL involves magnetic labeling of arterial blood below the imaged slab. Because ASL is able to provide measurement of reductions in cerebral blood flow (CBF) and volume (CBV) for the entire brain, as well as for specific regions, it has value for studies aimed at characterizing hemodynamic changes occurring with cognition and the aging brain. The BOLD response also can be used for this purpose. It tracks quite closely with ASL but is a less direct measure of blood flow.

2.3.2 Magnetic Resonance Spectroscopy (MRS)

MRS is used for measuring biochemical changes in the brain. MRS has primarily been used clinically for assessment of patients with brain tumors. It allows the comparison of the chemical composition of normal brain tissue with that of abnormal tissue found in a brain tumor or in other types of lesions. MRS can be performed with the same machine used to perform MRI. Whereas most MRS studies focus on the proton (^{1}H) environment, other targets exist, such as carbon (^{13}C) and phosphorus (^{31}P). More recent technological and methodological innovations, including higher field MRI scanners (e.g., 3T+), short echo time (TE), and edited approaches (MEGA-PRESS), as well as quantitative analytic methods, have revitalized interest in this methodology. These approaches allow quantification of a growing number of metabolites in the brain.

The most common and widely studied method is single-voxel MRS, in which the concentration of metabolites in a particular brain region of interest (ROI) is measured. Accordingly, the brain region that will be assessed must be specified prior to data collection. Other MRS approaches have been developed in recent years (2-D, 3-D, functional) that provide additional information beyond what can be derived from single-voxel MRS and ultimately may be very useful in studies of brain aging. However, since most aging

research to date has employed single-voxel MRS, our discussion will be limited to this approach.

In single-voxel MRS, the location of the voxel (i.e., ROI) is selected relative to the participant's structural MRI image, which is collected immediately before the MRS acquisition during a scanning session. The volume of the voxel can vary depending on the target anatomy but also the time available for acquisition and the sensitivity needed for the target metabolite. With all other parameters held constant, a larger voxel will yield greater signal. While an 8-cubic-centimeter voxel collected in under 5 minutes may be sufficient for n-acetyl aspartate imaging, a 27-cubic-centimeter voxel, collected for 10 or more minutes, is common for γ-aminobutyric acid (GABA) imaging. Additionally, an unsuppressed water measurement is often collected from the same anatomy to provide a reference for quantification of metabolite concentration.

The cerebral metabolites that have been most widely studied using proton MRS are n-acetyl aspartate (NAA), choline (Cho), creatine (Cr), myo-inositol (MI), glutamate-glutamine (Glx), and GABA. The concentration of each of these metabolites may vary within the brain, giving insight into local physiology and its relationship to aging and cognition.

The NAA measurement obtained from MRS is most often the result of the combined signal from NAA and neuronal N-acetylaspartylglutamate (NAAG), although the contribution of NAAG is generally assumed to be insubstantial and is commonly not considered when the data are interpreted. NAA is present in neuronal cell bodies and is often interpreted as a marker of neuronal density and viability. In the context of aging and neurodegenerative disease, NAA has been shown to decrease [1]. Recent reports suggest a relationship between NAA and intelligence [2].

MRS Cho signal is predominantly generated by glycerophosphocholine and phosphocholine with a smaller contribution from free choline. Choline measurement is widely interpreted as a marker of cell membranes and, in turn, cell density in healthy brains. It may reflect membrane turnover in disease and inflammation. Cho correlates with acetylcholine in rodent models [3], though caution is advised when extending this interpretation to humans.

Cr plays a central role in cellular energetics. Historically, Cr concentration has been assumed to be constant. For this reason, it has been used as the base for calculating the relative concentration of other metabolites, aiding in the interpretation of MRS data. Unfortunately, the constancy of Cr concentration has not been borne out by further investigation. Water-referenced approaches that allow for calculation of the relative concentration of metabolites (including Cr) have now become more common.

MI has been employed as a glial marker and is an osmolyte. Elevated MI has been interpreted as evidence of inflammation in the brain and has been reported in many populations, including heavy consumers of alcohol and patients with HIV infection [4–8] or Alzheimer's disease.

Glx reflects the combined signal from glutamate, glutamine, and, depending on the acquisition and analytic approach, a small contribution from GABA. Glutamate is the largest contributor to the Glx signal and Glx is often interpreted as glutamate. Glx increases in response to metabolic activity and is reduced in diseases associated with accelerated aging such as HIV, in which it has also been positively associated with cognitive function. Consideration of the role of glutamate in both neurotransmission and cellular metabolism, as well as the free exchange of glutamate between pools that serve these functions, is necessary when interpreting Glx findings.

GABA is the principal inhibitory neurotransmitter in the nervous system. Owing to comparatively low concentrations of GABA as compared with other metabolites, special methodology is required for its measurement. Generally, an "edited" MRS approach (MEGA-PRESS), requiring a long acquisition time and a large voxel, is employed. Additionally, macromolecules are often included in the measurement (commonly referred to as GABA+). These can be suppressed, though this further reduces the sensitivity of the measure.

A degree of caution is recommended for the interpretation of all MRS-quantified metabolites given that nearly all of them serve multiple physiological roles that can vary by tissue, cell type, and the relative quantities of gray matter, white matter, and cerebrospinal fluid in the voxel of interest.

3 Neuroimaging Evidence of Changes in the Aging Brain

There are structural, functional, metabolic, and physiological brain changes that occur in association with aging. Many questions remain about the mechanisms underlying these changes and the potential value of particular neuroimaging indices as clinical biomarkers. However, that aging-associated changes occur is indisputable, given the accumulated findings from neuroimaging and spectroscopy studies conducted over the past three decades. Furthermore, these changes are evident among aging adults without neurodegenerative disease or other neurological disorders and have been demonstrated with multiple neuroimaging and spectroscopy modalities. Aging-associated changes in the brain are discussed next, along with their relationship to cognitive performance and functional status.

3.1 Changes in Brain Structure

In clinical settings, MRI is most commonly used to identify major brain structural abnormalities resulting from stroke, tumor, degenerative diseases, or other neurological conditions that cause cortical or subcortical lesions. These abnormalities are typically quite apparent from visual inspection of the MRI. The prevalence of many of these brain disorders increases with aging. Neuroradiological assessments of the brain using MRI often report evidence of cortical atrophy that is more extensive than expected given the patient's age. In patients with AD and other neurodegenerative diseases, the MRI often shows unmistakable signs of atrophy by the time they convert to dementia. This atrophy includes the narrowing of cortical gyri, widening of sulci, and ventricular enlargement. Severe atrophy is usually indicative of neuropathology rather than "normal" brain aging. However, when atrophy is subtler, as is the case with normal brain aging and in the early stages of neurodegenerative disease, visual inspection is less reliable in detecting pathological states. For this reason, both the clinical assessment and methods for quantifying these changes in different locations are important.

Early neuroimaging studies that employed quantitative methods primarily focused on brain macrostructure. Typically, volumetric or morphometric changes in cortical and subcortical gray and white matter were measured, including changes occurring in specific brain regions and structures (e.g., the hippocampus). Another line of research focused on microvascular lesions occurring in cortical, deep subcortical, and periventricular white matter, evident as white matter hyperintensities (WMH) on FLAIR and

T2 imaging. Efforts to better assess white matter changes led to other neuroimaging methods (e.g., DTI) that enabled the characterization of white matter integrity, even in the absence of overt lesions. Using techniques such as DTI, there is now considerable evidence for aging-associated structural changes of white matter pathways.

3.1.1 Gray Matter Volume

Neuroimaging studies conducted over the past two decades have consistently shown that there are reductions in cortical volume over the adult life span. For example, we have found aging-associated reductions in total gray matter volume in a large international sample of adults aged 21–76 [9]. Aging was associated with reduced performance on measures of attention and executive functioning, as well as a reduction of gray matter volume in major frontal sub-regions (lateral, medial, orbital), the hippocampus, the amygdala, and the putamen. Regional frontal volumes predicted performance on tests of attention and executive functioning. There was an interaction between lateral frontal volume and age. Reduced frontal volume and greater age were associated with weaker executive performance.

Other studies conducted during this same time period found similar relationships between age and brain volume [10–17]. Considered together, the findings from these studies suggest particular vulnerability of the frontal cortex, especially the lateral prefrontal areas. A limitation of these findings is that they were primarily derived from cross-sectional studies. Thus, rate of brain aging could only be estimated from correlations with age, not directly on the basis of change over time. However, a few of these studies were longitudinal, providing more information about brain aging.

Reznick et al. assessed 92 nondemented older adults between 59 and 85 years of age using structural MRI at three time points: baseline and two and four years later. They found significant reductions in gray matter volumes over time [13]. The annual rate of total brain volume loss was approximately 5 cubic centimeters, while cortical gray matter loss was approximately 3 cubic centimeters and ventricular enlargement occurred at the rate of approximately 1.4 cubic centimeters per year. In this study, greatest volume changes were noted in frontal, cingulate, insular, and inferior parietal areas.

Raz and his colleagues conducted one of the first longitudinal studies, providing metrics of aging-associated volume changes in multiple cortical regions over five years in a sample of 72 adults without clinical evidence of neurodegenerative disease [18]. Volume reductions ranged from 0.32% to 0.91% annually with the greatest changes occurring in the lateral and orbital prefrontal and inferior parietal cortices, hippocampus, caudate, and cerebellum. Over a five-year period, the cumulative volume reduction ranged from 0.2 to 0.8 cubic centimeters across regions. Notably the entorhinal cortex did not show significant change.

Subsequent studies have generally shown similar findings. Ziegler et al. recently used data from the Alzheimer's Disease Neuroimaging (ADNI) cohort to estimate the longitudinal trajectory of volumetric changes as a function of age using Bayesian modeling [19]. Besides validating previous findings on aging-associated atrophy, these analyses showed how different fixed and random effects influence the trajectory of change. Individual differences among older adults with various demographic and clinical characteristics contributed to differences in trajectory. Madsen et al. mapped ventricular expansion to cortical gray matter changes in older adults from the ADNI cohort [20]. Percentage ventricular volume change at one- and two-year follow-up was associated with baseline cortical volume and thickness after controlling for demographic variables and diagnosis. Age was associated with reduced cortical volume and thickness and increased ventricular volume.

Ventricular enlargement is a cardinal feature of AD but it also occurs to a lesser extent with normal aging. In an effort to better understand the relationship between ventricular enlargement and the influence of amyloid-beta peptide in the CSF to reductions in cognitive functioning, we conducted a sub-study of older adults from the ADNI cohort [21]. CSF amyloid beta, tau, and phosphorylated tau, along with cortical and ventricular volume, were evaluated in 288 ADNI participants classified as being either normal aging controls ($n = 87$) or having MCI ($n = 136$) or mild AD ($n = 65$). Notably, among the normal aging group, ventricular volume was negatively associated with CSF amyloid beta (Aβ) levels among participants who were apolipoprotein (APOE) ε4 positive. In contrast, among participants with AD, ventricular volume was negatively associated with tau but not with Aβ among those who were ε4 positive. This finding suggested that Aβ effects among older adults at risk for AD occur at a preclinical stage, whereas increased tau level has a stronger relationship to ventricular volume once AD is evident. The apparent effect of the APOE ε4 genotype on the relationship of ventricular volume to Aβ and tau levels was interpreted as reflecting alterations in the clearance of Aβ and tau into the CSF over the course of disease. These findings also illustrate that aging-associated volumetric changes may be a manifestation of complex interactions among underlying disease mechanisms at different stages of cognitive decline and the importance of correctly classifying older adults with preclinical AD or who are at risk for AD.

Nissim et al. [22] found that cortical surface area was reduced in three frontal lobe regions (medial orbital, inferior, and superior frontal gyri) among adults with impaired working memory compared with those with normal working memory. Cortical thickness did not vary as a function of working memory performance. Therefore, impairment of working memory was associated with reduced frontal gray matter volume, but not cortical thickness, which is noteworthy given that reduced cortical thickness occurs with neurodegenerative tissue loss but tends not to occur with the typical cognitive changes associated with brain aging. In this same cohort, reduced hippocampal volume was associated with weaker overall cognitive performance (MoCA and NIH-Tool Box Fluid Cognition Composite Score), as well as deficits across multiple cognitive domains (episodic memory, working memory, and executive functioning). Accordingly, in the context of typical cognitive aging, hippocampal volume may be relevant not only to memory-related functions but also to working memory and executive functions.

There is now evidence of alterations in the shape of certain brain structures that may have functional significance beyond the effect of volume reductions [23–31]. These studies have shown aging-associated changes in structural shape among adults with and without neurodegenerative disease. Changes in thalamic shape have been reported with advanced age [23]. The greatest shape changes occur in the anterior, ventral anterior, and dorsomedial thalamic nuclei. Geradin et al., using vector machine algorithms for automated classification, achieved an 83% correct classification rate for distinguishing MCI from controls on the basis of hippocampal shape [25]. In another study, Xu et al. demonstrated that changes in hippocampal morphology and volume in

cognitively healthy older adults were strongly related to age, while age was not the driving factor among patients with AD and vascular dementia [27]. While there was significant atrophy among patients with AD and vascular dementia, reduced volume was unrelated to age.

3.1.2 White Matter Volume

In late life, people begin to experience a reduction in the volume of white matter. We previously demonstrated smaller total and regional white matter volumes among older adults compared with middle-aged and young adults that was associated with reduced neurocognitive functioning [32]. Raz et al. found that volume of the prefrontal white matter decreased by approximately 1 cubic centimeter over 5 years [18]. Aging-associated reductions in white matter volume have been shown to correlate with gray matter changes, although fewer studies have examined white matter volumetric changes and findings have been less consistent.

3.1.3 White Matter Hyperintensities

A much larger body of research exists on aging-associated increases in the quantity of white matter hyperintensities (WMH). Whereas extensive WMHs are rare in healthy young adults, they are relatively common among aging adults and quantity increases with age. Clinically, the presence of WMHs is often indicative of cerebrovascular disease causing small vessel infarction or hypoperfusion. Therefore, aging-associated increases in the quantity of WMH may reflect the increased prevalence of cerebrovascular disease with advancing age, coupled with the effects of vascular disease on the brain accumulated over the lifetime. Extensive WMHs are, however, not present in all healthy older adults. This is evident in Figure 4.1, as marked differences in the extent of subcortical and periventricular WMHs are seen in two people who are over the age of 85. Neither of these individuals had significant cognitive or function decline or any other evidence of neurodegenerative disease. Neither had a history of stroke or diagnosed cerebrovascular disease, though the individual with more extensive WMHs had a history of mild but controlled hypertension. The primary difference in their cognitive presentation was that the individual with more extensive WMHs exhibited greater slowing on timed tasks and greater, though mild, executive deficits.

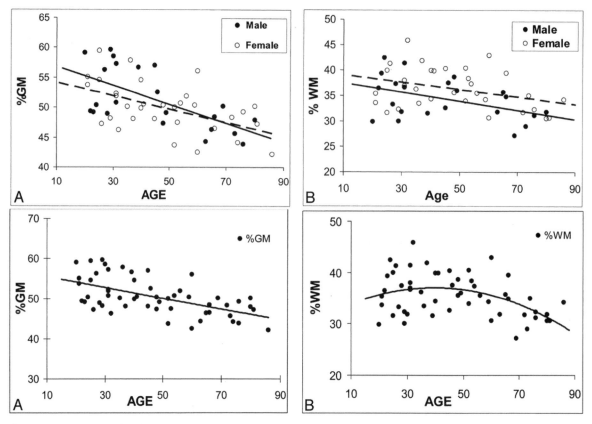

Figure 4.2 Cross-sectional results demonstrating aging-related reductions in cortical gray matter and white matter. Reprinted with permission from "Age-related total gray matter and white matter changes in normal adult brain. Part I: Volumetric MR imaging analysis." Yulin Ge, Robert I. Grossman, James S. Babb, Marcie L. Rabin, Lois J. Mannon, and Dennis L. Kolson. *American Journal of Neuroradiology*, September 2002. 23(8):1327–33.

3.1.4 White Matter Integrity

WMHs are not the only changes in the integrity of the brain's white matter to occur with advancing age. Reductions in the integrity of white matter are also evident through analysis of fractional anisotropy on diffusion tensor imaging (DTI) studies. The following section provides an overview of the effect of aging and aging-associated health conditions on white matter as determined with a variety of MR diffusion techniques.

Although gray matter atrophies throughout adulthood [11, 12, 15, 17, 18, 33–35], changes in white matter volume that occur with normal aging may be subtle. In one cross-sectional study, significant aging-related decrements in white matter volume were not observed when examined over the entire life span [36]. However, it is likely that an initial early-life increase in white matter volume occurs followed by a shift toward atrophy in late life [37]. The majority of cross-sectional and longitudinal studies of aging

demonstrate a decline of both gray and white matter in typical aging [38] (see Figure 4.2), which is accelerated with neurodegenerative disease [39]. A wide variety of methods has been utilized to study the integrity of white matter as a function of aging and new methods are still being developed and refined. The most common way to investigate white matter physical characteristics using DTI is through the creation of fractional anisotropy (FA) and mean diffusivity (MD) maps (further explained below). To a lesser degree, studies also utilize other features of the white matter microstructure, such as radial diffusivity (RD) and axial diffusivity (AD), which reflect myelination and axonal integrity of white matter, respectively. Other more recent metrics have been developed and are in the process of being validated for use, such as free water (FW) and neurite orientation dispersion and density imaging (NODDI), which will be discussed later in this chapter. FA is a measure of the degree to which the freedom of movement of a water molecule is constrained to certain directions. For example, within the straight portion of an axon, that molecule is entirely free to diffuse along the axis of the axon but has very limited ability to diffuse at a right angle to the axis because of the barrier posed by myelin investment. FA is by far the most commonly utilized and well-studied DTI metric in aging research because of the extent to which it captures overall white matter tissue integrity. It also has the benefit of simplicity of interpretation as its values fall on a scale from 0 to 1. Brownian, or random molecular, motion occurs in the cerebrospinal fluid (CSF) and is represented by an FA value of close to 0. However, FA can approach the theoretical limit of 1 in regions, such as the genu and splenium of the corpus callosum, where white matter fiber orientation is highly homogenous. Most studies demonstrate an aging-related reduction of FA values throughout the brain, a finding that is thought to represent demyelination. One early study demonstrated the strongest negative association between FA and aging to be in the genu of the corpus callosum and in the centrum semiovale [40]. A more recent study of 4,532 adults demonstrated widespread changes in FA with advancing age across all association, commissural, and limbic pathways [41].

Whereas FA captures the relative ease of diffusion in a particular direction, RD captures the absolute propensity for diffusion perpendicular to the axis of an axon. Aging-related demyelination, as reflected by increased RD, has been demonstrated in a number of white matter pathways [42] (Figure 4.3). Although increased RD appears to be widespread, some studies have suggested that specific regions are particularly affected, such as the frontal lobes and genu of the corpus callosum, where there is a higher proportion of thin or unmyelinated fibers [43, 44].

Several methods have been developed for investigating white matter integrity using DTI, one of which is tract-based spatial statistics (TBSS). Use of this method allows for the creation of a white matter skeleton common to all participants in a particular group or study. This enables voxel-wise comparisons of DTI metrics between groups, across time, or in relation to variables of interest, such as age. One longitudinal study of 203 adults utilized the TBSS approach at two time points separated by 3.6 years. The investigators found a number of aging-related declines in white matter integrity, including a decrease in FA and an increase in AD, RD, and MD

values [45]. These results were consistent with those of past cross-sectional studies of aging and white matter [46, 47] but also provided strong evidence that demyelination may be a primary source of decline in aging white matter given the magnitude of the increase in RD values with age.

A recently developed tool being utilized by DTI researchers is neurite orientation dispersion and density imaging [48] (NODDI). While this method has the disadvantage of requiring a proprietary MR image acquisition technique, which limits retrospective study of previously collected data, it has a number of potential advantages over currently used techniques. NODDI is able to quantify the density of dendrites and axons, collectively referred to as neurites, as a representation of complexity and function. Researchers have used staining techniques to determine that a reduction in neurite complexity or density can signal advancing age [49], which makes NODDI a useful noninvasive technique for estimating axon and dendrite complexity in vivo. A particular advantage of this technique is that it provides more specific information about the nature of microstructural change, as reductions in metrics such as FA can be a nonspecific indicator of neurite density reduction, increased neurite dispersion, or any of a number of other potential structural changes, such as loss of crossing fibers at a given voxel [50, 51]. Since the introduction of NODDI by Zhang et al. in 2012 [48], a number of researchers have utilized the technique to study aging. One particularly well-constructed investigation found decreasing gray matter orientation dispersion index (ODI) with aging across a number of neocortical regions [52]. Decreasing ODI also corresponded with concurrent reductions in functional resting state network connectivity, suggesting ODI was reflective of reduced neuronal density and functioning. Conversely, successful aging was associated with increased dispersion in the hippocampus and regions of the cerebellum. When taken together with histological studies suggesting that increased dendritic growth and branching in the hippocampus is a compensatory mechanism inherent to successful aging [53, 54], their results indicated that increases in ODI should occur with normal aging and any reductions would be reflective of potential neurologic disease. These findings are particularly intriguing as they suggest the NODDI method would be sensitive to hippocampus-selective neurologic disease, such as Alzheimer's disease [55].

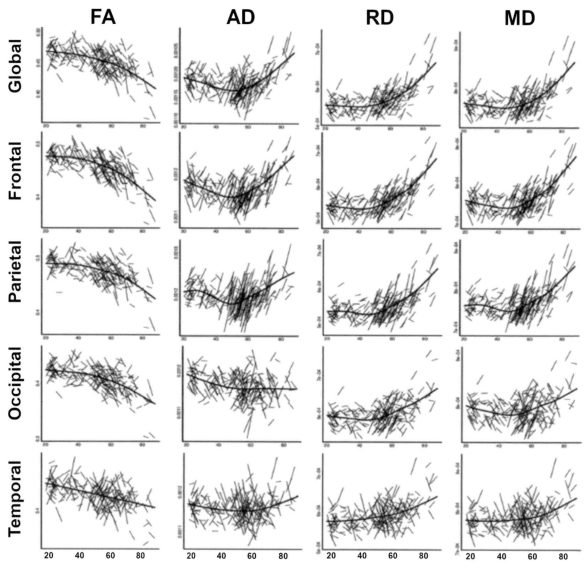

Figure 4.3 Acceleration of individual changes in fractional anisotropy (FA), axial diffusivity (AD), radial diffusivity (RD), and mean diffusivity (MD) with age. Results are displayed by global, frontal, parietal, occipital, and temporal regions of interest (ROI). Each measure represents an assumption-free general additive model as a function of age (ages 20–80) fitted to describe changes across the range of ages. Diffusivity values are in $mm^2 s^{-1} \times 10^{-3}$. Adapted from Sexton, C., Walhovd, K., Storsve, A., Tamnes, C., Westlye, L., Johansen-Berg, H., and Fjell, A., "Accelerated changes in white matter microstructure during aging: a longitudinal diffusion tensor imaging study." 2014. *The Journal of Neuroscience*, 34 (46):15425–36.

3.2 Changes in Brain Function

Aging-associated changes in functional brain response have been demonstrated on both task-dependent and resting state fMRI. The research on resting state fMRI in the context of aging is easier to summarize than research utilizing task-based fMRI, in large part because of greater uniformity in methods. The major differences between resting state fMRI studies involve the duration of imaging,

whether eyes were kept open or closed during the session, and the analytic approaches used to measure effects.

3.2.1 Resting State fMRI

Alterations in synaptic activity during the resting state have been shown to occur in the context of normal aging [56, 57]. The strength of functional connectivity among nodes within the DMN tends to decrease with aging. The degree of reduction in connectivity in this network also varies across the spectrum of cognitive health in older adults [56–59]. While reductions in the strength of connectivity within the DMN exist among older adults who are aging successfully and have preserved cognitive function, the magnitude of these reductions tends to be much less than those observed in patients with MCI or AD [56–58].

Aging-associated connectivity in the DMN during rest has been shown to be associated with cognitive performance. For the most part, reduced functional connectivity between nodes of the network (e.g., posterior cingulate cortex (PCC), insula, precuneus, and medial frontal) is associated with increased cognitive deficits and greater reductions in cognitive performance as adults reach advanced age [60]. In a study of older adults without MCI or AD, Lee et al. found that functional connectivity of the DMN differed depending on task type, performance level, and age [61]. Connectivity effects also differed between brain regions and between the cerebral hemispheres. In this study, "good" and "poor" cognitive performers were classified based on performance on three tests conducted outside the MRI (set-shifting, visual match-to-sample, and paired associate learning). The set shifting task was a variant of the Wisconsin Card Sorting Task. Poor cognitive performers showed age-dependent reductions in connectivity between the *right* insula and the PCC. In contrast, good cognitive performers showed decreased connectivity between the *left* insula and the PCC. Different effects were evident for other connections. Aging-associated decreases in connectivity between the left PCC, left medial prefrontal cortex, and anterior cingulate cortex (ACC) were observed. Functional connectivity between the left PCC and ACC was positively correlated with paired associate learning performance [56]. These results suggest that a complex relationship exists between functional connectivity patterns and the ability to perform specific cognitive tasks.

While the DMN has received the most attention in research utilizing rfMRI, aging-associated alterations during rest in other functional brain networks have also been observed, typically involving decreases in connectivity between nodes of particular networks. Joo et al. summarized recent studies addressing this topic and concluded that aging-associated reductions in functional connectivity occur across nodes of the salience network (comprised of the anterior insula and the dorsal anterior cingulate cortex) and the central executive network (which includes the dorsolateral prefrontal cortex and the lateral posterior parietal cortex) [22, 62] and that these correlate with severity of cognitive decline [63–65]. For example, in an rfMRI study that compared older adults aging normally with participants with neurodegenerative disease, the neural response of three separate functional networks (default, central executive, and salience) was shown to vary based on both age and cognitive status [63].

3.2.2 Task-Dependent fMRI

Many studies have demonstrated aging-associated changes involving both activation of specific ROIs and alterations in functional networks that occur when fMRI is acquired during cognitive task performance. However, these changes are more varied and more difficult to characterize than changes observed with rfMRI. This is due in part to the fact that many different cognitive paradigms have been studied with fMRI. The magnitude, direction (i.e., greater or lesser activation across conditions), and functional anatomic distribution of the neural response depends on task complexity and task demands. Whether or not a particular task can be performed with minimal errors also determines the nature of the functional brain response. For example, for tasks that can be performed in a nearly errorless manner, better performance is often associated with reduced extent of activation in the primary task-associated brain regions.

Two aging-associated effects have been demonstrated by Cabeza and his colleagues: (1) a posterior to anterior shift in fMRI activation (PASA), and (2) a hemispheric asymmetry reduction in older adults (HAROLD). Both of these effects involve shifts in the brain areas activated during cognitively demanding tasks. These effects are most evident during working memory tasks [66, 67] but have been observed with fMRI studies in a number of different cognitive domains. The PASA effect refers to a tendency for older adults to show greater frontal activation, even when tasks require significant involvement of posterior brain areas. The HAROLD effect reflects the fact that, with certain tasks, prefrontal activation is less lateralized in old adults than in young adults. Cabeza and colleagues interpreted the HAROLD effect as a compensatory neural mechanism that can counteract an aging-related decline in unilateral hemispheric functioning [68].

Finally, as people age, the amount of activation observed with fMRI studies employing a variety of cognitive task paradigms tends to increase, particularly in the context of high task complexity and a high demand for controlled effortful processing. The extent of activation also tends to expand beyond the primary functional brain regions that are engaged when younger people perform a task. These tendencies often reverse when there is a large area of brain damage that impedes task performance; in such cases, fMRI activation is diminished in the primary task-related brain regions. It is not clear whether the PASA effect, the HAROLD effect, and the tendency to more extensive engagement of cortical areas seen with aging are beneficial and indicative of successful compensation as a number of studies have failed to show that these effects are associated with better cognitive performance.

Aging-associated changes in task-dependent fMRI response have been shown across a number of cognitive domains. While it is beyond our scope to review this literature in detail, some of the major trends are worth noting.

3.2.2.1 Attention

The extent of synaptic activity revealed by fMRI during tasks requiring selective, focused, and sustained attention varies as a function of age [69–77]. Madden et al. found that aging effects were maximal on tasks requiring top-down attentional control [74]. Mitchell et al. showed that older and younger adults differ in extent of activation on tasks requiring "reflective" attention but not on "perceptual" attention tasks [73]. Reflective attention is focused on internal representations or associations [22], whereas perceptual attention is directed to external stimuli. When older adults focused on their memory of prior facial stimuli (reflective attention), they exhibited less deactivation within the attention network.

Aging-associated effects of reduced attentional resources on the learning and memory of associative relationships have also been examined using fMRI [76]. On tasks that make greater demands on attentional resources, older adults exhibit both impaired performance and reduced fMRI responses. However, on less attentionally demanding tasks, cognitive performance and imaging patterns in older and younger adults are similar. Significant reductions of activity in task-related areas necessary for relational memory encoding were observed in older adults as a function of attentional demand. The greatest effects were evident in ventrolateral and dorsolateral prefrontal areas, superior and inferior parietal regions, and the left hippocampus. These findings demonstrate the contribution of the prefrontal and parietal attentional systems to memory encoding occurring in the hippocampus and the influence of attentional demands on neural responses as a function of advancing age.

Aging-associated differences in activation of dorsal and ventral attentional networks are also evident on fMRI. The dorsal and ventral attentional networks are components of the frontal-parietal attentional system [37]. The dorsal network consists of the frontal eye fields and intra-parietal sulcus and is most active during the overt and covert orienting of attention (e.g., spatial search). The ventral network consists of the ventral frontal cortex and temporal-parietal junction. It is more lateralized to the right hemisphere and tends to exhibit maximal responses to behaviorally relevant stimuli that occur unexpectedly, particularly outside the current attentional focus. Kurth et al. demonstrated greater activation of the dorsal attention network in association with attention to external stimuli, regardless of age [75]. Increased activation of the dorsal attentional network also occurred as a function of short-term memory load in both young and older adults. Both observations suggest preservation of the response of this network with aging. However, older adults exhibited greater recruitment of areas outside this network when greater attentional demands were present. In contrast, reductions in activation of the ventral attentional network were observed among older adults, suggesting that this attentional system is more vulnerable to the effects of aging.

Aging-associated differences in synaptic activity have also been shown to occur as a function of selective attention. In a study by Geerligs et al. [78], a selective attention task was administered in which relevant and irrelevant information was presented simultaneously. Older adults exhibited slower responses due to distraction by irrelevant targets. Responses were associated with larger increases in activation and connectivity in the frontoparietal network (see also Chapter 12). The frontoparietal network is involved in attention, executive function, and working memory, particularly when there is a demand for cognitive control. It is comprised of the lateral prefrontal cortex and posterior parietal cortex [79]. Greater recruitment of areas surrounding the frontoparietal network occurred during target detection among older adults. Increased connectivity between this cognitive control network and somatosensory and motor areas was also found, which suggested that older adults required greater neural network activation for response selection and execution. Neural network activation in older adults also varies as a function of attentional capacity limitations, as shown in fMRI studies of dual-task performance [80, 81]. Attentional capacity and focus have also been shown to affect neural activation during dual-task performance by older adults [82]. In this study, greater activation of the occipital fusiform gyri bilaterally and the right pre- and postcentral gyri was associated with better working memory and response inhibition. Greater activation in left cerebellum and bilateral occipital fusiform gyri was associated with better digit span scores, while greater right pre- and postcentral gyrus activation was associated with less interference on the Stroop test. These effects appeared to have functional significance, as older adults with greater activation had better scores on a mobility index. Reduced activation of motor regions during this attention task was associated with an increased tendency for older adults to have falls. Thus, at advanced age, people who demonstrate greater network activation tend to have a greater capacity for divided attention and inhibition, whereas decreased activation in motor regions occurring during this divided attention task has negative functional consequences for mobility and the propensity for falling. These findings are akin to the ability to dual task, such that performing a cognitive task while engaging in motor activity reduces the ability to accurately perform the motor task in older adults.

3.2.2.2 Executive Functioning

Aging-associated changes in functional brain response have been demonstrated for several component processes of executive control, including inhibition and switching in studies employing task-based fMRI during Stroop, set shifting, and other attention-executive paradigms [83–86]. Stroop paradigms have been used to examine inhibitory control processes in the context of advancing age. Tam et al. found that the magnitude of neural activation during the Stroop test varied as a function of age and response time [87]. Healthy older adults with longer response latencies exhibit greater activation of the frontoparietal attentional regions, whereas younger adults with longer response latencies exhibit greater activation of the DMN. Fjell et al. found that longitudinal reductions in executive functioning performance over 3 years were associated with aging-associated reductions in structural integrity of a number of large white matter pathways [88]. Further, they noted that 82.5% of the variance in executive functioning decline was explained by a combination of functional and structural decline, suggesting that this decline in cognitive function performance was a consequence of aging-related disconnection.

Set shifting tasks elicit aging-associated differences in activation. Eich et al. found aging-related differences in switching costs. Older adults exhibited greater activation of both the dorsal and ventral attentional networks when there was greater switching cost [89]. However, there was also significant task-associated activation outside the ventral pathway, reflecting greater spread of activation. In another study, Hampshire et al. reported that older adults have inefficiencies in the strategy used to perform executive-attentional switching, along with a decrease in task-associated neural activity on fMRI task-related ROIs [77]. The task was to respond to the target object in a stimulus set consisting of two faces and two buildings, presented as two compound object pairs. Feedback (correct, incorrect) was provided and was used by the participants to determine the switching. Aging-associated reductions in activation in dorsolateral and ventrolateral prefrontal and posterior parietal ROIs were observed and reduced activation in these brain regions was associated with a decrement in performance in older adults.

3.2.2.3 Working Memory

Aging-associated changes in neural activation in task-associated brain regions during working memory paradigms have been shown in multiple studies [90–117]. The majority of these studies show evidence of increased activation in task-related ROIs with advanced age (e.g., dorsolateral prefrontal, parietal, supplementary motor, anterior cingulate cortices). The previously discussed aging-associated HAROLD effect – the shift in the balance of cortical activation from the left to the right hemisphere – was demonstrated in part using working memory paradigms [66]. Older adults exhibited greater shifts in activation to the nondominant hemisphere when task demands for working memory increased. Greater activation in frontal systems during tasks requiring working memory has also been shown in the majority of studies of older adults [66, 98, 118, 119]. However, in one study by Otsuka et al., the opposite effect was observed: there was decreased anterior cingulate activation among older adults that corresponded to reduced working memory performance [120]. This study involved a small sample size and the working memory task may have been too difficult for the older adults. When working memory tasks can be performed with reasonable accuracy, activation in frontal regions tends to increase with age. However, when demands are excessive and older adults become overwhelmed, they apparently do not engage fully.

Emery et al. compared young and old adults on an fMRI working memory paradigm and found that they differed in the magnitude and spatial extent of their neural responses [97]. In this study, task demands were adjusted so that performance was equivalent across age groups and the working memory condition was not more difficult than the control condition. In younger adults, manipulation-related increases in activation were limited to the core area of the working memory network, including left posterior prefrontal cortex (PFC) and bilateral inferior parietal cortices. In contrast, older adults showed more widespread activation, both within and outside this working memory network, with the greatest extra-regional activation in the bilateral PFC. These results suggest that activation and aging-related differences in lateral PFC engagement during working memory manipulation conditions may reflect strategy use and controlled processing demands or, alternatively, inefficient recruitment of the primary working memory–related areas.

3.2.2.4 Memory

There is now a relatively large fMRI research literature on the brain's neural response during memory encoding and retrieval, including a growing body of research focusing on aging-associated changes. The initial impetus for this work came from studies focused on the amnestic disturbances occurring in MCI and AD [121, 122], although increasingly, research has focused on aging effects in people without clinical evidence of these disorders who exhibit successful cognitive aging. Differences in task-associated regional activation between old and young adults have been demonstrated, although the brain regions showing these effects vary by memory type (e.g., episodic, prospective) and task demands

[106, 108, 111, 112, 123–130]. Several effects have been relatively consistent across studies. In contrast to AD, alterations in neural response of the hippocampus and entorhinal cortex are not observed in most studies involving healthy older adults. However, there are reports of aging-associated changes in cortical response. For example, posterior medial cortical areas (i.e., precuneus, retrosplenial, and posterior cingulate cortices) of the DMN were implicated in a study of the relationship between encoding and retrieval in people with early stage neurodegenerative disease and those with typical advanced aging [131]. Normally, during encoding, portions of this network exhibit reduced activation, but patients with early Alzheimer's disease do not exhibit this attenuation. Increased inferior parietal activation has been associated with better memory performance and decreased and less variable response times in older adults [132]. Aging-associated increases in the magnitude and extent of pre-frontal activation during memory encoding and retrieval have also been observed in the absence of improvements in performance [72, 99, 101, 104, 107, 109, 112, 117, 130, 133, 134], suggesting that top-down control processes become less efficient. The fact that, with advanced age, greater activation (magnitude and spatial extent) typically occurs in pre-frontal brain areas that are not highly correlated with stronger recall performance supports this possibility.

3.2.2.5 Other Cognitive Functions

Although aging-associated changes in cortical activation are evident across many cognitive domains, this is not the case for all cognitive functions. Cortical engagement associated with crystallized cognitive functions (e.g., language, semantics, and visual perception) is relatively stable across the life span. In a study conducted by Amanda Garcia in our laboratory [135], older adults (age up to mid-90s) performed normally on semantic tasks requiring judgments about the similarity in meaning of word pairs that varied in their associative relationships and concreteness. The angular gyrus and the anterior temporal lobe in both hemispheres were hubs when functional connectivity was examined. There were no significant aging-related changes in the activation of these or other areas on this task.

In another recent fMRI study of older adults conducted by Talia Seider in our laboratory [136], neural activation was assessed during three perceptual

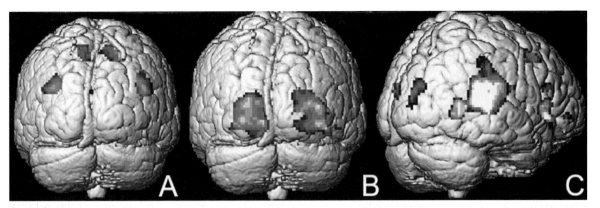

Figure 4.4 Activation observed in older adults on three perceptual tasks. (A) Location discrimination elicited activation in regions of the dorsal pathway (angular gyrus bilaterally, right precuneus, and left superior parietal lobule). (B) Shape discrimination elicited activation in the ventral pathway (left middle occipital gyrus, right middle temporal gyrus, and fusiform and lingual gyri). (C) Velocity discrimination elicited activation in the V5/MT (occipitotemporoparietal junction) and frontal areas; a large right hemisphere cluster with peak activity in the superior temporal gyrus; left middle occipital, cuneus, and supramarginal regions; and anterior right hemisphere regions with peak activity in the middle and inferior frontal gyri. These patterns were not different from those elicited in younger participants. A black and white version of this figure will appear in some formats. For the color version, please refer to the plate section.

discrimination tasks (location, shape, and velocity) using a match-to-sample paradigm. As is evident in Figure 4.4, each task activated brain regions known to constitute separate visual processing systems, including the ventral and dorsal visual pathways and area V5/MT (which supports movement perception). While there were some differences in response time as a function of age, the areas of activation, the magnitude of responses, and the functional connectivity between these areas and other brain regions remained remarkably stable, without evidence of aging-associated changes.

Findings showing selective stability of the BOLD fMRI response in semantic and visual paradigms provide strong evidence that aging is not associated with domain-nonspecific alterations in the brain's neural response.

3.2.3 Cerebral Perfusion

Normally, adequate blood flow to the brain is maintained via hemodynamic autoregulation, which in the past was widely believed to protect the brain from reductions in systemic perfusion. While hemodynamic autoregulation does provide considerable protection to the brain, cerebral blood flow tends to decrease as people reach advanced age. Reduced cerebral perfusion also occurs with alterations in hemodynamic regulatory functions that are common as people reach advanced age and there is evidence that hypoperfusion is associated with brain dysfunction [137–141].

Cerebral blood flow declines with advancing age [142]. While this may occur as a manifestation of aging-associated brain disorders [143–145], reductions in cerebral blood flow have been shown to exist among older adults without clinical evidence of neurodegenerative disease or other overt brain disorders [142, 146]. MRI studies employing ASL methods in the study of aging have revealed decreased regional cerebral blood flow and cerebral blood volume. Reduced cerebral flood flow in older adults has been shown to be associated with reduced cognitive function [147–149].

Currently, ASL is the MR-based approach most commonly used to characterize cerebral blood flow and cerebral blood volume. However, other approaches exist that can provide useful information. The BOLD response that is used primarily for fMRI is strongly driven by perfusion to regions that are the most metabolically active during specific cognitive tasks. fMRI during rest is strongly linked to cerebral perfusion as well, although because the BOLD signal must be analyzed as a function of two regions, it is not possible to derive a direct measure of cerebral blood flow from BOLD. Nonetheless, ASL and BOLD responses tend to track reasonably well together over time [150–152].

It is also worth noting that ASL can be used for functional neuroimaging investigations. Aging-associated changes in functional ASL response correlate with the BOLD response [153]. For example, brain

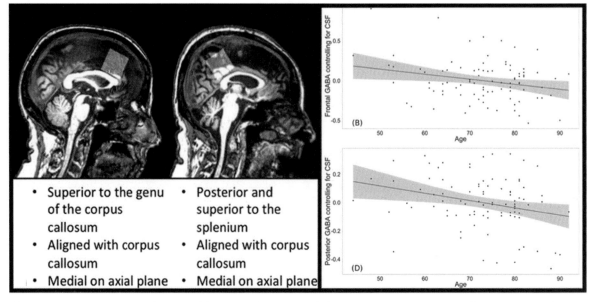

- Superior to the genu of the corpus callosum
- Aligned with corpus callosum
- Medial on axial plane

- Posterior and superior to the splenium
- Aligned with corpus callosum
- Medial on axial plane

Figure 4.5 Anterior and posterior locations of the MRS voxels are depicted, along with graphic representation of aging-associated change in GABA concentrations. It is unclear if these findings are driven by loss of GABAergic neurons, reduced GABA synthesis, or alterations of other pools of GABA (e.g., astrocytes); however, aging rodent models do indicate a reduction in the GABA synthesizing enzyme over the life span [163]. GABA concentrations were associated with cognitive performance such that older adults with greater concentrations of frontal GABA but not posterior GABA had superior performance. This finding persists when controlling for age, suggesting that it reflects aging-related changes and not age per se.

activation elicited by performance of the Stroop task yields comparable BOLD and ASL responses in the anterior cingulate, precuneous, insula, and parietal cortex [154, 155]. ASL studies conducted with induced hypercapnia, which produces maximal perfusion, exhibit particularly robust aging effects. With ASL, a "flow labeled" image is derived that is referenced to a control image in which the tissue signals are identical but the magnetization of the inflowing blood is different [156]. Arterial water is magnetically tagged before it arrives at that ROI and the image is acquired after sufficient delay to allow the tagged water to get to the ROI (inversion delay). Phase contrast MRI is another approach that characterizes the influence on cerebral blood volume of neck arterial and venous compliance (i.e., pulsitivity) before blood enters the brain [157–159]. This approach provides a way of linking systemic hemodynamic factors with cerebral perfusion, which is important given the fact that older adults exhibit decreased vascular compliance. We are currently conducting a study examining these effects in people over 85 years of age who are aging successfully.

3.2.4 Cerebral Metabolism

Changes in the brain's metabolic functions occur with aging. These changes can be assessed and quantified using magnetic resonance spectroscopy (MRS). Research has particularly focused on NAA and GABA.

Aging is associated with declines in NAA throughout the cortex. These widespread changes have been interpreted as evidence not only of tissue loss (reduced NAA-containing gray matter) but also of reduced neuronal metabolic activity [160].

In recent years, much attention has also focused on aging-associated changes in cortical GABA concentrations. Gao et al. [161] reported that cortical GABA decreases throughout adulthood, and recent work by our group has extended this into a large cohort of older adults (73.12 ± 9.9 years). We reported that cortical GABA concentrations continue to decrease into advanced age, even when an adjustment is made for CSF volume (atrophy adjustment) [162, 163] (see Figure 4.5).

Myo-inositol (MI) is a glucose metabolite that plays a role in neurotransmitter and steroid hormone receptor binding and contributes to the structure of a number of secondary intracellular messengers and membrane phospholipids. Increases in concentrations of MI have not been observed in the majority of studies of healthy aging, which typically employ measurement in a single voxel [164]. However, a recent study employing whole brain MRS imaging (MRSI) found aging-associated increases in MI and other metabolites, such as Cho and Cr, in cerebral white matter [165]. These metabolites are involved in glial function, neuroinflammation, cellular membrane turnover, and energy metabolism. It seems likely that earlier studies failed to find these effects because of methodological differences associated with single-voxel MRS and because they typically focused on cortical areas rather than white matter.

Carbon (^{13}C) and phosphorus (^{31}P) MRS have been used to a limited extent in studies of brain aging. MRS driven by metabolites containing carbon and phosphorus is potentially valuable because these elements are constituents of many compounds that play important roles in neuronal metabolism. Reductions in ATP and other phosphorus-based metabolites have been shown to occur in the aging brain, implicating changes in mitochondrial function [166–168]. Carbon-13 MRS has been used to characterize glucose metabolism in the brain [169–172], although to date there are minimal data regarding the effects of brain aging per se.

A degree of caution is recommended in the interpretation of all MRS-quantified metabolites, given that nearly all of these serve multiple physiological roles that can vary by tissue and cell type. A single MRS voxel can also capture multiple tissues, for example, gray matter, white matter, and CSF.

3.2.5 Positron Emission Tomography

Most of this chapter has focused on MRI methods for the study of cognitive function and the aging brain. Positron emission tomography (PET) and single photon emission computed tomography (SPECT), which employ radioactive ligands to elucidate physiological processes occurring in the brain, provide other important means for studying aging-associated changes. There are a large number of studies employing PET or SPECT so results will be summarized only briefly.

Direct measurement of regional cerebral metabolism can be achieved with PET and SPECT, whereas metabolic activity can only be indirectly assessed using MRI. These radiological methods can also be used to study neurotransmitter function and to quantify specific neurotransmitter receptors. For example, SPECT is commonly used to quantify the dopamine transporter, providing a measure of the quantity of dopaminergic axon terminals in the basal ganglia; significant reductions suggest Parkinson's disease [173–175]. In principle, a similar strategy can be used for investigating other neurotransmitter systems.

PET is also used to measure particular peptides (e.g., β-amyloid and tau protein) in the brain. The use of PET to quantify these peptides is relevant to the study of normal cognitive aging because excessive deposition of both is suggestive of AD. However, β-amyloid deposition commonly occurs with apparently normal aging and the distribution of deposits in AD does not coincide with the geography of AD pathology. Beta-amyloid has been viewed as a major neuropathological factor in AD since the mid-1980s [176]. Given that AD is often currently defined by the presence of abnormally high levels of β-amyloid in the brain, demonstrating deposition of this peptide may be of value in making a diagnosis of AD [177]. Tau is a soluble protein that serves to stabilize axonal microtubules. Microtubules provide the rails along which molecular motors run to transport everything from proteins to mitochondria along axons. Thus, tau plays a critical role in brain function. However, in AD, tau is hyperphosphorylated, rendering it susceptible to polymerization, which leads to the formation of neurofibrillary tangles [178]. While tau protein deposition has been linked to AD, tau accumulations occur in other brain disturbances, including chronic traumatic encephalopathy [179]. Accordingly, abnormal whole brain levels of tau observed in PET studies are not specific to any one etiology but, rather, are indicative of altered phosphorylation and neuropathology. The most common abnormalities observed at postmortem examination of aging brains are hyperphosphorylated tau, observed in both neurons and glia, and β-amyloid aggregation in the neuropil [180].

4 Conclusions

Neuroimaging provides a valuable tool for the study of brain aging. Currently, neurodiagnostic MRI is primarily used for the assessment of neurological disorders. However, based on the current mandate of the National Academy of Medicine, there is a need for greater attention to brain wellness. The goal is preventing, limiting, and ameliorating the neurobehavioral effects of brain aging before severe dysfunction has developed. To date, the neuroimaging approaches discussed in this chapter, for the most part, have not been used for this purpose. Multimodal neuroimaging employing MRI and MRS can provide information that bridges brain structure, function, and pathophysiology. Most existing neuroimaging research on cognitive and brain aging has focused on a single modality, whether it be cortical structure, white matter integrity, or functional brain response. The real power of these methods will emerge when data from multiple modalities are integrated to provide a complete picture of the health of an individual's aging brain.

With aging, there are changes in brain structure and function, along with metabolic and physiological changes (e.g., cerebral blood flow), that influence cognition. As discussed in this chapter, there are aging-related reductions of volume in specific regions of the cerebral cortex and subcortical nuclei, as well as in subcortical white matter. Individual differences exist in these rates of change, which appear to be influenced by a variety of factors. The shape of particular brain structures also changes with age, although this is a topic of research that requires more investigation. Changes in cortical thickness, in the absence of neurodegeneration, are not dramatic compared with changes in cortical surface area. It is probably reductions in the density of dendritic branching that account for aging-related reductions in surface area, as there is not a major loss of neurons, but rather changes in micro-architecture. Changes in functional brain responses also occur that can be detected using resting-state and task-dependent fMRI. Resting-state fMRI probably has more short-term potential as a clinical assessment tool because of the uniformity in the nature and temporal pattern of cerebral activity during scanning in the resting state. However, there are limits to what can be determined during the resting state. Ultimately, the implementation of standard tasks will be used for probing particular cognitive domains. There is considerable complexity in the nature of the neural response occurring across different tasks. Therefore, it will likely take additional research before task-dependent fMRI fulfills its potential. Changes in neural response occur with advanced age that involve a number of cognitive domains, including attention, executive functioning, working memory, and encoding and retrieval of memory. However, functional imaging patterns associated with functions such as language, semantics, and perception remain relatively constant through the lifetime.

Structural and functional imaging have historically received the most attention. Yet, from a clinical perspective, methods that enable the measurement of physiological and metabolic changes may have the greatest potential for elucidating the brain mechanisms underlying cognitive changes that occur with aging and for establishing targets for interventions. MRS that incorporates phosphorus and carbon metabolites would be extremely useful for characterizing specific metabolic changes. Cerebral blood flow measurement via ASL provides a noninvasive method for assessing cerebral perfusion changes. When these types of data are coupled with structural and functional neuroimaging, it becomes possible to track not only changes in brain structure and neural response over time, but also factors that may help to account for these declines. Although great progress has been made in neuroimaging over the past two to three decades, there is still much that remains to be learned. Establishing the upper limits of brain health in the oldest of old, successful and "super agers," remains a topic that needs additional studies. The use of imaging methods for detecting subtle pre-clinical brain changes among people at risk for developing neurodegenerative changes is another critical area of current and future inquiry. Furthermore, implementation of these approaches into the clinical arena is still in its infancy. In the sum, neuroimaging of cognitive and brain aging remains an open frontier.

References

1. Huang, W., et al., High brain myo-inositol levels in the predementia phase of Alzheimer's disease in adults with Down's syndrome: a 1H MRS study. *Am J Psychiatry*, 1999. **156**(12):1879–86.

2. Paul, E.J., et al., Dissociable brain biomarkers of fluid intelligence. *Neuroimage*, 2016. **137**:201–211.

3. Wang, X.C., et al., Correlation between choline signal intensity and acetylcholine level in different brain regions of rat. *Neurochem Res*, 2008. **33**(5):814–19.

4. Cohen, R.A., et al., Cerebral metabolite abnormalities in human immunodeficiency virus are associated with cortical and subcortical volumes. *J Neurovirol*, 2010. **16**(6):435–44.

5. Harezlak, J., et al., Persistence of HIV-associated cognitive impairment, inflammation, and neuronal injury in era of highly active antiretroviral treatment. *AIDS*, 2011. **25**(5):625–33.

6. Harezlak, J., et al., Predictors of CNS injury as measured by proton magnetic resonance spectroscopy in the setting of chronic HIV infection and CART. *J Neurovirol*, 2014. **20**(3):294–303.

7. Hua, X., et al., Disrupted cerebral metabolite levels and lower nadir CD4+ counts are linked to brain volume deficits in 210 HIV-infected patients on stable treatment. *Neuroimage Clin*, 2013. **3**:132–42.

8. Long, Z., et al., Vulnerability of welders to manganese exposure – a neuroimaging study. *Neurotoxicology*, 2014. **45**:285–92.

9. Zimmerman, M.E., et al., The relationship between frontal gray matter volume and cognition varies across the healthy adult lifespan. *Am J Geriatr Psychiatry*, 2006. **14**(10):823–33.

10. Bartzokis, G., et al., Age-related changes in frontal and temporal lobe volumes in men: a magnetic resonance imaging study. *Arch Gen Psychiatry*, 2001. **58**(5):461–5.

11. Raz, N., et al., Selective aging of the human cerebral cortex observed in vivo: differential vulnerability of the prefrontal gray matter. *Cereb Cortex*, 1997. **7**(3):268–82.

12. Raz, N., et al., Aging, sexual dimorphism, and hemispheric asymmetry of the cerebral cortex: replicability of regional differences in volume. *Neurobiol Aging*, 2004. **25**(3):377–96.

13. Resnick, S.M., et al., Longitudinal magnetic resonance imaging studies of older adults: a shrinking brain. *J Neurosci*, 2003. **23**(8):3295–301.

14. Scahill, R.I., et al., A longitudinal study of brain volume changes in normal aging using serial registered magnetic resonance imaging. *Arch Neurol*, 2003. **60**(7):989–94.

15. Sullivan, E.V., et al., Effects of age and sex on volumes of the thalamus, pons, and cortex. *Neurobiol Aging*, 2004. **25**(2):185–92.

16. Jernigan, T.L., et al., Effects of age on tissues and regions of the cerebrum and cerebellum. *Neurobiol Aging*, 2001. **22**(4):581–94.

17. Pfefferbaum, A., et al., A quantitative magnetic resonance imaging study of changes in brain morphology from infancy to late adulthood. *Arch Neurol*, 1994. **51**(9):874–87.

18. Raz, N., et al., Regional brain changes in aging healthy adults: general trends, individual differences and modifiers. *Cereb Cortex*, 2005. **15**(11):1676–89.

19. Ziegler, G., et al., Estimating anatomical trajectories with Bayesian mixed-effects modeling. *Neuroimage*, 2015. **121**:51–68.

20. Madsen, S.K., et al., Mapping ventricular expansion onto cortical gray matter in older adults. *Neurobiol Aging*, 2015. **36**(Suppl 1):S32–S41.

21. Metastasio, A., et al., Conversion of MCI to dementia: role of proton magnetic resonance spectroscopy. *Neurobiol Aging*, 2006. **27**(7):926–32.

22. Sabayan, B., et al., Cerebrovascular hemodynamics in Alzheimer's disease and vascular dementia: a meta-analysis of transcranial Doppler studies. *Ageing Res Rev*, 2012. **11**(2):271–7.

23. Hughes, E.J., et al., Regional changes in thalamic shape and volume with increasing age. *Neuroimage*, 2012. **63**(3):1134–42.

24. Yang, X., et al., Evolution of hippocampal shapes across the human lifespan. *Hum Brain Mapp*, 2013. **34**(11):3075–85.

25. Gerardin, E., et al., Multidimensional classification of hippocampal shape features discriminates Alzheimer's disease and mild cognitive impairment from normal aging. *Neuroimage*, 2009. **47**(4):1476–86.

26. Miller, M.I., et al., Collaborative computational anatomy: an MRI morphometry study of the human brain via diffeomorphic metric mapping. *Hum Brain Mapp*, 2009. **30**(7):2132–41.

27. Xu, Y., et al., Age effects on hippocampal structural changes in old men: the HAAS. *Neuroimage*, 2008. **40**(3):1003–15.

28. Scher, A.I., et al., Hippocampal shape analysis in Alzheimer's disease: a population-based study. *Neuroimage*, 2007. **36**(1):8–18.

29. Wang, L., et al., Abnormalities of hippocampal surface structure in very mild dementia of the Alzheimer type. *Neuroimage*, 2006. **30**(1):52–60.

30. Bouix, S., et al., Hippocampal shape analysis using medial surfaces. *Neuroimage*, 2005. **25**(4):1077–89.

31. Wang, L., et al., Changes in hippocampal volume and shape across time distinguish dementia of the Alzheimer type from healthy aging. *Neuroimage*, 2003. **20**(2):667–82.

32. Brickman, A.M., et al., Regional white matter and neuropsychological functioning across the adult lifespan. *Biol Psychiatry*, 2006. **60**(5):444–53.

33. Blatter, D.D., et al., Quantitative volumetric analysis of brain MR: normative database spanning 5 decades of life. *AJNR Am J Neuroradiol*, 1995. **16**(2):241–51.

34. Jernigan, T.L., G.A. Press, and J.R. Hesselink, Methods for measuring brain morphologic features on magnetic resonance images. Validation and normal aging. *Arch Neurol*, 1990. **47**(1):27–32.

35. Sullivan, E.V., et al., Sex differences in corpus callosum size: relationship to age and intracranial size. *Neurobiol Aging*, 2001. **22**(4):603–11.

36. Pfefferbaum, A., et al., A controlled study of cortical gray matter and ventricular changes in alcoholic men over a 5-year interval. *Arch Gen Psychiatry*, 1998. **55**(10):905–12.

37. Aasprang, A., et al., Ten-year changes in health-related quality of life after biliopancreatic diversion with duodenal switch. *Surg Obes Relat Dis*, 2016. **12**(8):1594–600.

38. Ge, Y., et al., Age-related total gray matter and white matter changes in normal adult brain. Part I: volumetric MR imaging analysis. *AJNR Am J Neuroradiol*, 2002. **23**(8):1327–33.

39. Driscoll, I., et al., Longitudinal pattern of regional brain volume change differentiates normal aging from MCI. *Neurology*, 2009. **72**(22):1906–13.

40. Pfefferbaum, A., et al., Age-related decline in brain white matter anisotropy measured with spatially corrected echo-planar diffusion tensor imaging. *Magn Reson Med*, 2000. **44**(2):259–68.

41. de Groot, M., et al., Tract-specific white matter degeneration in aging: the Rotterdam Study. *Alzheimers Dement*, 2015. **11**(3):321–30.

42. Davis, S.W., et al., Assessing the effects of age on long white matter tracts using diffusion tensor tractography. *Neuroimage*, 2009. **46**(2):530–41.

43. Aboitiz, F., et al., Age-related changes in fibre composition of the human corpus callosum: sex differences. *Neuroreport*, 1996. **7**(11):1761–4.

44. Bartzokis, G., Age-related myelin breakdown: a developmental model of cognitive decline and Alzheimer's disease. *Neurobiol Aging*, 2004. **25**(1):5–18; author reply 49–62.

45. Sexton, C.E., et al., Accelerated changes in white matter microstructure during aging: a longitudinal diffusion tensor imaging study. *J Neurosci*, 2014. **34**(46):15425–36.

46. Bennett, I.J., et al., Age-related differences in multiple measures of white matter integrity: a diffusion tensor imaging study of healthy aging. *Hum Brain Mapp*, 2010. **31**(3):378–90.

47. Westlye, L.T., et al., Life-span changes of the human brain white matter: diffusion tensor imaging (DTI) and volumetry. *Cereb Cortex*, 2010. **20**(9):2055–68.

48. Zhang, H., et al., NODDI: practical in vivo neurite orientation dispersion and density imaging of the human brain. *Neuroimage*, 2012. **61**(4):1000–16.

49. Jacobs, B., L. Driscoll, and M. Schall, Life-span dendritic and spine changes in areas 10 and 18 of human cortex: a quantitative Golgi study. *J Comp Neurol*, 1997. **386**(4):661–80.

50. Beaulieu, C., *The biological basis of diffusion anisotropy*, in *Diffusion MRI: From Quantitative Measurement to In-vivo Neuroanatomy*, H. Johansen-Berg and T.E.J. Behrens, editors. London: Academic Press, 2009, pp. 155–84.

51. Pierpaoli, C., et al., Diffusion tensor MR imaging of the human brain. *Radiology*, 1996. **201**(3):637–48.

52. Nazeri, A., et al., Functional consequences of neurite orientation dispersion and density in humans across the adult lifespan. *J Neurosci*, 2015. **35**(4):1753–62.

53. Flood, D.G., et al., Age-related dendritic growth in dentate gyrus of human brain is followed by regression in the "oldest old." *Brain Res*, 1985. **345**(2):366–8.

54. Pyapali, G.K. and D.A. Turner, Increased dendritic extent in hippocampal CA1 neurons from aged F344 rats. *Neurobiol Aging*, 1996. **17**(4):601–11.

55. Colgan, N., et al., Application of neurite orientation dispersion and density imaging (NODDI) to a tau pathology model of Alzheimer's disease. *Neuroimage*, 2016. **125**:739–44.

56. Sala-Llonch, R., D. Bartres-Faz, and C. Junque, Reorganization of brain networks in aging: a review of functional connectivity studies. *Front Psychol*, 2015. **6**:663.

57. Anthony, M. and F. Lin, A systematic review for functional neuroimaging studies of cognitive reserve across the cognitive aging spectrum. *Arch Clin Neuropsychol*, 2018. **33**(8):937–48.

58. Dennis, E.L. and P.M. Thompson, Functional brain connectivity using fMRI in aging and Alzheimer's disease. *Neuropsychol Rev*, 2014. **24**(1):49–62.

59. Ouchi, Y. and M. Kikuchi, A review of the default mode network in aging and dementia based on molecular imaging. *Rev Neurosci*, 2012. **23**(3):263–8.

60. Wang, L., et al., Amnestic mild cognitive impairment: topological reorganization of the default-mode network. *Radiology*, 2013. **268**(2):501–14.

61. Lee, A., M. Tan, and A. Qiu, Distinct aging effects on functional networks in good and poor cognitive performers. *Front Aging Neurosci*, 2016. **8**:215.

62. Onoda, K., M. Ishihara, and S. Yamaguchi, Decreased functional connectivity by aging is associated with cognitive decline. *J Cogn Neurosci*, 2012. **24**(11):2186–98.

63. Joo, S.H., H.K. Lim, and C.U. Lee, Three large-scale functional brain networks from resting-state functional MRI in subjects with different levels of cognitive impairment. *Psychiatry Investig*, 2016. **13**(1):1–7.

64. Cieri, F. and R. Esposito, Neuroaging through the lens of the resting state networks. *Biomed Res Int*, 2018. **2018**:5080981.

65. Chhatwal, J.P. and R.A. Sperling, Functional MRI of mnemonic networks across the spectrum of normal aging, mild cognitive impairment, and Alzheimer's disease. *J Alzheimers Dis*, 2012. **31** (**Suppl 3**):S155–S167.

66. Cabeza, R., et al., Task-independent and task-specific age effects on brain activity during working memory, visual attention and episodic retrieval. *Cereb Cortex*, 2004. **14**(4):364–75.

67. Paskavitz, J.F., et al., Recruitment and stabilization of brain activation within a working memory task; an FMRI study. *Brain Imaging Behav*, 2010. **4**(1):5–21.

68. Cabeza, R., et al., Aging gracefully: compensatory brain activity in high-performing older adults. *Neuroimage*, 2002. **17** (3):1394–402.

69. Spreng, R.N., et al., Attenuated anticorrelation between the default and dorsal attention networks with aging: evidence from task and rest. *Neurobiol Aging*, 2016. **45**:149–60.

70. Schmitz, T.W., et al., Distinguishing attentional gain and tuning in young and older adults. *Neurobiol Aging*, 2014. **35** (11):2514–25.

71. Russell, C., et al., Dynamic attentional modulation of vision across space and time after right hemisphere stroke and in ageing. *Cortex*, 2013. **49**(7):1874–83.

72. Oren, N., et al., How attention modulates encoding of dynamic stimuli in older adults. *Behav Brain Res*, 2018. **347**:209–18.

73. Mitchell, K.J., et al., Age differences in brain activity during perceptual versus reflective attention. *Neuroreport*, 2010. **21** (4):293–7.

74. Madden, D.J., et al., Adult age differences in the functional neuroanatomy of visual attention: a combined fMRI and DTI study. *Neurobiol Aging*, 2007. **28** (3):459–76.

75. Kurth, S., et al., Effects of aging on task- and stimulus-related cerebral attention networks. *Neurobiol Aging*, 2016. **44**:85–95.

76. Kim, S.Y. and K.S. Giovanello, The effects of attention on age-related relational memory deficits: fMRI evidence from a novel attentional manipulation. *J Cogn Neurosci*, 2011. **23**(11):3637–56.

77. Hampshire, A., et al., Inefficiency in self-organized attentional switching in the normal aging population is associated with decreased activity in the ventrolateral prefrontal cortex. *J Cogn Neurosci*, 2008. **20** (9):1670–86.

78. Geerligs, L., et al., Brain mechanisms underlying the effects of aging on different aspects of selective attention. *Neuroimage*, 2014. **91**:52–62.

79. Zanto, T.P. and A. Gazzaley, Fronto-parietal network: flexible hub of cognitive control. *Trends Cogn Sci*, 2013. **17**(12):602–3.

80. Van Impe, A., et al., Age-related changes in brain activation underlying single- and dual-task performance: visuomanual drawing and mental arithmetic. *Neuropsychologia*, 2011. **49** (9):2400–9.

81. Hartley, A.A., J. Jonides, and C.Y. Sylvester, Dual-task processing in younger and older adults: similarities and differences revealed by fMRI. *Brain Cogn*, 2011. **75**(3):281–91.

82. Nagamatsu, L.S., et al., The neurocognitive basis for impaired dual-task performance in senior fallers. *Front Aging Neurosci*, 2016. **8**:20.

83. Gauthier, C.J., et al., Absolute quantification of resting oxygen metabolism and metabolic reactivity during functional activation using QUO2 MRI. *Neuroimage*, 2012. **63**(3):1353–63.

84. Goodwin, J.A., et al., Quantitative fMRI using hyperoxia calibration: reproducibility during a cognitive Stroop task. *Neuroimage*, 2009. **47** (2):573–80.

85. Mildner, T., et al., Towards quantification of blood-flow changes during cognitive task activation using perfusion-based fMRI. *Neuroimage*, 2005. **27** (4):919–26.

86. Mohtasib, R.S., et al., Calibrated fMRI during a cognitive Stroop task reveals reduced metabolic response with increasing age. *Neuroimage*, 2012. **59**(2):1143–51.

87. Tam, A., et al., Effects of reaction time variability and age on brain activity during Stroop task performance. *Brain Imaging Behav*, 2015. **9**(3):609–18.

88. Fjell, A.M., et al., The disconnected brain and executive function decline in aging. *Cereb Cortex*, 2017. **27**(3):2303–17.

89. Eich, T.S., et al., Functional brain and age-related changes associated with congruency in task switching. *Neuropsychologia*, 2016. **91**:211–21.

90. Takeuchi, H., et al., Failing to deactivate: the association between brain activity during a working memory task and creativity. *Neuroimage*, 2011. **55** (2):681–7.

91. Oren, N., et al., Neural patterns underlying the effect of negative distractors on working memory in older adults. *Neurobiol Aging*, 2017. **53**:93–102.

92. Nyberg, L., et al., Neural correlates of variable working memory load across adult age and skill: dissociative patterns within the fronto-parietal network. *Scand J Psychol*, 2009. **50**(1):41–6.

93. Nagel, I.E., et al., Load modulation of BOLD response and connectivity predicts working memory performance in younger and older adults. *J Cogn Neurosci*, 2011. **23**(8):2030–45.

94. Luis, E.O., et al., Successful working memory processes and cerebellum in an elderly sample: a neuropsychological and fMRI study. *PLoS One*, 2015. **10**(7): e0131536.

95. Heinzel, S., et al., Prefrontal-parietal effective connectivity during working memory in older adults. *Neurobiol Aging*, 2017. **57**:18–27.

96. Hakun, J.G. and N.F. Johnson, Dynamic range of frontoparietal functional modulation is associated with working memory capacity limitations in older adults. *Brain Cogn*, 2017. **118**:128–36.

97. Emery, L., et al., Age-related changes in neural activity during performance matched working memory manipulation. *Neuroimage*, 2008. **42**(4):1577–86.

98. Grady, C.L., H. Yu, and C. Alain, Age-related differences in brain activity underlying working memory for spatial and nonspatial auditory information. *Cereb Cortex*, 2008. **18**(1):189–99.

99. Shing, Y.L., et al., Neural activation patterns of successful episodic encoding: reorganization during childhood, maintenance in old age. *Dev Cogn Neurosci*, 2016. **20**:59–69.

100. Cooper, C.M., et al., Memory and functional brain differences in a national sample of U.S. veterans with Gulf War Illness. *Psychiatry Res Neuroimaging*, 2016. **250**:33–41.

101. Wang, T.H., et al., The effects of age on the neural correlates of recollection success, recollection-related cortical reinstatement, and post-retrieval monitoring. *Cereb Cortex*, 2016. **26**(4):1698–714.

102. Cansino, S., et al., fMRI subsequent source memory effects in young, middle-aged and old adults. *Behav Brain Res*, 2015. **280**:24–35.

103. Maillet, D. and M.N. Rajah, Age-related differences in brain activity in the subsequent memory paradigm: a meta-analysis. *Neurosci Biobehav Rev*, 2014. **45**:246–57.

104. Mattson, J.T., et al., Effects of age on negative subsequent memory effects associated with the encoding of item and item-context information. *Cereb Cortex*, 2014. **24**(12):3322–33.

105. Angel, L., et al., Differential effects of aging on the neural correlates of recollection and familiarity. *Cortex*, 2013. **49**(6):1585–97.

106. Sambataro, F., et al., Normal aging modulates prefrontoparietal networks underlying multiple memory processes. *Eur J Neurosci*, 2012. **36**(11):3559–67.

107. Salami, A., J. Eriksson, and L. Nyberg, Opposing effects of aging on large-scale brain systems for memory encoding and cognitive control. *J Neurosci*, 2012. **32** (31):10749–57.

108. Ramsoy, T.Z., et al., Healthy aging attenuates task-related specialization in the human medial temporal lobe. *Neurobiol Aging*, 2012. **33**(9):1874–89.

109. Maillet, D. and M.N. Rajah, Age-related changes in the three-way correlation between anterior hippocampus volume, whole-brain patterns of encoding activity and subsequent context retrieval. *Brain Res*, 2011. **1420**:68–79.

110. Protzner, A.B., et al., Network interactions explain effective encoding in the context of medial temporal damage in MCI. *Hum Brain Mapp*, 2011. **32**(8):1277–89.

111. Trivedi, M.A., et al., fMRI activation changes during successful episodic memory encoding and recognition in amnestic mild cognitive impairment relative to cognitively healthy older adults. *Dement Geriatr Cogn Disord*, 2008. **26** (2):123–37.

112. Kircher, T., et al., Anterior hippocampus orchestrates successful encoding and retrieval of non-relational memory: an event-related fMRI study. *Eur Arch Psychiatry Clin Neurosci*, 2008. **258**(6):363–72.

113. Bangen, K.J., et al., Differential age effects on cerebral blood flow and BOLD response to encoding: associations with cognition and stroke risk. *Neurobiol Aging*, 2009. **30**(8):1276–87.

114. Han, S.D., et al., Verbal paired-associate learning by APOE genotype in non-demented older adults: fMRI evidence of a right hemispheric compensatory response. *Neurobiol Aging*, 2007. **28**(2):238–47.

115. Rand-Giovannetti, E., et al., Hippocampal and neocortical activation during repetitive encoding in older persons. *Neurobiol Aging*, 2006. **27** (1):173–82.

116. Vandenbroucke, M.W., et al., Interindividual differences of medial temporal lobe activation during encoding in an elderly population studied by fMRI. *Neuroimage*, 2004. **21**(1):173–80.

117. Morcom, A.M., et al., Age effects on the neural correlates of successful memory encoding. *Brain*, 2003. **126**(Pt. 1):213–29.

118. Cabeza, R., Hemispheric asymmetry reduction in older adults: the HAROLD model. *Psychol Aging*, 2002. **17**(1):85–100.

119. Park, D.C., et al., Working memory for complex scenes: age

differences in frontal and hippocampal activations. *J Cogn Neurosci*, 2003. **15**(8):1122–34.

120. Otsuka, Y., et al., Decreased activation of anterior cingulate cortex in the working memory of the elderly. *Neuroreport*, 2006. **17**(14):1479–82.

121. Corkin, S., Functional MRI for studying episodic memory in aging and Alzheimer's disease. *Geriatrics*, 1998. **53**(**Suppl 1**): S13–S15.

122. Clement, F. and S. Belleville, Test-retest reliability of fMRI verbal episodic memory paradigms in healthy older adults and in persons with mild cognitive impairment. *Hum Brain Mapp*, 2009. **30**(12):4033–47.

123. Dennis, N.A., H. Kim, and R. Cabeza, Age-related differences in brain activity during true and false memory retrieval. *J Cogn Neurosci*, 2008. **20**(8):1390–402.

124. Rajah, M.N. and A.R. McIntosh, Age-related differences in brain activity during verbal recency memory. *Brain Res*, 2008. **1199**:111–25.

125. Stevens, W.D., et al., A neural mechanism underlying memory failure in older adults. *J Neurosci*, 2008. **28**(48):12820–4.

126. Bai, F., et al., Abnormal functional connectivity of hippocampus during episodic memory retrieval processing network in amnestic mild cognitive impairment. *Biol Psychiatry*, 2009. **65**(11):951–8.

127. Spaniol, J. and C. Grady, Aging and the neural correlates of source memory: over-recruitment and functional reorganization. *Neurobiol Aging*, 2012. **33**(2):425 e3–18.

128. St Jacques, P.L., D.C. Rubin, and R. Cabeza, Age-related effects on the neural correlates of autobiographical memory retrieval. *Neurobiol Aging*, 2012. **33**(7):1298–310.

129. Sugarman, M.A., et al., Functional magnetic resonance imaging of semantic memory as a presymptomatic biomarker of Alzheimer's disease risk. *Biochim Biophys Acta*, 2012. **1822** (3):442–56.

130. Geddes, M.R., et al., Human aging reduces the neurobehavioral influence of motivation on episodic memory. *Neuroimage*, 2018. **171**:296–310.

131. Huijbers, W., et al., Explaining the encoding/retrieval flip: memory-related deactivations and activations in the posteromedial cortex. *Neuropsychologia*, 2012. **50** (14):3764–74.

132. MacDonald, S.W., et al., Increased response-time variability is associated with reduced inferior parietal activation during episodic recognition in aging. *J Cogn Neurosci*, 2008. **20**(5):779–86.

133. Foster, C.M., et al., Prefrontal contributions to relational encoding in amnestic mild cognitive impairment. *Neuroimage Clin*, 2016. **11**:158–66.

134. Pudas, S., et al., Longitudinal evidence for increased functional response in frontal cortex for older adults with hippocampal atrophy and memory decline. *Cereb Cortex*, 2018. **28**(3):936–48.

135. Garcia, A., *Functional activation and connectivity of the semantic network in older adults.* PhD diss., University of Florida, Gainesville, 2017.

136. Seider, T., *Seeing brain: an FMRI study of age-related changes in visual perception and discrimination.* PhD diss., University of Florida, Gainesville, 2017.

137. Alosco, M.L., et al., The synergistic effects of anxiety and cerebral hypoperfusion on cognitive dysfunction in older adults with cardiovascular disease. *J Geriatr Psychiatry Neurol*, 2015. **28**(1):57–66.

138. Alosco, M.L., et al., The adverse effects of reduced cerebral perfusion on cognition and brain structure in older adults with cardiovascular disease. *Brain Behav*, 2013. **3**(6):626–36.

139. Alosco, M.L., et al., The impact of hypertension on cerebral perfusion and cortical thickness in older adults. *J Am Soc Hypertens*, 2014. **8**(8):561–70.

140. Brickman, A.M., et al., Reduction in cerebral blood flow in areas appearing as white matter hyperintensities on magnetic resonance imaging. *Psychiatry Res*, 2009. **172**(2):117–20.

141. Zimmerman, B., et al., Cardiorespiratory fitness mediates the effects of aging on cerebral blood flow. *Front Aging Neurosci*, 2014. **6**:59.

142. Leoni, R.F., et al., Cerebral blood flow and vasoreactivity in aging: an arterial spin labeling study. *Braz J Med Biol Res*, 2017. **50**(4): e5670.

143. Du, A.T., et al., Hypoperfusion in frontotemporal dementia and Alzheimer disease by arterial spin labeling MRI. *Neurology*, 2006. **67** (7):1215–20.

144. Fleisher, A.S., et al., Cerebral perfusion and oxygenation differences in Alzheimer's disease risk. *Neurobiol Aging*, 2009. **30** (11):1737–48.

145. Alexopoulos, P., et al., Perfusion abnormalities in mild cognitive impairment and mild dementia in Alzheimer's disease measured by pulsed arterial spin labeling MRI. *Eur Arch Psychiatry Clin Neurosci*, 2012. **262**(1):69–77.

146. Gauthier, C.J., et al., Age dependence of hemodynamic response characteristics in human functional magnetic resonance imaging. *Neurobiol Aging*, 2013. **34**(5):1469–85.

147. De Vis, J.B., et al., Arterial-spin-labeling (ASL) perfusion MRI predicts cognitive function in

elderly individuals: a 4-year longitudinal study. *J Magn Reson Imaging*, 2018. **48**(2):449–58.

148. Hays, C.C., et al., Subjective cognitive decline modifies the relationship between cerebral blood flow and memory function in cognitively normal older adults. *J Int Neuropsychol Soc*, 2018. **24** (3):213–23.

149. Lee, C., et al., Imaging cerebral blood flow in the cognitively normal aging brain with arterial spin labeling: implications for imaging of neurodegenerative disease. *J Neuroimaging*, 2009. **19**(4):344–52.

150. Tancredi, F.B., I. Lajoie, and R.D. Hoge, Test-retest reliability of cerebral blood flow and blood oxygenation level-dependent responses to hypercapnia and hyperoxia using dual-echo pseudo-continuous arterial spin labeling and step changes in the fractional composition of inspired gases. *J Magn Reson Imaging*, 2015. **42**(4):1144–57.

151. Huppert, T.J., et al., Quantitative spatial comparison of diffuse optical imaging with blood oxygen level-dependent and arterial spin labeling-based functional magnetic resonance imaging. *J Biomed Opt*, 2006. **11**(6):064018.

152. Huppert, T.J., et al., A temporal comparison of BOLD, ASL, and NIRS hemodynamic responses to motor stimuli in adult humans. *Neuroimage*, 2006. **29**(2):368–82.

153. De Vis, J.B., et al., Age-related changes in brain hemodynamics; a calibrated MRI study. *Hum Brain Mapp*, 2015. **36**(10):3973–87.

154. Hoge, R.D., et al., Simultaneous recording of task-induced changes in blood oxygenation, volume, and flow using diffuse optical imaging and arterial spin-labeling MRI. *Neuroimage*, 2005. **25**(3):701–7.

155. Bowtell, J.L., et al., Enhanced task-related brain activation and resting perfusion in healthy older adults after chronic blueberry supplementation. *Appl Physiol Nutr Metab*, 2017. **42**(7):773–79.

156. Petersen, E.T., T. Lim, and X. Golay, Model-free arterial spin labeling quantification approach for perfusion MRI. *Magn Reson Med*, 2006. **55**(2):219–32.

157. Cebral, J.R., et al., Flow-area relationship in internal carotid and vertebral arteries. *Physiol Meas*, 2008. **29**(5):585–94.

158. Tain, R.W., B. Ertl-Wagner, and N. Alperin, Influence of the compliance of the neck arteries and veins on the measurement of intracranial volume change by phase-contrast MRI. *J Magn Reson Imaging*, 2009. **30**(4):878–83.

159. Teng, P.Y., A.M. Bagci, and N. Alperin, Automated prescription of an optimal imaging plane for measurement of cerebral blood flow by phase contrast magnetic resonance imaging. *IEEE Trans Biomed Eng*, 2011. **58** (9):2566–73.

160. Haga, K.K., et al., A systematic review of brain metabolite changes, measured with 1H magnetic resonance spectroscopy, in healthy aging. *Neurobiol Aging*, 2009. **30**(3):353–63.

161. Gao, F., et al., Edited magnetic resonance spectroscopy detects an age-related decline in brain GABA levels. *Neuroimage*, 2013. **78**:75–82.

162. Porges, E.C., et al., Impact of tissue correction strategy on GABA-edited MRS findings. *Neuroimage*, 2017. **162**:249–56.

163. Porges, E.C., et al., Frontal gamma-aminobutyric acid concentrations are associated with cognitive performance in older adults. *Biol Psychiatry Cogn Neurosci Neuroimaging*, 2017. **2**(1):38–44.

164. Rae, C.D., A guide to the metabolic pathways and function of metabolites observed in human brain 1H magnetic resonance spectra. *Neurochem Res*, 2014. **39** (1):1–36.

165. Ding, X.Q., et al., Physiological neuronal decline in healthy aging human brain – an in vivo study with MRI and short echo-time whole-brain (1)H MR spectroscopic imaging. *Neuroimage*, 2016. **137**:45–51.

166. Schmitz, B., et al., Effects of aging on the human brain: a proton and phosphorus MR spectroscopy study at 3T. *J Neuroimaging*, 2018. **28**(4):416–21.

167. Harper, D.G., et al., Brain levels of high-energy phosphate metabolites and executive function in geriatric depression. *Int J Geriatr Psychiatry*, 2016. **31**(11):1241–9.

168. Forester, B.P., et al., Age-related changes in brain energetics and phospholipid metabolism. *NMR Biomed*, 2010. **23**(3):242–50.

169. Duarte, J.M., F.M. Girault, and R. Gruetter, Brain energy metabolism measured by (13)C magnetic resonance spectroscopy in vivo upon infusion of [3-(13) C]lactate. *J Neurosci Res*, 2015. **93** (7):1009–18.

170. Maher, E.A., et al., *Metabolism of [U-13 C]glucose in human brain tumors in vivo. NMR Biomed*, 2012. **25**(11):1234–44.

171. Lei, H., et al., Direct validation of in vivo localized 13C MRS measurements of brain glycogen. *Magn Reson Med*, 2007. **57** (2):243–8.

172. Taylor, A., et al., Approaches to studies on neuronal/glial relationships by 13C-MRS analysis. *Dev Neurosci*, 1996. **18** (5-6):434–42.

173. Isaacson, S.H., et al., Clinical utility of DaTscan imaging in the evaluation of patients with parkinsonism: a US perspective. *Expert Rev Neurother*, 2017. **17** (3):219–25.

174. Kaasinen, V. and T. Vahlberg, Striatal dopamine in Parkinson disease: a meta-analysis of imaging studies. *Ann Neurol*, 2017. **82**(6):873–82.

175. Zou, J., et al., Position emission tomography/single-photon emission tomography neuroimaging for detection of premotor Parkinson's disease. *CNS Neurosci Ther*, 2016. **22** (3):167–77.

176. Wong, C.W., V. Quaranta, and G.G. Glenner, Neuritic plaques and cerebrovascular amyloid in Alzheimer disease are antigenically related. *Proc Natl Acad Sci U S A*, 1985. **82**(24):8729–32.

177. Jack, C.R., Jr., et al., Introduction to the recommendations from the National Institute on Aging–Alzheimer's Association workgroups on diagnostic guidelines for Alzheimer's disease. *Alzheimers Dement*, 2011. 7(3):257–62.

178. Goedert, M., et al., Multiple isoforms of human microtubule-associated protein tau: sequences and localization in neurofibrillary tangles of Alzheimer's disease. *Neuron*, 1989. 3(4):519–26.

179. McKee, A.C., et al., The spectrum of disease in chronic traumatic encephalopathy. *Brain*, 2013. **136** (Pt. 1):43–64.

180. Alafuzoff, I., *Minimal neuropathologic diagnosis for brain banking in the normal middle-aged and aged brain and in neurodegenerative disorders*, in *Handbook of Clinical Neurology*, B. Aminoff MJ, F, Swaab, DF, editors. New York: Elsevier, 2018, pp. 131–41.

Changes in Visuospatial, Visuoperceptual, and Navigational Ability in Aging

Gabrielle A. Hromas and Russell M. Bauer

Aging-related changes in visual perception are ubiquitous and well documented and are the source of major concern and disability among aging adults. With aging, many people, including those who are functioning effectively and not seen in geriatric or neurologic clinics, complain of difficulties in both elementary and complex perception that may affect their ability to read, find personal items on a cluttered table, or navigate the environment without resorting to compensatory strategies. This chapter provides a brief overview of the visuoperceptual and visuospatial changes that can occur with aging.

1 Theoretical Overview

Many of the other chapters in this book address changes in cognitive abilities associated with aging, such as processing speed and episodic memory. However, one critical question that has emerged in recent years is to what extent such changes are related to perceptual dysfunction. Aging can exert an effect on elemental sensory processing in every modality, including visual perception. Alterations of visual perception can be related to retinal, corneal, and lens-related changes that affect the quality of information presented to the brain. Aging-related changes in cortical and subcortical visual areas have both qualitative and quantitative effects on higher-level visual function. We will briefly examine the nature of these changes, beginning with structural and functional changes to the visual sensory system, and then discuss changes in cortical processing of information critical to the efficacy of perceptual, spatial, and navigational behavior in aging adults.

2 Aging-Related Optical Changes

Visual processing begins as light is focused by the cornea and the lens onto the retina, which contains the photoreceptors (rods and cones). The rods and cones act as light- and color-sensitive receptors and provide the basis for higher visual discrimination. The fovea, which is centrally located on the retina, is the point of highest visual acuity. Axons of retinal ganglion cells leave the retina at the optic disc and gather to form the optic nerve. Optic nerve fibers that come from portions of the retina lateral to the fovea of one eye cross at the optic chiasm and join the fibers coming from the portions of the retina medial to the fovea of the opposite eye, forming the left and right optic tracts. About 90% of the optic tract fibers synapse onto neurons located in the lateral geniculate nucleus (LGN) of the thalamus, which is comprised of six layers. The first two (magnocellular) layers are responsible for relaying information critical to motion and spatial analysis from the retina's parasol cells. The third through sixth layers of the LGN form the parvocellular layers, which are responsible for relaying information about form and color. The LGN projects to the primary visual cortex (V1) of the ipsilateral occipital lobe via the geniculo-calcarine pathway [1]. A minority of optic tract fibers bypass the LGN and go directly to the brachium of the superior colliculus, forming the extra-geniculate visual pathway. This pathway projects to the pretectal area (dorsal midbrain), which is involved in controlling pupil diameter in proportion to light intensity (the pupillary light reflex). Both the pretectal area and the superior colliculus (immediately caudal to it) play a role in directing ocular movements and visual attention toward stimuli. Pathways project from these areas to other portions of the brainstem and, via the pulvinar nucleus of the thalamus, to the lateral parietal cortex and frontal eye fields [1].

Aging has an effect on nearly every portion of the eye and, thus, has the potential for impairing visual detection and perception. It is tempting to attribute aging-related visual perceptual dysfunction to degradation of information resulting from changes of the eye [2]. However, aging-related alterations of perceptual function likely also involve aging-related changes of the brain [3].

Aging-related changes of the eye include decreased tear production from the lacrimal glands, weakening of the muscles that control the eye movements that maintain the two eyes in precise alignment, and weakening of the muscles controlling the eyelids [4]. The cornea also changes with aging; alterations of its curvature result in an atypical astigmatism. Increased thickness and opacity of the cornea can alter visual acuity [4]. The pupil shrinks in size and the iris becomes less reactive; these changes, together with increased thickness of the cornea, reduce the amount of light that reaches the retina [5]. With aging, the lens gradually yellows, increasing blue light absorption and affecting color vision. The lens hardens, inducing presbyopia, and cataracts often form [4]. The vitreous fluid between the lens and retina can condense, causing it to pull away from the retina in a condition known as posterior vitreous detachment. This, in turn, can lead to retinal tears or retinal detachment [4].

Finally, the retina, which is in the eye but is literally part of the brain, changes with aging, resulting in decreased visual acuity, changes in contrast sensitivity, and altered dark adaptation. The "outer segment" (rhodopsin-containing) portion of rod cells in the retina renew throughout life, but this renewal slows down when people reach 60–70 years of age. Cone cell membranes begin to be lost after about 40 years of age, resulting in decreased light absorption and alterations in blue-light reception. Up to 50% of retinal ganglion cells may be lost by the seventh decade of life. Macular degeneration, which commonly occurs with aging, is the leading cause of aging-associated blindness [4, 6].

Aging is associated with a general impairment of visual abilities in low light environments. This decreased visual ability persists even after adaptation to the dark. These changes often precede loss of rod photoreceptors (which are responsible for vision in dark conditions). One cause of poor dark vision is changes in the biochemical pathway that supports regeneration of rhodopsin (a light-sensitive retinal pigment). With impaired regeneration, dark adaptation abilities are slowed. Delayed dark adaptation could also be caused by metabolic changes within the ocular system that result in decreased access to vitamin A, which is important for keeping photoreceptors healthy. Structural changes in the cornea and the lens that cause light to scatter before reaching the retina also affect visual acuity in dark environments by increasing glare [7].

3 Aging-Related Neurological Changes

In addition to the changes in vision caused by aging-related optical disorders, there are many perceptual alterations that are caused by aging-related changes of the brain [8]. Changes in contrast threshold accumulate with aging and affect both central and peripheral vision. Spatial contrast sensitivity refers to the ability to detect changes in wavelength (including light–dark transitions). Abrupt spatial changes in luminance serve to define the edges of objects and transitions between objects and backgrounds. The level of contrast needed to define the edge of an object is called the "contrast threshold." Contrast threshold has been shown to increase with aging, even after controlling for changes in the eye [8]. Contrast sensitivity deficits in older adults worsen with increasing spatial frequency of contrast change. This could be related to normal aging-related cell death in the parvocellular layers of the LGN [5, 8]. Contrast sensitivity also decreases as luminance decreases.

It has long been known that aging reduces the speed of visual processes affecting critical flicker fusion, the frequency at which a flickering light appears to be constant to the observer [9]. This may have implications for the performance of older individuals on time-sensitive perceptual tasks. For example, the time to find items or to read or process a complex visual array may be prolonged. These changes may affect aging people in activities such as driving. Changes in vision are also often associated with declines in other cognitive domains (such as attention) (Chapter 10). Some researchers hypothesize that this decline is a part of the generalized cognitive slowing that normal adults experience with aging. They also posit that impairments in attentional disengagement and set-shifting contribute to aging-related deficits in visual processing speed [5].

Aging adults also show reductions in their ability to process motion. This deficit might impair performance on tasks in which motion cues are utilized to help define shape or form, and on collision prediction and prevention tasks, such as driving and ambulating in crowded environments, as well as other activities where relative motion and speed perception are critical. Older adults also show poor integration of local and global movement information. These declines seem to happen gradually with aging, and it is estimated that subjects over the age of 70 have motion thresholds twice as great as those of 30-year-olds. There also appears to be a gender difference, with females showing higher motion thresholds than males for reasons that are yet poorly understood [3]. The relative contribution of sensory/perceptual and higher order cognitive factors to these deficits has not been fully elucidated. Some researchers have posited that these changes are due to decline in the function of the magnocellular LGN, which projects to the motion-processing portions of the temporal lobe [8]. Cortical changes have also been cited as the cause of changes in motion perception. For example, aging-related increases in movement detection threshold (the amount of movement needed to give rise to the perception of motion) have been attributed to changes in the temporal lobe, particularly posterior portions of the middle temporal gyrus (MT), the medial superior portions of which are involved in motion analysis, including analysis of movement direction and speed.

The ability to perform eye movements (saccades and smooth pursuit movements) also declines with age. Specifically, individuals over the age of 75 exhibit significantly lower smooth pursuit gains (speed of adjustment of eye rotational velocity to the speed of the visual target), especially when pursuing faster moving stimuli. Saccades also have slower peak velocities, longer and more variable reaction times, and reduced accuracy. These phenomena could be the result of a multitude of normal aging-related changes, such as general cortical slowing, decreased attention, and neuronal changes in the frontal lobes (the site of neurons responsible for generating saccadic eye movements) [10].

4 Aging and Domain-Specific Visuoperceptual Changes

Thus far, we have discussed aging-related changes in sensory processing, emphasizing the effects of aging on the manner in which visual sensory information is collected. In this section, we consider aging-related changes in higher-order visuoperceptual processes, including object and face recognition. Given the previously described aging-related changes in visual acuity, contrast sensitivity, and perceptual processing speed, it stands to reason that higher-order perceptual skills such as face and object recognition and spatial navigation might suffer in kind.

There is substantial evidence of a link between cognitive and perceptual decline in aging. This phenomenon has been explained in four ways. The "common cause" hypothesis is that a third factor in aging is responsible for both cognitive and perceptual decline [11]. The "sensory deprivation" hypothesis posits perceptual decline as a primary aging-related phenomenon that leads to a degradation of higher cortical visual neuronal activity. The "cognitive load on perception" hypothesis is that perceptual dysfunction results from primary deficits in cognition. The "information degradation" hypothesis is that the perceptual system, because of problems in more elementary sensory processing, suffers from degraded input and thus does not bring sufficiently processed information to the brain to sustain normal perception [2]. Evidence favoring the "information degradation" hypothesis comes from experiments in which young and aging adults performed a digit cancellation task. Custom stimulus arrays were created such that critical contrast thresholds were matched across individuals, regardless of age. When such manipulations put young and old adults on equal footing, aging-related perceptual differences tend to disappear [12]. Having reviewed this literature critically, we favor a view that explains aging-related perceptual dysfunction as a complex by-product of both peripheral changes in structure and function of the sensory apparatus (what we have called "eye-to-brain" mechanisms) and aging-related impairments in cortical processors specialized for key domains of perceptual skill. In keeping with this view, our description of aging-related perceptual changes will separately consider how aging affects neuropsychologically relevant domains of perceptual function, including face recognition, form perception, object recognition, visuospatial perception and imagery, spatial memory, and environmental navigation.

4.1 Face Recognition

Older adults frequently complain of difficulties in recognizing previously familiar faces that do not reach the level of prosopagnosia but that affect social interaction in various ways [13, 14]. It has long been known that older adults show reduced performance on tasks of facial recognition memory, a deficit that cannot be explained by a conservative response bias designed to minimize the number of false positive recognitions [15]. In fact, older adults tend to show increased "false recognitions" of faces in contrast to an "I don't know" bias. This has been interpreted by some as reflecting an increasing reliance on familiarity instead of recollection (saying "yes" to an item that was not studied but that shares features or context with items that have been studied). Indeed, this effect is more likely related to an aging-related reduction in use of recollection as a strategy [16] or reduction in the capacity of the hippocampal system to support episodic memory encoding and recollection (Chapters 3 and 7) [17]. When learning new faces, older adults are less effective in encoding contextual cues (i.e., are less sensitive to the environment in which faces were encoded), and thus show a sort of "eyewitness" effect in which fewer internal details are recognized when faces are presented during the memory test, particularly at longer delays [18]. These data strongly suggest that aging-related disturbances in face recognition result from a combination of memory and perceptual factors.

On the perceptual side, the aging-related deficit in face recognition likely results from a combination of deficits in holistic processing, semantic access to information about the owner of the face, and deficits in proper name retrieval [19]. Deficits in global holistic processing involving facial feature configurations may be a consequence of reductions in contrast sensitivity, which involves integrated processing of multiple spatial frequency bands [20].

Perceiving and encoding faces depends critically on other components of configural processing: the processing of spatial relations among facial components, including the overall organization of facial features, their spatial relationships to one another, and the overall "gestalt" created by these relationships [21]. One way of investigating configural processing in face recognition tasks is to examine recognition of upside-down (inverted) faces, which particularly challenges this type of processing. The "face inversion effect" has been replicated numerous times in the literature and is widely regarded as the result of an impairment of second-order relational processing, including disruption of spatial analysis of the distance between features [22]. Older adults do not show the normal facial inversion effect, suggesting that their perception of upright faces is not dependent on configural processing [21]. However, in Chaby's [21] experiment, when facial features were modified vertically or horizontally (by manipulating distances between features), older adults showed a pattern of performance similar to that seen in young participants – they were able to detect vertical modifications but not horizontal ones. These results suggest that aging has an effect on configurational processing of faces, with relative preservation of vertical as compared to horizontal second-order processing [21].

4.2 Form Perception

Problems in integrating spatial and temporal cues in ambient vision may lead to significant changes in the ability to process two- and three-dimensional forms. In recognition experiments in which specific featural details of the to-be-identified stimuli are partially obscured by an opaque foreground object, older adults show differential vulnerability to reductions in featural detail, suggesting that aging-related declines in extracting contours are due to declines in spatial integration [3]. Failures in spatial integration can also affect the manner in which the visual system can recover information about shape from relative motion, and have been invoked to explain the particular difficulties aging adults have in judging shape from kinetic depth cues or motion parallax [23].

4.3 Object Recognition

Recognition of familiar objects is critical to survival and has been identified as an aspect of memory-guided perception that declines in normal aging [24, 25]. In animal models, studies have shown significant decline in delayed non-matching to sample performance in aged monkeys [26, 27], a finding traditionally interpreted as reflecting an aging-associated impairment in new learning (i.e., novelty detection). However, this task is also dependent on perception and encoding of object features necessary to discriminate the novel from the previously studied object, such that aging in perceptual (as opposed to mnemonic) functions may play a role.

Recent evidence suggests that the perirhinal cortex (PrC), a cortical region in the anterior medial temporal lobe, is particularly altered with aging. Although there is no loss of PrC neurons with aging, PrC principal cells are less responsive to object stimuli in older animals and a larger proportion of PrC cells are quiet during object exploration [28]. PrC function also suffers from the depletion of amino acids and polyamines necessary for normal function and synaptic plasticity [29]. In fact, it has been argued that aging rats perform difficult tasks of visual discrimination (i.e., tasks on which target and foil share many common features) in a way that is remarkably similar to young rats with PrC lesions [30]. Lesions of the PrC impair the ability to discriminate complex stimuli that share common features [31, 32]. For example, when monkeys are trained to discriminate between objects with many features in common, animals with PrC lesions are impaired relative to controls yet are able to perform normally if the rewarded and unrewarded stimuli do not share common featural elements [32]. As the PrC has extensive connections with frontal lobe, it is possible that these deficits result in part from frontally based reductions in top-down control of attention, resulting in the transmission of less detailed object information to the PrC.

The effect of featural overlap or similarity has been the focus of recent work that aims to understand the nature of aging-related changes in visual perception. In a series of elegant experiments in which featural overlap between rewarded and unrewarded stimuli was manipulated using artificially constructed Lego stimuli, Burke and colleagues have shown that, as the degree of featural overlap increased, more trials were required for the older rats to learn which object of the pair was associated with reward [33]. Once the response–reward association was learned, there were no age differences in memory for the association after a 48-hour delay. This finding ascribes perceptual, as opposed to mnemonic, functions to the PrC. It has been proposed that, as part of a perceptual network, the primary role of the PrC is to bind together complex conjunctions of stimulus features necessary for uniquely defining specific objects for use in both memory and perception [34]. These bound feature conjunctions are then transmitted via the PrC-entorhinal system to the hippocampus for episodic memory encoding. Although aging-related decline in perceptual function can explain these results, it is also possible that they are mnemonic in nature, related either (1) to deficits in early and late LTP, linked to hippocampal changes with aging (Chapters 3 and 15), or (2) to a degradation of dentate function, thereby markedly decreasing featural overlap between cortical representations instantiated as CA3 activity [17, 35].

Recent work with humans supports the notion that the functions of the PrC are likely to be conserved across species. This has significant potential implications for understanding aging-related memory and perceptual decline. In humans, the PrC is important in complex aspects of perception, including the ability to parse unique objects by processing feature conjunctions. In general, there is good correspondence with the animal work in that humans with medial temporal lesions extending to the PrC are able to make simple visual discriminations based on individual features. However, these patients exhibit impairments in object discrimination when the target and foil objects have a high number of overlapping features [36, 37]. It is important to note that many participants in human studies suffered extensive damage after herpes encephalitis, status epilepticus, or carbon monoxide poisoning, so it would be a mistake to uncritically attribute perceptual impairment entirely to damage in the MTL-hippocampal system.

Corroborative evidence for the role of the PrC in object recognition also comes from human functional imaging studies. Devlin and Price [38] used FDG PET to show perirhinal activation during an "oddity" task in which a unique object had to be discriminated from three foils. In an "easy" condition, the three foils were identical in every way, such that the discrimination could be performed by finding a distinctive feature of the unique object that made it different from the foils. In the "difficult" condition, the foils corresponded to the same object but it was shown from three different viewpoints, such that success at this task required the formation of an abstract, viewpoint-invariant representation. The PrC was active only in the "difficult" condition, suggesting its critical importance for integrating features to form this type of object representation. In subsequent work, Barense and colleagues [39] showed that PrC activation in "oddity" tasks was dependent on object "meaningfulness" (familiarity), suggesting that it may play a role in integrating visual and semantic aspects of perceived objects.

Recent work in our laboratory has shown that performance on perceptual tasks, such as the Devlin and Price "oddity" task described above, is not only age dependent but may also be sensitive to early pathological aging-related cognitive and memory changes that presage the development of dementia. Using the Devlin and Price [38] task, we [40] have shown that early reductions in visual discrimination ability are more sensitive than standardized episodic memory tasks in detecting the transition from normal cognitive aging to a stage of functioning that has been referred to as "pre-MCI" [41]. Individuals who meet research criteria for pre-MCI have subjective cognitive deficits with normal-range performance on cognitive assessments and, therefore, do not meet diagnostic criteria for MCI. The patients are, however, six times more likely to progress to aMCI or dementia than cognitively normal peers [42]. Therefore, impairment in PrC-related functions, such as object recognition, could be a sensitive indicator of early levels of cognitive impairment [43]. This impairment would be consistent with the finding that one of the sites of earliest appearance of tangle pathology in AD is the transentorhinal cortex, or Area 35 of the perirhinal cortex, a major source of input into the hippocampus [44–46]. The hippocampus is, of course, a critical structure in encoding episodic memory. Regional tau deposition has been shown to correlate with atrophy of bilateral PrC in early AD [47, 48], and tau deposition is a better predictor of future cognitive decline than is amyloid accumulation [49].

Although much more work is left to be done, research on aging-related changes in human object recognition suggests a primary effect of aging on the efficiency and selectivity of processing within the ventral visual stream, of which the PrC is a critical part. Using fMRI, Park et al. demonstrated aging-related decreases in selectivity of response in components of the ventral visual stream to four categories of visual stimuli, including faces, chairs, houses/places, and pseudowords [50]. While younger participants showed differentiated responses to these stimuli in regions of the inferotemporal cortex, parahippocampal gyrus, and fusiform area, older participants showed less selectivity, a pattern that Park et al. refer to as "dedifferentiation." This loss of selectivity could require older adults to utilize more attention-consuming compensatory strategies that require executive control to help complete perceptually demanding tasks [51, 52]. This could lead to performance decrements, since executive control itself is prone to aging-related decline (Chapter 12).

4.4 Visuospatial Perception

Spatial cognition refers to the ability to represent, organize, understand, and navigate the environment [53]. It involves small-scale processes concerned with identifying objects in space and utilizing them when performing everyday tasks. There are also large-scale processes involved in navigating the environment and remembering the absolute and relative location of key environmental features or landmarks [54]. Small-scale visuospatial abilities are typically assessed with neuropsychological tests designed to evaluate people's ability to perceive spatial relationships, scan environments, or mentally rotate objects in space. The brain computes two types of spatial relation representations. Categorical representations allow the assignment of a spatial relationship to an abstract category such as "above" or "to the right of." Coordinate representations allow the preservation of stimulus and location information in more precise metric detail that can be represented as, for example, distance in millimeters or inches. This distinction was first suggested by Kosslyn [55], who proposed that categorical representations were associated with left hemisphere processing, while coordinate representations were lateralized to the right hemisphere [55]. More recent research suggests that this is an overly simplistic view, with some studies revealing right vs. left hemispheric differences and others aligning the hippocampus with coordinate processing and the parietal lobe with categorical processing [56]. With regard to mnemonic function, both coordinate and categorical processing may be affected in proportion to involvement of the hippocampus, with coordinate processing more affected by anterior HC/PrC dysfunction and categorical processing more affected by posterior HC/PhG dysfunction. With regard to basic visuospatial perception, most available data suggest that age does not exert a significant effect, although older adults may require more time to make spatial judgments [57]. However, in line with ubiquitous evidence of hippocampal involvement in the aging process, there is evidence that coordinate spatial representations are more susceptible to aging-related decline [58].

Another hypothesized dichotomy relevant to the representation of spatial information in the brain is the difference between egocentric and allocentric frames of reference. The *egocentric* frame contains spatial information on the location of objects in the environment in relation to the viewer. These object-to-subject relations provide the basis for body-centered representations. The *allocentric* frame contains spatial information about the position of environmental objects relative to each other. It is therefore based on object-to-object relationships and involves the creation of a cognitive map of the environment independent of the individual's body, head, or eyes [59]. These two frames of reference are mediated by different neural systems. Some authors believe that the allocentric frame is supported primarily by portions of the medial temporal lobe, including hippocampal place cells, entorhinal grid cells, the parahippocampal region, and the retrosplenial cortex [60]. In contrast, the egocentric frame is supported by structures that represent movement and spatial coordination, including the caudate, the medial parietal lobe, and posterior parietal area A7 [61]. Efficient navigation involves the ability to shift back and forth between these frames, an ability that seems to be dependent on the posterior cingulate and retrosplenial regions, where these two frames likely interact [62, 63].

An unresolved issue in the literature is the precise relationship between the coordinate-categorical distinction and the distinction between egocentric and allocentric representation of object locations. Jager and Postma [64] suggested that these two distinctions may interact such that allocentric processing is associated with categorical coding of spatial relations, while egocentric processing is associated with coordinate coding. While some studies have suggested that categorical judgments are more accurate under allocentric than under egocentric processing conditions, thus supporting an interaction [65], others have suggested that these represent two independent mechanisms that depend on different subregions of the hippocampus and parietal cortex [56].

It has now been well established in both preclinical and human studies that aging affects navigational ability not by impairing a specific "navigational processor" but through a variety of mechanisms [66]. Older adults have deficits in perceiving the direction and speed of self-motion [67]. They also underestimate distances and have difficulty returning to the beginning of a path [68]. Additionally, reductions in spatial working memory [69] or vestibular dysfunction [70] can contribute to decline in navigational abilities. High-level sensory dysfunction can impair the computation of spatial information from incoming sensory systems, including optical flow – the apparent motion of objects and surfaces in a visual scene caused by observer motion. In addition, deficits in spatial memory or planning can affect the development of stable memory traces or the manner in which the environment is sampled during navigational tasks.

These deficits can affect the accuracy of existing spatial memory representations. Older adults may have additional problems in encoding and retrieving new long-term spatial memories [66](see also Chapters 3 and 7). For example, several studies using virtual adaptations of the Morris water maze show slower learning rates [71], less frequent location of the hidden platform using predominantly nonspatial strategies [72], and reduced accuracy in reproducing a map of the environment [73].

4.5 Mental/Spatial Imagery

In a typical imagery task, participants are asked to form a mental image of a stimulus, maintain that image in memory, rotate it in space, and scan it to perform a spatial ("where") or perceptual ("what") judgment. While early studies suggested that mental/spatial imagery processing abilities decline with aging, the bulk of the data now suggests that older adults show selective impairments in image generation and rotation, with preservation of image maintenance and scanning [54, 74]. These deficits have been linked to aging-related dysfunction in dorsolateral prefrontal cortex [75], and in general, aging-related changes in mental imagery have been attributed to reduction in executive or "top-down" processing. As individuals age, there is reduced selectivity in the category-specific regions of the ventral visual stream that are activated with specific types of imagery (e.g., fusiform face area for facial imagery, V5 for motion imagery). This decline is accompanied by reduced connectivity between these regions and the prefrontal cortex [76].

Aging-related degradation in imagistic representation of the environment may also extend to mental representation of actions (motor imagery), an important modality for planning and executing movements in relation to the environment [77]. Motor (also known as kinesthetic) imagery is an active cognitive process in which an action representation is internally produced in the absence of overt movement [78]. Several studies have suggested that motor imagery also declines with advancing age [79, 80]. For example, older adults were less accurate than younger adults in estimating distances needed to move in order to reach an object [81]. There is also evidence of aging-related increases in the size of the brain network activated when mentally walking through an imagined environment, suggesting that older adults need to recruit larger regions of the network during imagery in order to successfully process the image. Such increases were highly correlated with reductions in executive functions in the older group [82]. Aging-related decrements in mentally representing and planning movements may have critical implications for understanding and treating fall-related injury risk in older adults.

4.6 Spatial Memory

Older persons often complain of changes in spatial memory. For example, they often cannot remember the location of household objects and frequently report the experience of getting temporarily lost or disoriented in previously familiar surroundings. These complaints may also signal aging-related impairment in memory for spatial locations or in spatial working memory.

One common paradigm for assessing aging-related changes in spatial memory is to assess learning and recall of the location of objects in an array. In general, results from two decades of studies on aging and object location memory in older adults provide no evidence of a reduction in performance on tasks that assess memory for a small number of spatial locations. However, there is evidence of impairment when the number of locations increases, in other words, when working memory demands increase [83]. Preclinical studies of aging-related spatial memory function in rodents have found multiple alterations in hippocampal connectivity and plasticity (long-term potentiation) [84, 85]. In humans, functional imaging experiments have found reduced hippocampal activation during allocentric spatial memory tasks in older adults [86].

4.7 Environmental Navigation

An aging-related reduction in navigation ability has been widely reported in both preclinical and human studies, particularly affecting the ability to get around in novel as compared to familiar environments [87]. In the geriatric neuropsychology clinic, older adults, even those who do not complain of widespread cognitive decline, commonly report navigational challenges. Navigation ability is critical to quality of life in older adults, and the development of impairment in this ability can signal changes that greatly limit independence and freedom. Older adults perform similarly to younger adults when routes are familiar

or when the environment supports route-following through the presence of recognizable landmarks, but aging-related differences emerge when performance depends on memory for the route [54]. In these circumstances, older adults seem to have particular difficulty utilizing spatial strategies, often returning to previously incorrect locations or using landmark cues to find their way [88]. Younger adults typically outperform older adults on tasks that require an overall mental representation of space or the layout of an environment [89]. On virtual water maze tasks, older adults often perform similarly to rats with hippocampal lesions or of advanced age: they show longer paths to the virtual platform, spend less time adjacent to the platform, and make fewer successful trials in which the platform is located [89].

Most data suggest that allocentric navigation strategies are particularly susceptible to the effects of aging [59]. In a virtual Y-maze task in which participants were asked to navigate to previously learned locations, younger adults were evenly split between the use of egocentric (46%) and allocentric (54%) strategies. In contrast, the older adults were significantly biased toward using an egocentric strategy, with 83% selecting this approach [90]. Older adults also appear to have difficulty switching from an egocentric to an allocentric frame, but not vice versa [91].

Why does aging cause a decline in allocentric navigation and an impairment in switching between navigational reference frames? Connectivity patterns substantially define the functional domains of neurons throughout the brain. The PrC-entorhinal-anterior hippocampal system is substantially connected with anterior temporal and frontal cortices. It therefore logically provides major support for allocentric navigation, which involves locations of nearby objects as features of an object representation. The parahippocampal-entorhinal-posterior hippocampal system is substantially connected with parietal cortices. It therefore logically provides major support for egocentric navigation, which depends on the absolute representation of object location in a body-centered coordinate system. Thus, the aging-related decline in allocentric navigation and in switching between navigational frames may be related to the degradation of PrC function discussed early in this chapter.

The best-supported neurobiological theory suggests that the important role played by the hippocampal system in allocentric computations makes it critical in the creation of cognitive maps, which require integrating such computations with egocentric information arriving from other cortical areas [92]. It may be that the functional specialization of specific regions of the hippocampus for cognitive mapping is related to their specific connection, via parahippocampal-entorhinal pathways, with dorsal visual stream structures processing "where" (spatial) information. Several studies have now shown aging-related reductions in hippocampal, parahippocampal, medial temporal, and retrosplenial activation during spatial memory and navigation tasks in the elderly [86, 93]. The parahippocampal region further supports the encoding of landmarks and their locations [94]. Regarding the deficit in egocentric-to-allocentric switching, other structures are implicated, including the dorsolateral prefrontal cortex and the ascending noradrenergic system that arises from the locus coeruleus, a site of early accumulation of aging-related pathological changes [95, 96].

Because of a combination of aging-related changes, older adults (and aged animals) may also have deficits in route- and response-based navigation as well. Route learning differs from navigating based on cognitive mapping in that successful navigation depends on the recognition and sequencing of landmarks, the sequence of "relevant" landmarks (those that are associated, for example, with decisions like where to make turns), and directional information. Older adults are less accurate in linking directional knowledge to landmarks [97] and are less able to remember the sequence in which landmarks are encountered [98]. Together, these problems can impair the learning and retrieval of route information.

5 Rehabilitation of Aging-Related Perceptual Dysfunction

A small literature exists on the rehabilitation of aging-related visual perceptual dysfunction in older adults, including interventions designed to improve driving, attentional disorders/neglect [99], and reading performance [100]. The stroke literature contains several small-scale studies addressing the rehabilitation of anosognosia associated with hemi-attentional dysfunction [101], cortical blindness [102], and general impairment of visuoperceptual and visuospatial skills [103]. With some notable exceptions, the emphasis in this area has been on treating peripheral deficits such

as macular degeneration and less on treating disorders of higher visual function. There is a significant need for developing assessments and interventions in this area, as many rehabilitation professionals understand how aging-related perceptual dysfunction can significantly limit quality of life and mobility. It is time to transform this understanding into intervention.

The potential role of leading-edge rehabilitation techniques such as virtual environments [104] and location-based systems employing wearables and other personally owned GPS and related devices [105] hold great promise. Finally, in the area of visuoperceptual dysfunction, several studies have used perceptual learning approaches to treat aging-related deficits in face and object recognition [106], and this represents an area of future opportunity. Clinical neuropsychologists and neurologists would do well to translate their mechanism-based knowledge of perceptual and spatial dysfunction in the elderly into useful treatment approaches designed to reduce visuoperceptual-related disability in older individuals.

6 Summary and Conclusion

Age-related visuoperceptual and visuospatial dysfunction is commonly encountered in neuropsychology and neurology clinics, and such dysfunction has significant implications for quality of life in older individuals. Visuoperceptual and visuospatial dysfunction likely contribute to safety-related issues (e.g., falls) and contribute to loss of independence and disability in this population. Although these problems have been studied, the literature in this area is not nearly as developed, theoretically or practically, as is the literature on other aging-related cognitive changes such as episodic memory or executive function. It is clear that aging-related perceptual dysfunction exists, at least partially independently of cognitive changes in other domains, owing in part to susceptibility of high-level visuoperceptual areas to functional, structural, and pathological aging. Significant opportunities exist for neuropsychologists and neurologists to work with rehabilitation colleagues in occupational therapy and physical therapy to apply what is known about such changes to the development of rehabilitation and management efforts designed to mitigate the effects of such changes on safety, independence, and quality of life.

References

1. Blumenfeld H. *Neuroanatomy through Clinical Cases.* Sunderland, MA: Sinauer Associates; 2018.

2. Monge ZA, Madden DJ. Linking cognitive and visual perceptual decline in healthy aging: the information degradation hypothesis. *Neuroscience and Biobehavioral Reviews.* 2016;69:166–73.

3. Andersen GJ. Aging and vision: changes in function and performance from optics to perception. *Wiley Interdisciplinary Reviews Cognitive Science.* 2012;3 (3):403–10.

4. Salvi SM, Akhtar S, Currie Z. Ageing changes in the eye. *Postgraduate Medical Journal.* 2006;82:581–7.

5. Owsley C. Vision and aging. *Annual Review of Vision Science.* 2016;2:255–71.

6. Marshall J. The ageing retina: physiology or pathology. *Eye (London).* 1987;1:282–95.

7. van den Berg TJTP, van Rijn LJ, Kaper-Bongers R, Vonhoff DJ, Volker-Dieben HJ, Grabner G, et al. Disability glare in the aging eye: assessment and impact on driving. *Journal of Optometry.* 2009;2(3):112–18.

8. Spear PD. Neural bases of visual deficits during aging. *Vision Research.* 1993;33(18):2589–609.

9. Coppinger NW. The relationship between critical flicker frequency and chronologic age for varying levels of stimulus brightness. *Journal of Gerontology.* 1955;10 (1):48–52.

10. Moschner C, Baloh RW. Age-related changes in visual tracking. *Journal of Gerontology.* 1994;49 (5):M235–M238.

11. Lindenberger U, Baltes PB. Sensory functioning and intelligence in old age: a strong connection. *Psychology and Aging.* 1994;9(3):339–55.

12. Toner CK, Reese BE, Neargarder S, Riedel TM, Gilmore GC, Cronin-Golomb A. Vision-fair neuropsychological assessment in normal aging, Parkinson's disease and Alzheimer's disease. *Psychology and Aging.* 2012;27:785.

13. Boutet I, Meinhardt-Injac B. Age differences in face processing: the role of perceptual degradation and holistic processing. *The Journals of Gerontology Series B, Psychological Sciences and Social Sciences,* gbx172, https://doi.org/10.1093/geronb/gbx172.

14. Chaby L, Narme P. Processing facial identity and emotional expression in normal aging and neurodegenerative diseases. *Psychologie et Neuropsychiatrie du Vieillissement.* 2009;7:31–42.

15. Flicker C, Ferris SH, Crook T, Bartus RT. Impaired facial recognition memory in aging and dementia. *Alzheimer Disease and Associated Disorders.* 1990;4 (1):43–54.

16. Edmonds EC, Glisky EL, Bartlett JC, Rapcsak SZ. Cognitive mechanisms of false facial recognition in older adults. *Psychology and Aging.* 2012;27 (1):54–60.

17. Brickman AM, Khan UA, Provenzano FA, Yeung LK, Suzuki W, Schroeter H, et al. Enhancing dentate gyrus function with dietary flavanols improves cognition in older adults. *Nature Neuroscience.* 2014;12:1798–803.

18. Memon A, Bartlett J, Rose R, Gray C. The aging eyewitness: effects of age on face, delay, and source-memory ability. *The Journals of Gerontology Series B, Psychological Sciences and Social Sciences.* 2003;58(6):P338–P345.

19. Maylor EA. Recognizing and naming faces: aging, memory retrieval, and the tip of the tongue state. *Journal of Gerontology.* 1990;45(6):P215–P226.

20. Smith ML, Cottrell GW, Gosselin F, Schyns PG. Transmitting and decoding facial expressions. *Psychological Science.* 2005;16:184–9.

21. Chaby L, Narme P, George N. Older adults' configural processing of faces: role of second-order information. *Psychology and Aging.* 2011;26 (1):71–9.

22. Rossion B. Picture-plane inversion leads to qualitative changes of face perception. *Acta Psychologica.* 2008;128:274–89.

23. Andersen GJ, Atchley P. Age-related differences in the detection of three-dimensional surfaces from optic flow. *Psychology and Aging.* 1995;21:74–85.

24. Insel N, Ruiz-Luna ML, Permenter M, Vogt J, Erickson CA, Barnes CA. Aging in rhesus macaques is associated with changes in novelty preference and altered saccade dynamics. *Behav Neurosci.* 2008;122:1328–42.

25. Burke SN, Barnes CA. Senescent synapses and hippocampal circuit dynamics. *Trends in Neurosciences.* 2010;33:153–61.

26. Rapp PR, Amaral DG. Recognition memory deficits in a subpopulation of aged monkeys resemble the effects of medial temporal lobe damage. *Neurobiology of Aging.* 1991;12:481–6.

27. Shamy JL, Buonocore MH, Makaron LM, Amaral DG, Barnes CA, Rapp PR. Hippocampal volume is preserved and fails to predict recognition memory impairment in aged rhesus monkeys (*Macaca mulatta*). *Neurobiology of Aging.* 2006;27:1405–15.

28. Burke SN, Maurer AP, Nematollahi S, Uprety A, Wallace JL, Barnes CA. Advanced age dissociates dual functions of the perirhinal cortex. *Journal of Neuroscience.* 2014;34:467–80.

29. Liu P, Gupta N, Jing Y, Zhang H. Age-related changes in polyamines in memory-associated brain structures in rats. *Neuroscience.* 2008;155:789–96.

30. Burke SN, Ryan L, Barnes CA. Characterizing cognitive aging of recognition memory and related processes in animal models and in humans. *Frontiers in Aging Neuroscience.* 2012;4(15):1–13.

31. Bartko SJ, Winters BD, Cowell RA, Saksida LM, Bussey TJ. Perceptual functions of perirhinal cortex in rats: zero-delay object recognition and simultaneous oddity discriminations. *Journal of Neuroscience.* 2007;27:2548–59.

32. Bussey TJ, Saksida LM, Murray EA. Impairments in visual discrimination after perirhinal cortex lesions: testing "declarative" vs. "perceptual-mnemonic" views of perirhinal cortex function. *European Journal of Neuroscience.* 2003;17:649–60.

33. Burke SN, Wallace JL, Hartzell AL, Nematollahi S, Plange K, Barnes CA. Age-associated deficits in pattern separation functions of the perirhinal cortex: a cross-species consensus. *Behavioral Neuroscience.* 2011;125:836–47.

34. Murray EA, Bussey TJ. Perceptual-mnemonic functions of the perirhinal cortex. *Trends in Cognitive Sciences.* 1999;3:142–51.

35. Rolls ET, Treves A. *Neural Networks and Brain Function.* New York: Oxford University Press; 1998.

36. Barense MD, Rogers TT, Bussey TJ, Saksida LM, Graham KS. Influence of conceptual knowledge on visual object discrimination: insights from semantic dementia and MTL amnesia. *Cerebral Cortex.* 2010;20(11):2568–82.

37. Behrmann M, Lee AC, Geskin JZ, Graham KS, Barense MD. Temporal lobe contribution to perceptual function: a tale of three patient groups. *Neuropsychologia.* 2016;90:33–45.

38. Devlin JT, Price CJ. Perirhinal contributions to human visual perception. *Current Biology: CB.* 2007;17(17):1484–8.

39. Barense MD, Henson RN, Graham KS. Perception and conception: temporal lobe activity during complex discriminations of familiar and novel faces and objects. *Journal of Cognitive Neuroscience.* 2011;23(10):3052–67.

40. Gaynor LS, Curiel RE, Penate A, Rosselli M, Burke SN, Wicklund M, et al. Visual object discrimination impairment as an early predictor of mild cognitive impairment and Alzheimer's disease. *Journal of the International Neuropsychological Society.* 2019 May 21:1–11. Submitted.

41. Duara R, Loewenstein DA, Greig MT, Potter E, Barker W, Raj A, et al. Pre-MCI and MCI: neuropsychological, clinical, and imaging features and progression rates. *The American Journal of Geriatric Psychiatry: Official Journal of the American Association for Geriatric Psychiatry.* 2011;19(11):951–60.

42. Loewenstein DA, Greig MT, Schinka JA, Barker W, Shen Q, Potter E, et al. An investigation of PreMCI: subtypes and longitudinal outcomes. *Alzheimer's & Dementia: The Journal of the Alzheimer's Association.* 2012;8(3):172–9.

43. Fidalgo CO, Changoor AT, Page-Gould E, Lee AC, Barense MD. Early cognitive decline in older adults better predicts object than scene recognition performance. *Hippocampus.* 2016;26(12):1579–92.

44. Arriagada PV, Marzloff K, Hyman BT. Distribution of Alzheimer-type pathologic changes in nondemented elderly individuals matches the pattern in Alzheimer's disease. *Neurology.* 1992;42(9):1681–8.

45. Braak H, Braak E. Neuropathological stageing of Alzheimer-related changes. *Acta Neuropathologica.* 1991;82(4):239–59.

46. Khan UA, Liu L, Provenzano FA, Berman DE, Profaci CP, Sloan R, et al. Molecular drivers and cortical spread of lateral entorhinal cortex dysfunction in preclinical Alzheimer's disease. *Nature Neuroscience.* 2014;17(2):304–11.

47. Olsen RK, Yeung LK, Noly-Gandon A, D'Angelo MC, Kacollja A, Smith VM, et al. Human anterolateral entorhinal cortex volumes are associated with cognitive decline in aging prior to clinical diagnosis. *Neurobiology of Aging.* 2017;57:195–205.

48. Sone D, Imabayashi E, Maikusa N, Okamura N, Furumoto S, Kudo Y, et al. Regional tau deposition and subregion atrophy of medial temporal structures in early Alzheimer's disease: a combined positron emission tomography/magnetic resonance imaging study. *Alzheimer's and Dementia.* 2017;9:35–40.

49. Huber CM, Yee C, May T, Dhanala A, Mitchell CS. Cognitive decline in preclinical Alzheimer's disease: amyloid-beta versus tauopathy. *Journal of Alzheimer's Disease: JAD.* 2018;61(1):265–81.

50. Park DC, Polk TA, Park R, Minear M, Savage A, Smith MR. Aging reduces neural specialization in ventral visual cortex. *Proceedings of the National Academy of Sciences of the United States of America.* 2004;101(35):13091–5.

51. Park DC, Reuter-Lorenz P. The adaptive brain: aging and neurocognitive scaffolding. *Annual Review of Psychology.* 2009;60:173–96.

52. Reuter-Lorenz PA, Park DC. Human neuroscience and the aging mind: a new look at old problems. *The Journals of Gerontology Series B, Psychological Sciences and Social Sciences.* 2010;65(4):405–15.

53. Spence I, Feng J. Video games and spatial cognition. *Review of General Psychology.* 2010;14:92–104.

54. Klencklen G, Despres O, Dufour A. What do we know about aging and spatial cognition? Reviews and perspectives. *Ageing Research Reviews.* 2012;11(1):123–35.

55. Kosslyn SM, Koenig O, Barret A, Cave CB, Tang J, Gabrieli JDE. Evidence for two types of spatial representations: hemispheric specialization for categorical and coordinate relations. *Journal of Experimental Psychology Human Perception and Performance.* 1989;15:723–35.

56. Baumann O, Mattingley JB. Dissociable roles of the hippocampus and parietal cortex in processing of coordinate and categorical spatial information. *Frontiers in Human Neuroscience.* 2014;8:73.

57. Meadmore KL, Dror II, Bucks RS. Lateralisation of spatial processing and age. *Laterality.* 2008;14:1–13.

58. Bruyer R, Scailquin J-C, Coibion P. Dissociation between categorical and coordination spatial computations: modulation by cerebral hemispheres, tasks properties, mode of response, and age. *Brain and Cognition.* 1997;33:245–77.

59. Colombo D, Serino S, Tuena C, Pedroli E, Dakanalis A, Cipresso P, et al. Egocentric and allocentric spatial reference frames in aging: a systematic review. *Neuroscience and Biobehavioral Reviews.* 2017;80:605–21.

60. Zhang H, Ekstrom A. Human neural systems underlying rigid and flexible forms of allocentric spatial representation. *Human Brain Mapping.* 2013;34(5):1070–87.

61. Burgess N. Spatial cognition and the brain. *Annals of the New York Academy of Sciences.* 2008;1124:77–97.

62. Wolbers T, Hegarty M. What determines our navigational abilities? *Trends in Cognitive Sciences.* 2010;14(3):138–46.

63. Burgess N. Spatial cognition and the brain. *Annals of the New York Academy of Sciences.* 2008;1124:77–97.

64. Jager G, Postma A. On the hemispheric specialization for categorical and coordinate spatial relations: a review of the current evidence. *Neuropsychologia.* 2003;41(4):504–15.

65. Ruotolo F, van der Ham IJ, Iachini T, Postma A. The relationship between allocentric and egocentric frames of reference and categorical and coordinate spatial information processing. *Quarterly Journal of Experimental Psychology.* 2011;64:1138–56.

66. Lester AW, Moffat SD, Wiener JM, Barnes CA, Wolbers T. The aging navigational system. *Neuron.* 2017;95(5):1019–35.

67. Lich M, Bremmer F. Self-motion perception in the elderly. *Frontiers of Human Neuroscience.* 2014;8:681.

68. Adamo DE, Briceno EM, Sindone JA, Alexander NB, Moffat SD. Age differences in virtual environment and real world path integration. *Frontiers in Aging Neuroscience.* 2012;4:26.

69. Bates SL, Wolbers T. How cognitive aging affects multisensory integration of navigational cues. *Neurobiology of Aging.* 2014;35:2761–9.

70. Arshad Q, Seemungal BM. Age-related vestibular loss: current understanding and future research directions. *Frontiers in Neurology.* 2016;7:231.

71. Daugherty AM, Yuan P, Dahle CL, Bender AR, Yang Y, Raz N. Path complexity in virtual water maze navigation: differential associations with age, sex, and regional brain volume. *Cerebral Cortex.* 2015;25(9):3122–31.

72. Turner SM, Gaynor LS, Ellison CN, Dunn CB, Janus CM, Bauer RM. Qualitative measurement of spatial navigation task reveals reduced allocentric search strategy use in normal and abnormal aging. 16th Annual Meeting of the American Academy of Clinical Neuropsychology; June 21, 2018; San Diego, CA, 2018.

73. Moffat SD, Resnick SM. Effects of age on virtual environment place navigation and allocentric cognitive mapping. *Behavioral Neuroscience.* 2002;116(5):851–9.

74. Dror IE, Kosslyn SM. Mental imagery and aging. *Psychology and Aging.* 1994;9:90–102.

75. Raz N, Briggs SD, Marks W, Acker JD. Age-related deficits in generation and manipulation of mental images: II. The role of dorsolateral prefrontal cortex. *Psychology and Aging.* 1999;14(3):436–44.

76. Kalkstein J, Checksfield K, Bollinger J, Gazzaley A. Diminished top-down control underlies a visual imagery deficit in normal aging. *The Journal of Neuroscience: The Official Journal of the Society for Neuroscience.* 2011;31(44):15768–74.

77. Gabbard C. Mental representation for action in the elderly: implications for movement efficiency and injury risk. *Journal of Applied Gerontology: The Official Journal of the Southern Gerontological Society.* 2015;34(3):NP202–NP212.

78. Decety J, Grezes J. Neural mechanisms subserving the perception of human actions. *Trends in Cognitive Sciences.* 1999;3:172–8.

79. Cacola P, Roberson J, Gabbard C. Aging in movement representations for sequential

finger movements: a comparison between young, middle aged, and older adults. *Brain and Cognition.* 2013;82:1–5.

80. Zapparoli L, Invernizzi P, Gndola M, Verardi M, Berlingeri M, Sherna M, et al. Mental images across the adult lifespan: a behavioural and fMRI investigation of motor execution and motor imagery. *Experimental Brain Research.* 2013;224(4):519–40.

81. Gabbard C, Cacola P, Cordova A. Is there an advanced aging effect on the ability to mentally represent action? *Archives of Gerontology and Geriatrics.* 2011;53:206–9.

82. Allali G, van der Meulen M, Beauchet O, Rieger SW, Vuilleumier P, Assal F. The neural basis of age-related changes in motor imagery of gait: an fMRI study. *The Journals of Gerontology Series A, Biological Sciences and Medical Sciences.* 2014;69(11):1389–98.

83. Cherry KE, Park DC, Donaldson H. Adult age differences in spatial memory: effects of structural context and practice. *Experimental Aging Research.* 1993;19(4):333–50.

84. Jiang HK, Owyang V, Hong JS, Gallagher M. Elevated dynorphin in the hippocampal formation of aged rats: relation to cognitive impairment on a spatial learning task. *Proceedings of the National Academy of Sciences of the United States of America.* 1989;86:2948–51.

85. Kadar T, Silbermann M, Brandeis R, Levy A. Age-related structural changes in the rat hippocampus: correlation with working memory deficiency. *Brain Research.* 1990;512:113–20.

86. Antonova E, Parslow D, Brammer M, Dawson GR, Jackson SHD, Morris RG. Age-related neural activity during allocentric spatial memory. *Memory* 2009;17:125–43.

87. Devlin AS. *Mind and Maze: Spatial Cognition and Environmental Behavior.* Westport, CT: Greenwood Press; 2001.

88. Moffat SD, Zonderman AB, Resnick SM. Age differences in spatial memory in a virtual environment navigation task. *Neurobiology of Aging.* 2001;22(5):787–96.

89. Moffat SD. Aging and spatial navigation: what do we know and where do we go? *Neuropsychology Review.* 2009;19(4):478–89.

90. Rodgers MK, Sindone JA, 3rd, Moffat SD. Effects of age on navigation strategy. *Neurobiology of Aging.* 2012;33(1):202 e15–22.

91. Harris MA, Wiener JM, Wolbers T. Aging specifically impairs switching to an allocentric navigation strategy. *Frontiers in Aging Neuroscience.* 2012;4:29.

92. O'Keefe J, Nadel L. *The Hippocampus as a Cognitive Map.* New York: Oxford University Press; 1978.

93. Moffat SD, Elkins W, Resnick SM. Age differences in the neural systems supporting human allocentric spatial navigation. *Neurobiology of Aging.* 2006;27(7):965–72.

94. Janzen G, Wagensveld B, van Turennout M. Neural representation of navigational relevance is rapidly induced and long lasting. *Cerebral Cortex.* 2007;17:975–81.

95. Allard S, Gosein V, Cuello AC, Ribeiro-de-Silva A. Changes with aging in the dopaminergic and noradrenergic innervation of rat neocortex. *Neurobiology of Aging.* 2011;32:2244–53.

96. Grudzien A, Shaw P, Weintraub S, Bigio E, Mash DC, Mesulam MM. Locus coeruleus neurofibrillary degeneration in aging, mild cognitive impairment, and early Alzheimer's disease. *Neurobiology of Aging.* 2007;28:327–35.

97. Zhong JY, Moffat SD. Age-related differences in associative learning of landmarks and heading directions in a virtual navigation task. *Frontiers in Aging Neuroscience.* 2016;8:122.

98. Wiener JM, Kmecova H, de Condappa O. Route repetition and route retracing effects of cognitive aging. *Frontiers in Aging Neuroscience.* 2012;4:7.

99. Umarova RM. Adapting the concepts of brain and cognitive reserve to post-stroke cognitive deficits: implications for understanding neglect. *Cortex; A Journal Devoted to the Study of the Nervous System and Behavior.* 2017;97:327–38.

100. Pijnacker J, Verstraten P, van Damme W, Vandermeulen J, Steenbergen B. Rehabilitation of reading in older individuals with macular degeneration: a review of effective training programs. *Neuropsychology, Development, and Cognition Section B, Aging, Neuropsychology and Cognition.* 2011;18(6):708–32.

101. Starkstein SE, Jorge RE, Robinson RG. The frequency, clinical correlates, and mechanism of anosognosia after stroke. *Canadian Journal of Psychiatry/ Revue canadienne de psychiatrie.* 2010;55(6):355–61.

102. Stoerig P. Functional rehabilitation of partial cortical blindness? *Restorative Neurology and Neuroscience.* 2008;26(4–5):291–303.

103. Cooke DM, McKenna K, Fleming J. Development of a standardized occupational therapy screening tool for visual perception in adults. *Scandinavian Journal of Occupational Therapy.* 2005;12(2):59–71.

104. Riva G, Rizzo A, Alpini D, Attree EA, Barbieri E, Bertella L, et al. Virtual environments in the diagnosis, prevention, and intervention of age-related diseases: a review of VR scenarios proposed in the EC VETERAN Project. *Cyberpsychology & Behavior: The Impact of the Internet, Multimedia and Virtual Reality on Behavior and Society.* 1999;2(6):577–91.

105. Pulido Herrera E. Location-based technologies for supporting elderly pedestrian in "getting lost" events. *Disability and Rehabilitation Assistive Technology.* 2017;12(4):315–23.

106. Maniglia M, Cottereau BR, Soler V, Trotter Y. Rehabilitation approaches in macular degeneration patients. *Frontiers in Systems Neuroscience.* 2016;10:107.

Chemosensory Function during Neurologically Healthy Aging

Jennifer J. Stamps

1 Introduction

Both taste and olfactory function are known to decline with aging and much more significantly with neurodegenerative diseases. Taste variation in general, either genetic or pathologic, is known to have predictive value for health status across the life span [1–6]. Olfactory function may be an accurate gauge for overall health, particularly during aging. Large epidemiological studies have found olfactory dysfunction to be an independent risk factor for death for older adults [7] and one of the strongest predictors of 5-year mortality, independently and more significantly than heart disease or cancer [8]. The hazard ratios for mortality for those scoring in the first, second, and third quartiles of an odor identification test compared with those in the fourth quartile were 3.81, 1.75, and 1.58 [9]. Impairment of odor identification is also significantly associated with the risk of developing cognitive impairment within the following five years [10]. The chemical senses are particularly vulnerable to insult due to the intimate interaction between olfactory and gustatory receptors and the outside world. Upper respiratory infections, viruses, medications, head trauma, environmental toxins, radiation therapy, and inflammation can damage the olfactory epithelium and/or the cranial nerves responsible for conveying taste and smell information from the periphery [11, 12]. As we age, the effects of damage on these networks from these various causes accrue, creating difficulties in teasing apart the specific effects of aging. Both the peripheral taste and olfactory receptors rely on constant cell renewal, which is known to slow with aging. The central processing of taste and smell also deteriorates in aging, even in cognitively healthy older adults.

Olfaction declines more with aging than taste [13], likely because taste is conveyed by three cranial nerves and damage to one or two can be compensated by the others. However, functional loss of one taste nerve can significantly diminish flavor perception even when whole mouth taste perception remains intact [14]. Retronasal olfaction enables perception of flavor volatiles from the mouth, as opposed to orthonasal olfaction, which enables perception of odor volatiles outside the body. Taste and oral touch interact with retronasal olfaction to produce the multimodal perception of flavor. Elderly people often complain of a loss or change in the flavor of foods and they demonstrate difficulty differentiating among food odors [15]. Unperceived loss of individual taste nerve function may combine with a general decline in olfactory function, causing an additive effect on the impairment of flavor perception, reducing the pleasure obtained from food, and resulting in a decline in intake. A loss of taste or oral somatosensory function can cause a dissociation between orthonasal and retronasal olfactory ability, and therefore each should be independently clinically assessed.

Gaps remain in our understanding of molecular and cellular mechanisms underlying olfaction, gustation, and neurogenesis and in how these mechanisms are affected by aging. Technological advances, however, are helping advance our knowledge. Likewise, our understanding of chemical sensory perception has advanced alongside technological improvements in human psychophysics – the mathematical measurement of conscious experience [16]. In addition to the population data that have been available on olfactory function, recent epidemiological studies on taste function throughout the life span have now better informed us on the prevalence of taste and smell perception decrements with aging.

2 Gustation and Oral Somatosensation

2.1 Basic Anatomy

Both taste and oral touch are vital functions and are uniquely mediated by three cranial nerves. Each nerve is responsible for transporting taste and/or touch information to the brain from discrete populations of papillae within the oral cavity [17]. Mushroom-shaped fungiform papillae (FuP), each containing 0–18 taste buds, are scattered over the apex and anterior sides of the tongue and are innervated by the chorda tympani branch of the facial nerve (CN VII) to mediate taste sensations [18]. These same papillae are innervated by the lingual nerve of the mandibular division of the trigeminal nerve. These fibers terminate in mechano-, thermo-, and pain receptors, as well as polymodal nociceptors, to mediate touch sensation [19]. Filling in the spaces between the fungiform papillae are heavily keratinized, cone-shaped filiform papillae, devoid of taste buds, that cover the entire surface of the anterior two-thirds of the tongue and help to grip food, spread saliva, and clean the mouth [20]. Foliate papillae (FoP) are vertical folds located on the posterolateral edges of the tongue; they are innervated by both the chorda tympani branch of CN VII and the lingual branch of the glossopharyngeal nerve (CN IX). Eight to twelve large, round circumvallate papillae (CvP) across the posterior tongue are also innervated by CN IX. FoP and CvP contain hundreds of taste buds along the walls of their troughs. Taste buds along the boundary of the hard and soft palate are innervated by the greater superficial petrosal branch of CN VII and those in the larynx and esophagus by the internal branch of the superior laryngeal branch of the vagus nerve (CN X). Transfer of both taste and somatosensory information from the CvP and from the larynx and esophagus is accomplished by taste-specific neurons and general sensory neurons with mechano- and thermo-receptors, and polymodal nociceptors in CN IX and X [18]. Differential expressions of transient receptor potential cation channels on these general sensory neurons are responsible for their functional heterogeneity: perception of various textures, temperature, irritants, and viscosity [21, 22]. Neural pathways mediating taste and oral touch are closely adjacent all the way from the periphery to the cerebral cortex.

Taste buds within the taste papillae contain about 50–100 cells divided into basal cells, the progenitors for new taste receptor cells, and three types of bipolar taste receptor cells whose receptors are housed within microvilli that protrude out of a taste pore of the papillae. Tastants dissolve into the mucosal lining of the tongue and into saliva so they can be carried to taste receptors within the pore, both G-protein–coupled receptors and ion channel receptors. All taste papillae contain all three types of bipolar taste receptor cells responsive to the four basic taste qualities: sweet, salty, sour, and bitter. The taste receptor cells do not have axons. Most are linked by synapses at their base, relaying taste information to the terminals of the cranial nerves, most likely using adenosine triphosphate as the neurotransmitter [23]. Individual taste nerve fibers may be classified as "sweet-best," "salt-best," etc. However, they respond to multiple tastant qualities and some also respond to tactile and temperature stimuli. Yet taste is "analytic": lemonade tastes sweet and sour, not a synthesis of the two tastes [24]. This topic is reviewed in detail by Smith and Margolskee [25] and by Chaudhari and Roper [26, 27].

The fibers of the cranial nerves for taste terminate in the nucleus tractus solitarius (NTS) in the medulla. From there, the second-order neurons project to the ventral posteromedial nucleus of the thalamus (VPM) via the central tegmental tract. The signal continues via the internal capsule to primary taste cortex, defined by cortical targets of VPM projections. These include the ipsilateral dorsal anterior insular-opercular cortex, the caudolateral orbitofrontal cortex (OFC), and the precentral gyrus, in an extension of primary somatosensory cortex [28, 29]. A second, primary projection carries hedonic and visceral information from the NTS in the medulla to regions in the ventral forebrain, including the nucleus accumbens, lateral hypothalamus, amygdala, and nucleus of the stria terminalis. This projection contributes to autonomic function, the control of feeding, and the hedonic response to taste [17, 23, 30, 31]. Secondary cortical taste areas in primates include the caudolateral OFC and posterior parietal cortex, where both gustatory and olfactory signals are received by bimodal neurons [32]. The OFC also receives taste afferents from the lateral hypothalamus that mediate satiety. Top-down modulation of taste responses also occurs via efferents from taste cortex to the rostral NTS [17].

For oral somatosensation, the sensory neurons, whose receptors are within the taste papillae, project via the trigeminal (FuP), glossopharyngeal (FoP and CvP), and vagal ganglia (epiglottis, larynx, pharynx) to various levels of the trigeminal sensory nuclear complex in the brain stem. The trigeminal nucleus transmits pain, temperature, and touch sensation via two ascending pathways in the trigeminothalamic tract to thalamic nuclei, including the contralateral VPM of the thalamus, where taste fibers also project. VPM neurons mediating pain and temperature sensation project to the insula, just posterior to the taste projections from the VPM. General sensory fibers sent to other thalamic nuclei also project to the anterior cingulate cortex. VPM neurons mediating touch sensation project to the primary somatosensory cortex [33]. In primates, uni-, bi-, and tri-modal neurons that respond to taste, temperature, capsaicin, and viscosity are found in the OFC [34]. The insular cortex also co-encodes multiple physical and chemical properties of stimuli placed in the mouth. For example, increased temperature on the anterior tongue induces a perception of sweetness [35] by activating transient receptor potential cation channel subfamily M member 5 (TRPM5) channels, which respond to temperatures over 40°C, and to capsaicin [36], and are also important for sweet and bitter taste transduction [37].

2.2 Variations in Gustatory Abilities Independent of Age: Genes and Environmental Insults

Dramatic individual variation in taste ability was first noted in 1931 when phenylthiocarbamide was spilled, a plume of it filled a lab, and some noticed a bitter taste while others noticed nothing [38]. Tasters of that chemical and a safer congener, 6-n-propylthiouracil (PROP), are born with one or both dominant alleles for the Ta2r38 bitter gene on chromosome 7 [39]. Nontasters of PROP are born with two recessive alleles. Tasters of PROP who also have a high density of fungiform papillae are supertasters [40]. There is a 3.3-fold range in the number of FuP and a 14-fold range in the number of taste pores among healthy young adults [41]. The more FuP, the more intense the taste of sweet, salty, sour, and bitter stimuli [42–45]. Because FuP also house trigeminal nerve endings, the intensity of oral irritants like capsaicin and carbonation and other somatosensory stimuli, such as the sense of creaminess, also increase with higher fungiform density [46–48].

Mediation of taste via the chorda tympani branch of CN VII is especially vulnerable as this structure can be damaged as a result of injections for routine dental anesthesia, otitis media, head trauma, third molar extractions, diabetes, and other systemic diseases.

Other known causes of chorda tympani damage include hyperemesis during pregnancy, gastroesophageal reflux disease, upper respiratory infections, and radiation therapy for cancer [49–53]. Tonsillectomies and radiation therapy for head and neck cancer are the only known causes of CN IX damage [49, 54, 55]. Smokers have fewer FuP compared with nonsmokers and FuP density correlates with pack years of smoking [56]. Smoking can damage the trigeminal nerve and, because the nerve endings of its lingual branch form little baskets around the taste buds, when they die and wither away, the taste buds and inevitably the whole FuP also wither away. Shingles, caused by herpes zoster, has also been associated with trigeminal nerve damage [57].

2.3 Effects of Aging on Gustation and Oral Somatosensation

2.3.1 Mechanical Breakdown

The capacity to regenerate taste receptor cells that are continuously dying off in the periphery declines with aging, even among the healthy. Taste receptor cells continuously regenerate throughout life with an average turnover rate of 8–12 days in the young [58]. Components of taste progenitor/stem cells and signal transduction molecules important for cell fate, differentiation, and migration are being identified [59], and many of these components are also found to decline with aging, adversely affecting taste bud homeostasis in a number of different ways. For example, older mice show a decrease in the proliferating population of the stem cells that differentiate into all three types of taste receptor cell within the circumvallate (CvP) and foliate (FoP) papillae [60–62]. Aged mice also have significantly lower mRNA expressions of key signal transduction molecules in the CVP and FuP [63].

In humans, the average number of taste buds within CvP in the elderly is reduced by 30–50% [64, 65]. A study quantifying taste buds within FuP of humans found no significant differences across the life span between 2 and 90 years old [66]. While the number of taste buds within FuP does not decline with aging, the quantity of FuP does decrease [45, 67]. Controlling for taster status (nontaster, medium taster, supertaster) and other confounding variables, our laboratory also found that the number of FuP on the tip of the tongue decreases with aging [68]. In addition, a significant deterioration of FuP shape and of the vascularization of the anterior tongue has been observed among participants over 60 years old, and these changes have correlated with taste acuity [69].

2.3.2 Loss of Neurotrophic Support and Vital Nutrients

Another likely cause for a degradation of taste papillae is the waning of neurotrophic support [70]. For example, brain-derived neurotrophic factor (BDNF) is highly expressed throughout the gustatory and olfactory pathways from the peripheral to the central structures [71]. Many large cross-sectional studies have revealed a decline in plasma BDNF with increasing age [72–74]. A corroborating longitudinal study of healthy agers also found that plasma BDNF levels were inversely correlated with age [75]. Taste bud development depends on BDNF [76]. Taste receptor cells that express BDNF receptors are specifically innervated by CN VII axons in the chorda tympani and, accordingly, FuP are sensitive to a decline in BDNF levels [77, 78]. Neurotrophic factors 3 and 4 are also important for taste and oral somatosensory function and show aging-associated decreases [79–82]. Endurance exercises involving the legs can prevent declines in neurotrophins like BDNF [83].

Nutrients play a role in chemosensory functions. Stewart-Knox et al. [84] found that older participants with higher erythrocyte zinc concentrations had a greater sensitivity for salt and those with lower serum zinc had a decreased sensitivity to sour. No relationship was found in younger participants. The same group found that 30 mg/day of a zinc supplement improved salt taste acuity in people over 70 years old [85]. Older people with taste disorders were found to have lower salivary concentrations of zinc and manganese and higher salivary concentrations of copper than older people without taste disorders [86]. In a study of 408 participants, a significantly higher percentage of those over 65 years of age had low serum zinc levels, and zinc supplementation improved taste perception in 70% of all participants [87].

2.3.3 Dehydration and Loss of Stimulus Carrier

In order to be tasted, a nonvolatile compound must be carried in the saliva to the taste pores of the papillae. Due to decreased hydration and the effects of some medications, aging people may experience reduced salivary secretion and changes in the composition of saliva, changes that can impede gustation

[88–90]. A meta-analysis of 47 studies concluded that stimulated and unstimulated whole mouth and submandibular and sublingual salivary flow significantly decreases after the age of 60 regardless of medications being taken [91]. While this decrease was evident in nonmedicated older people [92], xerostomia is also directly proportional to the total number of medications taken per day [93], and some medications, like those with anticholinergic side effects, have much greater effects than others [94]. The number of medications taken increases as people age, and more than 250 drugs have been reported to affect the sense of taste [11, 95].

The speed of salivary flow determines electrolyte concentrations because the faster the flow, the less the time for electrolytic exchange. Changes in the inorganic composition of saliva have been found with aging. A significant increase of salivary sodium was found in males over 40 years of age, while calcium, phosphate, and potassium were found to trend upward with increasing age, starting after age 40 in people of both sexes [96–98]. These changes in the ionic background of the oral cavity could contribute to changes in taste perception with age. Other detectable changes in saliva, like DNA methylation patterns (an epigenetic effect) and protein carbonyl levels, can actually be used to accurately predict the age of the donor [99, 100].

2.3.4 *Central Network Breakdown*

Once a taste compound has been absorbed into saliva and carried to taste receptor cells, which transmit the message from the periphery via the taste nerves to the brain stem, taste perception becomes dependent on primary and secondary central connections and structures [101]. EEG and fMRI studies have provided evidence for aging-related changes in the functions of central taste systems. Topographical analyses of EEG-recorded gustatory event-related potentials from 128 scalp electrodes delineated five distinct topographical maps involved in taste processing of the basic tastants, each presented at a medium concentration to healthy young adults. The time course of evolution of one of these maps significantly changed with aging, and another map all but disappeared in older adults [102]. In an fMRI study, the dorsomedial nucleus of the thalamus, the posterior insular cortex, and the right amygdala were significantly less activated in older than younger participants, and the only tastant that elicited activity above baseline levels in these aging participants was sour. In contrast to the aging participants, the younger group exhibited an increase in activity in response to all tastants. As with the psychophysical studies, the differences between the young and old groups were larger at the lowest and highest concentrations of tastants. No differences between the young and old groups were found in activity in the NTS or the VPM nucleus of the thalamus, suggesting that aging does not affect information transmission from the periphery but does affect higher level taste processing, especially in the primary and secondary somatosensory areas [103]. Another fMRI study found that, while no aging-related differences were measured in taste or pleasantness intensity ratings of sucrose during hunger or satiety, fMRI activation in response to sucrose was significantly lower in both hunger states in middle-aged adults and in the elderly compared with the young in a number of brain regions, most notably the insula and prefrontal cortex, regions important for sensory and reward processing [104, 105].

2.3.5 Prevalence of the Loss of Taste Perception with Aging

How do these morphological and chemical changes and alterations in neurobiological processing correlate with, and predict, functional impairments? A study of 1,312 participants, 25–75 years old, found that roughly 15% of women of all ages and 23–28% of men, particularly those of advanced age, could not identify all four tastants. Sweet was the most often correctly identified tastant and sour the least often [106]. In a study of 761 healthy participants aged 5–89 years (mean = 35.8), using two methods, threshold recognition and whole mouth identification, hypogeusia was found in 5%, ageusia was very rare, and all four tastants were correctly identified 94% of the time. A weak, negative correlation was found with age [107]. The National Social Life, Health, and Aging Project (NSHAP) chemosensory study, which specifically targeted older, community-dwelling US adults (57–85 years, N = 3,005), found that 14.8% had severe impairment of whole mouth taste identification. Better scores were independently linked with lower age, female gender, fewer medications, and a higher level of education [108]. The second NSHAP study was a global sensory study on a subset of the participants from the original taste study (N = 1,301). They found taste, measured only by whole mouth identification, to be the most effected sensory

modality, with 74% of those between 57 and 85 years old being unable to correctly identify all four tastants [109]. In contrast, large population-based studies of young participants' taste identification ability found that between 0.84% [110] and 4% [111] had impairment.

Population-based studies that utilized somewhat different measurements of gustatory function, taste recognition threshold, and supra-threshold taste intensity have demonstrated greater aging-related impairment in taste. A Japanese study of 2,015 participants, divided into young (24–32 years old), young-old (69–71 years old), and old-old (79–81 years old) groups, found that, with the exception of sweet, whole mouth taste recognition thresholds increased significantly with age, and that women had significantly lower thresholds than men in both older groups. At the highest concentration, all young participants correctly detected the four basic tastes, but in the young-old and old-old groups, 1.3% and 3.5% missed sweet, 6.3% and 18.8% missed sour, 6.7% and 13.2% missed salty, and 29.2% and 37.9% missed bitter [112]. These results are congruent with those of the US population-based studies described above and another comprehensive study of taste quality confusions across the life span [113]. As in the US studies, gender and cognitive health were major factors affecting taste function in the older groups, along with alcohol consumption, hypertension, number of teeth, salivary flow, and years of education [114]. These same researchers conducted the only reported longitudinal study of taste function in an aging population by conducting follow-up exams 3 years later on 328 of the 621 old-old participants from the study above. After 3 years, a third of the participants had decreased sensitivity for sweet, sour, and bitter, while two-thirds had decreased sensitivity for salty. Males showed a more significant decline than females for sweet and sour, and all participants with lower cognitive testing scores showed a significant decline in salty perception [115]. However, a study of *supra-threshold* whole mouth taste intensity, measured via the generalized labeled magnitude scale [116], involving 2,374 participants aged 21–84 years, found that while being female and having a higher level of education was associated with higher taste intensity ratings for each of the four tastants, no consistent relationship was found with aging [117]. These results are in line with the findings of smaller studies that found that taste identification declines with aging, taste detection and recognition thresholds increase, but little change occurs in supra-threshold taste intensity ratings.

2.3.6 Perceptual Changes with Aging

The simplest test of taste function is threshold testing with electrogustometry [118]. A gradually increasing electrical current is delivered to the tongue until the individual reports a sensation. Many studies have found a trend toward increased thresholds with aging [119–122] but only a few have found significant increases in differences between the youngest and oldest groups [119, 123]. Most electrogustometry studies have also concluded that women tend to have greater taste acuity than men [122, 123] and that taste acuity at the hard and soft palates is more affected by aging than acuity at the tongue tip [123]. While electrogustometry quantifies the sensitivity of the taste nerve innervating the area where the anode is placed, it does not assess the person's ability to detect or identify any of the four basic tastes.

Absolute concentration thresholds for detecting a taste difference between two solutions and for actually identifying the difference can be established through a number of quantitative methods [124, 125]. Many studies have found lower detection thresholds in the young compared with the old for all four basic tastes but, unfortunately, the reported differences vary from two- to nine-fold, in part because of methodological differences [126–133]. Additionally, some studies did not control for such confounds as taster type, the number and type of medications taken by participants, or medical history. In studies that analyzed gender effects, older women were found to detect all four tastes at lower concentrations than older men [128], or to detect just salty [134], or just salty and sour [135], at lower concentrations than older men [126, 130]. Sensitivity to salty and bitter have most often been found to decline significantly with aging, and the aging-related ionic changes in saliva discussed earlier have been suggested to contribute to increased salty thresholds [126, 127, 131–133, 136]. Sensitivity to salty was also found to depend on the medium in which it is tested. For example, salt detection thresholds were 7–10 times higher in tomato soup than in water for all age groups, and both the middle-aged group and the elderly group required approximately twice the concentration of salt as did the young group to detect it [137].

While measurement of absolute concentration thresholds is useful for assessing the physiologic function of the taste system, perceived intensity of taste is not a linear function of concentration [138] and absolute threshold data cannot be generalized to supra-threshold sensations, those perceived above threshold levels [129, 139]. Therefore, measurement of supra-threshold functions is needed to study impairments that are relevant to everyday perception of taste, as well as to investigate genotype effects and predict dietary behavior [140–142]. Supra-threshold function can be assessed through magnitude estimation [143]. For example, a study participant can be asked to assess the intensity of a given taste relative to that of a control intensity [144, 145]. Magnitude matching requires participants to rate the sensation of interest and a sensation of a different sensory modality on a common scale, thus providing an outside standard insensitive to the variable of interest in a study, in this case, of taste, thereby enabling valid comparisons of sensory experiences between different age groups [146, 147].

To compare different age groups, Bartoshuk et al. [132] asked participants to "magnitude match" the perceived intensity of water and weak, moderate, and strong taste stimuli to decibels of sound at a tone predetermined to be unaffected by aging. Dilute solutions of each of the basic tastes were matched to sounds of varying intensity by younger and older participants. It was found that the two groups matched moderate and strong taste solutions to the same sound levels. Thus, despite the elevated taste thresholds in the older group, the perceived intensities of tastes encountered most often in everyday life were not affected by aging. Other studies have generally corroborated these findings, suggesting that whole mouth taste intensity is relatively stable across the life span [148–153]. However, some discrepancies have been found with sour and bitter [151, 154] and with lower concentrations of tastants [135, 155]. With aging, bitter perception appears to differentially decline and salty sensation less so, while sweet perception remains constant. One potential reason for a whole mouth reduction in bitter perception could be that bitter taste nerve fibers are thin and unmyelinated and therefore more susceptible to damage [156]. Aging has greater effects on physiologic function, as assessed by measuring absolute concentration thresholds, than it does on levels of sensation encountered in everyday experiences, assessed via supra-threshold measurements.

There is no consistent evidence that the modest aging-related differences in perception of taste intensity, particularly for salty and bitter, have any impact on the likability of certain tastes or concentrations or any ramifications for food intake [157]. Furthermore, both perception and likability are strongly influenced by context. For example, older people may prefer saltier mashed potatoes or chicken broth [158, 159], but their salt preferences in soup or tomato juice do not differ from those of young individuals [160, 161]. Mojet et al. found that, when the nose was clipped, aging-related differences in taste perception disappeared [155]. This suggests that aging-related taste decrements are at least partly due to a decrement in intensity of retronasal olfactory cues (see below). Consistent with this interpretation, a study of healthy older women found that the 37 of the 80 who had olfactory dysfunction also had a lower preference for bitter/sour foods (e.g., citrus) and pungent foods, and an increased intake of sweet foods [162]. Thus, olfactory impairments, specifically retronasal olfactory impairments, rather than relatively minor taste impairments, are more likely to cause changes in food preference and intake.

Because we know that anesthetizing a single taste nerve can decrease retronasal olfactory intensity by 50% [14], a more significant decline in flavor perception than in whole-mouth taste would be expected to result from the loss of function of individual taste nerves. A stark clinical example comes from a patient I tested who had a stroke involving his NTS precisely where CNs VII and IX, but not CN X, send taste information. He tasted nothing on the areas of the tongue innervated by CNs VII or IX. However, because the area where CN X innervates the NTS was spared, his whole mouth taste intensity ratings were normal for every tastant. Unfortunately, despite intact whole mouth taste and above average orthonasal olfactory function, chocolate was the only odor out of 25 tested that he could perceive retronasally. This profound loss of retronasal olfaction caused anhedonia, dramatic weight loss, and malnutrition.

Integration of input from CNs VII, IX, and X maintains whole mouth taste even when a loss of input from any individual nerve occurs. Therefore, even patients with extensive areas of damage can appear to be nearly normal on a conventional, whole mouth taste test, a phenomenon known as "taste constancy" [163–165]. This happens because the loss of function of one taste or sensory nerve innervating a particular area of the tongue causes disinhibition of the remaining intact nerves that innervate other areas of the tongue [166]. The location of the taste or somatosensory sensations is not evident to the person, just the intensity [167]. The loss of individual taste nerve function is common and can occur at any age; however, spatial testing of the tongue is required to detect this loss [168].

Localized loss of taste and touch sensation restricted to the area of innervation of one of the three cranial nerves for taste or oral touch is found to occur more often with aging than whole mouth decrements. Studies employing spatial tongue tests have reported aging-related localized taste loss, mostly from the CvP innervated by CN IX and primarily for bitter [150]. This loss appears to be caused by the accumulated effects of environmental insults. In females, it is also associated with menopause [169].

Studies of aging effects on oral somatosensory function have reported increased two-point discrimination thresholds and impaired discrimination of tactile and vibratory sensations on the lip in participants over 80. However, no aging-associated changes in stereognostic ability, proprioception, thermal or somesthetic sensitivity, vibrational sensitivity, or two-point discrimination thresholds were found on the tongue or palate [170]. Detection thresholds for capsaicin (a burning irritant) also do not show any aging-associated decline [171]. Trigeminal sensory receptors are also located in the nasal cavity. Studies have shown no aging-related changes in detection thresholds for CO_2 [172], no aging-related declines in supra-threshold intensity of CO_2 [139, 172], no decline in trigeminal lateralization thresholds for butanol [173], and no impairment of ability to discriminate relative to ability to identify irritant qualities across different types of odorants with irritant properties [174]. As with behavioral measurements, aging-associated decreases in the amplitudes of chemosensory event-related potentials are more prominent in response to pure olfactory stimuli than nasal trigeminal stimuli [175].

2.3.7 Conclusions on Taste and Oral Touch during Aging

Population-based studies have demonstrated that 14.8% of older US adults have severe impairment in whole mouth taste identification and 74% were unable to correctly identify all four basic tastes. Bitter taste is affected the most, followed by sour and salty, while only 3.5% of the very old misidentify sweet.

Neural network degeneration rather than peripheral loss of function may be the major contributor to impairment in taste identification. Epidemiological studies also report significantly elevated taste recognition thresholds except for sweet and have found that, overall, older women have better taste recognition sensitivity than older men. Smaller studies have revealed elevated detection and recognition taste thresholds with aging, especially for bitter and salty, and more so in men than in women. Other than for limited evidence of minor, quality-specific decrements, mainly for bitter, supra-threshold taste intensity (assessed in magnitude estimation studies) appears to be relatively stable across the life span. When localized supra-threshold intensity is measured from discrete areas of innervation by the different cranial nerves mediating taste and oral touch sensation, CvP function, subserved by CN IX, appears to be the most vulnerable to aging effects. This is consistent with the results of studies of molecular, cellular, and morphological changes that occur with aging. These changes include a decrease in the proliferating population of the stem cells that differentiate into all three taste receptor cell types within the CvP, lower mRNA expression of key signal transduction molecules in the CvP, and a 30–50% decline in the average number of taste buds within the CvP of humans over 70 years old. Unlike the changes in intake and health shown to result from more profound taste damage and loss of taste perception, the minor aging-associated taste decrements have not been found to cause significant detrimental changes in taste preferences or intake. Studies of oral touch show only minor, aging-related decrements. The capacity of oral taste and touch systems for maintenance of constancy of taste and oral touch in spite of damage suggests that both systems are important throughout the life span for avoiding potentially noxious or poisonous substances and for incentivizing ingestion of substances vital for brain function and energy like fat, sugar, and salt [176, 177].

The universal finding from all lines of research on the topic of taste function in aging, including anatomical studies, molecular studies, imaging studies, and behavioral studies, is that variance within a particular age group increases as age increases. This variance suggests that with aging, some individuals maintain taste function better than others. Avoiding upper respiratory infections, certain medications, head trauma, and other sources of cranial nerve damage,

as well as maintaining levels of neurotrophins like BDNF through exercise, and sustaining a diet rich in nutrients like zinc and magnesium, may help to preserve both taste and smell function late into life.

3 Olfaction

3.1 Basic Anatomy

The olfactory system enables the perception of at least a trillion different and unpredictable odors that a human might encounter in a lifetime [178]. Odorant molecules are warmed and moistened in the mucosa of the nasal turbinates or the mouth. They are guided to the olfactory epithelium in the nasopharynx via the orthonasal route during inhalation and via the retronasal route during exhalation while chewing and swallowing. Odorant molecules are organic, volatile molecular compounds that differ in carbon chain link, functional groups, and chirality. Single-atom differences can be detected by the olfactory system. In contrast to taste receptor cells, which are modified epithelial cells that synapse on first-order taste nerves, olfactory sensory neurons are bipolar neurons. A particular chemical attribute of an odor molecule docks onto an odor-binding pocket of a G-protein–coupled receptor, which resides atop one of the 10–30 cilia floating in the mucus on the dendritic knob of an olfactory sensory neuron within the olfactory epithelium [179, 180]. Each olfactory sensory neuron expresses one type of olfactory receptor coded by one of approximately 400 functional olfactory receptor genes. This is the largest gene family in the human genome, underscoring how vital olfaction is for success of the organism [181, 182].

Thousands of olfactory sensory neuron axons of the same olfactory receptor type coalesce to form an olfactory nerve. The olfactory nerve then traverses the cribiform plate at the base of the skull and converges onto a specified pair of glomeruli on the medial and lateral sides of the olfactory bulb [183]. A glomerulus houses a mitral or a tufted cell. Among the mitral and tufted cells are interneurons that provide local and distal coordinated inhibition of other glomerular units scattered throughout the olfactory bulb [184–186]. This enables the enhancement of signal-to-noise ratios and synchronization of the activated mitral cells [187]. When all the olfactory receptors responding to all the particular chemical groups of an odor molecule transmit their signal to their particular glomeruli, a glomerular activation signature pattern specific to that odor is elicited across the olfactory bulb, much like notes played across a piano to form a chord. This constitutes the spatial representation of that odor, an "odor image" [188–190].

The axons of the mitral and tufted cells of the olfactory bulb bundle together to form the olfactory tract, which directly distributes the extracted features of the odor stimulus to the many pyramidal cells across olfactory cortex. This is the only sensory pathway that bypasses the thalamus. The mitral and tufted cells project directly to the nucleus accumbens, the piriform cortex, the amygdala, the entorhinal cortex, and the insula [191–193]. The piriform cortex functions much like the association cortices of other sensory systems except that it processes olfactory information. The piriform cortex has a highly autoassociative architecture and has reciprocal connections with many other regions, such as the orbitofrontal cortex, the entorhinal cortex, the nucleus accumbens, and the amygdala [194–197]. As in other association cortices, learning occurs in the piriform cortex [198] and pattern completion occurs when molecular components of an odor are missing [199]. The piriform cortex rapidly adapts to constant odors and is especially activated by changes in its input. Also, as in other sensory association cortices, synaptic strengths change with repeated exposure, thereby instantiating odor memory, which can be matched to subsequent input [200]. The main function of these microcircuits is to form an odor object from an input that reflects a multitude of diverse stimuli [201].

Most olfactory efferent fibers from the piriform cortex, the nucleus accumbens shell, and the amygdala project directly to the orbitofrontal cortex (OFC), which has reciprocal connections with these structures [194–197]. In this way, the deciphered odor image is linked to representations of emotional meaning and valence [202, 203]. Pleasant odors and flavors activate the left medial rostral OFC, while unpleasant ones activate the left lateral OFC [204, 205]. Lesions of the OFC impair both orthonasal and retronasal olfactory identification of odors [206]. Just as the thalamus is not a relay between CN I and primary olfactory cortex, it does not act as a gateway between primary olfactory cortex and neocortex either. Most humans are not aware of the vital importance of olfaction, unless they lose it, but the processing

privileges of this sensory system are suggestive of its importance in human life, most clearly manifest in flavor perception and retronasal olfaction.

While both orthonasal and retronasal olfactory routes lead odor molecules to the same olfactory epithelium, retronasal olfaction is perceived and centrally processed differently because it is linked to processing of taste and oral somatosensation [207]. The strong association between retronasal olfaction, taste, and oral somatosensation creates the "oral capture" of retronasal olfaction, the perception that the flavor sensation is coming from the mouth and not the nose [208, 209]. For example, chocolate actually tastes only sweet and a little bitter. The flavor of chocolate is a retronasal olfactory percept. An orange and a strawberry both taste sweet and sour, and feel juicy, fibrous, and cool, but without retronasal olfaction, they are indistinguishable. Older people commonly complain of losing taste but, on testing, prove to have preserved taste but impaired retronasal olfaction.

Retronasal olfaction is the foremost sensory modality of flavor perception with taste and oral touch providing both positive and negative influences. For example, adding sweet taste can increase the retronasal olfaction of strawberry [210–212], a phenomenon exploited by food companies. The addition of flavor volatiles can increase or decrease the perceived taste of a food or beverage [213, 214]. Particular volatiles within fruits can increase their perceived sweetness independent of their sugar concentration [215–218]. Just as the OFC, the insula, and adjacent frontal operculum have multimodal neurons that respond to temperature, texture, and taste, these major integration areas also have bimodal neurons for taste and retronasal olfaction whose responses can be conditioned to learned associations [29, 32]. A large percentage of posterior piriform neurons also selectively respond to taste stimuli [219] and the NTS has bimodal neurons for smell and taste [220].

3.2 Variations in Olfactory Abilities Independent of Age: Genes and Environmental Insults

As with gustation, olfactory function reflects considerable genetic variation. Autosomal dominant congenital anosmia can occur but the prevalence is low [221]. On the other hand, odorant-specific hyposmia and anosmia is common and has been documented for dozens of different odors [222–226]. For example, 30% of the population is specifically anosmic to androstenone and the perception of its odor quality and valence varies dramatically among the 70% who can smell it [227–229].

Olfactory receptors constitute the only neuronal receptors located outside the skull and completely exposed to the environment. This direct, chemical interaction with the environment allows the olfactory system to function as the most accurate and sensitive mass spectrometer in the world. Unfortunately, it also creates a unique vulnerability to environmental toxins, foreign substances, viruses, and other infectious agents. In fact, upper respiratory infections are the most common cause of loss of olfactory function. In addition, the thin, unmyelinated axons of the olfactory receptors must travel through the holes of the cribiform plate of the ethmoid bone at the base of the skull to connect with the olfactory bulb. This makes them particularly vulnerable to head trauma, a common cause of loss of smell, often severe. Chronic nasal and sinus diseases causing epithelial inflammation or polyps can cause olfactory loss by obstructing airflow and preventing odor volatiles from reaching olfactory receptors. Aging and several neurodegenerative diseases, such as Parkinson's disease (PD) and Alzheimer disease (AD), can also cause loss of olfactory function [230].

3.3 Effects of Aging on Olfaction

3.3.1 Mechanical Breakdown

As with taste receptor cells, olfactory sensory neurons are short lived and are continuously replaced from a population of basal cells layered within the olfactory epithelium. Unfortunately, the number of adult stem cells and their proliferative potential appear to decline with aging [231]. The subventricular zone within the lateral ventricle is the main neurogenic stem cell niche for the brain (other than the dentate nucleus of the hippocampus) and the olfactory bulb provides a significant drive for stem cell production. Olfactory function depends on the constant rostral migration of progenitors from the subventricular zone to the olfactory bulbs and epithelium [232]. During aging, this important neurogenic niche becomes more restricted in area and astrocytes increase and neuroblasts decline [233].

A human study of 121 cadavers aged 0–91 years, none with intracranial disease, examined the integrity of the glomeruli within the olfactory bulbs to infer the quantity of olfactory nerve fibers. Glomeruli declined by an average of 1% per year and 73% had been lost by age 91 [234]. A later study found the same 1% per year loss of glomeruli with aging and a decline in mitral cells from a youthful average of 38,000–18,000 in middle age and 11,000 at advanced age [235]. Both studies suggested that, while a progressive decline in glomeruli clearly occurs with aging, nasal disease may be the major determinative factor in the loss of olfactory nerve fibers because of the large variation in atrophy in individuals within the same age group and because, occasionally, complete atrophy was found in the olfactory bulb of younger people.

Animal studies that eliminate the confounds of environmental toxins and infectious agents can provide information on aging in the relative absence of external factors. One such study in mice found that the volumes of the olfactory bulb cell layers did not change, stereotypic glomerular convergence of olfactory sensory neuron axons in the olfactory bulb was maintained, and the quantity of projection neurons and interneurons remained stable. However, a significant decline in afferent and local circuit synapses was noted within the glomerular layer of the olfactory bulb [236]. Whether this loss of synapses is due to a loss of olfactory sensory neurons in the olfactory epithelium, a decline in axonal branching, or changes in synaptic dynamics remains unknown [236]. Another similar murine study did find more diffuse axon targeting of glomeruli by olfactory sensory neurons in older mice [237].

Naessen determined in human cadavers free of intracranial or intranasal disease that the zonal distribution of olfactory sensory neurons between layers of supporting cells and basal cells in the olfactory epithelium in the fetus was lost with aging and that total degeneration of the olfactory epithelium with complete loss of olfactory sensory neurons was predominantly seen in the elderly, although significant individual variation was noted. This study also found that with aging, olfactory epithelium was increasingly replaced with respiratory epithelium [238]. Another human study of cadavers, free from confounding causes of loss, corroborated these findings [239]. Nakashima et al. concluded that much of the degeneration may be the result of an accumulation of damage from upper respiratory infections and that perhaps the continuous renewal of olfactory sensory neurons, found to occur in response to such environmental insults [240], may be what actually deteriorates with aging [239]. Results of studies of rodents provide support for this hypothesis [241–243]. Similar to the effects of aging on taste cell turnover, the actively proliferative globose basal cells were greatly reduced, while the quiescent, reserve population of progenitors, the horizontal basal cells, remained unaffected by aging [242]. Unfortunately, this reserve population is unresponsive to the progressive loss of olfactory sensory neurons and is stimulated only in response to acute injury of the olfactory epithelium, independent of age [244, 245] (see also review by Schwob et al. [246].

Qualitative aging-associated changes in the olfactory pathway may also affect olfactory function. Calcium imaging was utilized to measure odor-induced responses from 621 olfactory sensory neurons recovered from olfactory epithelium biopsies of 440 humans either ≤45 years of age or ≥60 years of age [246]. The number of viable olfactory sensory neurons per biopsy was not different between the two age groups. However, all the odorant-responsive cells from the younger group responded to only one odorant, while 24.6% of cells from the older group responded to both odorants. This decline in selectivity correlated with poorer odor detection. It could reflect the loss of afferent and local circuit synapses, as found in the glomerular layer of the olfactory bulbs of older mice, or the loss of olfactory nerve fibers found to occur more often in the glomeruli of older humans, as described above [234–236]. Paradoxical decreases in intracellular Ca^{2+} in response to odor stimulation, rather than the expected increases, also occurred in the neurons from the older group [247]. Axonal mistargeting of glomeruli [243], possibly related to changes in olfactory receptor gene expression, is another potential cause of these aging-associated changes [248].

To a substantial extent, aging-related changes in olfactory function reflect epigenetic changes, which alter gene expression. Only 4.3% of olfactory receptor genes were differentially expressed in the oldest mice compared with the youngest [249]. In contrast, significant downregulation was found for 589 genes associated with cellular responses to axonal injury, transduction pathways that regulate neurogenesis and angiogenesis, multiple extracellular matrix proteins, as well as cellular processes underlying extracellular matrix and collagen fibril organization important for the olfactory epithelial progenitor cell

niche. Insulin-like growth factor 1 (IGF-1), a crucial neurotrophin for the maintenance of the olfactory system, was also significantly downregulated. This downregulation would hinder tissue regeneration and homeostasis of the lamina propria of the olfactory epithelium, which is indeed thinner in aging mice and humans. Conversely, a significant upregulation was found for 389 genes associated with olfactory signal transduction and steroid hormone biosynthesis. Genes encoding cytokines of the senescence-associated secretory phenotypes, like interleukin 6 (IL-6), were also upregulated. Having high IL-6 and low IGF-1 would cause a decline in differentiation and maturation of olfactory progenitor cells into mature olfactory sensory neurons [242]. These phenomena parallel aging-associated changes in the taste system, where mRNA expression levels of genes encoding taste receptor cells appear to be stable across the life span while genes implicated in epithelial maintenance and signal transduction are significantly downregulated [63].

3.3.2 Loss of Neurotrophic Support and Vital Nutrients

Neurotrophic factors are essential for preservation of olfactory function. BDNF is vital for immature olfactory receptor neuron survival and function, and when it is diminished, olfactory function is compromised [250]. BDNF declines with aging but this loss can be prevented with leg-based exercise [83]. IGF-1 is the only neurotrophin for which gene expression in the olfactory epithelium declines with aging, and supplementation has been suggested as a potential treatment to restore olfactory functional loss [242]. The production of vascular endothelial growth factor (VEGF) is also reduced with aging [251]. VEGF is another important stimulant for neurogenesis [252]. There are VEGF receptors in the olfactory epithelium of adult humans and VEGF influences the migration of olfactory epithelium neural progenitor cells [253]. It is also essential to the maturation of adult-borne neurons in the olfactory bulb [254].

As with taste, zinc plays an important role in olfaction, modulating ion channels and amino acid receptors expressed by the olfactory bulb [255]. Zinc is an essential trace metal necessary for cellular growth and development and it is an important component of multiple enzyme systems, including carbonic anhydrase VI, which is vital for taste and smell function. On the other hand, excessive zinc can promote apoptotic cell death and lead to anosmia.

Theophylline, a drug that inhibits apoptosis via its effect on tumor necrosis factor α and its receptors, has been reported to increase smell function in hyposmic patients [256]. Vitamin B12 deficiency may cause a complete loss of both taste and smell [257]. A larger study of patients with vitamin B12 deficiency found that 56.4% were hyposmic and 5.1% were anosmic [258]. This can be mitigated with B12 injections or sublingual tablets, but it is unknown how much function can be recovered. Vitamins B6 and A have also been implicated in chemosensory loss. Retinoic acid, a metabolic product of vitamin A, is a signaling molecule that modulates the genesis, growth, and stability of olfactory epithelial cells, olfactory bulb interneurons, and slowly dividing subventricular zone neural precursor cells [259].

3.3.3 Dehydration and Loss of Stimulus Carrier

Like taste molecules transported by saliva, odor volatiles are captured by the mucus that additionally serves as the medium for movement of the cilia that house the olfactory receptors on the dendrites of olfactory sensory neurons. Changes in mucosal composition and decreases in mucosal secretion often result in changes in the motility of the cilia and impaired enzymatic degradation and clearance of both odor volatiles and environmental toxins that can impede olfaction [90, 260, 261]. These changes parallel those in saliva, discussed above, that impact taste function. In addition, the enzymatic system of the olfactory mucosa responsible for solubilizing odorants so they can bind to olfactory receptors becomes less efficient with aging, more so for some odorants than others [262–264]. This may contribute to the heterogeneity of functional loss seen in odor identification studies involving older humans. In a large study of healthy individuals, an in vitro test of ciliary beat frequency used to monitor mucociliary clearance in the nose found no significant changes over an age range of 20–80 years. However, variance did significantly increase with age [265].

3.3.4 Central Network Breakdown

In a study of brains from 39 nondemented people aged 51–88 years and cognitively tested premortem, within a year of death, neurofibrillary tangles were found in the entorhinal and perirhinal cortex, the anterior olfactory nucleus, the periamygdaloid cortex, and in the hippocampal CA1 field, all of which are involved in some aspect of olfactory processing,

including the encoding and recall of memories with an olfactory component. At least a few tangles were found in all of these brains beginning in the sixth decade, and the extent of these neurofibrillary tangles increased exponentially with aging [266]. Functional neuroimaging studies suggest that there is also a loss of function in brain regions involving olfaction that occurs with normal aging. In response to orthonasally presented food and nonfood odors, older adults showed significantly less activation in primary olfactory areas, that is, the piriform cortex, the amygdala, and the entorhinal cortex, than did young adults [267]. The same group did a functional neuroimaging study of connectivity between individual voxels of regions of interest during an olfactory task. They found that activation in the piriform cortex, insula, and right parahippocampal cortex and hippocampus was highly correlated with activation in the orbitofrontal cortex of young participants, whereas in older participants this correlation was not observed [268]. Corroborating these neuroimaging studies, a cross-sectional evoked potential study reported that both the N1/P2 early components of olfactory event-related potentials (reflecting sensory processing) and the later P3 component (reflecting attentional allocation and stimulus evaluation) [269] decreased in amplitude and increased in latency with aging. The magnitude of these changes in evoked potentials increased continuously from the second decade of life through the seventh [270].

3.3.5 Epidemiology of Olfactory Functions with Aging

Large population-based, self-report studies of olfactory function, like the National Geographic survey of 1.2 million free-living Americans [228] and the 1994 Disability Supplement to the National Health Interview Survey of 107,469 Americans [271], estimated the prevalence of chronic olfactory problems at 0.8% [228] and 1.42% [271], respectively. Prevalence increased with age up to 4.6% in those 75 years and older [271]. However, large population-based studies of measured olfactory function have found a higher prevalence of dysfunction. The Beaver Dam, Wisconsin, study of 2,400 people found the overall prevalence of odor identification impairment to be 24.5%. It increased to 62.5% in those 80–97 years old, and in this group, sensitivity of self-report was 12% for women and 18% for men [272]. A study to normalize the University of Pennsylvania Smell Identification Test (UPSIT), a multiple choice scratch-n-sniff test, involved 1,900 participants and included a sample of elderly participants from long-term care facilities [273]. These investigators found that over 50% of people 65–80 years old, and over 75% of those over 80, were significantly impaired at odor identification [273]. Unfortunately, these population-based studies did not discriminate those participants with dementia from the cognitively healthy elderly, and therefore a large-scale population study on olfactory loss due to healthy aging per se is not available.

3.3.6 Perceptual Changes with Aging

Smaller studies that have screened for dementia have found significant changes in olfactory perception during healthy aging. Odor thresholds, like taste thresholds, are elevated in older people compared with young people. However, unlike taste and auditory perception, which are most effected at low stimulus amplitudes, olfactory detection and recognition thresholds are elevated uniformly across concentrations, and the increases in threshold correspond to supra-threshold intensity ratings, at least for some odorants [274]. There is general agreement that odor detection and recognition thresholds increase with age, indicating decrements in sensitivity, that women tend to have lower odor thresholds than men, and that threshold increases vary from 2- to 9-fold depending on the experimental method used, the odorant used, and the particular group of participants, reflecting the increased variance that occurs with increasing age with all measures of olfactory function [11, 275–278]. Molecular differences between odorants also affect the variance in threshold increases with aging. For example, just as a taste compound with higher molecular weight has a higher taste detection threshold in the elderly [132], the molecular weight of odor volatiles correlates positively with olfactory detection thresholds in older participants [278, 279]. The effect of molecular weight may help to explain the finding that the enzymatic process in the olfactory mucosa that solubilizes odor volatiles for olfactory receptor binding declines with aging for some odorants but not for others [263]. Losing sensitivity to just a few odors can have serious consequences. Natural gas is odorless. Therefore, mercaptan is added so that gas leaks can be detected; however; 45% of older people, compared with 10% of younger people, are not able to detect the odor of the safety standard level of mercaptan [280]. And what if

it is a bulky pyrazine from a favorite flavor that is no longer detected by the older person [278]? In a test of retronasal odor detection, only 33% of middle-aged and 20% of elderly participants were able to detect marjoram flavor in a soup medium compared with 88% of the young participants [140].

In contrast to taste perception, odor detection thresholds are somewhat predictive of magnitude estimation intensity ratings of supra-threshold stimuli. These stimuli, which are above detection thresholds, are more relevant to everyday experience. Magnitude matching studies across the life span consistently show an aging-related decline of 5–10% in odor intensity estimation ratings across different supra-threshold concentrations. Not all odors are equally affected. Estimates vary from odor to odor, and both pleasant and unpleasant odors are affected [13, 274, 280–282]. Similar results were found when comparing supra-threshold retronasal olfactory magnitude estimates of intensity with estimates of sound intensity in young and old participants [283]. However, we found, in both a large study of more than 300 participants and four foods and a smaller study of 70 participants and 15 foods, that the overall orthonasal and retronasal intensity ratings of the older participants were not significantly different from those of the younger participants [284]. Potential reasons for not corroborating the small but significant declines in intensity ratings found in earlier studies include our larger sample size and the extensive cognitive evaluation of the older participants in the smaller study, establishing that the participants were high-functioning and free of incipient dementia. In these studies, we used the updated Global Sensory Intensity Scale, which involves magnitude matching but utilizes cross-modality matching and a 100-point scale with ratio properties [285].

Schiffman and Warwick measured odor discrimination, the ability to differentiate one odor from each of nine different odorants, among participants between 10 and 80 years of age. They found a significant drop in performance starting in the seventh decade [282]. A study of 3,282 participants in four age groups, ranging from 5 to >55 years, used an "odd man out" triangle test to test odor discrimination ability. The investigators found a small but significant difference between the 36- to 55-year-old group and the >55-year-old group [286]. Gender differences typically are not apparent in odor discrimination tasks. Older people have also been found to have greater difficulty discriminating odors retronasally [287, 288]. A study that used six odors at two concentrations, presented over 120 trials, asked participants aged 18–88 years to decide if odors presented two at a time were the same or different in quality regardless of intensity. Discrimination declined significantly between each age group from 0.95 in the young to 0.89 in the middle-aged and 0.78 in the elderly at the lower concentration [289]. Relatively minor decrements in discrimination could be associated with the finding that olfactory sensory neurons of young people are highly selective in response to odors, whereas the olfactory sensory neurons of older people lack that specificity and often respond to multiple odors [247]. Providing a list of the names of the odorants enhanced discrimination in all age groups, and discrimination ability correlated with measures of olfactory identification, including consistency of naming, whether correct or incorrect. Whereas aging-related decline in discrimination ability is fairly uniform across olfactory stimuli, the ability to identify odors varies among odor stimulants [289].

In studies that tested multiple olfactory functions within the same participant group, aging-related impairments were most marked for odor detection thresholds, followed by identification, discrimination, and intensity ratings using magnitude estimation, which were least affected [275, 286, 289]. There is a consensus that all of these olfactory functions, as with the anatomical integrity of the olfactory epithelium and the olfactory bulb, decline continuously across the entire life span, often starting before adulthood, and that the rate of decline is greater in males than females (odor discrimination excepted) [273, 276, 286, 289–291].

Aging-related impairment also occurs on higher-order olfactory tasks such as odor identification [273], odor recall memory, and odor recognition memory [292]. These tasks are more reliant on central nervous system functions. A large, longitudinal study found that poorer performance on odor identification predicts cognitive decline within five years in populations that show no evidence of cognitive impairment at baseline [293]. Again, there was high variability in the older groups. Whereas Stevens and Cain noted only a gradual decline with advancing age in threshold sensitivity and olfactory discrimination on their seven-odor identification test, they found no significant difference between young and middle-aged

participants but significantly worse performance in the oldest group [140, 275]. Retronasal odor identification, the ability to identify the flavor of a wide variety of blended foods, also significantly declined in old age [287, 294]. The normalization studies for the University of Pennsylvania Smell Identification Test (UPSIT) suggest that aging-related decline of odor identification begins in the sixth decade [273], although a more challenging test, involving 80 odors from their actual source and no cues, revealed a more continuous decline from the early 20s onward and raised the possibility of a ceiling effect constraining other odor identification studies [274, 291]. A study of 221 males and 166 females between 19 and 95 years of age that carefully separated healthy participants from those being treated for medical conditions or taking prescription medications found that older participants had lower scores on the UPSIT, higher rates of anosmia, and more chemosensory complaints than the young. However, they also found that those being treated for medical problems had scores only slightly lower than the healthy participants, suggesting that aging-related declines were mainly due to normal aging [295].

A longitudinal study of 481 healthy older persons measured odor identification and five domains of cognitive function every year for three years. At baseline, odor identification scores correlated with function in each cognitive domain. Perceptual speed and episodic memory function among those in the lowest 10th percentile for odor identification declined more than twice as rapidly as in those in the 90th percentile. Participants in the 10th percentile were significantly more likely to have developed mild cognitive impairment at the 5-year follow-up analysis. Semantic memory, working memory, and visuospatial ability did not correlate with odor identification ability [296]. In a follow-up to this investigation, postmortem studies were performed on 129 of the 166 participants who died. Scores on the odor identification task correlated with extent of AD pathology. A composite measure of amyloid plaques and neurofibrillary tangles in the entorhinal cortex, CA1 field of the hippocampus, and the subiculum accounted for > 12% of the variation in odor identification, controlling for dementia and semantic memory function. The density of tangles was inversely related to odor identification, and after controlling for tangles, a similar effect for amyloid burden was attenuated [297]. Imaging studies conducted in cognitively healthy older adults have found that UPSIT scores correlate with postcentral gyrus cortical thickness, volume of the right amygdala, and gray matter volume of the perirhinal and entorhinal cortices bilaterally, providing further support for the hypothesis that olfactory dysfunction is a preclinical indicator of neurodegeneration [298].

The UPSIT and its derivatives are multiple choice tests and provide no information as to why the person made the odor identification error. Possible error types include anosmia, when the odor is not detected; anomia, when the odor is detected and properly described but cannot be correctly named; and associative agnosia, a perceptual recognition deficit whereby the odor is detected and discriminated from others but is not accurately recognized and described. In an open-choice odor identification task of 15 real food items, younger participants (average age 25.8) were compared with older participants (average age 73.3) who underwent an extensive battery of cognitive tests to ensure that they were not cognitively impaired. The younger participants were significantly better than the older, cognitively healthy participants at identifying odors orthonasally and retronasally. The ability to identify an odor retronasally was generally better than the ability to do so orthonasally in both age groups [284]. The older and younger participants did not differ in their types of errors, the most common being anosmia and associative agnosia.

Olfactory memory impairments, observed in the elderly and to a greater extent in patients with neurodegenerative diseases such as AD, implicate portions of the Papez circuit and the hippocampal system in particular in smell memory. A study testing the memory of young and older participants for the faces of previous American presidents and vice presidents, engineering symbols they were shown, and everyday odors they smelled in a previous session, found that episodic olfactory memory was the most significantly affected by aging [299]. Studies measuring the local field potentials in the olfactory bulb, piriform cortex, entorhinal cortex, and the dentate gyrus of the hippocampus of rats [300] and guinea pigs [301] suggest a direct polysynaptic olfactory pathway to the dentate gyrus. They further demonstrate that patterned stimulation of the olfactory input that mimics sniffing patterns during odor discrimination induces a diffuse activation of both ipsi- and contralateral hippocampi, followed by the entorhinal cortices. The olfactory deficits that occur as a result of normal aging are amplified in patients with AD, who on average

perform below the 25th percentile for their age group [11]. Impairment in the recognition and identification of odorants [302] as well as the memory of odorants [303] is very prominent in the earliest phases of this disease.

3.3.7 The Effects of Retronasal Olfactory Function on Nutritional Status

Decreased gustatory ability, olfactory ability, or both may adversely affect diet and nutrition as a loss of flavor perception may result in an unhealthy decline in intake, increasing the risk of malnutrition in the elderly. Male weight under 63.9 kg (141 lb) or female weight under 51.8 kg (114 lb) is associated with an approximately two-fold increase in mortality in older adults [304]. In general, elderly people with dementia weigh less and have lower body mass indices (BMI) than those without, and common causes leading to both AD and weight loss are suspected [305, 306].

In fMRI studies, many of the brain areas associated with craving and that are components of the reward circuit are less active in elderly subjects during flavor perception tests [307, 308]. One behavioral study that assessed flavor perception in aging humans found that retronasal olfaction tends to decline more than orthonasal olfaction [309]. A synergism between taste impairment and a general decline in olfactory function could be one casual factor for the decline in food pleasure and intake often observed in the elderly. We examined orthonasal and retronasal olfaction using food items that varied in olfactory, taste, and trigeminal intensity to determine the effects of different sensory modalities on the loss of flavor perception. For this study we included 40 younger (18–39 years old) participants; 35 older, healthy participants (60–91 years old); 21 participants with AD; and 23 participants with PD. The objective was to determine if clinical taste impairment diminishes flavor perception and if there is a point at which a decline in olfaction combines with taste impairment to diminish flavor perception even further. The participants had a wide range of functional loss from different, individual areas of innervation of the cranial nerves mediating taste and oral somatosensation. They also varied significantly in their orthonasal and retronasal olfactory function. We found that all tested taste variables except for sweet intensity ratings on the FuP and CvP and all tested oral somatosensory variables were significantly lower in those who perceived less intense retronasal olfaction at any fixed intensity level of orthonasal olfaction. This finding was independent of age and disease status. Among the older, healthy participants, the 27 who were well nourished, when compared with four who were not (measured with the Mini-Nutritional Assessment, MNA) [310], had significantly higher orthonasal and retronasal olfactory identification scores, significantly higher Mini-Mental Statues Exam scores, and significantly higher salt intensity ratings on the CvP. In the AD and PD participant groups, we conducted binary logistic regression analyses and determined that the best predictor of being classified as nourished or as at-risk/malnourished by the MNA in either AD or PD was the percentage correct on the retronasal odor identification task. For the participants with AD, the intensity ratings from the fungiform papillae and the average intensity rating of oral somatosensation of the 15 tested foods also significantly contributed to nutritional status. Disease severity was an additional contributor to nutritional status in those with PD. None of the measures of orthonasal olfactory function had any predictive value for nutritional status [311].

3.3.8 Conclusions on the Effects of Aging on Olfactory Functions

An average loss of 1% per year in olfactory nerve fibers within the glomeruli begins in the first year of life and totals 73% in old age [234, 235]. Odor detection and recognition thresholds, odor discrimination, and, to some extent, odor identification also exhibit a gradual, monotonic decline in early adulthood that continues, with ever increasing variation, into old age. The spotty displacement of olfactory epithelium by respiratory epithelium, the breakdown of the enzymatic processes in the olfactory mucosa that solubilize some odorant molecules but not others, and the decline in afferent and local circuit synapses within the olfactory bulb help to explain the fact that some odors are affected more than others during normal aging. Central processes underlying olfactory function also deteriorate, as reflected in smaller amplitudes and longer latencies of olfactory event-related potentials. fMRI studies also reveal that engagement of olfactory structures of the central nervous system decreases, as reflected in decreased activity in primary and secondary olfactory cortices. Because retronasal olfaction reflects the combined central nervous system processing of olfactory, gustatory, and oral somatosensory input, it can be affected differently by aging than orthonasal olfaction. Retronasal olfaction is the most important function for the appreciation of flavor and maintenance of adequate nutrition.

4 Main Conclusions

Regions of the brain important for taste, smell, and their integration are commonly affected during healthy aging and even more so in the setting of neurodegenerative diseases [312, 313]. Anatomical, physiological, and psychophysical studies have revealed aging-related decline in the olfactory and gustatory systems. There is slowing of cell regeneration and atrophy and loss of connectivity of the primary structures. Detection thresholds are elevated while supra-threshold intensity measurements (magnitude estimation) show modest to no changes depending on tastant and odorant concentration. Identification is often the most impaired function. Variation of function is much higher with aging and self-assessment of impairment is not reliable. Another consensus view from decades of research is that aging takes a greater toll on olfaction than on taste [13]. However, as with taste loss, olfactory loss with aging is often a reflection of accrued environmental insults and disease. Therefore, the effects of pure aging are difficult to determine. While decrements in taste may intuitively seem to be the most influential on food preferences and dietary intake, quality of life in the realm of food enjoyment and nutritional intake derives largely from the ability to perceive flavor, which is substantially the product of retronasal olfaction.

References

1. Getchell TV, Doty RL, Bartoshuk LM, Snow JB, eds. *Smell and taste in health and disease.* New York: Raven Press; 1991.

2. Prescott J, Tepper BJ, eds. *Genetic variation in taste sensitivity.* New York: Marcel Dekker; 2004.

3. Hutchins HL, Healy NA, Duffy VB. PROP bitterness associates with dietary fat behaviors and risk for cardiovascular disease (CVD) in middle-aged women. *Chem Senses.* 2003; 28:551–63.

4. Duffy VB, Peterson JM, Bartoshuk LM. Associations between taste genetics, oral sensation and alcohol intake. *Physiol Behav.* 2004 Sep 15;82(2–3):435–45.

5. Basson MD, Bartoshuk LM, Dichello SZ, Panzini L, Weiffenbach JM, Duffy VB. Association between 6-n-propylthiouracil (PROP) bitterness and colonic neoplasms. *Dig Dis Sci.* 2005 Mar;50(3):483–9.

6. Bartoshuk LM, Duffy VB, Hayes JE, Moskowitz HR, Snyder DJ. Psychophysics of sweet and fat perception in obesity: problems, solutions and new perspectives. *Philos Trans R Soc Lond B Biol Sci.* 2006 Jul 29;361(1471):1137–48.

7. Wilson RS, Yu L, Bennet DA. Odor identification and mortality in old age. *Chem Senses.* 2011;36:63–7.

8. Pinto JM, Wroblewski KE, Kern DW, Schumm LP, McClintock MK. Olfactory dysfunction predicts 5-year mortality in older adults. *PLoS ONE.* 2014 Oct;9(9): e107541.

9. Devanand DP, Lee S, Manly J, Andrews H, Schupf N, Masurkar A, et al. Olfactory identification deficits and increased mortality in the community. *Ann Neurol.* 2015 Sep;78(3):401–11.

10. Schubert CR, Carmichael LL, Murphy C, Klein BEK, Klein R, Cruickshanks KJ. Olfaction and the 5-year incidence of cognitive impairment in an epidemiological study of older adults. *J Am Geriatr Soc.* 2008 Aug;56(8):1517–21.

11. Schiffman SS, Gatlin CA. Clinical physiology of taste and smell. *Annu Rev Nutr.* 1993;13:405–36.

12. Bartoshuk LM, Catalanotto F, Hoffman H, Logan H, Snyder DJ. Taste damage (otitis media, tonsillectomy and head and neck cancer), oral sensations, and BMI. *Phys Behav.* 2012 Jul;107:516–26.

13. Stevens JC, Bartoshuk LM, Cain WS. Chemical senses and aging: taste versus smell. *Chem Senses.* 1984;9:167–79.

14. Snyder DJ, Clark CJ, Catalanotto FA, Mayo V, Bartoshuk LM. Oral anesthesia specifically impairs retronasal olfaction. *Chem Senses.* 2007 Apr;32:A15

15. Schiffman S, Pasternak M. Decreased discrimination of food odors in the elderly. *J Gerontol.* 1979 Jan;34(1):73–9.

16. Fechner GT. *Elemente der psychophysik 1860.* Translation: Rand B, ed. Leipzig: Breitkopf and Härtel; 1912.

17. Simon SA, de Araujo IE, Gutierrez R, Nicolelis MAL. The neural mechanisms of gustation: a distributed processing code. *Nat Rev Neurosci.* 2006 Nov;7:890–901.

18. Pritchard TC, Norgren R. Gustatory system. In: Paxinos G, Mai JK, eds. *The human nervous system.* 2nd ed. Amsterdam: Elsevier; 2004, pp. 1171–96.

19. Perl E. Function of dorsal root ganglion neurons: an overview. In: Scott SA, ed. *Sensory neurons: diversity, development, and plasticity.* New York: Oxford University Press; 1992, pp. 3–23.

20. Iwasaki S. Evolution of the structure and function of the vertebrate tongue. *J Anat.* 2002 Jul;201(1):1–13.

21. Julius D, Basbaum AI. Molecular mechanisms of nociception. *Nature.* 2001;413:203–10.

22. Clapham DE. TRP channels as cellular sensors. *Nature.* 2003;426:517–24.

23. Herness S. The neurobiology of gustation. In: Johnson LR, Kaunitz JD, Said HM, Merchant JL, Ghishan FK, Wood JD, eds. *Physiology of the gastrointestinal tract.* 5th ed. New York: Academic Press; 2012, pp. 741–67.

24. Hollingworth HL, Poffenberger AT Jr. *The sense of taste.* New York: Moffat, Yard; 1917.

25. Smith DV, Margolskee RF. Making sense of taste. *Scientific American.* 2001 Mar:32–9.

26. Chaudhari N, Roper SD. The cell biology of taste. *J Cell Biol.* 2010 Aug;190(3):285–96.

27. Roper SD, Chaudhari N. Taste buds: cells, signals and synapses. *Nat Rev Neurosci.* 2017 Aug;18 (8):485–97.

28. Pritchard TC, Hamilton RB, Morse JR, Norgren R. Projections of thalamic gustatory and lingual areas in the monkey, Macaca fascicularis. *J Comp Neurol.* 1986 Feb;244(2):213–28.

29. Scott TR, Plata-Salaman CR. Taste in the monkey cortex. *Physiol Behav.* 1999;67:489–511.

30. Hadley K, Orlandi RR, Fong KJ. Basic anatomy and physiology of olfaction and taste. *Otolaryngol Clin North Am.* 2004 Dec;37 (6):1115–26.

31. Zaidi FN, Todd K, Enquist L, Whitehead MC. Types of taste circuits synaptically linked to a few geniculate ganglion neurons. *J Comp Neurol.* 2008 Dec;511 (6):753–72.

32. Rolls ET, Bayliss LL. Gustatory, olfactory, and visual convergence within the primate orbitofrontal cortex. *J Neurosci.* 1994;14:5437–52.

33. Haines DE. *Neuroanatomy: An atlas of structures, sections, and systems.* 7th ed. Philadelphia: Lippincott Williams & Wilkins, Wolters Kluwer; 2008.

34. Kadohisa M, Rolls ET, Verhagen JV. Orbitofrontal cortex: neuronal representation of oral temperature and capsaicin in addition to taste and texture. *Neuroscience.* 2004;127:207–21.

35. Bartoshuk LM, Rennert K, Rodin J, Stevens JC. Effects of temperature on the perceived sweetness of sucrose. *Physiol Behav.* 1982 May;28(5):905–10.

36. Talavera K, Yasumatsu K, Voets T, Droogmans G, Shigemura N, Ninomiya Y, et al. Heat activation of TRPM5 underlies thermal sensitivity of sweet taste. *Nature.* 2005;438:1022–5.

37. Perez CA, Margolskee RF, Kinnamon SC, Ogura T. Making sense with TRP channels: store-operated calcium entry and the ion channel Trpm5 in taste receptor cells. *Cell Calcium.* 2003;33:541–9.

38. Blakeslee AF, Fox AL. Our different taste worlds. *J Heredity.* 1932;23:97–107.

39. Kim UK, Jorgenson E, Coon H, Leppert M, Risch N, Drayna D. Positional cloning of the human quantitative trait locus underlying taste sensitivity to phenylthiocarbamide. *Science.* 2003;299:1221–5.

40. Bartoshuk LM, Duffy VB, Miller IJ. PTC/PROP tasting: anatomy, psychophysics, and sex effects. *Physiol Behav.* 1994;56:1165–71.

41. Miller IJ Jr, Reedy FE Jr. Quantification of fungiform papillae and taste pores in living human subjects. *Chem Senses.* 1990;15:281–94.

42. Smith DV. Taste intensity as a function of area and concentration: differentiation between compounds. *J Exp Psychol* 1971;87:163–71.

43. Miller IJ Jr, Reedy FE Jr. Variations in human taste bud density and taste intensity perception. *Physiol Behav.* 1990;47:1213–19.

44. Prutkin JM, Duffy VB, Etter L, Fast K, Gardner E, Lucchina LA, et al. Genetic variation and inferences about perceived taste intensity in mice and men. *Physiol Behav.* 2000;261 (1):161–73.

45. Just T, Wilhelm Pau H, Witt M, Hummel T. Contact endoscopic comparison of morphology of human fungiform papillae of healthy subjects and patients with transected chorda tympani nerve. *Laryngoscope.* 2006 Jul;116:1216–22.

46. Prescott J, Swain-Campbell N. Responses to repeated oral irritation by capsaicin, cinnamaldehyde, and ethanol in PROP tasters and nontasters. *Chem Senses* 2000;25:239–46.

47. Duffy VB, Lucchina LA, Bartoshuk LM. Genetic variation in taste: potential biomarker for cardiovascular disease risk? In: Prescott J, Tepper B, eds. *Genetic variation in taste sensitivity.* New York: Marcel Dekker; 2003, pp. 197–229.

48. Tepper B, Nurse B. Fat perception is related to PROP taster status. *Physiol Behav.* 1997;61(6):949–54.

49. Bartoshuk LM, Catalanotto F, Hoffman H, Logan H, Snyder DJ. Taste damage (otitis media, tonsillectomy and head and neck cancer), oral sensations and BMI. *Physiol Behav.* 2012 Nov;107 (4):516–26.

50. Sipiora ML, Murtaugh MA, Gregoire MB, Duffy VB. Bitter taste perception and severe vomiting during pregnancy. *Physiol Behav.* 2000;69:259–67.

51. Duffy VB, Fast K, Lucchina LA, Bartoshuk LM. Oral sensation and cancer. In: Berger AM, Portenoy RK, Weissman D, eds. *Principles and practice of palliative care and supportive oncology.* 2nd ed. Philadelphia: Lippincott Williams & Wilkins; 2002, pp. 178–93.

52. Bartoshuk LM, Snyder DJ, Grushka M, Berger AM, Duffy VB, Kveton JF. Taste damage: previously unsuspected consequences. *Chem Senses.* 2005;30(Suppl 1):i218–i219.

53. Logan HL, Bartoshuk LM, Fillingim RM, Tomar ST, Mendenhall W. Metallic taste phantoms predicts oral pain among 5-year survivors of head and neck cancer. *Pain* 2008;140:323–31.

54. Bartoshuk LM, Kveton J, Yanagisawa K, Catalanotto F. Taste loss and taste phantoms: A role of inhibition in taste. In: Kurihara K, Suzuki N, Ogawa H, eds. *Olfaction and taste XI.* New York: Springer-Verlag; 1994, pp. 557–60.

55. Goins MR, Pitovski DZ. Posttonsillectomy taste distortion: a significant complication. *Laryngoscope.* 2009;114:1206–21.

56. Pavlidis P, Gouveris C, Kekes G, Maurer J. Changes in electrogustometry thresholds, tongue tip vascularization, density and form of the fungiform papillae in smokers. *Eur Arch Otorhinolaryngol.* 2014 Aug;271 (8):2325–31.

57. Millar EP, Troulis MJ. Herpes zoster of the trigeminal nerve: the dentists' role in diagnosis and treatment. *Canadian Dental J.* 1994;60:450–3.

58. Beidler LM, Smallman RL. Renewal of cells within taste buds. *J Cell Biol.* 1965 Nov;27 (2):263–72.

59. Barlow LA, Klein OD. Developing and regenerating a sense of taste. *Curr Topics Dev Biol.* 2015;111:401–19.

60. Feng P, Huang L, Wang H. Taste bud homeostasis in health, disease, and aging. *Chem Senses* 2014;29:3–16.

61. Takeda N, Jain R, Li D, Li L, Lu MM, Epstein JA. Lgr5 identifies progenitor cells capable of taste bud regeneration after injury. *PLoS One.* 2013;8:e66314.

62. Yee KK, Li Y, Redding KM, Iwatsuki K, Margolskee RF, Jiang P. Lgr5-EGFP marks taste bud stem/progenitor cells in posterior tongue. *Stem Cells.* 2013;31:992–1000.

63. Narukawa M, Kurokawa A, Kohta R, Misaka T. Participation of the peripheral taste system in aging-dependent changes in taste sensitivity. *Neuroscience.* 2017;358:249–60.

64. Arey LB, Tremaine MJ, Monzingo FL. The numerical and topographical relations of taste buds to human circumvallate papillae throughout the life span. *Anat Rec.* 1935;64:9–25.

65. Mochizuki Y. An observation of the numerical and topographical relation of taste buds to circumvallate papillae of Japanese. *Okajimas Folia Anat Jpn.* 1937;15:595–608.

66. Arvidson K. Location and variation in number of taste buds in human fungiform papillae. *Eur J Oral Sci.* 1979 Dec;87 (6):435–42.

67. Pavlidis P, Gouveris H, Anogeianaki A, Koutsonikolas D, Anogianakis G, Kekes G. Age-

85

related changes in electrogustometry thresholds, tongue tip vascularization, density, and form of the fungiform papillae in humans. *Chem Senses.* 2013;38:35–43.

68. Stamps JJ, Mayo V, Snyder D, Bartoshuk LM. Taste changes during healthy aging. Manuscript in preparation.

69. Negoro A, Umemoto M, Fukazawa K, Terada T, Sakagami M. Observation of tongue papillae by video microscopy and contact endoscopy to investigate their correlation with taste function. *Auris Nasus Larynx.* 2004;31:255–9.

70. Winkler S, Garg AK, Mekayarajjananonth T, Bakaeen LG, Khan E. Depressed taste and smell in geriatric patients. *J Amer Dental Assoc.* 1999;130:1759–65.

71. Murer MG, Yan Q, Raisman-Vozari R. Brain-derived neurotrophic factor in the control human brain, and in Alzheimer's disease and Parkinson's disease. *Prog Neurobiol.* 2001 Jan;63 (1):71–124.

72. Lommatzsch M, Zingler D, Schuhbaeck D, Schloetcke K, Zingler C, Schuff-Werner P, et al. The impact of age, weight, and gender on BDNF levels in human platelets and plasma. *Neurobiol Aging.* 2005;26:115–23.

73. Ziegenhorn AA, Schulte-Herbrüggen O, Danker-Hopfe H, Malbranc M, Hartung HD, Anders D, et al. Serum neurotrophins – a study on the time course and influencing factors in a large old age sample. *Neurobiol Aging.* 2007;28:1436–45.

74. Erickson KI, Kim JS, Suever BL, Voss MW, Francis BM, Kramer AF. Genetic contributions to age-related decline in executive function: a 10-year longitudinal study of COMT and BDNF polymorphisms. *Front Hum Neurosci.* 2008;2:11.

75. Golden E, Emiliano A, Maudsley S, Windham BG, Carlson OD, Egan JM, et al. Circulating brain-derived neurotrophic factor and indices of metabolic and cardiovascular health: data from the Baltimore Longitudinal Study of Aging. *PLoS ONE.* 2010 Apr;5 (4):e10099.

76. Zhang C, Brandemihl A, Lau D, Lawton A, Oakley B. BDNF is required for the normal development of taste neurons *in vivo. NeuroReport.* 1997 Mar;8 (4):1013–17.

77. Gardiner J, Barton D, Vanslambrouck JM, Braet F, Hall D, Marc J, et al. Defects in tongue papillae and taste sensation indicate a problem with neurotrophic support in various neurological diseases. *Neuroscientist.* 2008 Jun;14 (3):240–50.

78. Sun C, Krimm R, Hill DL. Maintenance of mouse gustatory terminal field organization is dependent on BDNF at adulthood. *J Neurosci.* 2018 Jun; 0.1523/JNEUROSCI.0802-18.2018.

79. Bergman E, Ulfhake B, Fundin BT. Regulation of NGF-family ligands and receptors in adulthood and senescence: correlation to degenerative and regenerative changes in cutaneous innervation. *Eur J Neurosci.* 2000 May;12:2694–706.

80. Stucky CL, Shin J-B, Lewin GR. Neurotrophin-4: a survival factor for adult sensory neurons. *Current Biol.* 2002 Aug;12:1401–4.

81. Nosrat IV, Agerman K, Marinescu A, Ernfors P, Nosrat CA. Lingual deficits in neurotrophin double knockout mice. *J Neurocytol.* 2004;33:607–15.

82. Ito A, Nosrat C. Gustatory papillae and taste bud development and maintenance in the absence of TrkB ligands BDNF and NT-4. *Cell Tissue Res.* 2009 Jul;337:349–59.

83. Cotman CW, Berchtold NC, Christie LA. Exercise builds brain health: key roles of growth factor cascades and inflammation. *Trends Neurosci.* 2007;30:464–72.

84. Stewart-Knox BJ, Simpson EEA, Parr H, Rae G, Polito A, Intorre F. Zinc status and taste acuity in older Europeans: the ZENITH study. *Eur J Clin Nutr.* 2005;59: S31–S36.

85. Stewart-Knox B J, Simpson EEA, Parr H, Rae G, Polito A, Intorre F, et al. Taste acuity in response to zinc supplementation in older adults. *Brit J Nutr.* 2008;99:129–36.

86. Watanabe M, Asatsuma M, Ikui A, Ikeda M, Yamada Y, Nomura S, et al. Measurements of several metallic elements and matrix metalloproteinases (MMPs) in saliva from patients with taste disorders. *Chem Senses.* 2005;30:121–5.

87. Ikeda M, Ikui A, Komiyama A, Kobayashi D, Tanaka M. Causative factors of taste disorders in the elderly, and therapeutic effects of zinc. *J Laryngol Otol.* 2008;122:155–60.

88. Bradley RM, Beidler LM. Saliva: its role in taste function. In: Doty RL, ed. *The handbook of olfaction and gustation.* 2nd ed. New York: Marcel Dekker; 2003, pp. 639–50.

89. Ferry M. Strategies for ensuring good hydration in the elderly. *Nutr Rev.* 2005 Jun;63(6 Pt 2): S22–S29.

90. Fortes MB, Owen JA, Raymond-Barker P, Bishop C, Elghenzai S, Oliver SJ, et al. Is this elderly patient dehydrated? Diagnostic accuracy of hydration assessment using physical signs, urine, and saliva markers. *J Am Med Dir Assoc.* 2015 Mar;16(3):221–8.

91. Affoo RH, Foley N, Garrick R, Siqueira WL, Martin RE. Meta-analysis of salivary flow rates in young and older adults. *J Am Geriatr Soc.* 2015;63:2142–215.

92. Yeh CK, Johnson DA, Dodds MW. Impact of aging on human salivary gland function: a community-based study. *Aging Clin Exp Res.* 1998;10:421–8.

93. Singh ML, Papas A. Oral implications of polypharmacy in the elderly. *Dent Clin N Am.* 2014;58:783–96.

94. Ship JA, Pillemer SR, Baum BJ. Xerostomia and the geriatric patient. *J Am Geriatr Soc.* 2002;50:535–43.

95. Turner MD, Ship JA. Dry mouth and its effects on the oral health of elderly people. *J Am Dent Assoc.* 2007 Sept;138(1):S15–S20.

96. Becks H, Wainwright WW. Human saliva. XL. The effect of activation on salivary calcium and phosphate. *J Dental Res.* 1941;20:637–48.

97. Becks H. Human saliva. XIV. Total calcium content of resting saliva of 650 healthy individuals. *J Dental Res.* 1943;22:397–402.

98. Grad B. Diurnal age, and sex changes in the sodium and potassium concentrations of human saliva. *J Gerontol.* 1954;9:276–86.

99. Hong SR, Jung SE, Lee EH, Shin KJ, Yang WI, Lee HY. DNA methylation-based age prediction from saliva: high age predictability by combination of 7 CpG markers. *Forensic Sci Int Genet.* 2017 Jul;29:118–25.

100. Wang Z, Wang Y, Liu H, Che Y, Xu Y, E L. Age-related variations of protein carbonyls in human saliva and plasma: is saliva protein carbonyls an alternative biomarker of aging? *Age (Dordr).* 2015 Jun;37(3):9781.

101. Tandon S, Simon SA, Nicolelis MAL. Appetitive changes during salt deprivation are paralleled by widespread neuronal adaptations in nucleus accumbens, lateral hypothalamus, and central amygdala. *J Neurophysiol.* 2012;108(4):1089–105.

102. Iannilli E, Broy F, Kunz S, Hummel T. Age-related changes of gustatory function depend on alteration of neuronal circuits. *J Neurosci Res.* 2017 Oct;95(10):1927–36.

103. Hoogeveen HR, Dalenberg JR, Renken RJ, ter Horst GJ, Lorist MM. Neural processing of basic tastes in healthy young and older adults – an fMRI study. *NeuroImage.* 2015;119:1–12.

104. Green E, Jacobson A, Haase L, Murphy C. Can age-related CNS taste differences be detected as early as middle age? Evidence from fMRI. *Neuroscience.* 2013;232:194–203.

105. Jacobson A, Green E, Haase L, Szajer J, Murphy C. Age-related changes in gustatory, homeostatic, reward, and memory processing of sweet taste in the metabolic syndrome: an fMRI study. *Perception.* 2017 Mar–Apr;46(3–4):283–306.

106. Vennemann MM, Hummel T, Berger K. The association between smoking and smell and taste impairment in the general population. *J Neurol.* 2008 Aug;255(8):1121–6.

107. Welge-Lüssen A, Patrick Dörig P, Wolfensberger M, Krone F, Hummel T. A study about the frequency of taste disorders. *J Neurol.* 2011 Oct;258:386–92.

108. Boesveldt S, Tessler Lindau S, McClintock MK, Hummel T, Lundström JN. Gustatory and olfactory dysfunction in older adults: a national probability study. *Rhinol.* 2011 Aug;49(3):324–30.

109. Correia C, Lopez KJ, Wroblewski, KE, Huisingh-Scheetz M, Kern DW, Chen RC, et al. Global sensory impairment among older adults in the United States. *J Am Geriatr Soc.* 2016 Feb;64(2):306–13.

110. Pribitkin E, Rosenthal M, Cowart BJ. Prevalence and causes of severe taste loss in a chemosensory clinic population. *Ann Otol Rhinol Laryngol.* 2003;112:971–8.

111. Deems DA, Doty RL, Settle G, Moore-Gillon V, Shaman P, Mester AF, Kimmelmann CP, Brightman VJ, Snow JBJ. Smell and taste disorders, a study of 750 patients from the University of Pennsylvania smell and taste center. *Arch Otolaryngol Head Neck Surg.* 1991;117:519–28.

112. Yoshinaka M, Ikebe K, Uota M, Ogawa T, Okada T, Inomata C, et al. Age and sex differences in the taste sensitivity of young adult, young-old and old-old Japanese. *Geriatr Gerontol Int.* 2016;16:1281–8.

113. Doty RL, Chen JH, Overend J. Taste quality confusions: influences of age, smoking, PTC taster status, and other subject characteristics. *Perception.* 2017;46(3–4):257–67.

114. Uota M, Ogawa T, Ikebe K, Arai Y, Kamide K, Gondo Y, et al. Factors related to taste sensitivity in elderly: cross-sectional findings from SONIC study. *J Oral Rehab.* 2016;43:943–52.

115. Ogawa T, Uota M, Ikebe K, Arai Y, Kamide K, Gondo Y, et al. Longitudinal study of factors affecting taste sense decline in old-old individuals. *J Oral Rehab* 2017;44:22–9.

116. Bartoshuk LM, Duffy VB, Green BG, Hoffman HJ, Ko CW, Lucchina LA, et al. Valid across-group comparisons with labeled scales: the gLMS versus magnitude matching. *Physiol Behav.* 2004;82(1):109–14.

117. Fischer ME, Cruickshanks KJ, Schubert CR, Pinto A, Klein BEK, Klein R, et al. Taste intensity in the Beaver Dam Offspring Study. *Laryngoscope.* 2013 Jun;123(6):1399–404.

118. Krarup B. A method for clinical taste examinations. *Acta Oto-Laryngol.* 1958;49:294–305.

119. Bull TR. Taste and chorda tympani. *J Laryngol Otology.* 1965;79:479–93.

120. Miyoshi Y, Kimura T, Nakane H. Studies on the clinical gustatory examination: modified Krarup's method. *J Otolaryng.* 1968;71:139–40.

121. Hughs G. Changes in taste sensitivity with advancing age. *Gerontol Clin.* 1969;11:224–30.

122. Coats AC. Effects of age, sex, and smoking on electrical taste threshold. *Ann Otol.* 1974;83:365–9.

123. Nilsson B. Taste acuity of the human palate. Studies with electrogustometry on subjects in different age groups. *Acta Odontol Scand.* 1979;37:217–34.

124. Di Lorenzo PM, Chen JY, Rosen AM, Roussin AT. Tastant. In: Binder MD, Hirokawa N, Windhorst U, eds. *Encyclopedia of neuroscience.* Berlin: Springer; 2009.

125. Pfaffmann C, Bartoshuk LM, McBurney DH. Taste psychophysics. In: Beidler LM, ed. *Taste. Handbook of sensory physiology (Chemical Senses · Part 2),* vol. 4/2. Berlin: Springer; 1971.

126. Cooper RM, Bilash I, Zubek JP. The effect of age on taste sensitivity. *J Gerontol.* 1959;14:56–8.

127. Hermel J, Schönwetter SV, Samueloff S. Taste sensation and age in man. *J Oral Med.* 1970;25:39–42.

128. Finkentscher R, Rosenburg B, Spinar H, Bruchmuller B. Loss of taste in the elderly: sex differences. *Clin Otolaryngology.* 1977;2:183–9.

129. Bartoshuk LM. The psychophysics of taste. *Am J Clin Nutr.* 1978 Jun;31(6):1068–77.

130. Murphy C. The effects of age on taste sensitivity. In: Han SS, Coons DH, eds. *Special senses in aging.* Ann Arbor, MI: University of Ann Arbor, Institute of Gerontology; 1979, pp. 21–33.

131. Weiffenbach JM, Baum BJ, Burghauser R. Taste thresholds: quality specific variation with human aging. *J Gerontol* 1982;37:372–7.

132. Bartoshuk LM, Rifkin B, Marks LE, Bars P. Taste and aging. *J Gerontol.* 1986;41:51–7.

133. Mojet J, Christ-Hazelhof E, Heidema J. Taste perception with age: generic or specific losses in threshold sensitivity to the five basic tastes? *Chem Senses.* 2001;26:845–60.

134. Hyde RJ, Feller RP. Age and sex effects on taste of sucrose, NaCl, citric acid and caffeine. *Neurobiol Aging.* 1981 Winter;2(4):315–18.

135. Cowart BJ. Relationships between taste and smell across the adult life span. *Ann NY Acad Sci.* 1989;561:39–55.

136. Schiffman SS, Gatlin LA, Frey AE, Heiman SA, Stagner WC, Cooper DC. Taste perception of bitter compounds in young and elderly persons: relation to lipophilicity of bitter compounds. *Neurobiol Aging.* 1994 Nov;15(6):743–50.

137. Stevens JC, Cain WS, Demarque A, Ruthruff AM. On the discrimination of missing ingredients: aging and salt flavor. *Appetite.* 1991;16:129–40.

138. Moscowitz HR. Magnitude estimation: notes on what, how, when, and why to use it. *J Food Qual.* 1977 Dec;3:195–227.

139. Stevens SS. To honor Fechner and repeal his law. *Science.* 1961;133:80–6.

140. Stevens JC, Plantinga A, Cain WS. Reduction of odor and nasal pungency associated with aging. *Neurobiol Aging.* 1982;3:125–32.

141. Stevens JC, Cain WS. Changes in taste and flavor in aging. *Crit Rev Food Sci Nutr.* 1993;33(1):27–37.

142. Reed DR, Bartoshuk LM, Duffy V, Marino S, Price RA. Propylthiouracil tasting: determination of underlying threshold distributions using maximum likelihood. *Chem Senses.* 1995;20:529–33.

143. Hall MJ, Bartoshuk LM, Cain WS, Stevens JC. PTC taste blindness and the taste of caffeine. *Nature.* 1975 Feb;253(5491):442–3.

144. Stevens JC. Cross-modality validation of subjective scales for loudness, vibration, and electric shock. *J Exper Psychol.* 1959;57:201–9.

145. Luce RD, Steingrimsson R, Narens L. Are psychophysical scales of intensities the same or different when stimuli vary on other dimensions? Theory with experiments varying loudness and pitch. *Psychol Rev.* 2010;117(4):1247–58.

146. Stevens JC, Marks LE. Cross-modality matching functions generated by magnitude estimation. *Percept Psychophys.* 1980;27:379–89.

147. Bartoshuk LM, Duffy VB, Fast K, Green BG, Prutkin JM, Snyder DJ. Labeled scales (e.g., category, Likert, VAS) and invalid across-group comparisons. What we have learned from genetic variation in taste. *Food Qual Pref.* 2002;14:125–38.

148. Weiffenbach JM, Cowart BJ, Baum BJ. Taste intensity perception in aging. *J Gerontol.* 1986 Jul;41(4):460–8.

149. Chauhan J, Hawrysh ZJ. Suprathreshold sour taste intensity and pleasantness perception with age. *Physiol Behav.* 1988;43:601–7.

150. Bartoshuk LM. Taste: robust across the age span? *Ann NY Acad Sci.* 1989;561:65–76.

151. Murphy C, Gilmore MM. Quality specific effects of aging on the human taste system. *Percept Psychophys.* 1989;45:121–8.

152. Warwick ZS, Schiffman SS. Sensory evaluations of fat–sucrose

and fat–salt mixtures; relationship to age and weight status. *Physiol Behav.* 1990;48:633–6.

153. Weiffenbach JM, Tylenda CA, Baum JB. Oral sensory changes in aging. *J Gerontol.* 1990;45:121–5.

154. Enns MP, Hornung DE. Comparisons of the estimates of smell, taste and overall intensity in young and elderly people. *Chem Senses.* 1988;13(1):131–9.

155. Mojet J, Heidema J, Christ-Hazelhof E. Taste perception with age: genetic or specific losses in supra-threshold intensities of five taste qualities. *Chem Senses* 2003:28:397–413.

156. Renehan WE, Jin Z, Zhang X, Schweitzer L. Structure and function of gustatory neurons in the nucleus of the solitary tract: II. Relationships between neuronal morphology and physiology. *J Comp Neurol.* 1996;367:205–21.

157. Drewnowski A, Henderson SA, Driscoll A, Rolls BJ. Salt taste perceptions and preferences are unrelated to sodium consumption in healthy older adults. *J Am Diet Assoc.* 1996;96:471–4.

158. Pangborn RM, Braddock KS, Stone LJ. Ad libitum mixing to preference versus hedonic scaling: salts in broth and sucrose in lemonade. Presented at the Association for Chemoreception Sciences (AChems), Sarasota, FL; April 1983.

159. Zallen E, Hooks LB, O'Brien K. Salt taste preferences and perceptions of elderly and young adults. *J Am Diet Assoc.* 1990;90:947–50.

160. Little AC, Brinner L. Taste responses to saltiness of experimentally prepared tomato juice samples. *J Am Diet Assoc.* 1984;21:1022–7.

161. Chauhan J. Pleasantness perception of salt in young vs elderly adults. *J Am Diet Assoc.* 1989;89:834–5.

162. Duffy VB, Backstrand JR, Ferris AM. Olfactory dysfunction and related nutritional risk in free-living, elderly women. *J Am Diet Assoc.* 1995 Aug;95(8):879–84; quiz 885–6.

163. MacCarthy-Leventhal E. Post radiation mouth blindness. *Lancet.* 1959;19:1138–9.

164. Miller IJ, Bartoshuk LM. Taste perception, taste bud distribution, and spatial relationships. In: Getchell TV, Doty RL, Bartoshuk LM, Snow JB, eds. *Smell and taste in health and disease.* New York: Raven Press; 1991, pp. 205–33.

165. May M, Schaitkin BM. *The Facial Nerve.* 2nd ed. New York: Thieme; 2000.

166. Halpern BP, Nelson LM. Bulbar gustatory responses to anterior and to posterior tongue stimulation in the rat. *Am J Physiol.* 1965;209:105–10.

167. Todrank J, Bartoshuk LM. A taste illusion: taste sensation localized by touch. *Physiol Behav.* 1991;50:1027–31.

168. Bartoshuk LM, Desnoyers S, O'Brien M, Gent JF, Catalanotto FC. Taste stimulation of localized tongue areas: the Q-tip test. *Chem Senses.* 1985;10(3):453.

169. Weiffenbach JM, Duffy VB, Fast K, Cohen ZD, Bartoshuk LM. Bitter-sweet age, sex and PROP (6-n-propylthiouracil) effects: a role for menopause? *Chem Senses* 2000;25:639.

170. Calhoun KH, Gibson B, Hartley L, Minton J, Hokanson JA. Age-related changes in oral sensation. *Laryngoscope.* 1992 Feb;102 (2):109–16.

171. Fukunaga A, Uematsu H, Sugimoto K. Influences of aging on taste perception and oral somatic sensation. *J Gerontol.* 2005;60A(1):109–13.

172. Stevens JC, Cain WS. Aging and the perception of nasal irritation. *Physiol Behav.* 1986;37(2):323–8.

173. Wysocki CJ, Cowart BJ, Radil T. Nasal trigeminal chemosensitivity across the adult life span. *Percept Psychophys.* 2003 Jan;65 (1):115–22.

174. Laska M. Perception of trigeminal chemosensory qualities in the elderly. *Chem Senses.* 2001;26:681–9.

175. Hummel T, Barz S, Pauli E, Kobal G. Chemosensory event-related potentials change with age. *EEG Clin Neurophysiol.* 1998;108:208–17.

176. Silver WL. The common chemical sense. In: Finger TE, Silver WL, eds. *The neurobiology of taste and smell.* New York: John Wiley; 1987, pp. 65–87.

177. Bartoshuk LM, Snyder DJ. The affect of taste and olfaction: the key to survival. In: Barret LF, Lewis MA, Haviland-Jones JM, eds. *Handbook of emotions.* 4th ed. New York: Guilford Press; 2016, pp. 235–52.

178. Bushdid C, Magnasco MO, Vosshall LB, Keller A. Humans can discriminate more than 1 trillion olfactory stimuli. *Science.* 2014;343:1370–72.

179. Zhao H, Ivic L, Otaki JM, Hashimoto M, Micoshiba K, Firestein S. Functional expression of a mammalian odorant receptor. *Science* 1998;279:237–42.

180. Singer MS. Analysis of the molecular basis for octanal interactions in the expressed rat I7 olfactory receptor. *Chemical Senses* 2000;25:155–65.

181. Buck LB, Axel R. A novel multigene family may encode odorant receptors: a molecular basis for odor recognition. *Cell.* 1991;65:175–87.

182. Nimura Y, Nei M. Evolution of olfactory receptor genes in the human genome. *PNAS.* 2003 Oct:100(21):12235–40.

183. Bozza T, Feinstein P, Zheng C, Mombaerts P. Odorant receptor

expression defines functional units in the mouse olfactory system. *J Neurosci.* 2002;22:3033–43.

184. Maresh A, Rodriguez Gil D, Whitman MC, Greer CA. Principles of glomerular organization in the human olfactory bulb – implications for odor processing. *PLoS ONE.* 2008;3:e2640.

185. Shepherd GM, Chen WR, Willhite DC, Migliore M, Greer CA. The olfactory granule cell: from classical enigma to central role in olfactory processing. *Brain Research Rev* 2007;55:373–82.

186. Willhite DC, Nguyen KT, Masurkar AV, Greer CA, Shepherd GM, Chen WR. Viral tracing identifies distributed columnar organization in the olfactory bulb. *PNAS* 2006;103:12592–7.

187. Migliore M, Shepherd GM. Dendritic action potentials connect distributed dendrodendritic microcircuits. *J Comp Neurosci.* 2008;24:207–21.

188. Stewart WB, Kauer JS, Shepherd GM. Functional organization of the rat olfactory bulb analyzed by the 2-deoxyglucose method. *J Comp Neurol.* 1975;185:715–34.

189. Matsumoto H, Kobayakawa K, Kobayakawaa R, Tashiro T, Sakano H, Mori K. Spatial arrangement of glomerular molecular-feature clusters in the odorant-receptor class domains of the mouse olfactory bulb. *J Neurophysiol.* 2010;103:3490–500.

190. Shepherd GM. Outline of a theory of olfactory processing and its relevance to humans. *Chem Senses.* 2005;30(Suppl 1):i3–i5.

191. Stamps JJ, Yamurlu K, Deng JV, Shaw G. Uniquely human primary olfactory connection to the nucleus accumbens via the medial olfactory tract. In submission.

192. Carmichael ST, Clugnet MC, Price JL. Central olfactory connections in the macaque monkey. *J Comp Neurol.* 1994;346:403–34.

193. Turner BN, Gupta KC, Mishkin M. The locus and cytoarchitecture of the projection areas of the olfactory bulb in *Macaca mulatta*. *J Comp Neurol* 1978 Feb;177 (3):381–96.

194. Carmichael ST, Price JL. Limbic connections of the orbital and medial prefrontal cortex in macaque monkeys. *J Comp Neurol.* 1995;363:615–41.

195. Öngür D, Ferry AT, Price JL. Architectonic subdivision of human orbital and medial prefrontal cortex. *J Comp Neurol.* 2003;460:425–49.

196. Nieuwenhuys R, Voogd J, van Huijzen C. Telencephalon: introduction and olfactory system. In: *The Human Central Nervous System.* 4th ed. Berlin: Springer; 2008, pp. 337–59.

197. Rigoard P, Buffenoir K, Jaafari N, Giot JP, Houeto JL, Mertens P, et al. The accumbofrontal fasciculus in the human brain: a microsurgical anatomical study. *Neurosurgery.* 2011;68:1102–11.

198. Kanter ED, Haberly LB. NMDA-dependent induction of long-term potentiation in afferent and association fiber systems of piriform cortex in vitro. *Brain Res.* 1990;525:175–9.

199. Barnes DC, Hofacer RD, Zaman AR, Rennaker RL, Wilson DA. Olfactory perceptual stability and discrimination. *Nat Neurosci.* 2008;11:1368–80.

200. Fletcher ML, Wilson DA. Experience modifies olfactory acuity: acetylcholine-dependent learning decreases behavioral generalization between similar odorants. *J Neurosci.* 2000;114:32–41.

201. Wilson DA, Stevenson RJ. *Learning to smell: olfactory perception from neurobiology to behavior.* Baltimore: Johns Hopkins University Press; 2006.

202. Kringlebach, M.L. The human orbitofrontal cortex: linking reward to hedonic experience. *Nature Rev Neurosci.* 2005;6:691–702.

203. Gottfried JA. What can an orbitofrontal cortex-endowed animal do with smells? *Ann NY Acad Sci.* 2007;1121:102–20.

204. de Araujo IE, Rolls ET, Kringelbach ML, McGlone F, Phillips N. Taste-olfactory convergence, and the representation of the pleasantness of flavor, in the human brain. *Eur J Neurosci.* 2003;18:2059–68.

205. Rolls ET, Kringelbach ML, de Araujo IE. Different representations of pleasant and unpleasant odors in the human brain. *Eur J Neurosci.* 2003;18:695–703.

206. Jones-Gotman M, Zatorre RJ. Olfactory identification deficits in patients with focal cerebral excision. *Neuropsychologia.* 1988;26:387–400.

207. Shepherd G. Smell images and the flavour system in the human brain. *Nature.* 2006;444:316–21.

208. Murphy C, Cain WS, Bartoshuk LM. Mutual action of taste and olfaction. *Sens Proc.* 1977;1:204–11.

209. Rozin P. "Taste and smell confusions" and the duality of the olfactory sense. *Perception & Psychophys.* 1982;31:397–40ł.

210. Solms J, King BM, Wyler R. Interactions of flavor compounds with food components. In: Charalambous G, ed. *Quality of foods and beverages.* Cambridge, MA: Academic Press; 1981, pp. 7–18.

211. Voilley A, Beghin V, Charpentier C, Peyron D. Interactions between aroma substances and macromolecules in a model wine. *Lebens Wiss Technol-Food Sci Technol.* 1991;24:469–72.

212. Roberts DD, Elmore JS, Langley KR, Bakker J. Effects of sucrose, guar gum, and

carboxymethylcellulose on the release of volatile flavor compounds under dynamic conditions. *J Agr Food Chem.* 1996;44:1321–6.

213. Cliff M, Noble AC. Time-intensity evaluation of sweetness and fruitiness and their interaction in a model solution. *J Food Sci.* 1990 Mar;55(2):450–4.

214. Stevenson RJ, Prescott J, Boakes RA. Confusing tastes and smells: How odours can influence the perception of sweet and sour tastes. *Chem Senses.* 1999;24(6):627–35.

215. Tieman D, Bliss P, McIntyre LM, Blandon-Ubeda A, Bies D, Odabasi AZ, et al. The chemical interactions underlying tomato flavor preferences. *Curr. Biol.* 2012 Jun;22:1–5.

216. Schwieterman ML, Colquhoun TA, Jaworski EA, Bartoshuk LM, Gilbert JL, et al. Strawberry flavor: diverse chemical compositions, a seasonal influence, and effects on sensory perception. *PLoS ONE.* 2014 Jun;9(2):e88446.

217. Gilbert JL, Guthart MJ, Gezan SA, Pisaroglo de Carvalho M, Schwieterman ML, Colquhoun TA, et al. Identifying breeding priorities for blueberry flavor using biochemical, sensory, and genotype by environment analyses. *PLoS ONE.* 2015 Sept;10 (9):e0138494.

218. Colquhoun TA, Schwieterman ML, Snyder DJ, Stamps JJ, Sims CA, Odabasi AZ, et al. Laboratory demonstration of volatile-enhanced-sweetness. *Chem Senses.* 2015;40:622–3.

219. Maier JX, Wachowiak M, Katz DB. Chemosensory convergence on primary olfactory cortex. *J Neurosci.* 2012 Nov;32 (48):17037–47.

220. Van Buskirk RL, Erickson RP. Odorant responses in taste neurons of the rat NTS. *Brain Res.* 1977;135:287–303.

221. Ghadami M, Morovvati S, Majidzadeh-A K, Damavandi E,

222. Nishimura G, Kinoshita A, et al. Isolated congenital anosmia locus maps to 18p11, 23-q12.2. *J Med Genet.* 2004;41:299–303.

222. Blakeslee AF. Unlike reaction of different individuals to fragrance in verbena flowers. *Science.* 1918;48:298–9.

223. Amoore JE, Venstrom D, Davis AR. Measurements of specific anosmia. *Percept Mot Skills.* 1968;26:143–64.

224. Whissell-Buechy D, Amoore JE. Odour-blindness to musk: simple recessive inheritance. *Nature.* 1973;242:271–3.

225. Menashe I, Abaffy T, Hasin Y, Goshen S, Yahalom V, Luetje CW, et al. Genetic elucidation of human hyperosmia to isovaleric acid. *PLoS Biol.* 2007:5(11): e284.

226. Knaapila A, Keskitalo K, Kallela M, Wessman M, Sammalisto S, Hiekkalinna T, et al. Genetic component of identification, intensity and pleasantness of odours: a Finnish family study. *Eur J Hum Genet.* 2007;15:596–602.

227. Wysocki CJ, Beauchamp GK. Ability to smell androstenone is genetically determined. *Proc Natl Acad Sci USA.* 1984 Aug;81 (15):4899–902.

228. Wysocki CJ, Gilbert AN. National Geographic Smell Survey. Effects of age are heterogenous. *Ann NY Acad Sci.* 1989;561:12–28.

229. Wysocki CJ, Dorries K, Beauchamp GK. Ability to perceive androstenone can be acquired by ostensibly anosmic people. *PNAS.* 1989;86:7976–8.

230. Deems DA, Doty RL, Settle G, Moore-Gillon V, Shaman P, Mester AF, et al. Smell and taste disorders, a study of 750 patients from the University of Pennsylvania Smell and Taste Center. *Arch Otolaryngol Head Neck Surg.* 1991;117(5):519–28.

231. Jones DL, Rando TA. Emerging models and paradigms for stem

cell ageing. *Nat Cell Biol.* 2011;13:506–12.

232. Curtis MA, Kam M, Nannmark U, Anderson MF, Axell MZ, Wikkelso C, et al. Human neuroblasts migrate to the olfactory bulb via a lateral ventricular extension. *Science.* 2007 Mar;315(5816):1243–9.

233. Luo J, Daniels SB, Lennington JB, Notti RQ, Conover JC. The aging neurogenic subventricular zone. *Aging Cell.* 2006 Feb;5(2):139–52.

234. Smith CG. Age incidence of atrophy of olfactory nerves in man. *J Comp Neurol.* 1942;77:589–94.

235. Meisami E, Mikhail L, Baim D, Bhatnagar KP. Human olfactory bulb: aging of glomeruli and mitral cells and a search for the accessory olfactory bulb. *Ann NY Acad Sci.* 1998 Nov;855:708–15.

236. Richard MB, Taylor SR, Greer CA. Age-induced disruption of selective olfactory bulb synaptic circuits. *PNAS.* 2010 Aug;107 (35):15613–18.

237. Costanzo RM, Kobayashi M. Age-related changes in p2 odorant receptor mapping in the olfactory bulb. *Chem Senses.* 2010 Jun;35 (5):417–26.

238. Naessen R. An enquiry on the morphological characteristics and possible changes with age in the olfactory region of man. *Acta Otolaryngol.* 1971 Jan;71 (1):49–62.

239. Nakashima T, Kimmelman CP, Snow JB. Structure of human fetal and adult olfactory neuroepithelium. *Arch Otolaryngol.* 1984 Oct;110:641–6.

240. Graziadei PP, Monti-Graziadei GA. Neurogenesis and plasticity of the olfactory sensory neurons. *Ann NY Acad Sci.* 1985;457:127–42.

241. Loo AT. Youngentob SL, Kent PF, Schwob JE. The aging olfactory epithelium: neurogenesis, response to damage, and odorant-

induced activity. *Int J Devl Neurosci.* 1996;14(7–8):881–900.

242. Ueha R, Shichino S, Ueha S, Kondo K, Kikuta S, Nishijima H, et al. Reduction of proliferating olfactory cells and low expression of extracellular matrix genes are hallmarks of the aged olfactory mucosa. *Front Aging Neurosci.* 2018 Mar;10:1–13.

243. Child KM, Herrick DB, Schwob JE, Holbrook EH, Jang W. The neuroregenerative capacity of olfactory stem cells is not limitless: implications for aging. *J Neurosci.* 2018 Aug;38(31):6806–24.

244. Holbrook EH, Szumowski KE, Schwob JE. An immunochemical, ultrastructural, and developmental characterization of the horizontal basal cells of rat olfactory epithelium. *J Comp Neurol.* 1995;363:129–46.

245. Brann JH, Ellis DP, Ku BS, Spinazzi EF, Firestein S. Injury in aged animals robustly activates quiescent olfactory neural stem cells. *Front Neurosci.* 2015;9:367.

246. Schwob JE, Jang W, Holbrook EH, Lin B, Herrick DB, Peterson JN, et al. Stem and progenitor cells of the mammalian olfactory epithelium: taking poietic license. *J Comp Neurol.* 2017 Mar;525 (4):1034–54.

247. Rawson NE, Gomez G, Cowart BJ, Kriete A, Pribitkin E, Restrepo D. Age-associated loss of selectivity in human olfactory sensory neurons. *Neurobiol Aging.* 2012 Sept;33(9):1913–19.

248. Mombaerts P, Wang F, Dulac C, Chao SK, Nemes A, Mendelsohn M, et al. Visualizing an olfactory sensory map. *Cell.* 1996;87:675–86.

249. Khan M, Vaes E, Mombaerts P. Temporal patterns of odorant receptor gene expression in adult and aged mice. *Mol Cell Neurosci.* 2013 Nov;57:120–9.

250. Buckland ME, Cunningham AM. Alterations in the neurotrophic factors BDNF, GDNF, and CTNF

in the regenerating olfactory system. *Ann NY Acad Sci.* 1998;855:260–5.

251. Rivard A, Fabre J-E, Silver M, Chen D, Murohara T, Kearney M, et al. Age-dependent impairment of angiogenesis. *Circulation.* 2018 Mar;99:111–20.

252. Jin K, Zhu Y, Sun Y, Mao XO, Xie L, Greenberg DA. Vascular endothelial growth factor (VEGF) stimulates neurogenesis in vitro and in vivo. *PNAS.* 2002;99:11946–50.

253. Ramírez-Rodríguez GB, Perera-Murcia GR, Ortiz-López L, Vega-Rivera NM, Babu H, García-Anaya M, et al. Vascular endothelial growth factor influences migration and focal adhesions, but not proliferation or viability, of human neural stem/ progenitor cells derived from olfactory epithelium. *Neurochem Int.* 2017 Sep;108:417–25.

254. Licht T, Eavri R, Goshen I, Shlomai Y, Mizrahi A, Keshet E. VEGF is required for dendritogenesis of newly born olfactory bulb interneurons. *Development.* 2010;137:261–71.

255. Blakemore LJ, Trombley PQ. Zinc as a neuromodulator in the central nervous system with a focus on the olfactory bulb. *Front Cell Neurosci.* 2017 Sept; 11:297.

256. Henkin RI, Velicu I, Schmidt L. An open-label controlled trial of theophylline for treatment of patients with hyposmia. *Am J Med Sci.* 2009 Jun;337(6):396–406.

257. Mundt B1, Krakowsky G, Röder H, Werner E. Loss of smell and taste within the scope of vitamin B 12 deficiency. *Psychiatr Neurol Med Psychol.* 1987 Jun;39 (6):356–61.

258. Derin S, Koseoglu S, Sahin C, Sahan M. Effect of vitamin B12 deficiency on olfactory function. *Allergy Rhinol.* 2016 Apr;6 (10):1051–5.

259. Rawson NE, LaMantia AS. Once and again: retinoic acid signaling

in the developing and regenerating olfactory pathway. *J Neurobiol.* 2006 Jun;66 (7):653–76.

260. Hahn I, Scherer PW, Mozell MM. A mass transport model of olfaction. *J Theor Biol.* 1994;167:115–28.

261. Zhao K, Scherer PW, Hajiloo SA, Dalton P. Effect of anatomy on human nasal air flow and odorant transport patterns: implications for olfaction. *Chem Senses.* 2004;29:365–79.

262. Getchell ML, Getchell TV. Fine structural aspects of secretion and extrinsic innervation in the olfactory mucosa. *Microsc Res Tech.* 1992 Oct;23(2):111–27.

263. Leclerc S, Heydel JM, Amossé V, Gradinaru D, Cattarelli M, Artur Y, et al. Glucuronidation of odorant molecules in the rat olfactory system: activity, expression and age-linked modifications of UDP-glucuronosyltransferase isoforms, UGT1A6 and UGT2A1, and relation to mitral cell activity. *Brain Res Mol Brain Res.* 2002 Nov;107(2):201–13.

264. Yoshikawa K, Wang H, Jaen C, Haneoka M, Saito N, Nakamura J, et al. The human olfactory cleft mucus proteome and its age-related changes. *Scientific Reports.* 2018 Nov;8:17170.

265. Edelstein DR. Aging of the normal nose. *Laryngoscope.* 1996 Sept:106 (S81):1–25.

266. Price JL, Morris JC. Tangles and plaques in nondemented aging and "preclinical" Alzheimer's disease. *Ann Neurol.* 1999;45:358–68.

267. Cerf-Ducastel B, Murphy C. fMRI brain activation in response to odors is reduced in primary olfactory areas of elderly subjects. *Brain Res.* 2003;986:39–53.

268. Murphy C, Cerf-Ducastel B, Calhoun-Haney R, Gilbert PE, Ferdon S. ERP, fMRI and functional connectivity studies of

brain response to odor in normal aging and Alzheimer's disease. *Chem Senses.* 2005;30(Suppl 1): i170–i171.

269. Donchin E, Karis D, Bashore TR, Coles MGH, Gratton G. Cognitive psychophysiology and human information processing. In: Coles MGH, Donchin E, Porges SW, eds. *Psychophysiology: systems, processes, and applications.* New York: Guilford Press; 1986, pp. 244–67.

270. Murphy C, Morgan CD, Geisler MW, Wettera S, Covington JW, Madowitza MD, et al. Olfactory event-related potentials and aging: normative data. *Int J Psychophysiol.* 2000;36:133–45.

271. Hoffman HJ, Ishii EK, MacTurk RH. Age-related changes in the prevalence of smell/taste problems among the United States adult population: results of the 1994 Disability Supplement to the National Health Interview Survey (NHIS). *Ann NY Acad Sci.* 1998;855:716–22.

272. Murphy C, Schubert CR, Cruickshanks KJ, Klein BEK, Klein R, Nondahl DM. Prevalence of olfactory impairment in older adults. *JAMA.* 2002;288 (18):2307–12.

273. Doty RL, Shaman P, Dann M. Development of the University of Pennsylvania Smell Identification Test: a standardized microencapsulated test of olfactory function. *Physiol Behav.* 1984;32:489–502.

274. Cain WS, Stevens JC. Uniformity of olfactory loss in aging. *Ann NY Acad Sci.* 1989;561:29–38.

275. Stevens JC, Cain WS. Old-age deficits in the sense of smell as gauged by thresholds, magnitude matching, and odor identification. *Psychol Aging.* 1987;2(1):36–42.

276. Venstrom D, Amoore JE. Olfactory threshold in relation to age, sex, or smoking. *J Food Sci.* 1968;33:264–5.

277. Schiffman SS, Moss J, Erickson RP. Thresholds of food odors in the elderly. *Exp Aging Res.* 1976;2:389–98.

278. Schiffman SS, Leffingwell JC. Perception of odors of simple pyrazines by young and elderly subjects: a multidimensional analysis. *Pharmacol Biochem Behav.* 1981;14:787–98.

279. Sinding C, Puschmann L, Hummel T. Is the age-related loss in olfactory sensitivity similar for heavy and light molecules? *Chem Senses.* 2014;39:383–90.

280. Stevens JC, Cain WS, Weinstein DE. Aging impairs the ability to detect gas odor. *Fire Technol.* 1987;23(3):198–204.

281. Stevens JC, Cain WS. Age-related deficiency in the perceived strength of six odorants. *Chem Senses.* 1985;10(4):517–29.

282. Schiffman SS, Warwick ZS. Changes in taste and smell over the life span: their effect on appetite and nutrition in the elderly. In: Friedman MI, Tordoff MG, Kare MR, eds. *Chemical senses, appetite, and nutrition.* New York: Dekker; 1991, pp. 341–65.

283. Stevens JC, Cain WS. Smelling via the mouth: effect of aging. *Percept Psychophys.* 1986;40(3):142–6.

284. Stamps JJ, Bartoshuk LM. Orthonasal and retronasal olfaction during healthy aging: supra-threshold intensity and identification. Manuscript in preparation.

285. Snyder DJ, Puentes LA, Sims CA, Bartoshuk LM. Building a better intensity scale: which labels are essential? *Chem Senses.* 2008;33: S142.

286. Hummel T, Kobal G, Gudziol H, Mackay-Sim A. Normative data for the "Sniffin' Sticks" including tests of odor identification, odor discrimination, and olfactory thresholds: an upgrade based on a group of more than 3,000 subjects. *Eur Arch Otorhinolaryngol.* 2007;264:237–43.

287. Schiffman SS. Food recognition by the elderly. *J Gerontol.* 1977;32:586–92.

288. Schiffman SS, Pasternak M. Decreased discrimination of food odors in the elderly. *J Gerontol.* 1979;34(1):73–9.

289. De Wijk RA, Cain WS. Odor quality: discrimination versus free and cued identification. *Perception Psychophys.* 1994;56(1):12–18.

290. Cain WS, Gent JF, Goodspeed RB, Leonard G. Evaluation of olfactory dysfunction in the Connecticut Chemosensory Clinical Research Center. *Laryngoscope.* 1988;98(1):83–8.

291. Murphy C, Cain WS. Odor identification: the blind are better. *Physiol Behav.* 1986;37:177–80.

292. Murphy C, Nordin S, Acosta L. Odor learning, recall and recognition memory in young and elderly adults. *Neuropsychol.* 1997;11(1):126–37.

293. Olofsson JK, Rönnlund M, Nordin S, Nyberg L, Nilsson L-G, Larsson M. Odor identification deficit as a predictor of five-year global cognitive change: interactive effects with age and ApoE-ε4. *Behav Genet.* 2009;39:496–503.

294. Murphy C. Cognitive and chemosensory influences on age-related changes in the ability to identify blended foods. *J Gerontol* 1985;40:47–52.

295. Ship JA, Weiffenbach JM. Age, gender, medical treatment, and medication effects on smell identification. *J Gerontol: MED SCI.* 1993;48(1):M26–M32.

296. Wilson RS, Arnold SE, Tang Y, Bennett DA. Odor identification and decline in different cognitive domains in old age. *Neuroepidemiol.* 2006;26:61–7.

297. Wilson RS, Arnold SE, Schneider JA, Tang Y, Bennett DA. The relationship between cerebral Alzheimer's disease pathology and odour identification in old age.

J Neurol Neurosurg Psychiatry. 2007;78:30–5.

298. Segura B, Baggio HC, Solana E, Palacios EM, Vendrell P, Bargalló N, et al. Neuroanatomical correlates of olfactory loss in normal aged subjects. *Behav Brain Res.* 2013;246:148–53.

299. Cain WS, Murphy CL. Influence of aging on recognition memory for odors and graphic stimuli. *Ann NY Acad Sci.* 1987;510:212–15.

300. Kay LM. Two species of gamma oscillations in the olfactory bulb: dependence on behavioral state and synaptic interactions. *J Integr Neurosci.* 2003 Jun;2 (1):31–44.

301. Uva L, de Curtis M. Propagation pattern of entorhinal cortex subfields to the dentate gyrus in the guinea-pig: an electrophysiological study. *Neurosci.* 2003;122(3):843–51.

302. Koss E, Weiffenbach JM, Haxby JV, Friedland RP. Olfactory detection and identification performance are dissociated in early Alzheimer's disease. *Neurol.* 1988;38(8):1228–32.

303. Gilbert PE, Barr PJ, Murphy C. Differences in olfactory and visual memory in patients with pathologically confirmed Alzheimer's disease and the Lewy body variant of Alzheimer's disease. *J Int Neuropsychol Soc.* 2004 Oct;10(6):835–42.

304. Fried LP, Kronmal RA, Newman AB. Risk factors for 5-year mortality in older adults: the Cardiovascular Health Study. *JAMA* 1998;279:585–92.

305. Fabiny AR, Kiel DP. Assessing and treating weight loss in nursing home patients. *Clin Geriat Med* 1997;13:737–51.

306. Buchman AS, Wilson RS, Bienias JL, Shah RC, Evans DA, Bennett DA. Change in body mass index and risk of incident Alzheimer's disease. *Neurol.* 2005;65:892–7.

307. Pelchat ML, Johnson A, Chan R, Valdez J, Ragland JD. Images of desire: food-craving activation during fMRI. *Neuroimage.* 2004;23:1486–93.

308. Volkow ND, Wise RA. How can drug addiction help us understand obesity? *Nature Neurosci.* 2005;8:555–60.

309. Duffy VB, Cain WS, Ferris AM. Measurement of sensitivity to olfactory flavor: application in a study of aging and dentures. *Chem Senses.* 1999;24:671–7.

310. Langkamp-Henken B. Usefulness of the MNA in the long-term and acute-care settings within the United States. *J Nutr Health Aging.* 2006;10(6):502–6.

311. Stamps JJ, Bartoshuk LM, Heilman KM. Taste, orthonasal and retronasal olfaction, and the nutritional consequences during Alzheimer's and Parkinson's diseases. Manuscript in preparation.

312. Lerch JP, Pruessner JC, Zijdenbos A, Hampler H, Teipel SJ, Evans AC. Focal decline of cortical thickness in Alzheimer's disease identified by computational neuroanatomy. *Cerebral Cortex.* 2005;15:995–1001.

313. Gomez-Isla T, Hollister R, West H, Mui S, Growdon JH, Petersen RC, et al. Neuronal loss correlates with but exceeds neurofibrillary tangles in Alzheimer's disease. *Ann Neurol.* 1997;41:17–24.

Memory Changes in the Aging Brain

Glenn J. Larrabee

Normal aging is characterized by linear declines in both physical and mental abilities that are associated with the passage of time, rather than with disease or injury [1]. This chapter focuses on normal aging-related changes in memory, considered in the context of aging-related changes in other cognitive skills. This review will be based on normative data for memory tests focusing on aging-related changes in performance. As such, the chapter provides information that is useful in clinical applications of memory testing procedures.

1 Definitions

To begin, a basic definition of learning is the acquisition of knowledge or skills through experience, study, or instruction, whereas memory refers to the ability to recall or recognize an experience, knowledge, or information that has been acquired through learning [2]. During learning, the brain encodes and stores information, which can be retrieved in the course of multiple learning trials or at varying periods of delay following the period of initial learning [3]. Cognition is a broader construct that encompasses a number of domains of mental function, including perception, attention, memory, symbolic representation (language), and executive processing, including decision-making, reasoning, and problem-solving [3]. These elements of cognition comprise the major domains assessed in a comprehensive neuropsychological evaluation [4, 5].

Memory has been conceptualized in terms of stages differing in duration and amount of information retained [3, 6]: (1) sensory memory: information held for fractions of a second (iconic for visual, echoic for auditory), (2) short-term memory: information held for up to a few seconds, in limited amounts (7 ± 2 items) and lost without rehearsal, also known as working memory, and (3) long-term memory: enduring storage of information about both recent

and remote events or knowledge. This knowledge can be in many domains, such as language (e.g., speaking, reading, and writing), visuospatial (face recognition, emotional facial recognition, location, object and movement recognition), nonverbal auditory (e.g., environmental sounds, emotional prosody, music, and voice recognition), as well as object recognition in other modalities such as touch, smell, and taste.

Long-term memory can be characterized as declarative or nondeclarative [3, 6]. Declarative or explicit memory capacity provides the basis for conscious retrieval or recognition of information or episodes, whereas nondeclarative memory refers to implicit or procedural memory, for example, skills, procedures, habits, or classically conditioned responses occurring outside conscious awareness. Declarative memory can be further divided into semantic memory for knowledge or facts that is noncontextual (i.e., not associated with a particular time or setting), and episodic memory for contextual information (acquired at a specific place and time). For example, remembering what the Enola Gay was may be an episodic memory for someone who was a teenager at the time of the end of World War II but would likely be in semantic memory for a modern teenage history buff.

2 Chapter Outline

The plan for the remainder of this chapter is to first consider the boundaries of what has been considered to be normal aging-related changes in long-term memory. This will be followed by discussion of aging-related changes in declarative memory (semantic and episodic), memory stages (short-term or working memory and long-term memory), and the major cognitive processes important in long-term memory processes, including learning, delayed recall, forgetting rates, and recognition. This chapter will also discuss the effects of aging on the factor analytic structure of memory tests in the context of other cognitive test scores. In this chapter, I will not be discussing nondeclarative, implicit, or procedural memory (discussed in Chapter 11). Nor will I be discussing classical conditioning.

Data to be presented derive from age-cohort normative data for clinical measures of short-term/working memory (see also Chapter 12) and long-term memory (episodic and semantic). Data analysis involves comparing each successive age cohort to the normative performance of young adults. Effect sizes for the mean performance of successive age cohorts are derived from comparison to the young adult mean and standard deviation (SD), converted to a T score metric (mean = 50, SD = 10). For example, if an 80-year-old group's mean performance falls 1 SD below the young adult mean, the mean score assigned for that group is 40: (50 − [10 × 1]); if performance is 0.5 SD below young adults, the T score is 45. Analysis of normative data sets from clinical tests for purposes of studying age-related changes in cognition is well accepted [1]. Here it involves compiling estimates of age-related differences relative to young adult norms for traditional clinical memory tests. This procedure has also been used to study aging effects on tests designed to tap everyday memory abilities such as name–face recall, memory for object location, and facial recognition memory [7].

3 Normal versus Abnormal Aging-Related Changes in Long-Term Memory

Attempts to specify the boundaries between normal and abnormal aging-related changes in long-term memory date to the work of the Canadian psychiatrist V. A. Kral [8–10]. Based on mental status testing and follow-up over a 4-year period, he identified a form of senescent forgetfulness in 18% of the residents of a retirement home, characterized as the inability to recall episodic data (details of an experience such as a name, date, or place), but spared recall of the experience itself. He also observed that the participant might retrieve the forgotten information at a later date, suggesting that inconsistent retrieval from long-term memory storage was a core feature. After finding that the mortality of these forgetful persons was no different four years later than that of persons of similar age without this type of forgetfulness, and that their memory disorder did not progress, Kral

concluded that this type of senescent forgetfulness was "benign." By contrast, Kral found that 30% of the same elderly population presented with total failure to retrieve any information about events from the recent past. These persons had increased mortality compared with the "benign" forgetful group, as well as progressive cognitive decline, and these people frequently required institutionalization due to their progressive dementia, leading Kral to identify them as having "malignant" senescent forgetfulness.

Larrabee, Levin, and High [11] attempted to specify the psychometric characteristics of "benign" senescent forgetfulness (BSF) with a variety of measures of verbal and visual learning and memory, as well as measures of non-memory cognitive functions. They were able to identify a subgroup of forgetful elderly who differed from their age peers in memory ability but were not demented. Over a one-year follow-up, these forgetful elderly people did not show evidence of further decline in memory or other cognitive functions. Moreover, they did not differ on P300 auditory evoked potential testing, conducted to rule out an underlying neurophysiologic basis to their reduced memory performance [12].

In the mid-1980s, a new construct for characterization of aging-associated change in memory function appeared: age-associated memory impairment (AAMI; [13]). Criteria for a diagnosis of AAMI included age greater than 50 years, documentation of complaints of aging-related change in memory function compared with young adult years, evidence of performance in the bottom 16% of young adult levels of memory function that could not be accounted for by below average intellectual ability (minimum raw score of at least 32, equivalent to a scaled score of 9 on the Wechsler Adult Intelligence Scale Vocabulary subtest), absence of depression (Hamilton Depression Rating Scale score of <13), absence of evidence for dementia (Mini-Mental Status Examination score of 24 or higher), and absence of neurologic, psychiatric, and medical diseases known to impact cognition. By definition, AAMI incorporated both subjects experiencing the natural, aging-associated decline in long-term memory function and subjects experiencing what Kral had identified as BSF. That is, some of the subjects with AAMI who underperformed younger adults on memory testing also underperformed their age-matched peers. Therefore, Blackford and LaRue [14] proposed expanding the AAMI criteria to further identify subjects who had worse performance on memory testing compared with young adults *and* age-matched peers. They termed this disorder "Late Life Forgetfulness." This recommendation defined two subgroups of AAMI: (1) those subjects who had age-consistent memory impairment (performance within ± 1 SD of age peer performance on 75% of the tests administered), and (2) late life forgetfulness (performance between 1 and 2 SD below age-peer performance on 50% of more of tests administered). Blackford and LaRue surmised that the majority of cases that Kral would have identified as persons with benign senescent forgetfulness would have met criteria for late life forgetfulness.

While the construct of AAMI generated a significant amount of research [15], AAMI drew increasing criticism in the 1990s because of the heterogeneity of clinical memory tests and varying sensitivity of these tests to aging effects [16]. At the same time, interest shifted to a new construct, mild cognitive impairment (MCI; [17]), intended to identify a group of subjects who had memory decline compared with age-peers but who were not demented and did not have decline in other cognitive abilities or show deterioration in activities of daily living. In the original paper, MCI was defined by memory function at or below −1.5 SD compared with age-appropriate normative data, in the absence of dementia, as defined by a Verbal and Performance IQ that fell within 0.5 SD of normal control subjects. Petersen and colleagues [17] followed their MCI subjects over a 4-year period and found conversion to AD at a rate of 12% per year, contrasted with the incidence of AD in normal elderly individuals of 1–2% per year. The authors conjectured that MCI may represent the earliest stages of AD and, thus, was of both theoretical and practical importance [17].

Since the publication of the original paper on MCI, there has been extensive investigation of this disorder and its relationship to AD, as well as other conditions characterized by changes in memory and other cognitive functions. This research is summarized nicely in the book by Smith and Bondi [18], who themselves have contributed extensive empirical research on MCI (Smith was a co-author on the original MCI paper [17]). Smith and Bondi also reviewed the aging-associated memory impairments discussed above and grouped them into (1) "normal aging" (which included Kral's BSF, AAMI, and Blackford and LaRue's ACMI) and (2) an "abnormal state"

(which included Kral's malignant senescent forgetfulness and Blackford and LaRue's late life forgetfulness, as well as MCI). The extensive body of research reviewed by Smith and Bondi has led to refined criteria for the diagnosis of MCI and the use of multiple measures of memory and other cognitive abilities to define subtypes of MCI, including amnestic and non-amnestic variants.

Moving on from discussion of the border zone between normal and abnormal changes in long-term memory, I will now discuss aging-related changes in the various forms of memory. As noted earlier, these changes will be considered in comparison to normal subjects, who are in their mid- to late 20s.

4 Aging-Related Changes in Memory and Other Cognitive Abilities

Table 7.1 displays aging-associated changes in long-term verbal and visual/nonverbal memory, working memory, processing speed, spatial/perceptual cognition, and semantic memory. Data were selected from the published normative data for the Wechsler Memory Scale III (WMS-III; [19]) and the Wechsler Adult Intelligence Scale-III (WAIS-III; [20]). The third version of Wechsler's tests of memory and intelligence was selected rather than the more current fourth edition due to the continuity in memory tasks for the WMS-III across the entire adult age range of 25–89, and due to the continuity of normative data for the Letter-Number Sequencing Test, a measure of short-term or working memory, across this same range. Similar continuity was not available for the fourth edition of the scales.

The following subtests were selected for comparison: Logical Memory II and Verbal Paired Associates II as measures of long-term episodic verbal memory, Visual Reproduction II as a measure of long-term episodic visual memory, Vocabulary and Information subtests as measures of semantic memory, Block Design and Matrix Reasoning as measures of spatial cognition, Digit Span and Letter-Number Sequencing as measures of verbal working memory, and Digit Symbol and Symbol Search as measures of processing speed. For each of these WMS-III and WAIS-III subtests, the raw score performance of subjects in the 25- to 29-year-old range that corresponded to 50th percentile performance was selected as the mean for this age group. The standard deviation was determined by taking the average of the difference between

Table 7.1 Aging-associated changes in verbal and visual episodic memory, semantic memory, working memory, processing speed, and spatial cognition (T scores based on age 25–29 cohort data)

Domain	Age 30–34	Age 35–44	Age 45–54	Age 55–64	Age 65–69	Age 70–74	Age 75–79	Age 80–84	Age 85–90
Verbal episodic memory[a]	50.0	50.0	48.6	45.0	43.0	42.5	40.1	38.0	36.5
Visual episodic memory[b]	50.0	48.3	45.4	40.9	35.0	33.9	33.9	30.9	28.5
Semantic long-term memory[c]	51.9	53.6	55.3	52.1	52.1	52.1	51.1	47.3	47.1
Verbal working memory[d]	49.4	49.4	47.8	45.0	45.0	42.2	42.2	40.0	37.8
Processing speed[e]	48.9	47.9	44.4	39.0	35.7	34.5	31.8	28.3	25.5
Spatial cognition[f]	49.8	48.8	45.6	43.6	40.4	38.7	38.0	36.1	35.3

[a] Based on WMS-III Logical Memory II and Verbal Paired Associates II; [b] based on WMS-III Visual Reproduction II; [c] based on WAIS-III Information and Vocabulary subtests; [d] based on WAIS-III Digit Span and Letter Number Sequencing subtests; [e] based on WAIS-III Symbol Search and Digit Symbol subtests; [f] based on WAIS-III Block Design and Matrix Reasoning. See references [19, 20].

this score and raw score values falling 1 SD above and 1 SD below it. Each successive age cohort raw score mean was compared with the mean score and standard deviation of the 25–29 cohort to determine the z score associated with the distance of that age cohort raw score mean from the mean of the 25–29 age cohort. These z scores were transformed to T scores (mean of 50, SD of 10), and the average T score was determined for the subtest pairs comprising each cognitive domain (with the exception of Visual Long-Term Memory, which was based on WMS-III Visual Reproduction II alone). Since the T scores are based on distance from the young adult mean in young adult standard deviation units, they can also readily yield effect size measures (Cohen's d); thus, a T score of 45 represents Cohen's d of −0.5 (45 − 50/10), a T score of 40 represents Cohen's d of −1.0, and a T score of 30 represents a Cohen's d of −2.0.

Although cross-sectional comparisons as a function of age have been criticized for magnifying aging-related differences in ability, in comparison to smaller changes seen in longitudinal evaluation of the same cohort assessed repeatedly over time, recent research has suggested that the difference between the results of these two approaches is substantially due to practice effects/test familiarity for persons examined in longitudinal designs [21]. In other words, the practice effects/instrument familiarity effects attenuate aging-related changes in longitudinal studies relative to cross-sectional data by inflating performance on retesting.

Table 7.1 shows progressive decline in long-term verbal and visual episodic memory that is most apparent starting with the age 45–54 cohort. The same is seen for verbal working memory and spatial cognition. By contrast, decline is apparent earlier, starting at the 35–44 age cohort, for processing speed. By the oldest age cohort, 85–90, effect sizes are maximal for processing speed, followed by visual memory, with large but relatively smaller declines in long-term verbal episodic memory, verbal working memory, and spatial cognition. Of interest, long-term semantic memory shows little decline in association with advancing age. Indeed, long-term semantic memory ability actually increases in association with advancing age relative to the performance of 25- to 29-year-old subjects, with higher mean values for successive age cohorts through the 75–79 age group; similar findings have been reported by others [1]. Of course, if a semantic ability measure includes a time component, for example, letter fluency (generating words starting with a specific letter of the alphabet), or semantic category fluency tests (e.g., animal naming in 60 sec), age effects are more pronounced due to the processing speed component, and such measures may share associations with both semantic memory and processing speed (see Table 3; [22]). Performance on letter and, to a lesser extent, category fluency tests also depends on frontal-executive function, aging-related decline in which is detailed in Chapter 12.

The greater decline in visual episodic memory and processing speed compared with verbal episodic memory that is apparent in Table 7.1 may be a function of the memory tests used. There are three basic verbal learning and memory paradigms: text recall, paired associate learning (the Logical Memory and Verbal Paired Associate Learning measures in Table 7.1), and tests of learning and retention of a supra-span list of words [4, 5]. A supra-span word list contains a number of items that is beyond the typical span that can be recalled after a single presentation (e.g., 7 ± 2 items). Supra-span list learning tasks such as the California Verbal Learning Test-II (CVLT-ll) [23], the Rey Auditory Verbal Learning Test (AVLT) [24], and the Verbal Selective Reminding Test (VSRT; [25]), tend to show greater age effects. In a comparison of normative data from these three tasks for long delay free recall, the CVLT-II performance of the 80- to 89-year-old cohort, males and females combined, corresponded to a T score of 34.05 relative to 20- to 29-year-old performance [23], AVLT performance to a score of 24.8 [24], and VSRT performance to a score of 11.9 [25]. Again, recall that the lower the T score the more pronounced the decline in performance.

Although the CVLT-II T score for long delay free recall for the oldest cohort is only slightly lower than the T score for the oldest cohort in Table 7.1 (data based on Logical Memory and Verbal Paired Associate delayed recall), the values for the AVLT and VSRT are substantially lower, with the VSRT delayed recall showing the greatest aging-associated decline in performance, even exceeding that shown for processing speed. The differential sensitivity of the CVLT-II, AVLT, and VSRT to aging-associated changes is likely a direct consequence of the amount of organization and structure that is inherent in the test items, and how these items are presented for learning and recall. The CVLT-II is comprised of 16 words, and, although these words are presented in a random order, they come from four different semantic categories (e.g., tools, fruits, clothing, spices), providing inherent organization to the test stimuli. Furthermore, the entire list is repeated each time and the test assesses immediate recall, short delay recall, short delay cued recall, long delay free recall, and long delay cued recall. The short delay cued recall trials arguably serve as a re-presentation of the test stimuli. Indeed, perusal of the CVLT-II normative data reveals slightly higher long delay free recall performance compared with short delay free recall, supporting this inference.

The AVLT is comprised of 15 unrelated words that are presented on every learning trial. Lack of words grouped in categories and absence of a short delay cued recall trial make the AVLT less structured than the CVLT.

Last, the VSRT is comprised of 12 unrelated words, but the entire word list is not provided on each learning trial; rather, during the repetition trial subjects are provided only with the words that they did not recall on the preceding trial, yet they still are asked to provide all 12 words on the list. As a consequence, the VSRT, despite using a 12-word list compared with 15 for the AVLT and 16 for the CVLT-II, shows the greatest aging-associated decline in long-term verbal episodic memory.

Visual memory is typically assessed using two types of tests: recognition memory (yes/no recognition of recurring vs. nonrecurring abstract visual stimuli, such as the Continuous Visual Memory Test, CVMT; [26, 27], or forced choice recognition of faces previously or not previously seen [28]) and design reproduction from memory, such as the Visual Reproduction subtest of the WMS-III [19] or the Rey Complex Figure [29]. For people in their 80s, when compared with young adults, there are pronounced declines in CVMT performance (T score of 19.1) and Rey Figure performance (T score 16.7). Aging-related declines, however, are less pronounced for the Visual Reproduction Test (T score 28.5; Table 7.1).

The magnitude of aging-associated changes in delayed recall shown in Table 7.1, and discussed in relation to the CVLT-II, AVLT, VSRT, and CVMT, is matched by the degree of aging-associated decline over the learning/acquisition trials of these tests. This raises the question as to what accounts for the decline in delayed recall. Is this a problem with encoding and immediate retrieval during learning trials, or is it a problem of memory storage and retrieval 30 or more minutes after encoding? Haaland, Price, and LaRue [30] evaluated these processes for Logical Memory and Visual Reproduction using the complete data from the WMS-III standardization sample. They found that aging-associated decline in delayed recall and recognition was largely explained by poorer initial learning rather than impaired retrieval or accelerated forgetting. They concluded that comparable aging effects for decline in both immediate and delayed memory reflected the effects of encoding more than retrieval or storage of new information.

Table 7.2 Performance by females on the California Verbal Learning Test-II[a]

Age cohort	Trial 5 mean recall	Long delay mean free recall	Difference	Recognition hits	False positives	Recognition discriminability
20–29	14.0	12.5	1.5	16	1	3.4
30–44	13.5	13.0	.5	16	1	3.4
45–59	13.0	11.5	1.5	15	2	3.0
60–69	12.0	10.5	1.5	15	2	3.0
70–79	11.5	9.5	2.0	15	2.5	2.8
80–89	10.5	9.0	1.5	15	4	2.6

[a] See [23].

Table 7.3 Performance by males on the California Verbal Learning Test-II[a]

Age Cohort	Trial 5 mean recall	Long delay mean free recall	Difference	Recognition hits	False positives	Recognition discrimination
20–29	13.0	11.5	1.5	15	1	3.2
30–44	13.0	11.5	1.5	15	2	3.2
45–59	11.0	9.5	1.5	14	2.5	2.6
60–69	10.0	8.5	1.5	14	3.5	2.6
70–79	10.0	7.5	2.5	14	3.5	2.4
80–89	8.0	6.5	1.5	14	6.0	2.0

[a] See [23].

5 Learning, Delayed Recall, Forgetting, and Recognition in Long-Term Episodic Memory

Table 7.2 displays the normative data for women and Table 7.3 the same data for men on the CVLT-2 for learning trial 5, long delay free recall, the difference between the two, raw score values for recognition hits, false positive recognition, and recognition discriminability associated with performances falling at the 50th percentile for the following age cohorts: 20–29, 30–44, 45–59, 60–69, 70–79, and 80–89. Data are presented separately because of sex effects, with women performing better than men across the age range. However, there is no apparent interaction of age with gender: differences appear to be the same for trial 5 score minus long delay score and for recognition hits for both sexes and all age groups (e.g., men do not show an increasing difference in association

with advancing age). The data are striking in showing a fairly consistent mean difference between raw scores defining the mean level of performance for each age cohort on trial 5 versus long delay free recall: 1.5 words for both men and women (with the exception of the 70–79 cohort). Indeed, the correlation between the trial 5 and long delay recall scores in Tables 7.2 and 7.3 is 0.963 for females and 0.981 for males. Moreover, the recognition hits, despite showing sex effects (women performing better than men), show little decline with age. Mean raw scores associated with the 50th percentile for women are a perfect 16 of 16 for the two youngest age cohorts and 15 of 16 for the four oldest cohorts. For men, the mean raw recognition score is 15 out of 16 for the two youngest cohorts, and 14 out of 16 for the four oldest cohorts. By contrast, there appears to be a greater association between age and false positive errors made on the recognition trial of the CVLT-II. The same is true for discriminability, a signal detection measure based on both recognition hits and false alarms (in this computation, the higher the recognition hits and lower the false positive errors, the larger the discriminability score).

These data suggest two things about aging-associated changes. First, although there are linear declines in both the amount learned and the amount remembered, the amount remembered is the direct result of the amount learned. In other words, with advancing age in normal individuals, men and women, there is no accelerated loss of learned information. This is similar to what Haaland et al. [30] reported for WMS-III Logical Memory and Visual Reproduction tests and suggests that, with aging, the major memory deficits are problems with encoding rather than storage or retrieval. Second, Tables 7.2 and 7.3 reflect a significantly increasing discrepancy between long delay free recall versus nearly perfect recognition across the age range, implying that aging-associated decline in long-term memory is due to retrieval problems. This inference must be given additional consideration, however. First, this conclusion is not supported by the close similarity of the difference between trial 5 and long delay recall in Tables 7.2 and 7.3. On average, normally aging adults are recalling nearly as much as they initially learned, showing essentially 88% retention for young adult males declining slightly to 81% for males in their 80s. The same is true of females. Both males and females show a stable loss, on average of about 1.5 words from trial 5 to long delay free recall on the CVLT-11. Thus, if persons are recalling as much as they learned, how can this represent a retrieval deficit? Similarly, a problem in storage is ruled out by the lack of evidence for accelerated forgetting comparing trial 5 with long delay free recall.

Tables 7.2 and 7.3 give a more complete picture of older peoples' recognition memory performance on the CVLT-II. Despite minimal aging-related changes on recognition hits, more pronounced declines in association with age are apparent for false positive recognition and for the signal detection measure recognition discriminability, which combines both hits (true positives) and false positives (false alarms). Increase in false positive errors would not necessarily be inconsistent with encoding problems during learning trials, but recognition memory would need to be assessed immediately following the learning trials and compared with delayed recognition to determine whether this is related primarily to encoding processes as opposed to storage or retrieval processes. Again, the stable differences between trial 5 and long delay in Tables 7.2 and 7.3 suggest reduced encoding is the basis for aging-related decline in verbal episodic memory.

Similar data exist for visual memory, as demonstrated by the normative data for the Rey Complex Figure Test [29]. Since the Rey Complex Figure is presented only once for a copy administration, followed by immediate recall and then delayed recall, the immediate reproduction raw score represents the amount learned. From age 20–24 to age 80–89, there is no difference between the raw score defining the 50th percentile for immediate recall and the score representing the 50th percentile for delayed recall despite significant aging-related changes in both immediate and delayed reproduction of the Rey Figure. This lack of difference between age groups indicates that visual memory at delayed recall is directly related to and accounted for by the amount learned, with no evidence of accelerated forgetting in association with normal aging. Again, this finding suggests that aging-related declines are primarily a product of initial encoding of the stimuli. The amount recognized (maximum score 24; 12 target and 12 distractor items) that defines the 50th percentile in each successive cohort shows little variation, from around 21.5 (out of 24) for the 20- to 24-year-old cohort to 19.5 for the 80- to 89-year-old cohort. In other words, on average, normal adults over the 20–89 age range correctly discriminate actual Rey Figure elements versus distractors at accuracy rates that range between 81% and 90%. These values can be directly compared with CVLT-II data in Tables 7.2 and 7.3, by adding Total Hits + 32 – False Positives for each age cohort in these tables. The resulting mean total correct scores on recognition (hits and false positives) range between 90% and 98% for women and between 83% and 96% for men, across the age range studied.

6 Effects of Normal Aging on the Factor Structure of Memory Test Procedures

It has been long established that factor analysis is a useful method for determining the construct validity of both individual tests and collections of tests representing different cognitive and sensorimotor domains of performance. Construct validity refers to the degree to which a test is a valid measure of an underlying construct. Factor analysis captures patterns of correlation among observed variables, reduces a larger number of observed variables into a smaller number of factors, provides an operational definition for an underlying process (e.g., verbal episodic memory) by using observed variables (memory test scores), and can be used to test theories about the underlying process [31, 32]. Factor analysis statistically analyzes the pattern of intercorrelations among a set of variables. Variables that are intercorrelated with one another but relatively independent of other subsets of variables are combined into factors. The basic assumption is that results of tests loading on a particular factor (i.e., correlating with that factor) are explained by this factor. For example, if a test is truly a measure of long-term verbal episodic memory, it should load on the same factor as other tests known to be measures of verbal episodic memory, one that is distinct from factors correlating with verbal short-term memory, processing speed, and long-term semantic memory. The practical utility of tests of short- and long-term episodic and semantic memory would be enhanced by demonstrations of the same factor structure throughout the adult age range.

The effects of aging on factor analyses of memory tests and other measures of cognitive function have been examined in two different ways. One way has been to conduct confirmatory factor analysis to directly compare factor structure in different age cohorts. In one investigation using the performance of normal subjects on computer-simulated measures of everyday verbal working memory (telephone dialing), long-term verbal episodic memory (grocery list learning, first and last name paired associate learning), and long-term visual episodic memory (face memory, object location recall), grouped in age-cohorts of 50–58, 59–67, and 68–79, confirmatory factor analysis showed reasonable fit for a model assuming invariance of the pattern of loadings, the loadings themselves, and the covariances among the factors as a function of age [33].

Another way to evaluate similarity of factor structure has been to conduct two separate factor analyses, one on raw (or age-uncorrected) score performance and the other on scores that have been residualized for the effects of age. The age residualization process predicts performance on all of the test scores by age, saves the residuals remaining after removing the effects of age, and then factor analyzes the scores that have had the effects of age statistically removed.

Table 7.4 Factor analysis of delayed recall and delayed recognition raw scores and scores residualized for age

Test[a]	Factor 1	Factor 2	Factor 3	Factor 4
Serial Digits	0.41/ 0.40		0.61/ 0.61	
EPAT	0.47/ 0.44			
VSRT	0.73/ 0.72			
Visual Reprod	0.68/ 0.65	0.33/ 0.29		
CRM	0.56/ 0.55			
CVMT	0.55/ 0.51			
Mental Control			0.50/ 0.51	
Digit Span			0.66/ 0.66	
PASAT		0.34/ 0.34	0.51/ 0.50	
Trails B		−0.61/ −0.58		
Block Design	0.35/ 0.28	0.66/ 0.63		
Object Assembly		0.69/ 0.70		
Information				0.78/ 0.77
Vocabulary				0.80/ 0.79

[a] EPAT = Expanded Paired Associate Test; VSRT = Verbal Selective Reminding Test; Visual Reprod = WMS Visual Reproduction Delay; CRM = Continuous Recognition Memory; CVMT = Continuous Visual Memory Test; PASAT = Paced Auditory Serial Addition Test; Mental Control = Wechsler Memory Scale Mental Control subtest. Only loadings of 0.30 and higher for at least one member of the pair are displayed, raw score followed by age-residualized score. See [34].

Table 7.4 depicts the results of a factor analysis of patient data for clinical cases ranging in age from 16 to 70 [34]. The first score depicted for each factor loading in Table 7.4 is the score based on raw score performance, whereas the second score is based on test scores residualized for age. These data, based on delayed recall and delayed recognition performance, clearly show no difference in the factor structure (the only difference reported by these authors was the order of extraction of factors 3 and 4). The data in Table 7.4 also nicely demonstrate both short-term memory and long-term verbal episodic memory, as well as separate factors for verbal and visual long-term episodic memory (combined) versus semantic memory. Factor 1 is a long-term verbal and visual episodic memory domain, combined, factor 2 is processing speed and spatial cognition, combined, factor 3 is verbal working memory and concentration, and factor 4 is long-term semantic memory.

The same factor structure for simulated everyday memory has been reported in analyses comparing raw scores on simulated everyday memory tests with scores residualized for age [35]. Factor analyses were conducted on the performances of normal persons between 18 and 78 years of age on computer-simulated everyday memory tests, including immediate recall of telephone numbers and name–face associations, recognition of faces, object location recall, and reaction time in a simulated driving task. Factors were reported defining long-term verbal and visual episodic memory, vigilance, processing speed, and verbal and visual working memory for both raw scores and scores residualized for age [35].

7 Concluding Observations

This chapter has reviewed aging-associated changes in short- and long-term episodic memory, as well as aging-associated changes in episodic versus semantic memory processes. Changes in both short- and long-term memory are substantial and can be compared with aging-associated decline in other cognitive functions. The greatest declines are seen in visual memory and processing speed. Maximal aging-associated declines in episodic long-term verbal memory are seen with supra-span list-learning tests such as the Auditory Verbal Learning Test and the Verbal Selective Reminding Test, likely because of the greater demand on long-term memory encoding and retrieval processes associated with these tests (i.e., they are more difficult and provide less encoding support relative to the California Verbal Learning Test-II). Analysis of California Verbal Learning Test-II words provided on learning trial 5, long delay free recall, and recognition, for both males and females separately, shows pronounced age-related declines in Trial 5 and long delay

free recall, but the differences between these two free recall trials is essentially constant across the age range. Similar data exist for immediate versus delayed reproduction difference scores for the Rey Complex Figure Test. In other words, there is no accelerated forgetting occurring in the context of normal aging, and the aging-associated decline in long delay recall/reproduction is essentially fully accounted for by the amount of material learned initially. These findings replicate those of Haaland and colleagues [30], suggesting that aging-associated declines in verbal and visual episodic learning and memory are due to aging-associated changes in encoding processes. Recognition performances at delay for both the California Verbal Learning Test-II and the Rey Complex Figure Test remain close to ceiling and do not show much change in performance across the adult age range. While it is tempting to interpret the superior level of recognition to long delay recall as due to problems with memory retrieval processes, this does not explain the absence of change between learning trials and delayed recall on both the CVLT-II and the Rey Complex Figure. Last, the stability of factor structure over the adult age range shows that tests of working memory/short-term memory, long-term verbal and visual memory, as well as semantic memory are measuring the same constructs with advancing age.

The focus of the present chapter was on normal aging-related changes in memory function as reflected in the performance of normal subjects on clinically available tests of memory and other cognitive functions. It is only by knowing the parameters of normal function that we can then consider what is abnormal. Age is quite obviously a critical variable in determining the boundaries of what is normal ability. The DSM-V [36] has specified performance criteria for determination of a mild neurocognitive disorder as performance between 1 and 2 SD below appropriate norms, with major neurocognitive disorder defined as greater than 2 SD below the mean. Perusal of Table 7.1 shows that mean long-term verbal episodic memory scores falling between 1 and 2 SD below the young adult mean (T score of 30–40) occur in over 50% of normal elderly, aged 75 or older. Over 50% of 80- to 90-year-olds perform at a T score of 30 or lower relative to young adult norms on long-term visual episodic memory. Failure to account for these normal aging-related decrements could lead to problems of misdiagnosis, suggesting an acquired impairment, when these scores actually define the 50th percentile for normal persons aged 80–90.

References

1. Salthouse TA. *Major Issues in Cognitive Aging.* New York: Oxford University Press, 2010.

2. Hilgard ER, Bower GH. *Theories of Learning.* Englewood Cliffs, NJ: Prentice-Hall, 1975.

3. Purves D, et al. *Principles of Cognitive Neuroscience* (2nd ed.). Sunderland: Sinauer Associates, 2013.

4. Lezak MD, Howieson DB, Bigler ED, et al. *Neuropsychological Assessment* (5th ed.). New York: Oxford University Press, 2012.

5. Strauss E, Sherman EMS, Spreen OA. *Compendium of Neuropsychological Tests* (3rd ed.). New York: Oxford University Press, 2006.

6. Bauer RM, Reckess GZ, Kumar A, et al. Amnesic disorders. In: Heilman KM, Valenstein E (eds). *Clinical Neuropsychology* (5th ed.). New York: Oxford University Press, 2012; 504–581.

7. Larrabee GJ, Crook TH. Estimated prevalence of age-associated memory impairment derived from standardized tests of memory function. *Int Psychogeriat* 1994; **6**: 95–104.

8. Kral VA. Neuro-psychiatric observations in an old people's home. Studies of memory dysfunction in senescence. *J Gerontol* 1958; **13**:169–176.

9. Kral VA. Senescent forgetfulness: Benign and malignant. *J Canad Med Assoc* 1962; **86**:257–260.

10. Kral VA. Memory loss in the aged. *Diseases Nerv Sys* 1966; **27** (suppl.): 51–54.

11. Larrabee GJ, Levin HS, High WM. Senescent forgetfulness: A quantitative study. *Develop Neuropsychol* 1986; **2**: 373–385.

12. Loring DW, Levin HS, Papanicolaou AC, et al. Auditory evoked potentials in senescent forgetfulness. *Int J Neurosci* 1984; **24**: 133–141.

13. Crook TH, Bartus RT, Ferris SH, et al. Age-associated memory impairment: Proposed diagnostic criteria and measures of clinical change – report of a National Institute of Mental Health work group. *Develop Neuropsychol* 1986; **2**: 261–276.

14. Blackford RC, LaRue A. Criteria for diagnosing age-associated memory impairment: Proposed improvements from the field. *Develop Neuropsychol* 1989; **5**: 295–306.

15. Larrabee GJ. Age-associated memory impairment: Definition and psychometric characteristics. *Aging Neuropsychol Cognition* 1996; **3**: 118–131.

16. Smith GE, Ivnik RJ, Petersen RC, et al. Age-associated memory impairment diagnoses: Problems of reliability and concerns for terminology. *Psychol Aging* 1991; **6**: 551–558.

17. Peterson R, Smith G, Waring S, et al. Mild cognitive impairment: Clinical characterization and outcome. *Arch Neurol* 1999; **56**: 303–308.

18. Smith GE Bondi MW. *Mild Cognitive Impairment and Dementia: Definitions, Diagnosis and Treatment.* New York: Oxford University Press, 2013.

19. Wechsler D. *WMS-III. Wechsler Memory Scale Third Edition. Administration and Scoring Manual.* San Antonio: Psychological Corporation, 1997.

20. Wechsler D. *WAIS-III. Wechsler Adult Intelligence Scale Third Edition. Administration and Scoring Manual.* San Antonio: Psychological Corporation, 1997.

21. Salthouse TA. Why are there different age relations in cross-sectional and longitudinal comparisons of cognitive functions? *Current Directions Psychol Sci* 2014; **23**: 252–256.

22. Larrabee GJ. Association between IQ and neuropsychological test performance: Commentary on Tremont, Hoffman, Scott and Adams (1988). *Clin Neuropsychologist* 2000; **14**:139–145.

23. Delis DC, Kramer JH, Kaplan E, Ober BA. *CVLT-II. California Verbal Learning Test. Second Edition. Adult Version. Manual.* San Antonio: Psychological Corporation, 2000.

24. Schmidt M. *Rey Auditory and Verbal Learning Test. A Handbook.* Los Angeles: Western Psychological Services, 1996.

25. Larrabee GJ, Trahan DE, Curtiss G, et al. Normative data for the Verbal Selective Reminding Test. *Neuropsychol* 1988; **2**: 173–182.

26. Trahan DE, Larrabee GJ. *Continuous Visual Memory Test. Professional Manual.* Odessa: Psychological Assessment Resources, 1988.

27. Trahan DE, Larrabee GJ. *Continuous Visual Memory Test. Supplemental Normative Data for Children and Older Adults.* Odessa: Psychological Assessment Resources, 1997.

28. Warrington EK. *Recognition Memory Test.* Los Angeles: Western Psychological Services, 1984.

29. Meyers JE, Meyers KR. *Rey Complex Figure Test and Recognition Trial. Professional Manual.* Odessa: Psychological Assessment Resources, 1995.

30. Haaland KY, Price L, LaRue A. What does the WMS-III tell us about memory changes with normal aging? *J Internat Neuropsych Soc* 9: 89–96.

31. Larrabee GJ. Test validity and performance validity: Considerations in providing a framework for development of an ability-focused neuropsychological battery. *Arch Clin Neuropsychol* 29: 695–614.

32. Tabachnick BG, Fidell LS. *Multivariate Statistics* (4th ed.).

Needham Heights: Allyn and Bacon, 2001.

33. Tomer A, Larrabee GJ, Crook TH. The structure of everyday memory in adults with age-associated memory impairment. *Psychol Aging* 9: 606–615.

34. Larrabee GJ, Curtiss G. Construct validity of various verbal and visual memory tests. *J Clin Exper Neuropsychol* 17: 536–547.

35. Crook TH, Larrabee GJ. Interrelationships among everyday memory tests: Stability of factor structure with age. *Neuropsychol* 2: 1–12.

36. American Psychiatric Association. *Diagnostic and Statistical Manual of Mental Disorders* (5th ed.) (DSM-5). Washington, DC: American Psychiatric Publishing, 2013.

Aging-Related Alterations in Language

Stephen E. Nadeau

1 Introduction

One of the banes of advancing age is progressive difficulty with word finding. This is but the most conspicuous example of aging-related deterioration of function that spans all domains of language function. Everyone who experiences such language problems immediately fears an incipient dementing process. It is not possible to rule this out but there are other possible causes.

In the first section of this chapter, I will briefly review studies of age-related impairment in a broad spectrum of language functions, salient because of their methodology, size, or the insight they provide (for comprehensive reviews, see [1, 2]). In the second section – the major focus of this chapter – I will review potential mechanisms underlying age-related decline in language function. The focus will be on alterations in neural function and neural systems across the life span rather than on psychological or linguistic explanations.

2 Domains of Language Knowledge

Knowledge is represented in the brain as the strength of neural connections [3]. There are many domains of neural connectivity underlying language function (Table 8.1). Most obviously, there is the connectivity underlying semantic knowledge, our knowledge of the world and the objects within it. There is also the connectivity supporting our knowledge of the sequential order of the phonemes in the languages we speak [4, 5]. Patterns of neural activity involving the substrates for semantic knowledge (concept representations) become manifest as spoken word forms through connections linking substrates for semantic knowledge and phonologic sequence knowledge, commonly understood as lexical knowledge. Connectivity between auditory association cortices and substrates for semantic knowledge provides the basis

for comprehension of heard words. There is now a vast literature on selective impairment in grammatical morphology (case, gender, number, person, tense, aspect, and mood markers) in patients with Broca's aphasia. As I have noted elsewhere [3], this literature strongly suggests a neural network supporting grammatic morphologic sequence knowledge. Impairment in grammatic morphologic function in agrammatic patients reflects the combination of loss of this sequence knowledge and loss of knowledge represented in the connectivity between association cortices, particularly frontal, and the presumably perisylvian substrate for this morphologic sequence knowledge. Recently, employing techniques of diffusion tensor tractography, we have provided evidence of two perisylvian repositories of sequence knowledge, one linking auditory association cortices to Broca's region via the supramarginal gyrus, the other linking auditory association cortices to Broca's region via mid/anterior superior temporal gyrus and a white matter pathway traversing the external and extreme capsules [6]. We presume that both pathways support both phonologic and morphologic sequence knowledge but that, by virtue of the patterns of input they are exposed to during language acquisition (lexical-semantic and grammatic, respectively), the circumsylvian (supramarginal) network has an advantage in acquiring phonological sequence knowledge, whereas the transsylvian mid/anterior temporal pathway has an advantage in acquiring morphologic sequence knowledge. We have also found evidence of extensive connectivity (yet another knowledge domain) between almost the entire frontal convexity cortex and Broca's region [7] that presumably enables the selection of grammatic morphemes from the portfolio provided by the substrate for morphologic sequence knowledge.

Yet another domain of language knowledge, one presumably involving frontal convexity cortex and its

Table 8.1 Domains of language knowledge

Core
  Phonologic sequence*
  Semantic*
  Semantic-phonologic* (lexical – word form)
  Acoustic-semantic* (lexical)
Grammar
  Grammatic morphologic sequence
  Semantic-morphologic* (lexical – grammatic morphology)
  Sentence-level word order (syntax)
  Syntactic morphologic
Ancillary
  Visual-semantic* (naming to confrontation)
  Visual-phonologic* (naming to confrontation)

Note: Asterisks denote knowledge domains reviewed in Section 3 of this chapter.

links to postcentral cortices, enables the sequential ordering of concept representations and their modifications, that is, syntax. Connectivity between frontal cortex and perisylvian cortices (another knowledge domain) provides the basis for selection of words of purely grammatic significance, such as complementizers (she knew *that* he would go) and conjunctions.

Finally, there are two domains of knowledge that are essential to naming to confrontation, one enabling the translation of visual representations into concept representations, thence to phonologic/articulatory motor representations, the other enabling direct translation of visual representations into phonologic/articulatory motor representations. Differential damage to the former results in nonoptic aphasia [8], and to the latter, optic aphasia [9, 10].

Unfortunately, we lack data on age-related changes in a number of these knowledge domains. Only those denoted by an asterisk in Table 8.1 will be reviewed in the next section. Space does not allow consideration of such language-related functions as reading, writing, and spelling.

3 Aging-Related Changes in Specific Domains of Language Knowledge

3.1 Semantics

Tests of vocabulary probe semantic knowledge. Arguably, the purest test of vocabulary is synonym judgment because it does not require translation of a concept representation into a phonologic representation. It is often said that, unlike other domains of language knowledge, vocabulary continuously increases over the life span. This turns out not to be strictly correct. Bowles and Salthouse [11] reported performance on synonym judgment, antonym judgment, the Wechsler Adult Intelligence Scale vocabulary test, and the Woodcock Johnson picture vocabulary test for 3,512 adults who had participated in at least one of 18 prior studies that included one or more vocabulary tests. Performance on synonym judgments tests was representative. Performance improved in more or less linear fashion between ages 23 and 55, plateaued through age 75, and declined thereafter. However, the magnitude of the changes was modest. The gain between ages 23 and 55 was 0.9 SD. The loss between ages 75 and 85 was 0.4 SD. Consistent with these findings, Marini et al. [12] found that, in a study of picture description involving 69 participants aged 20–84, only those in the 75–84 age group exhibited an increased tendency to produce semantic paraphasic errors.

3.2 Lexicon
3.2.1 Word Finding Difficulty
Schmitter-Edgecombe and colleagues [13] studied responses to the Test of Word Finding in Discourse in 26 young (mean 18.93 years), 26 middle-aged (66.29), and 26 old-old (79.9) adults. They measured average number of substitutions (e.g., "She bought a windmill" (instead of "pinwheel")) and word reformulations (e.g., "He is, she is catching a butterfly"), as well as time fillers, insertions, and delays, per "T-unit" (in effect, a sentence). Middle-aged and old-old participants produced approximately twice the rate of substitutions and reformulations.

Salthouse and Mandell [14] examined the tip of the tongue (TOT) experience in 718 adults, age range 23–83, in naming to definition, description of places and people, and naming of famous faces (politicians and celebrities). A TOT state occurs when respondents are unable to produce a word even as they are certain that they know it. It has been shown that subjects in TOT states are able to name the initial phoneme and estimate the number of syllables with far greater than chance accuracy [4]. There was no age effect on TOT incidence with naming to definition. However, age accounted for 6–11% of the variance in TOT incidence with naming to description and

7–14% of the variance in naming of famous faces. Evrard [15] provided further evidence of the particular problem with proper nouns. In a study of 33 young (25.9 ± 4.85 years), 30 middle-aged (45.39 ± 6.68), and 33 older participants (63.59 ± 6.45), he tested naming latency and TOT incidence for photographs of everyday objects and very famous faces. Naming latency was greater for famous faces (approximately 2,000 milliseconds) than for everyday objects (1,300 milliseconds) but there was no age effect. However, while there was no age-related difference in TOT incidence for everyday objects (<2%), TOT incidence for very famous faces was 8.9% among the young and 18.3% among the older participants. Rendell et al. [16], in a study of 20 young (21.25 ± 3.02 years), 20 young-old (66.85 ± 1.35), and 20 old-old (73.4 ± 2.76) participants involving naming of 36 famous faces and 36 unfamiliar objects, found no age-related change in proportions of objects named correctly. However, there was a substantial decline in ability to name faces the participants recognized, from 64% to 46% correct (age × stimulus type interaction effect: p = 0.002). On the basis of further analyses, Rendell et al. concluded that the difference in object and face naming may have been related to a difference in familiarity. However, James [17] found more TOTs for names than for biographical information among older adults for photographs of celebrities judged to be familiar.

3.2.2 Naming to Confrontation

As I have noted, naming can occur via a single step, a direct route linking visual representations to phonologic/articulatory motor representations (in which case naming occurs without reference to meaning), or via a two-step indirect route from visual representations to semantic representations and thence to phonologic/articulatory motor representations (a third domain of knowledge). Both routes, hence both sets of knowledge, are likely used simultaneously and it is not possible to determine which is rate limiting.

Many studies of changes in the lexicon have employed the Boston Naming Test (BNT). Zec et al. [18], in a cross-sectional study of 1,111 participants, compared BNT performance (without cueing) across four decades (50–89) and as a function of education (less than high school, high school, greater than high school). Higher education was associated with an approximately 3.5–5 item better performance with no evidence of an age × education interaction effect. Participants in the lowest age group (50–59) on

average named four more items than those in the highest age group (80–89). When the analysis was limited to the 194 participants who had no evidence of dementia five or more years later, there was still a negative correlation of BNT performance with age (r = 0.15), although it was about half that of the remainder of the participants (see also [19]). Cross-sectional studies are susceptible to cohort effects: the learning experience of older subjects through the course of a lifetime is likely to have been different from that of younger subjects. In this respect, longitudinal studies are to be preferred. However, longitudinal studies pose risks of practice effects and their results could be biased by differential dropout across age groups. With these caveats in mind, the results of a second study of 541 participants by Zec et al. [20], this one longitudinal, are of interest. This study excluded participants who achieved criteria for dementia or amnestic mild cognitive impairment during the follow-up period. Mean annual rate of change in the 50–59 age group was +0.13, in the 60–69 group 0, in the 70–79 group −0.15, and in the 80–89 group, −0.15 (i.e., 1.5 words per decade). These are very modest changes. Tabor Connor et al. [21] reported BNT performance with semantic and phonological cueing in a longitudinal study of 236 participants aged between 30 and 90. They found a decline between ages 50 and 90 of 11% (6.6 items) with a slight acceleration over the age range. This study suggests that the value of semantic and phonological cueing declines more steeply with age than does uncued naming.

3.3 Phonological Sequence

I know of no data bearing directly on the integrity of phonological sequence knowledge over the life span. However, MacKay and James [22] carried out a reading experiment that sheds some light on this knowledge domain. Thirty-two young (19.1 ± 1.2 years) and 32 older (72.4 ± 3.1) adults were enrolled in a single word-naming task in which participants had to change /p/ to /b/ or vice versa. The older adults tended to make more omission errors, for example, stimulus-(target) → response: bans-(pans) → pan; preach-(breach) → beach, and sequential errors, usually anticipatory, for example, laps-(labs) → baps, but occasionally perseverative, for example, peg-(beg) → peb. All participants preserved strong sequences, for example, laps → labs, with maintenance of the

/s/ → /z/ phonetic transformation. However, older participants more often simply failed to make the /p/ → /b/ substitution in this situation.

3.4 Comprehension (Acoustic-Semantic [Lexical] Knowledge)

Auditory comprehension remains stable up to approximately age 65, at which point it progressively declines, exhibiting a total decline of about 1 SD by age 85 [23].

3.5 Syntax

Kemper and Sumner [24], in a cross-sectional study, assessed syntactic complexity during discourse about an influential person or interesting experience that had an effect on life in 100 young (22.8 ± 2.4 years) and 100 elderly (76.4 ± 6.2) adults. Syntactic complexity was operationally defined by "D-level," an ordinal scale ranging from 0 (simple, one-clause sentences) to 7 (complex sentences with multiple forms of embedding and subordination). They found a modest decline in D-level with age, from 2.5 to 2.0. ($p < 0.05$). In a second study, involving 30 participants aged 65–75 and followed for up to 15 years, Kemper and colleagues [25] found that syntactic complexity was maintained to about age 75 and then declined substantially thereafter.

3.6 Grammatic Morphology

There do not appear to be any published studies on the impact of aging on the integrity of grammatic morphologic sequence knowledge. Investigation of verb past tense formation might be a useful line of inquiry. Kavé and Levy [26] reported a study that probed the domain of semantic morphologic knowledge, that is, the integrity of the connectivity enabling selection of grammatic morphemes in a manner that is appropriate to the thematic roles of verb arguments. Verb representations, in the process of their association with noun concept representations, modify those representations to simultaneously incorporate the action and define thematic roles. To one degree or another, depending on how richly inflected the language is, this process engages specific grammatic morphologic representations from the substrate for morphologic sequence knowledge. Kavé and Levy looked at subject–verb agreement in gender marking in 48 young (23.04 ± 1.71 years) and

48 elderly (74.48 ± 4.33) speakers of Hebrew, a richly inflected language. The dependent measure was latency to read gender-congruent and gender-incongruent verbs in sentence context. Congruent and incongruent latencies in the young group were 637 and 660 milliseconds, respectively. In the elderly group, they were 934 and 989 milliseconds, respectively. The age × congruence interaction was statistically significant ($p < 0.05$), indicating that the members of the elderly group were significantly slower in dealing with incongruency. The authors also found that, in a lexical decision task involving pseudo-verbs with existent roots and pseudo-verbs with nonexistent roots, both older and younger adults were relatively slower in rejecting those with existent roots; however, there was an age × condition interaction effect such that older adults were significantly slower.

Marini et al. [12] found that in a narrative picture description task administered to 69 adults ranging in age from 20 to 84, members of the oldest age group (75–84) made significantly more paragrammatic errors. This could reflect either degradation of phonologic sequence knowledge or defective selection of grammatic morphemes.

3.7 Narrative Discourse

Narrative discourse depends largely on the definition of narrative goals as distributed representations and the orderly selection and modification of distributed concept representations commensurate with these goals. Wright et al. [27], in a study of 30 young (aged 23.67 ± 2.70) and 30 older participants (76.90 ± 4.51) involving narration from a picture story book without text, found that the two groups produced the same number of propositions. They also found, replicating an earlier study by Kemper and Sumner [24], that old participants used approximately 50% more words to relate the stories. They did not provide statistical data that might yield insight into the contributors to this age-related reduction in efficiency. However, they did provide a representative discourse sample from two participants, one young, one old. Review of these samples suggests that the older participant was more stimulus bound, devoting many words to specific details of the pictures and including many more sentences inferring motives and goals that were not particularly relevant to the overall narrative goal.

Marini et al. [12], in a study of 69 Italian participants aged 20–84 quantitatively assessing picture description, found that those in the 75–84 age group demonstrated reduced local coherence (the extent to which each utterance of the story was conceptually related to the utterance preceding it), an increase in errors of local coherence (errors involving anaphorical pronouns and number and gender agreement between pronouns and noun phrases across utterances), and a significant reduction in global coherence (the degree to which the main or essential propositions of a story were present in the correct order). They also found a gradual decline in lexical informativeness across the life span (the ratio of content and function words that were directly relevant to the narrative to total number of words produced).

Older adults, in repeatedly recomposing a spoken narrative from an eight-frame cartoon, unlike younger subjects, do not improve the succinctness of their narrative, defined by reduction in total words used and increase in words uttered per second, and their narratives have lower information content [28]. Older adults show a much greater tendency to relate information that has already been provided, contradict themselves, and show inconsistency in referents (e.g., pronouns).

Older adults are as good as younger adults at improving the efficiency of their verbal guidance to a partner in selecting one picture from an array of four as they and the partner gain experience with the stimulus sets, so long as they are able to benefit from cues (verbal evidence of comprehension) provided by the partner [29]. However, when guidance has to be provided to the familiar partner in the absence of cues from that partner, older adults are significantly less effective than younger participants in creating a narrative guidance strategy that takes advantage of the commonality of knowledge that the guider and partner had previously established.

4 Possible Mechanisms of Age-Related Decline in Language Function

4.1 Degenerative

In studies of aging effects on cognitive function, auditory or visual stimuli are designed to overcome mild deficits in hearing or vision and participants with noncompensable deficits are excluded. However, in daily life, hearing and visual impairment and defects in perceptual processing that reduce signal to noise ratio can lead to imprecise engagement of cerebral

representations of these stimuli, hence degradation of response, and there is good evidence that the potentially deleterious effect of impairment in perception has been broadly underestimated and inadequately controlled in studies of various domains of language function [1]. In particular, even mild age-related impairment in auditory acuity can have substantial effects on auditory electrophysiology at the brain-stem level, and both hearing loss and age are associated with impairment in auditory cortical processing with consequent deficits in auditory comprehension [23, 30].

Mild impairment in cognitive function can of course reflect the earliest stages of well-known dementing processes such as Alzheimer's disease, microvascular disease related to underlying risk factors such as hypertension, frontotemporal lobar degeneration (primary progressive aphasia), Parkinson's disease, and diffuse Lewy body disease. Although Alzheimer's disease remains the most common underlying cause of cognitive impairment up to age 100 and beyond, cerebral arteriolosclerosis (not necessarily related to underlying risk factors) and two more recently defined entities, primary age-related tauopathy (PART) and hippocampal sclerosis of aging/cerebral age-related TDP-43 with sclerosis (CARTS), become progressively more prevalent after age 80 [31, 32] (see Chapter 2, this volume). Most patients exhibit multiple pathologies at autopsy. The cognitive profile of these more recently defined entities remains poorly defined and language function has not been characterized in any detail. There is some evidence that PART presents as memory impairment in the absence of other cognitive decline, whereas CARTS, although it may start with memory impairment, tends to follow a trajectory resembling frontotemporal lobar degeneration [33]. Cerebral arteriolosclerosis has been linked to impairment in BNT performance and category fluency [34]. The rate of progression of these disorders is unknown and it is possible that incipient pathology could become manifest during the 70s and 80s.

4.2 Aging-Related Alteration of Neural Function

Neural function can decline over the life span in the absence of identifiable pathology as a consequence of processes that might best be viewed as ontogenetic or epigenetic (see Chapter 3). These processes most clearly affect memory acquisition but could have some bearing on aging-related changes in language function.

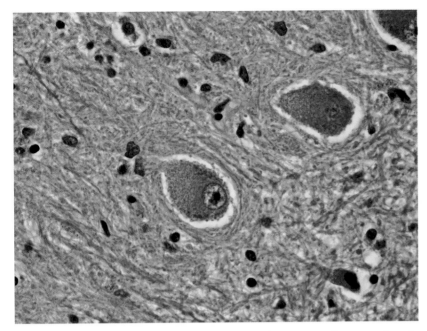

Figure 2.2 Two neurons containing granular yellowish lipofuscin pigment (dentate nucleus of cerebellum).

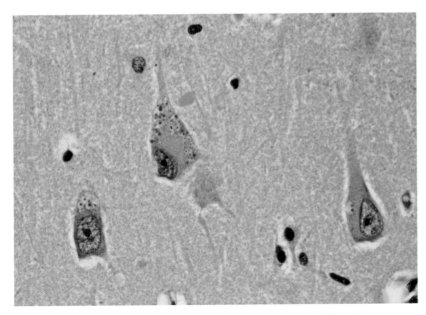

Figure 2.3 Three CA1 neurons showing granulovacuolar degeneration (H&E stain).

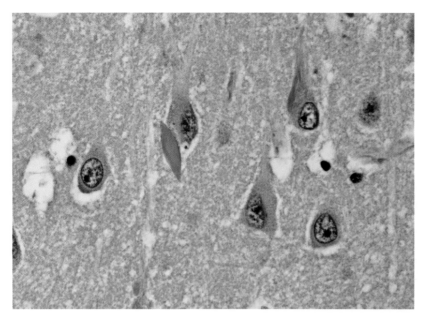

Figure 2.4 Hirano body: eosinophilic rod-shaped structure in close proximity to a hippocampal pyramidal neuron (H&E stain).

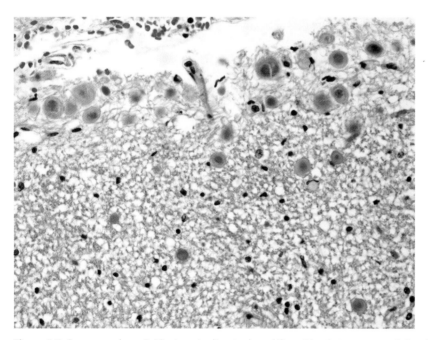

Figure 2.5 Corpora amylacea: 5–20 micron in diameter basophilic entities that are concentric lamellated structures commonly located in subpial, perivascular, and subependymal regions (H&E stain).

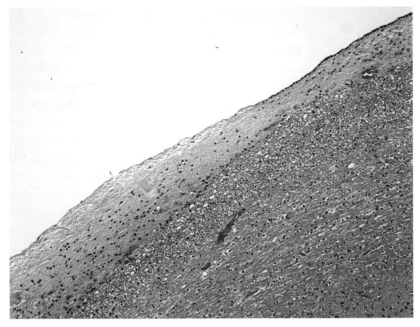

Figure 2.6 Subependymal reactive gliosis (center and lower left of image) that occurred in an area of ependymal denudation (H&E stain).

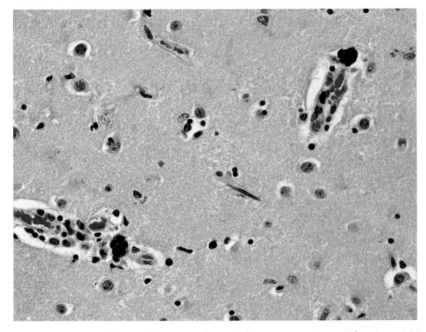

Figure 2.7 Perivascular hemosiderin accumulation (dark concretions – bottom left and top right) seen frequently in the basal ganglia with aging (H&E stain).

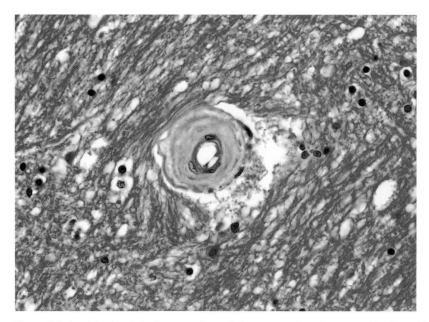

Figure 2.8 Arteriolosclerosis, hyaline type, of a small deep penetrating white matter blood vessel (H&E stain).

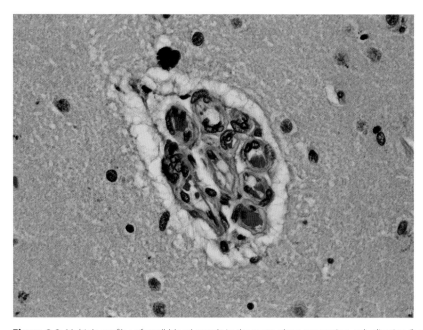

Figure 2.9 Multiple profiles of small blood vessels in the same plane suggesting reduplication (basal ganglia; H&E stain).

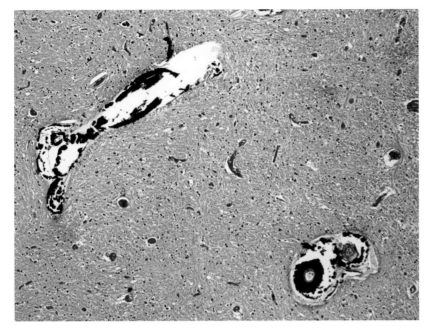

Figure 2.10 Blood vessels of the globus pallidus showing extensive calcification (H&E stain).

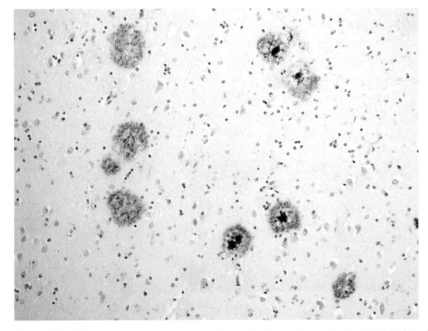

Figure 2.11 Diffuse (left) and neuritic plaques (right, with Aβ-amyloid cores). The patient had no detectable neurofibrillary tangles or Lewy body pathology and was cognitively intact ("pathological aging") (immunohistochemistry for Aβ-amyloid).

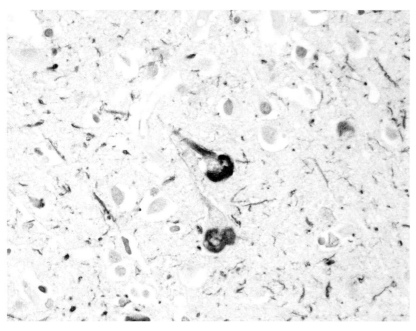

Figure 2.12 Tau-immunoreactive neurofibrillary tangles and neuropil threads in neurons of the transentorhinal cortex. The patient was 88 years old and had no apparent diffuse or neuritic plaques or Lewy body pathology ("primary age-related tauopathy").

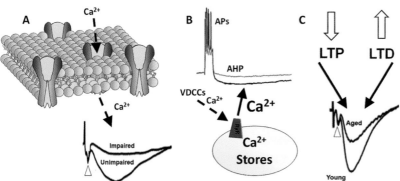

Figure 3.1 Senescent physiology due to a shift in Ca^{2+} regulation. (A) A decrease in Ca^{2+} influx through the NMDA receptor-gated channel of aged cognitively impaired animals is observed as a decrease in the NMDA receptor synaptic response for a given number of afferents activated. (B) During the generation of action potentials (APs), the depolarization activates voltage-dependent Ca^{2+} channels (VDCCs) in the membrane, and the Ca^{2+} influx through VDCCs acts on ryanodine receptors (RyR) on intracellular Ca^{2+} stores to increase Ca^{2+}-induced Ca^{2+} release (CICR). The Ca^{2+} from CICR activates sensitive potassium channels in the membrane to increase the amplitude of the after-hyperpolarization (AHP) in impaired (dark trace) relative to unimpaired (gray trace) animals. The larger after-hyperpolarization reduces cell burst activity and contributes to altered synaptic plasticity. (C) The shift in Ca^{2+} alters the balance of kinase and phosphatase activity, impairing LTP and facilitating induction of LTD. Altered synaptic plasticity promotes a decrease in synaptic transmission through the hippocampus, particularly for aged memory impaired animals. The open arrow heads in panels A and C indicate the fiber potential that precedes the synaptic responses.

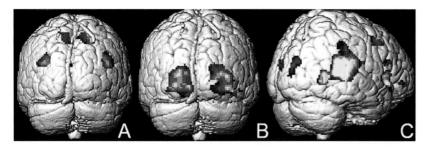

Figure 4.4 Activation observed in older adults on three perceptual tasks. (A) Location discrimination elicited activation in regions of the dorsal pathway (angular gyrus bilaterally, right precuneus, and left superior parietal lobule). (B) Shape discrimination elicited activation in the ventral pathway (left middle occipital gyrus, right middle temporal gyrus, and fusiform and lingual gyri). (C) Velocity discrimination elicited activation in the V5/MT (occipitotemporoparietal junction) and frontal areas; a large right hemisphere cluster with peak activity in the superior temporal gyrus; left middle occipital, cuneus, and supramarginal regions; and anterior right hemisphere regions with peak activity in the middle and inferior frontal gyri. These patterns were not different from those elicited in younger participants.

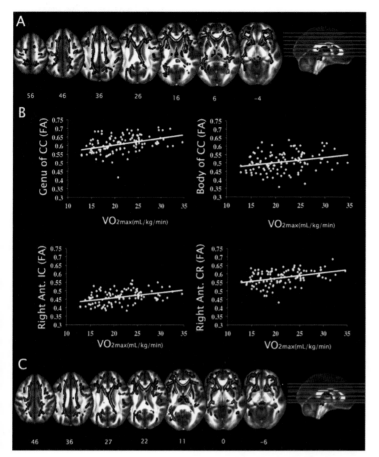

Figure 16.1 Relationship between fitness and white matter integrity in older adults. Shown are significant associations between cardiorespiratory fitness (CRF), fractional anisotropy (FA), and mean spatial working memory performance from Experiment 1 (of 2). (A) Clusters of voxels where fitness was significantly associated with FA. Warm-colored voxels show positive associations, cool-colored voxels demonstrate negative associations. Side panels indicate slice placements. Age, gender, and years of education were included as covariates. The z-plane coordinates of each slice, in MNI space, are presented at the bottom. For visualization purposes, tbss_fill was used to dilate statistical maps. (B) For illustration purposes, scatterplots and best-fit lines are shown for the relationship between CRF and FA in selected regions. (C) Spatial distribution of indirect path voxel clusters. Cyan-colored voxel clusters show a positive indirect effect, brown voxel clusters indicate a negative indirect effect. Ant, anterior; CC, corpus callosum; Ext, external; FA, fractional anisotropy; IC, internal capsule. From Oberlin et al. 2016 [10].

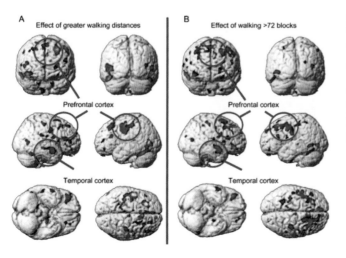

Figure 16.2 Brain regions associated with greater levels of walking. (A) Brain regions showing an association between greater amounts of physical activity (blocks walked) at baseline and greater gray matter volume. Statistical map is thresholded with a false discovery rate of p = 0.05 and a minimum cluster threshold of 100 contiguous voxels. (B) Brain regions showing greater volume in the highest activity quartile of the sample (>72 blocks walked in 2 weeks) compared with the bottom three quartiles. There were no reliable differences in brain volume among the bottom three quartiles. From Erickson et al., 2010 [57].

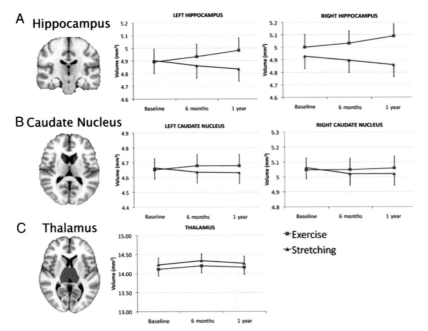

Figure 16.3 An exercise intervention increases the size of the hippocampus in older adults. (A) Example of hippocampus segmentation and graphs demonstrating a significant increase in hippocampus volume for the aerobic exercise group and a decrease in volume for the stretching control group. (B) Example of caudate nucleus segmentation and graphs demonstrating the change in volume for both groups. (C) Example of thalamus segmentation and graph demonstrating the change in volume for both groups. None of the changes was significant for the caudate or thalamus. From Erickson et al. 2011 [60].

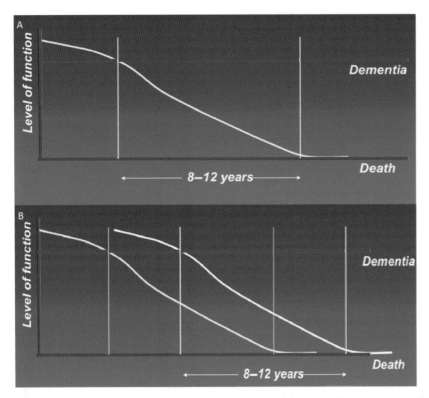

Figure 19.1 (A) Averaged natural history of cognitive/functional decline in Alzheimer's disease. The first vertical yellow line represents the onset of detectable symptoms; the second (white) line indicates approximate time of death. (B) Effect of a successful prevention or disease-modifying delay strategy. The curve of deterioration will be shifted to the right, delaying the onset of initial symptoms and subsequent decline to dementia. At the time when a person would have died if untreated, they would have only mild to moderate symptoms. If symptom onset is delayed by, e.g., 5 years, AD prevalence will be reduced 40% or more several decades later, and more people would die of a competing mortality with milder or no symptoms. If the delay in onset were extended to 10 years, the majority of cases of AD would be prevented, since the prevalence increases with age greater than 70 and thus most treated people would die of a competing mortality while cognitively normal or much less severely impaired.

4.3 Exogenous Noise

Cognitive impairment, including language dysfunction, can be caused by any of a number of factors, several of which become more prevalent with advanced age. These include migraine, restful sleep deprivation (particularly due to restless leg syndrome/ periodic limb movements of sleep and obstructive sleep apnea), fatigue, central nervous system active drugs, and distraction related to pain or situational stress. The potential impact of these factors has received scant attention in studies of language change with aging.

4.4 Mechanistic

In the following sections I will consider potential explanations for alterations of language function over the life span that stem from foundational properties of neural networks and neural systems and their ontogenesis.

4.4.1 Endogenous Neural Network Noise

The evidence of aging effects on orthographic-phonologic sequence transduction provided by the experiment of MacKay and James [22] (see Section 3.3 above, "Phonological Sequence") suggests that, with aging, neural networks – at least pattern associator networks supporting domains of sequence knowledge – have diminished capacity for dampening perturbation-induced noise. In the MacKay and James study, this resulted in a tendency to omit terminal phonemes that are both inconsistently used and unstressed, such as the plural "s" marker; to slip from less frequently used consonant clusters to simple consonants (e.g., breach → beach); and to make sequential errors as multiple phonemes remain in play while the network settles into the final sequence (e.g., laps → baps). Strong sequences, for example, lap/s/ and lab/z/, were preserved simply because the alternatives, lap/z/ and lab/s/, do not exist in the English phonological sequence lexicon. Neurophysiologic studies, including human electrocorticography, have in fact shown that aging is accompanied by an increase in baseline neural activity – neural noise [35].

Increases in neural noise could also contribute to the slowing of processing observed in nearly all studies of aging effects by virtue of resultant slowing of the process of settling into stable representations (attractor states; see below).

4.4.2 Neighborhood Density

Knowledge is accumulated throughout the life span on the basis of individual experiences and incorporated into cerebral cortex as changes in synaptic connection strengths, either directly (as in procedural and implicit memory acquisition) or via the hippocampal system (episodic memory acquisition). This encoding of knowledge in neural connectivity enables the generation of concept representations, which are population encoded (distributed), as patterns of features, but ultimately, as patterns of neural activity involving very large numbers of cortical micro-columns and billions of neurons [3]. The mathematical function of cortical activity is a surface in an N-dimensional hyperspace. To understand how this might look, we can do a thought experiment, taking a three-dimensional slice of the corresponding energy landscape, just as we might take a two-dimensional slice of a three-dimensional loaf of bread. In Figure 8.1, I have created such a slice in the general vicinity of mammals. The basin/sub-basin/sub-sub-basin organization of the surface reflects the mathematical properties of the underlying neural network, which provides the basis for a propensity to settle into attractor basins. The location of any one point of the surface on the z-axis represents the strength of encoding in neural connectivity, which is defined by extent of features shared with other concepts, frequency, and age of acquisition. Distance along the radial axis represents atypicality. At the very center of the large basin, the mammal basin is a representation of a prototypic mammal – something for which there is no exemplar. However, there are mammals, such as dogs, that would generally be regarded as highly typical mammals. Near the edge of the mammal basin are sub-basins corresponding to atypical mammals, such as platypuses and whales. Whales have a deep attractor sub-basin because we frequently consider them. Within sub-basins, there are sub-sub-basins, for example, corresponding to types of dogs. The variable θ signifies only that sources of atypicality vary; for example, whales are atypical in a different way than platypuses.

The usefulness of this mathematical conceptualization becomes fully apparent when we consider what happens to the surface depicted in Figure 8.1 in the context of semantic dementia. Because displacement along the z-axis is defined by strength of representation in neural connectivity, with loss of neurons and

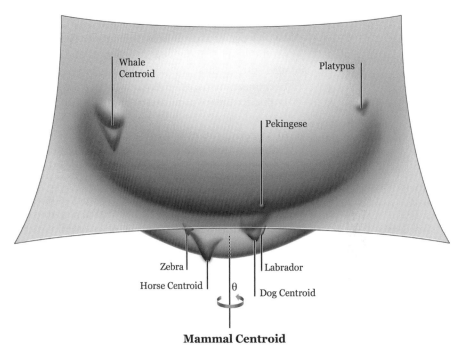

Mammal Centroid

Figure 8.1 Mathematical surface representing the energy landscape of population activity in the vicinity of mammals distributed over semantic cortices. From Nadeau SE. *The Neural Architecture of Grammar*. Cambridge, MA: MIT Press, 2012, with permission.

connections, the effect will be vertical attenuation of the whole manifold – in effect, it will become shallower. More atypical basins (e.g., platypus), as well as small sub-sub-basins (e.g., Pekinese and Labrador), will disappear. Other sub-basins will become shallower, such that the system will not necessarily settle into one of them even though perceptual input specifies that sub-basin. For example, a patient looking at a zebra may slip to the sub-basin closer to the centroid of the mammal basin and call it a horse – a coordinate semantic error. Or that same patient may slip all the way to the mammal centroid and call it a mammal or an animal (the latter preferred because of the basic level effect [36]) – a superordinate semantic error. Both phenomena are commonly observed in patients with semantic dementia.

Let us assume that in normal aging, the association cortices encoding semantic knowledge are intact. However, over the course of a lifetime, a large amount of knowledge has been accumulated. For example, an older person, when asked about members of the cat family, might respond not just with house cats, lions, tigers, leopards, and cheetahs, but also with ocelots, jaguars, panthers, bobcats, lynxes, snow leopards, servals, caracals, and margays. In other words,

the semantic cat neighborhood becomes considerably more crowded (in contrast to the sparse neighborhood featured in Figure 8.1). Semantic neighborhood density is greater in the elderly [37]. An older person might also know of more features shared between semantic neighbors. The more features shared between a given exemplar and its neighbors, the broader its attractor basin (the extreme breadth of the mammal attractor basin reflects the astounding number of features that mammals hold in common). Given increased neighborhood density and broader attractor basins, there will tend to be greater overlap between neighboring basins, and the latency to descend into the particular attractor basin specified by perceptual input, rather than a near neighbor that shares many features, will tend to increase. There will also tend to be more non-responses that occur when the threshold for one discrete phonological representation is not met, and an increase in the propensity for semantic and phonological slips. Psychological studies have shown that near semantic neighbors tend to compete with the exemplar, prolonging response latency, whereas more distant neighbors tend to promote the exemplar, presumably by virtue of priming via shared features [38, 39]. Mean distance between

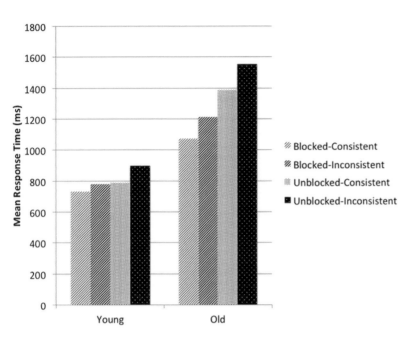

Figure 8.2 Aging effects on test performance on a modified Hayling test. Data from Tournier I, Postal V, Mathey S. Investigation of age-related differences in an adapted Hayling task. *Archives of Gerontology and Geriatrics.* 2014;59:599–606.

related words in semantic space has been shown to be a strong predictor of word recognition and semantic priming [40, 41].

What is the evidence of such effects in aging? Tournier et al. [42] employed a variation of the Hayling Test in a study of 30 young (20.68 ± 1.89 years) and 31 older (69.61 ± 7.35) participants matched for education. In the Hayling Test, participants are presented with sentences to which they have to provide a semantically consistent or inconsistent response. For example:

The child is crying for his . . . (mother)

The child is crying for his . . . (planet)

Tournier and colleagues changed the administration of the test in several ways to overcome some of its methodological shortcomings. To test for the possible role of strategy formation, they presented both the traditional blocked version and an unblocked version. Because search for a semantically inappropriate response can impose demands above and beyond those related to the feature of inappropriateness, they actually provided an inappropriate word. Finally, they allowed the participants to read the sentences on their own so that results would not be affected by differences in reading speed. For each sentence, both appropriate and inappropriate responses were provided, participants were cued as to which type to give, and the dependent variable was response latency. The

results are presented in Figure 8.2. Older participants were slower across the board, and they were relatively slower in the unblocked condition, which prevents the use of a response strategy. However, in both the blocked and unblocked conditions, older participants showed a particular disadvantage in the inconsistent condition, the condition in which semantic neighborhood effects would be more likely to be exerting an effect (in the consistent condition, the appropriate response receives heavy semantic priming from the preceding sentence). As noted above, semantic neighborhood density is greater in old subjects [37]. This would make the task more difficult for the elderly, explaining, at least in part, their poorer performance.

Whereas semantic neighborhoods are defined by extent of semantic features shared between concept representations, phonologic sequence neighborhoods are defined by extent of phonological sequence shared between representations.[1] Sommers and Danielson

---

[1] Phonological sequence neighborhoods should not be confused with phonological neighborhoods (discussed below), which are defined by the number of words that share a phonological sequence, a word being neurally defined as a semantic representation and the corresponding phonological sequence representation that is generated by virtue of the connectivity between the substrates for semantic and phonological sequence knowledge [43].

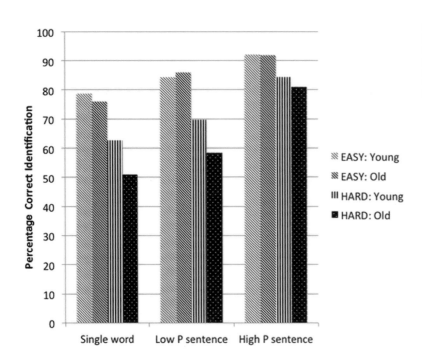

Figure 8.3 Phonemic context effects on lexical discrimination as a function of age. Data from Sommers MS, Danielson SM. Inhibitory processes and spoken word recognition in young and older adults: the interaction of lexical competition and semantic context. *Psychology and Aging*. 1999;14:458–72.

[44] (see also Taler et al. [45]) reported a study of phonemic context effects on lexical discrimination in 22 young (20 ± 2.1 years) and 20 elderly (75.5 ± 4.2) participants balanced for education and WAIS vocabulary. They defined phonemic similarity (corresponding to phonological sequence similarity) in traditional fashion as words differing from the target by addition, deletion, or substitution of a single phoneme. The increase in knowledge in the course of a lifetime should result in greater crowding of phonological sequence neighborhoods no less than semantic neighborhoods, plus the entities in these phonological sequence neighborhoods should have more semantic neighbors, which would come into play through bottom-up/top-down interaction effects. They posed three experimental conditions: (1) single words (SW), for example, "path"; (2) low probability (LP) sentences, for example, "She was thinking about the *path*"; and (3) high probability (HP) sentences, for example, "She was walking along the *path*." Index words were classified as easy or hard. Easy words were characterized by a mean phonemic neighborhood density of 9.1 (range 1–42) and a mean phonemic neighborhood frequency of 43.5 per million. Hard words were characterized by a mean phonemic neighborhood density of 28 and a mean phonemic neighborhood frequency of 455.8 per million. In order to

separate phonemic context effects from other possible contributions to item difficulty, stimuli were presented in the context of speech-shaped white noise ("pink noise") titrated in intensity to achieve equal young and old performance with easy words within each of the three contexts (SW, LP, HP). Listeners were asked to write down the word they thought was presented, or the last word in the sentence. The results are displayed in Figure 8.3. Performance with easy words was equal for young and old participants across all conditions, indicating that the authors achieved their aim in adding pink noise. There was no difference in the high neighborhood density (hard) word performance of young and old subjects when response was strongly aided by a sentence context that semantically primed the correct response (HP sentences). However, performance with hard words by both young and old was much poorer in the SW and LP conditions (in which there was no potential for semantic priming) and performance by old participants was significantly worse than by young participants (age × lexical difficulty × context interaction effect p < 0.001). Furthermore, the probability of producing a phonemic neighbor was higher in the elderly in SW and LP contexts. These results parallel an earlier study by Sommers [46] that found age-related deficits in perception of words in high-density phonological neighborhoods. Sommers and Danielson suggested their results might be explained by age-related decline in inhibitory control, supporting this argument by demonstrating correlations between performance in SW and LP conditions and performance on an auditory Stroop task, which was significantly poorer in the elderly (see Section 4.4.6 below, "Balance of Volitional and Reactive Intention"). However, as for semantic neighborhood effects, age-related differences in phonemic neighborhood density might also account for the results.

Newman and German [47], in a study of naming of pictures, sentence completion, and naming to definition in 1,075 individuals across the life span, reported roughly comparable results. Performance was worse with words from dense phonological neighborhoods. However, the effect was more marked among adolescents.

Phonological neighborhood effects, traditionally defined, may differ in the elderly. There is a strong consensus that in speech perception and word recognition tasks, phonologically related words compete [43, 48]. On the other hand, in speech production tasks, which have predominantly involved the tip of the tongue (TOT) phenomenon, words with dense phonological neighborhoods (i.e., many semantic entities that share word phonology) have generally shown a processing advantage [43, 48]. However, Vitevitch and Sommers [48] could not replicate this finding in a study of participants aged greater than 65, either in a TOT task or in latency of naming to confrontation. This difference could reflect the interaction of age-related differences in phonological sequence knowledge, on the one hand, and the links to semantic knowledge, which provide the basis for phonological neighborhood effects, on the other. More critically, these studies have not taken into account the ways in which regularities in phonological sequence experience might be wired into neural network connectivity [3] and the likelihood that in the phonologic sequence knowledge domain, regularities in particular word segments, for example, rhymes, may be preeminent in defining neighbor closeness. Thus, bat, fat, gnat, hat, mat, pat, sat, stat, tat, and vat may be closer phonological neighbors of cat than are caught, kit, kite, cot, coot, cute, and cut, even though members of each group differ by a single phoneme. In this view, members of rhyme neighborhoods might compete with the target, as do near semantic neighbors, whereas non-rhyme neighbors

might promote the target, as with more distant semantic neighbors. Notably, Newman and German [47] found that across the life span, words with high phonotactic probability (i.e., words that share phonemes and phoneme pairs characterized by high biphone probability) are produced more accurately (see also Vitevitch and Luce [49, 50]). Measures of biphone probability capture the effects of all regularities in phonological sequence but they might not adequately prioritize certain sequence regularities, for example, rhyme effects, that might be salient. Experimental capture of these effects might account for the failure of words with dense phonological neighborhoods to confer a processing advantage on TOT tasks in the elderly.

4.4.3 Age of Acquisition

Controlling for frequency, words acquired earlier in life are produced with greater reliability and at shorter latencies [51, 52] and they are relatively spared in aphasia [53–55] and dementia [56]. Age of acquisition effects persist through the lifetime and may become more marked after age 60 [47]. The mechanisms underlying age of acquisition effects remain uncertain. Psychological explanations have included differences in cumulative frequency of use and differences in time spent in lexical memory [57]. A neural hypothesis, formulated by Ellis and Lambon Ralph [51], is that the age of acquisition effect reflects the evolution in the magnitude of change in neural network connectivity that occurs with the learning of items over the course of the training life span of the network – that is, the evolution of its plasticity. They tested this hypothesis in an extensive series of training simulations employing a three-layer parallel distributed processing (PDP) network (100 input units, 50 intermediate units, 100 output units). Connection weights were initially set to small random values and adjusted during training in the direction of a maximum of +1 or a minimum of −1. A large set of abstract representations was fed to the input units and the network had to make a systematic change in each input pattern, which was expressed as a pattern across the output units. The network learned how to make this change through a training technique known as back propagation. Back propagation involves comparison of actual network output with target output, followed by slight adjustment of network connections strengths in proportion to their contribution to the error – the discrepancy between actual and targeted output pattern. In the course of repeatedly cycling through a training set, the network asymptotically approached optimal production of the desired output patterns for the entire training set. "Early" representation sets were trained during the initial 250 epochs (cycles through the set being trained), at which point (or later) training of "late" representation sets was initiated and sustained for at least 500 epochs (in association with continued training of the "early" set). The investigators found that the accuracy of production achieved with training of late sets was always less than that achieved with early sets, no matter how long training was sustained (out to 100,000 epochs). Furthermore, the later a training set was introduced, the lower the ultimate accuracy, again, no matter how large the number of training epochs. The larger the training set (the "vocabulary" of the network), the worse the ultimate performance, but disproportionately so for late sets. Late-trained sets were more vulnerable to network damage (and, by inference, noise).

The authors sought to determine why this occurred. They discovered that the magnitude of the error measure that drove learning declined over time as the activity of units in the intermediate layer of the network evolved, through the course of training, from an average of 0.5 (on a scale of 0–1, at which point error signal was maximal at 0.25) in the direction of 0 or 1, at which points the error signal was zero. That is, the more items previously trained, whether because of the size of the trained vocabulary or the point in time at which a given training set was introduced, the smaller the connection weight changes that occurred with learning of a new item – in essence, the less the "neuroplasticity" of the network. The smaller weight changes in turn made the production of late acquired items more susceptible to network damage and, by inference, to network noise.

It might fairly be argued that this dynamic was an artifact of the back-propagation algorithm. This criticism is hard to address because, whereas back propagation is a simple and powerful computer algorithm for training networks in simulations, we have yet to achieve a computer-realizable algorithm that captures the complexities involved in encoding of episodic memory by the hippocampal system and subsequent consolidation of these memories, to the extent that they can be consolidated, as declarative memory in cerebral cortex. On the other hand, the fundamental insight achieved by Ellis and Lambon Ralph has found extraordinary confirmation in empirical studies of human subjects. It is also congruent with the emerging concept of synaptic homeostasis [58], which is now supported by almost innumerable experimental studies. Learning during wakefulness corresponds to increases or decreases in synaptic strengths within neural systems implicated in learning experiences. Eventually, this will lead to saturation of neural connectivity as, over time, synaptic strengths are driven to maximal or minimal values. Not only does this steadily reduce learning capacity but it also decreases the ability to selectively encode more important memories. The synaptic homeostasis hypothesis is that during wakefulness, there is, in aggregate, an overall strengthening of synaptic connectivity, while during non-REM sleep, there occurs a normalization of synaptic connectivity defined by comprehensive downgrading of synaptic connections' strengths, constrained by a "survival of the fittest" process in which neural connectivity that is most implicated in the day's knowledge acquisition *and* implicated in existing long-term memory will be least weakened, or even strengthened, while neural connectivity that does not share these attributes will be differentially weakened. Thus, both capacity for further learning (neuroplasticity) and capacity for prioritization of knowledge to be retained are preserved. In this conceptualization, age of acquisition effects could reflect the fact that, given a sustained capacity for prioritization of memories based on reconciliation of existing memories with new experience, early acquired memories, by virtue of lifelong repeated reengagement and by virtue of being least affected by uncompensated saturation of neural connectivity, will be at an advantage.

Age of acquisition effects (and frequency effects) are gradually extinguished by the development of regularities in the knowledge accumulated by a network [52]. They are thus maximal for networks that support arbitrary mapping, for example, naming to confrontation (translation from representations of word meaning into representations of word sound), intermediate for networks with substantial regularities (e.g., semantics), and minimal to zero for networks with transparent mapping, for example, orthography to phonology (reading aloud), particularly in languages with fully transparent orthography. Age of acquisition effects could not readily account for age-related differences in performance on standardized batteries tapping bodies of knowledge already acquired by mid-life, such as the BNT, but they could contribute to difficulties with lexical access in conversation and the generation of TOT states during conversation when that access to a late acquired exemplar was being sought.

4.4.4 Selective Engagement

Selective engagement is the bringing online of selected representations in selected neural networks, by eliciting alterations in the pattern of neural activity, alterations in the likelihood of neural firing, or selection of inputs that will produce neural firing [59, 60]. Selective engagement is a general term that encompasses the many mechanisms by which the brain allocates resources. These include mechanisms underlying working memory and attention [61]. Working memory is not attention because it does not involve the focusing of sensory resources on a particular stimulus. However, it may rely on the same or similar underlying neural mechanisms.

Working memory capacity declines with age. Cansino et al. [62], in a study of 1,500 participants aged 21–80, found an age-related and roughly linear decline in d-prime on visual and verbal 1-back tests of approximately 15%, and on 2-back tasks, approximately 45%. Response latency on the 1-back task increased approximately 25%, and on the 2-back task, 15%, over the course of the life span tested. Age accounted for 6% and 14% of the variance in d' and response latency for the 1-back and 2-back tasks, respectively. Kemper and Sumner [24], in a study of 100 young (22.8 ± 2.4 years) and 100 elderly (76.4 ± 6.2) participants, found that digit span forward declined from 9.9 in the young group to 7.8 in the elderly group, and digit span backward declined from 8.2 to 5.4.

Letter and category fluency tests are complex tasks that tap both working memory and episodic memory capacities. Kavé and Knafo-Noam [63], in a study of 1,212 Hebrew speakers aged 5–86, found that letter fluency increased steadily up to age 23, remained stable until about age 72, and then declined 0.5 SD in the 75- to 86-year-old group. Category fluency also peaked in the early 20s but remained stable only into the mid-30s, declining more or less linearly by 0.5 SD by the early 70s, and then more precipitously, by a further 0.75 SD, in the 75- to 86-year-old group. Age accounted for 38% of the variance in phonemic fluency and 47% of the variance in semantic fluency.

Age-related simplification of syntax correlates strongly with decline in working memory capacity, as measured by digit span forward and backward [24, 25]. Even production of a simple sentence involving a three-argument verb (e.g., "The man gave the woman a rose") requires simultaneous maintenance of three separate distributed concept representations. More complex sentences, and the addition of anaphora (e.g., use of the article "the," which demands recall of what "the" refers to) add further to the memory load. Sentences containing complement-taking verbs impose greater demands on working (and episodic) memory. Older adults perform less well when obliged to produce such sentences [64].

Could decline in working memory capacity contribute to decline in performance associated with increasing semantic neighborhood density? We have long had data at the cellular level on the effect of frontal input to postcentral cortices, most clearly demonstrated in attentional tasks [60]. Recent studies suggest that declines in working memory (selective engagement) have coherent population level effects – rendering semantic attractor basins shallower [65] (see Chapter 14), thereby producing response failures that are phenomenologically comparable to those observed in semantic dementia. Increases in neural noise [35] would have a similar effect.

I have previously noted, citing language, magnitude estimation, and hemispatial neglect literature, that concept representations are not veridical [66]. They are most likely to be in error when they depend on knowledge deriving from limited experience – hence the tendency to underestimate large magnitudes and overestimate small magnitudes. Representations also reflect the degree to which the knowledge substrates supporting them are engaged. For example, patients with left hemispatial neglect bisect lines toward the right because, as a result of neglect-associated defective cortical engagement, they really do perceive the objectively elongated portion of the line to the left of their mark as being equal to the portion of the line to the right. In this circumstance, because of defective engagement, the right hemisphere attractor basin corresponding to line perception is smaller and shallower. In like manner, declines in working memory function (age associated or otherwise) might be associated with reduction in the breadth and depth of attractor basins associated with language representations.

4.4.5 Memory: Proper Nouns Revisited

Proper nouns constitute a unique domain. Most crucially, proper noun names represent labels, and thus they, in and of themselves, do not connote a portfolio of features potentially shared by many other objects. Some proper nouns refer to an individual, for example, Meryl Streep or the Brooklyn Bridge, that by association only is characterized by a host of features. Others, for example, "Egypt," connote an association of variously unrelated features and, in this respect, likely resemble abstract nouns in their mode of cerebral representation [3]. We routinely assess this class of proper nouns with tests of associative memory, for example, the Pyramids and Palm Trees test. There do not appear to have been any studies of differential aging effects on these two classes of proper nouns. In the following, I will focus on proper nouns corresponding to individual people or objects.

Knowledge of individual proper nouns is distinguished from our knowledge of common objects by links to specific places, settings, or times. All declarative knowledge is initially instantiated as episodic memory in neural connectivity involving hippocampal cornu amonis (CA) neurons linked to long-loop connections between the cerebral cortex and the hippocampal system [67–70]. Over time, this knowledge is gradually incorporated into cerebral cortical connectivity to the extent that it shares features with other cortical representations (the process of memory consolidation). However, place- and time-specific information cannot be so incorporated and, thus, remains perpetually hippocampally dependent. Hence the selective loss of autobiographical memory with acquired hippocampal lesions [71]. For these reasons, one might expect lexical access to proper nouns to decline in parallel with the deterioration in episodic memory observed with aging (see Chapter 7).

There may be other factors that contribute to the particular problems with proper noun access observed with aging. Semantic neighborhood density is particularly high for proper nouns [72] and presumably increases with age, hence there is greater benefit from homophone priming of proper names in elderly subjects [73]. Limbic function may also change with aging. Proper nouns, unlike common nouns, are commonly linked to the emotional aspects of our experience with them.

4.4.6 Balance of Volitional and Reactive Intention

Language function is automatic [3]. What is not automatic is the creation of a narrative plan and the orderly engagement and modification of distributed concept representations in the execution of that plan. This process of narrative plan execution can run amok in at least two ways, neither producing aphasia. First, because of executive dysfunction, the goal of communication may be poorly defined or poorly translated into narrative plan. Second, the execution of any plan involves a balance between reactive intention and volitional or intentional intention. Reactive intention corresponds to the generation of a plan as a distributed representation in frontal cortex that is elicited by activity in postcentral cortex via anterior–posterior connectivity [74]. This connectivity was first defined by Chavis and Pandya [75] (see also [76, 77]) and since has drawn much attention in the guise of mirror neuron networks [78]. Reciprocal frontal-postcentral projections may provide the substrate for working memory. Reactive intentional plans reflect well-learned strategies for dealing with everyday contingencies and are invaluable in enabling us to deal with the routine demands of life. For example, little or no planning is needed for routine driving until decisions have to be made (e.g., a turn at a particular intersection that is not part of one's daily routine) or unexpected events occur. Volitional intention derives more exclusively from frontal cortical activity and involves the generation of plans that are tailor-made to deal with novel events or situations. Narrative may solely be a product of volitional intention, but it may be, to one degree or another, susceptible to digressions driven by associations of concept representations that are in play or by intervening perceptions. Up to a point, such digressions may add color to narrative or reflect the response of the speaker to feedback from her audience. However, beyond this point, digressions begin to seriously disrupt the narrative stream. Narrative therefore necessarily involves a precise albeit varying balance between volitional and reactive intention. Aging may be associated with degradation of narrative strategy formation and execution because of a general shift that favors reactive over volitional intention. Age-associated declines in working memory function, detailed above, could also reflect a pathological shift toward reactive intention. There is compelling evidence of such a shift in aging-related changes in Stroop test performance.

The Stroop test is commonly viewed as simply a test of inhibition. However, it is actually a very good test of the balance between reactive and volitional intention. The reactive intentional response to the word "red" written in green is "red" whereas the volitional intentional response is "green." A large number of studies have demonstrated aging-related decline in performance on the interference condition of the Stroop test, whether defined by response latency/total test time [79–82] – even when corrected for processing speed [79, 82] – or defined by response errors [81, 82]. This evidence of pathological imbalance between reactive and volitional intention may help to explain the age-related impairments in narrative described in the first section of this chapter.

The results of the studies of Kavé and Levy [26] involving gender marking of verbs and lexical decision regarding pseudo-verbs with existent/nonexistent roots (see Section 3.6 above, "Grammatic Morphology") might also be best interpreted as the results of the effect of a pathological imbalance between volitional and reactive intention that favors reactive intention – hence greater latency to overcome the more automatic, reactively generated response and select the competing volitionally generated response.

It is also possible that these various impairments simply reflect deterioration of executive function (see also Chapter 12). However, it is a major challenge to differentiate the effects of intrinsic deterioration of function from the consequences of defective frontal engagement: witness attention-deficit hyperactivity disorder, in which deficits in executive function can be substantially addressed by improving frontal engagement using a pharmacological agent [83, 84]. It is possible that, at least to some degree, executive deficits of aging might be ameliorated by pharmacologic treatment [85] (but see also [86]).

4.4.7 Ontogenesis of Language Networks

A total of 10 papers published in the 1970s and 1980s found that patients with Wernicke's aphasia were, on average, nine years older than patients with Broca's aphasia (see in particular [87–90]) and that the relative frequency of Wernicke's aphasia steadily increases with age. Basso et al. [87] ruled out the possibility that this might have been due to differences in the average location of lesions, usually stroke, in younger and older patients. Miceli et al. [90] found a similar difference in patients with brain tumors.

Brown and Jaffe [91] suggested that these findings pointed to ontogenesis of language function over the life span, an interpretation that received strong support from all the studies that followed. Obler et al. [92], echoing this concept, suggested increased "automaticity of motor and sequential aspects of language."

A more granular explanation, based in neural connectivity, may be possible. In 2012, I posited the existence of a second pathway linking auditory association cortex with Broca's region, one providing relatively greater support for grammatic morphological sequence knowledge (the long recognized posterior circum-sylvian network linking auditory association cortex and Broca's region presumably providing the major substrate for phonological sequence knowledge) [3]. Since then, we have provided evidence from diffusion tensor imaging studies of the existence of both pathways. Innumerable cognitive neuropsychological studies provide strong evidence that the brain supports phonological and grammatical morphological sequence knowledge in perisylvian networks [3, 4]. Parallel distributed processing research has demonstrated that simple three-layer networks can support sequence knowledge [5, 93]. The major question that remains is the length of sequences that might be supported in this way by perisylvian networks. Plaut et al. and Seidenberg et al. provided proof of the concept with the onset-nucleus-coda sequences of single syllable words. It seems eminently plausible that such networks (perhaps endowed with explicit mechanisms for encoding sequence, e.g., simple recurrent networks [3]) might support single-word phonemic sequences that include consonant clusters, multisyllabic words, affixed words, and simple phrases, and the aphasia literature provides strong evidence of disruption of these sequences with perisylvian lesions.

The hypothesis I have proposed is that, over the course of the life span, such sequence knowledge expands to provide the basis for ever-longer sequences, perhaps including simple sentences and clauses [3], even as frontal cortex continues to provide the major substrate for sequential organization and modification of concept representations. On this basis, language sequence might be relatively preserved even with large frontal lesions that, in younger patients, produce Broca's aphasia. In this setting, serious disruptions of sequence would tend to occur mainly with posterior lesions that severely damage the major substrate for multi-morphemic sequence knowledge and its connectivity to the substrate for concept representations, yielding Wernicke's aphasia, either because of loss of this knowledge in the dominant hemisphere or inadequately developed knowledge in the nondominant hemisphere.

Can this expanding repertoire of phonological and morphological sequence knowledge account in any way for aging-related degradation of language function? Possibly so. If, with aging, there is a shift in the balance of volitional and reactive intention, as discussed in the previous section, this could lead to overreliance on postcentral systems. The consequence for language would be overreliance on the repertoire of sequences reinforced through a lifetime of speaking with associated loss of flexibility in adapting sentence structure to the unique demands of the conversational moment. Unfortunately, we lack empirical evidence of aging-related impairment in syntactic function beyond that relatable to impairment in working memory.

4.4.8 Language Use

If language use in speaking, reading, and writing contributes to maintenance or even enhancement of synaptic connectivity underlying language function, presumably via Hebbian mechanisms, then reductions of language use in advanced age could contribute to the decline in language function [94]. Social activity and time spent in cognitively challenging tasks would seem to represent reasonable surrogate measures of daily language use given the absence of direct measures. There have been many longitudinal studies that have tested the predictive value of these measures on subsequent cognitive decline. Unfortunately, the conclusions of these studies have been decidedly mixed, even as the reasons for the disparities remain unclear. The results of only large, recent studies with robust methodology will be summarized. Bourasa et al. [95] used latent growth curve models to estimate the effect of baseline social participation (volunteer work and participation in sports or social clubs, religious organizations, political or community organizations) in 19,832 participants in the Survey of Health, Aging, and Retirement in Europe study. The cognitive measures were category fluency and immediate and delayed word recall. There was a significant relationship between baseline social participation and the slope of decline in category fluency. The effect of a 1 SD difference in social participation was roughly equivalent to the effect of 10 years of aging. James

et al. [96], in a study of 1,100 participants from the Rush Memory and Aging Project, used a somewhat broader measure of social participation (going to restaurants, sporting events, off-track betting, or playing bingo; going on day trips; doing volunteer work; visiting relatives or friends; and participating in social or religious organizations). Outcome measures include a composite semantic measure (15-item BNT, verbal fluency not otherwise specified, and a test of reading). In a fully adjusted model, baseline social participation was significantly (negatively) correlated with subsequent decline in semantic function.

However, Brown et al. [97], in a series of multilevel growth models applied to four published longitudinal studies (total N = 3,723), found no relationship between baseline social participation (defined more or less as in the study of James et al. [96]) and subsequent change in a "fluency" measure (write as many synonyms as possible to a set of target words) or performance on a recognition vocabulary test. Likewise, they found no relationship between baseline engagement in cognitively stimulating activities and subsequent change in cognitive test performance [98]. McGue and Christensen [99] found, in an analysis of more than 1,000 pairs of like-sex twins from the Longitudinal Study of Aging Danish Twins, that baseline social activity did not predict change in cognitive function (category fluency, forward and backward digit span, immediate and delayed recall from a 12-item list). Furthermore, in a sub-analysis of monozygotic twins discordant for baseline level of social activity, they found that the less active twin was no more likely to experience cognitive decline than the highly active twin.

In balance, these studies do not provide a strong case for age-related decline in language use as an important explanatory variable for decline in language function. The analysis by McGue and Christensen [99] suggests that there are genetic factors that account for the empirical association between baseline social activity and cognitive decline and that, when these factors are removed, as in their monozygotic twin study, the association disappears.

4.4.9 White Matter Conduction Velocities

A consistent finding in the aging literature is that processing speed declines. This is evident in Figure 8.2. There may be multiple factors that contribute to this. I have already cited the increased time it may take for networks to settle into attractor basins in semantically dense neighborhoods and the potential effects of increased neural noise. Another factor may be speed of neural conduction. Language function depends on extensive back and forth transmission between pre- and postcentral cortices and between the hemispheres, as well as in the neuropil of the gray matter. Transcallosal conduction velocities in elderly participants (age 73 ± 7.5) have been found to be 77–81% of those in younger participants (22.4 ± 3) [100]. Similarly, central motor conduction velocities in the elderly (70+ years) have been found to be 81% of those in participants aged 20–29 [101].

Prolonged conduction times may have cascade effects because they necessitate more prolonged maintenance of the distributed representations currently at play in the processes of language production and comprehension. Language function depends on both working memory and episodic memory to maintain these representations [3]. Working and episodic

memory have a complementary relationship, episodic memory becoming progressively more important with longer processing times and greater memory loads [102]. Age-related impairment in working memory likely necessitates even greater reliance on episodic memory in language production and comprehension – an unfortunate reliance given the even greater decline in episodic memory function observed over the life span (see Chapter 7).

Prolongation of conduction times could also have differential hemispheric effects. There is reason to believe that one of the fundamental properties that distinguishes right and left hemisphere function is a greater extent of left hemisphere cortex dedicated to networks supporting sequential knowledge (e.g., phonology, grammatic morphology, phrase structure rules, sentence-level sequence (syntax) and praxis) [103]. Such sequence knowledge is less likely to be important for the sorts of gestalt processing long

Table 8.2 Potential mechanisms of aging-related decline in language function unrelated to dementia

Mechanism	Consequence
Increased baseline neural activity	Increased susceptibility to provoked phonological slips
	Exacerbation of neighborhood density effects
	Increased response latency
Increasing semantic and phonological neighborhood density	Anomia in spontaneous language and naming to confrontation
	Increased response latency
Age of acquisition	Increasing risk of anomia for late-acquired words
Deterioration of selective engagement (attention and working memory)	Exacerbation of neighborhood density effects
	Simplification of syntax
Deterioration of episodic memory function	Differential impairment in proper noun access
Shift of balance between volitional and reactive intention toward reactive	Decline in selective engagement
	Decline in Stroop test performance
	Age-related changes in narrative discourse
	Deterioration of grammatic morphology
+ontogenic change in language networks	Loss of syntactic flexibility and adaptability
Decrease in white matter conduction velocity	Increased response latency
	Increased reliance on declining episodic memory
	Differential impairment in right hemisphere function

associated with the right hemisphere, for example, visuospatial function, facial recognition, affective experience, affective prosody, and personality. Much sequence knowledge may be adequately supported by networks characterized by relatively short white matter connections, for example, the phonologic and grammatic morphologic sequence knowledge that is supported predominantly by left perisylvian cortex. On the other hand, visuospatial function may depend on a representation of the entire spatial world, thus requiring engagement of the entire parietal and linked frontal association cortices and requiring use of many long white matter pathways. For this reason, aging-related declines in white matter conduction velocities may differentially disadvantage functions particularly engaging the right hemisphere and, likewise, cognitive processes that particularly depend on callosal transmission.

5 Conclusion

The studies reviewed here provide unequivocal evidence of declining performance involving all language domains across the adult life span. This becomes most conspicuous after the age of 75, but some impairments, most notably problems with lexical access, become apparent considerably earlier. There is little doubt that the results of essentially all studies of aging effects on language function reflect inadvertent recruitment of some participants who were in the earliest stages of a dementing process. However, it is equally clear that this is not the whole story, unless the earliest stages of the dementing processes that start to become prevalent after age 90 (e.g., PART and CARTS) commonly begin in the 60s. These considerations, combined with accumulating evidence from psychological and neuropsychological studies, suggest that there are a variety of other mechanisms, not intrinsically pathological, that account in substantial part for age-related alterations in language function (Table 8.2). Some, including increases in neighborhood density, age of acquisition effects, and ontogenesis of language networks, appear to be directly related to fundamental mechanisms of human brain function. These are mechanisms that are responsible for the staggering cognitive capacity of the human brain – but also, in a sense, reflect a Faustian bargain by Nature as they have built-in limitations that eventually become apparent as we age. Others, for example, the shift from volitional to reactive intention and increased baseline neural activity, with all their potential adverse consequences (Table 8.2), may be susceptible to pharmacologic intervention.

References

1. Burke DM, Shafto MA. Language and aging. In: Craik FIM, Salthouse TA, editors. *Handbook of Aging and Cognition*. Mahwah, NJ: Lawrence Erlbaum; 2007, pp. 373–443.

2. Write HH. *Cognition, Language and Aging*. Amsterdam: John Benjamins; 2016.

3. Nadeau SE. *The Neural Architecture of Grammar*. Cambridge, MA: MIT Press; 2012.

4. Nadeau SE. Phonology: a review and proposals from a connectionist perspective. *Brain Lang.* 2001;**79**:511–79.

5. Plaut DC, McClelland JL, Seidenberg MS, Patterson K. Understanding normal and impaired word reading: computational principles in quasi-regular domains. *Psychol Rev.* 1996;**103**:56–115.

6. Bohsali A, Gullett J, Mareci T, Crosson B, Fitzgerald D, White K, et al. Structural connectivity of Broca's region. *Neurology.* 2016;**86** [16 Supplement]:I7.004.

7. Bohsali AA, Gullett JM, Mareci T, FitzGerald DB, Crosson B, White K, et al. *Frontal Lobe Language Pathways*. Chicago: Society for Neuroscience; 2015.

8. Shuren J, Heilman KM. Non-optic aphasia. *Neurology.* 1993;**43**:1900–7.

9. Beauvois MF, Saillant B. Optic aphasia for colours and colour agnosia: a distinction between visual and visuo-verbal impairments in the processing of colours. *Cogn Neuropsychol.* 1985;**2**:1–48.

10. Lhermitte F, Beauvois MF. A visual-speech disconnexion syndrome. Report of a case with optic aphasia, agnosic alexia and colour agnosia. *Brain.* 1973;**96**:695–715.

11. Bowles RP, Salthouse TA. Vocabulary test format and differential relations to age. *Psychol Aging.* 2008;**23**:366–76.

12. Marini A, Boewe A, Caltagirone C, Carlomagno S. Age-related differences in the production of textual descriptions. *J Psycholinguist Res.* 2005;**34**:439–63.

13. Schmitter-Edgecombe M, Vesneski M, Jones DWR. Aging and word-finding: a comparison of spontaneous and constrained naming tests. *Arch Clin Neuropsychol.* 2000;**15**:479–93.

14. Salthouse TA, Mandell AR. Do age-related increases in tip-of-the-tongue experiences signify episodic memory impairments? *Psychol Sci.* 2013;**24**:2489–97.

15. Evrard M. Ageing and lexical access to common and proper nouns in picture naming. *Brain Lang.* 2002;**81**:174–9.

16. Rendell PG, Castel AD, Craik FIM. Memory for proper names in old age: a disproportionate impairment? *Q J Exp Psychol.* 2005;**58A**:54–71.

17. James LE. Specific effects of aging on proper name retrieval: now you see them, now you don't. *J Gerontol B Psychol Sci.* 2006;**61B**: P180–P183.

18. Zec RF, Burkett NR, Markwell SJ, Larsen DL. A cross-sectional study of the effects of age, education and gender on the Boston Naming Test. *Clin Neuropsychol.* 2007;**21**:587–616.

19. MacKay A, Connor LT, Storandt M. Dementia does not explain correlation between age and scores on Boston Naming Test. *Arch Clin Neuropsychol.* 2005;**20**:129–33.

20. Zec RF, Markwell SJ, Burkett NR, Larsen DL. A longitudinal study of confrontation naming in the "normal" elderly. *J Int Neuropsychol Soc.* 2005;**11**:716–26.

21. Tabor Connor L, Spiro A, Obler LK, Albert ML. Change in object naming ability during adulthood. *J Gerontol B Psychol Sci Soc Sci.* 2004;**59**:203–9.

22. MacKay DG, James LE. Sequencing, speech production, and selective effects of aging on phonological and morphological speech errors. *Psychol Aging.* 2004;**19**:93–107.

23. Sommers MS, Hale S, Myerson J, Rose N, Tye-Murray N, Spehar B. Listening comprehension across the adult lifespan. *Ear Hear.* 2011;**32**:775–81.

24. Kemper S, Sumner A. The structure of verbal abilities in young and old adults. *Psychol Aging.* 2001;**16**:312–22.

25. Kemper S, Thompson M, Marquis J. Longitudinal change in language production: effects of aging and dementia on grammatical complexity and propositional content. *Psychol Aging.* 2001;**16**:600–14.

26. Kavé G, Levy Y. The processing of morphology in old age: evidence from Hebrew. *J Speech Lang Hear Res.* 2005;**48**:1442–51.

27. Wright HH, Capilouto GJ, Srinivasan C, Fergodiotis G. Story processing ability in cognitively healthy younger and older adults. *J Speech Lang Hear Res.* 2011;**54**:900–17.

28. Saling LL, Laroo N, Saling MM. When more is less: failure to compress discourse with re-telling in normal aging. *Acta Psychol [Amst].* 2012;**139**:220–4.

29. Horton WS, Spieler DH. Age-related differences in communication and audience design. *Psychol Aging.* 2007;**22**:281–90.

30. Bidelman GM, Villafuerte JW, Moreno S, Alain C. Age-related changes in the subcortico-cortical encoding and categorical perception of speech. *Neurobiol Aging.* 2014;**35**:2526–40.

31. Nelson PT, Trojanowski JQ, Abner EL, Al-Janabi OM, Jicha GA, Schmitt FA, et al. "New old pathologies": AD, PART, and cerebral age-related TDP-43 with sclerosis [CARTS]. *J Neuropathol Exp Neurol.* 2016;**75**:482–98.

32. Neltner JH, Abner EL, Jicha GA, Schmitt FA, Patel E, Poon LW, et al. Brain pathologies in extreme old age. *Neurobiol Aging.* 2016;**37**:1–11.

33. Blass DM, Hatanpaa KJ, Brandt J, Rao V, Steinberg M, Troncoso JC, et al. Dementia in hippocampal sclerosis resembles frontotemporal dementia more than Alzheimer disease. *Neurology.* 2004;**63**:492–7.

34. Kryscio RJ, Abner EL, Nelson PT, Benbnett D, Schneider J, Yu L, et al. The effect of vascular neuropathology on late-life cognition: results from the SMART Project. *J Prev Alzheimers Dis.* 2016;**3**:85–91.

35. Voytek B, Kramer MA, Case J, Lepage KQ, Tempesta ZR, Knight RT, et al. Age-related changes in 1/f neural electrophysiological noise. *J Neurosci.* 2015;**23**:13257–65.

36. Rogers TT, McClelland JL. *Semantic Cognition: A Parallel Distributed Processing Approach.* Cambridge, MA: MIT Press; 2004.

37. Conley P, Burgess C. Age effects on a computational model of memory. *Brain Cogn.* 2000;**43**:104–8.

38. Mirman D, Magnuson JS. Attractor dynamics and semantic neighborhood density: processing is slowed by near neighbors and speeded by distant neighbors. *J Exp Psychol Learn Mem Cogn.* 2008;**34**:65–79.

39. Mirman D. Effects of near and distant semantic neighbors on word production. *Cogn Affect Behav Neurosci.* 2011;**11**:32–43.

40. Buchanan L, Burgess C, Conley P. Overcrowding in semantic neighborhoods: modeling deep dyslexia. *Brain Cogn.* 1996;**30**:111–14.

41. Burgess C, Conley P. Developing semantic representations for proper nouns. In: *Proceedings of the Cognitive Science Society.* Hillsdale, NJ: Erlbaum; 1998, pp. 185–90.

42. Tournier I, Postal V, Mathey S. Investigation of age-related differences in an adapted Hayling task. *Arch Gerontol Geriatr.* 2014;**59**:599–606.

43. Vitevitch MS, Luce PA. Phonological neighborhood effects in spoken word perception and production. *Ann Rev Linguist.* 2016;**2**:75–94.

44. Sommers MS, Danielson SM. Inhibitory processes and spoken word recognition in young and older adults: the interaction of lexical competition and semantic context. *Psychol Aging.* 1999;**14**:458–72.

45. Taler V, Aaron GP, Steinmetz LG, Pisoni DB. Lexical neighborhood density effects on spoken word recognition and production in healthy aging. *J Gerontol Psychol Sci.* 2010;**65B**:551–60.

46. Sommers MS. The structural organization of the mental lexicon and its contribution to age-related declines in spoken word recognition. *Psychol Aging.* 1996;**11**:333–41.

47. Newman RS, German DJ. Life span effects of lexical factors on oral naming. *Lang Aphasia.* 2005;**48**:123–56.

48. Vitevitch MS, Sommers MS. The facilitative influence of phonological similarity and neighborhood frequency in speech production in younger and older adults. *Mem Cogn.* 2003;**31**:494–504.

49. Vitevitch MS, Luce PA. Probabilistic phonotactics and neighborhood activation in spoken word recognition. *J Mem Lang.* 1999;**40**:374–408.

50. Vitevitch MS, Luce PA. Increases in phonotactic probability facilitate spoken nonword repetition. *J Mem Lang.* 2005;**52**:193–204.

51. Ellis A, Lambon Ralph MA. Age of acquisition effects in adult lexical processing reflect loss of plasticity in maturing systems: insights from connectionist networks. *J Exp Psychol Learn Mem Cogn.* 2000;**26**:1103–23.

52. Lambon Ralph MA, Ehsan S. Age of acquisition effects depend on the mapping between representations and the frequency of occurrence: empirical and computational evidence. *Visual Cogn.* 2006;**13**:928–48.

53. Hinton GE, Shallice T. Lesioning an attractor network: investigations of acquired dyslexia. *Psych Rev.* 1991;**98**:74–95.

54. Hodges JR, Graham N, Patterson K. Charting the progression in semantic dementia: implications for the organization of semantic memory. *Memory.* 1995;**3**:463–95.

55. Rogers TT, Lambon Ralph MA, Garrard P, Bozeat S, McClelland JL, Hodges JR, et al. Structure and deterioration of semantic memory: a neuropsychological and computational investigation. *Psych Rev.* 2004;**111**:205–35.

56. Catling J, South F, Dent K. The effect of age of acquisition on older individuals with and without cognitive impairments. *Q J Exp Psychol.* 2013;**66**:1963–73.

57. Morrison CM, Hirsh KW, Chappell T, Ellis AW. Age and age of acquisition: an evaluation of the cumulative frequency hypothesis. *Eur J Cogn Psychol.* 2002;**14**:435–59.

58. Tononi G, Cirelli C. Sleep and the price of plasticity; from synaptic and cellular homeostasis to memory consolidation and integration. *Neuron.* 2014;**81**:12–34.

59. Desimone R, Duncan D. Neural mechanisms of selective visual attention. *Ann Rev Neurosci.* 1995;**18**:193–222.

60. Moran J, Desimone R. Selective attention gates visual processing in extrastriate cortex. *Science.* 1985;**229**:782–4.

61. Nadeau SE, Crosson B. Subcortical aphasia. *Brain Lang.* 1997;**58**:436–58.

62. Cansino S, Hernández-Ramos E, Estrada-Manilla C, et al. The decline in verbal and visuospatial working memory across the adult life span. *Age Aging.* 2013;**35**:2283–302.

63. Kavé G, Knafo-Noam A. Lifespan development of phonemic and semantic fluency: universal increase, differential decrease. *J Clin Exp Neuropsychol.* 2015;**37**:751–63.

64. Kemper S, Herman R, Lian C. Age differences in sentence production. *J Gerontol Psycholog Sci.* 2003;**58B**:P260–P268.

65. Rolls ET, Deco G. Stochastic cortical neurodynamics underlying the memory and cognitive changes in aging. *Neurobiol Learn Mem.* 2015;**118**:150–61.

66. Nadeau SE. Attractor basins: a neural basis for the conformation of knowledge. In: Chatterjee A, Coslett HB, editors. *The Roots of Cognitive Neuroscience.* Oxford: Oxford University Press; 2014, pp. 305–33.

67. Alvarez P, Squire LR. Memory consolidation and the medial temporal lobe: a simple network model. *Proc Natl Acad Sci USA.* 1994;**91**:7041–5.

68. McClelland JL, McNaughton BL, O'Reilly RC. Why there are complementary learning systems in the hippocampus and neocortex: insights from the successes and failures of connectionist models of learning and memory. *Psych Rev.* 1995;**102**:419–57.

69. Rolls ET, Treves A. *Neural Networks and Brain Function.* New York: Oxford University Press; 1998.

70. Squire LR, Zola-Morgan S. The medial temporal lobe memory system. *Science.* 1991;**253**:1380–6.

71. Vargha-Khadem F, Gadian DG, Watkins KE, Connelly A, Van Paesschen W, Mishkin M. Differential effects of early hippocampal pathology on episodic and semantic memory. *Science.* 1997;**277**:376–80.

72. Cohen G, Burke DM. Memory for proper names: a review. *Memory.* 1993;**1**:249–63.

73. Burke DM, Locantore JK, Austin AA, Chae B. Cherry pit primes Brad Pitt. Homophone priming effects on young and older adults' production of proper names. *Psychol Sci.* 2004;**15**:164–70.

74. Nadeau SE, Heilman KM. Frontal mysteries revealed. *Neurology.* 2007;**68**:1450–3.

75. Chavis DA, Pandya DN. Further observations on corticofrontal connections in the rhesus monkey. *Brain Res.* 1976;**117**:369–86.

76. Goldman-Rakic PS. Cellular and circuit basis of working memory in prefrontal cortex of nonhuman primates. *Prog Brain Res.* 1990;**85**:325–36.

77. Ongür D, Price JL. The organization of networks within the orbital and medial prefrontal cortex of rats, monkeys and humans. *Cereb Cortex.* 2000;**10**:206–19.

78. Rizzolatti G, Craighero L. The mirror-neuron system. *Ann Rev Neurosci.* 2004;**27**:169–92.

79. Adólfsdóttir S, Wollschlaeger D, Wehling E, Lundervold AJ. Inhibition and switching in healthy aging: a longitudinal study. *J Int Neuropsychol Soc.* 2017;**23**:90–7.

80. Aschenbrenner AJ, Balota DA. Interactive effects of working memory and trial history on Stroop interference in cognitively healthy aging. *Psychol Aging.* 2015;**30**:1–8.

81. Hankee LD, Preis SR, Piers RJ, Beiser AS, Devine SA, Liu Y, et al. Population normative data for the CERAD word list and Victoria Stroop Test in young- and middle-aged adults: cross-sectional analyses from the Framingham Heart Study. *Exp Aging Res.* 2016;**42**:315–28.

82. Troyer AK, Leach L, Strauss E. Aging and response inhibition:

normative data for the Victoria Stroop Test. *Neuropsychol Dev Cogn B Aging Neuropsychol Cogn.* 2006;**13**:20–35.

83. Adler LA, Solanto M, Escobar R, Lipsius S, Upadhyaya H. Executive functioning outcomes over 6 months of atomoxetine for adults with ADHD: relationship to maintenance of response and relapse over the subsequent 6 months after treatment. *J Atten Disord.* 2016. DOI 10.1177/10870547166644.

84. Bron TI, Bijlenga D, Boonstra AM, Breuk M, Pardoen WFH, Beekman ATF, et al. OROS-methylphenidate efficacy on specific executive functioning deficits in adults with ADHD: a randomized, placebo-controlled cross-over study. *Eur Neuropsychopharmacol.* 2014;**24**:519–28.

85. Jäkälä P, Riekkinen M, Sirviö J, Koivisto E, Kejonen K, Vanhanen M, et al. Guanfacine but not clonidine improves planning and working memory performance in humans. *Neuropsychopharmacol.* 1999;**20**:460–70.

86. van Dyck CH. Guanfacine treatment for prefrontal cognitive dysfunction in elderly subjects. 2014; Clinicaltrials.gov: NCT00935493.

87. Basso A, Bracchi M, Capitani E, Laiacona M, Zanobio ME. Age and evolution of language area functions. A study of adult stroke patients. *Cortex.* 1987;**23**:475–83.

88. Brown JW, Grober E. Age, sex, and aphasia type. Evidence for a regional cerebral growth process underlying lateralization. *J Nerv Ment Dis.* 1983;**171**:431–4.

89. Kertesz A, Sheppard A. The epidemiology of aphasic and cognitive impairment in stroke. Age, sex, aphasia type, and laterality differences. *Brain.* 1981;**104**:117–28.

90. Miceli G, Caltagirone C, Gainotti G, Masullo C, Silveri MC, Villa G.

Influence of age, sex, literacy and pathologic lesion on incidence, severity and type of aphasia. *Acta Neurol Scand.* 1981;**64**:370–82.

91. Brown JW, Jaffe J. Hypothesis on cerebral dominance. *Neuropsychologia.* 1975;**13**:107–10.

92. Obler LK, Albert ML, Goodglass H, Benson DF. Aphasia type and aging. *Brain Lang.* 1978;**6**:318–22.

93. Seidenberg MS, McClelland JL. A distributed, developmental model of word recognition and naming. *Psych Rev.* 1989;**96**:523–68.

94. Hultsch DF, Hertzog C, Small BJ, Dixon RA. Use it or lose it: engaged lifestyle as a buffer of cognitive decline in aging? *Psychol Aging.* 1999;**14**:245–63.

95. Bourassa KJ, Memel M, Woolverton C, Sbarra DA. Social participation predicts cognitive functioning in aging adults over time: comparisons with physical health, depression, and physical activity. *Aging Ment Health.* 2015;**21**:133–46.

96. James BD, Wilson RS, Barnes LL, Bennett DA. Late-life social activity and cognitive decline in old age. *J Int Neuropsychol Soc.* 2011;**17**:998–1005.

97. Brown CL, Gibbons LE, Kennison RF, Robitaille A, Lindwall M, Mitchell MB, et al. Social activity and cognitive functioning over time: a coordinated analysis of four longitudinal studies. *J Aging Res.* 2012; 2012:287438.

98. Mitchell MB, Cimino CR, Benitez A, Brown CL, Gibbons LE, Kennison RF, et al. Cognitively stimulating activities: effects on cognition across four studies with up to 21 years of longitudinal data. *J Aging Res.* 2012; 2012:461592.

99. McGue M, Christensen K. Social activity and healthy aging: a study

of aging Danish twins. *Twin Res Hum Genet*. 2007;**10**:255–65.

100. Davidson T, Tremblay F. Age and hemispheric differences in trancallosal inhibition between motor cortices: an ipsilateral silent period study. *BMC Neurosci*. 2013;**14**:62.

101. Shibuya K, Park SB, Geevasinga N, Huynh W, Simon NG, Menon P, et al. Threshold tracking transcranial magnetic stimulation: effects of age and gender on motor cortical function. *Clin Neurophysiol*. 2016;**127**:2355–61.

102. Shrager Y, Levy DA, Hopkins RO, Squire LR. Working memory and the organization of brain systems. *J Neuroscience*. 2008;**28**:4818–22.

103. Nadeau SE. Hemispheric asymmetry: what, why, and at what cost? *J Int Neuropsychol Soc*. 2010;**27**:1–3.

Chapter

9

Changes in Emotions and Mood with Aging

Erin Trifilio, John B. Williamson, and Kenneth M. Heilman

1 Introduction

Emotions are one of the major factors that determine our actions, our interactions, and our quality of life. Aging is associated with many changes in the brain. Some might assume that these changes inevitably lead to negative outcomes, especially in terms of emotional and psychological well-being. Although this may be true for a few people, healthy neurological aging is not necessarily associated with a reduction of positive emotions or an upregulation of negative ones. Of course, neurodegenerative disorders, cerebrovascular disease, or other brain injuries and diseases may negatively affect emotional processing. Further, many environmental, occupational, and psychosocial factors might influence the emotions and moods of aging individuals.

Whereas people know what the word "emotion" means, the entity is difficult to define. One of the terms used as a synonym is "feelings." However, a feeling is a sensory perception most often induced by touch, and, unlike the feelings a person gets from touching, emotions are often not directly related to incoming sensory information. Instead, for the most part, emotions are internally produced. There is still much debate about how the brain and body produce emotions; however, we know that emotional experiences represent complex neurological phenomena that involve cortical cognitive networks, portions of the limbic system, the autonomic nervous system, and even portions of the endocrine system and other body organs.

Emotional functions can be divided into two major domains: emotional behaviors and emotional experiences. Emotional behaviors may be transient or prolonged. Prolonged emotional experiences and behaviors are called moods. We have divided this chapter into four major sections that will discuss the influence of aging on (1) emotional communication, (2) emotion feelings and experiences, (3) moods, and (4) regulation of emotions.

Although it has been suggested that emotional experience and expression remain intact in old age and that older adults have better emotion regulation skills than younger people, emotional changes do occur with aging [1]. Ross et al. [2] divided emotions into primary (e.g., happy, sad, angry, fearful (anxious), surprise, disgust, and neutral) and social (e.g., embarrassed). In this chapter, we will focus on alterations of primary emotions that occur with aging.

2 Emotional Communication

2.1 Emotional Perception

2.1.1 Faces

2.1.1.1 Observations

The ability to correctly identify verbal and nonverbal emotional expressions is a critical aspect of communication. Impairments of emotional communication might induce interpersonal problems, reducing social competence and quality of life. Ruffman et al. [3] performed a meta-analysis of 28 data sets including 705 older adults and 962 younger adults to learn if there are age differences in recognition of emotional facial expressions. Older adults appeared to have increased difficulty recognizing some emotions, such as anger, fear, and sadness. This difficulty could create particular difficulties with emotional communication [4, 5].

Women of all ages are more accurate than men in perceiving emotional facial expressions [6]. Differences in visual scanning patterns may, at least in part, explain this gender difference. For example, Sullivan et al. [7] examined visual scanning patterns in men and women across the life span and reported that women attend more to the top half of the face while men attend more to the bottom of the face. Further, the tendency for women to attend more to the top half of the face correlated with their ability to correctly label emotional faces. The findings of Krendl

127

et al. [8] suggest that these differences may be moderated by overall cognitive ability. For example, sex-related differences in facial emotional recognition in aging adults appear to be attenuated among those with greater cognitive impairment, although this may be the case only for older men [9].

English and Cartensen [10] investigated the effect of perceiver emotional state and time of assessment on subjective emotional experience as a function of arousal. Older adults reported more positive emotions at the beginning and end of the day and this effect was greatest for low arousal emotions (e.g., calm, content, relaxed). These findings demonstrate the delicate interplay of situational emotional state and arousal with aging-related changes in emotion perception. In addition, Stanley and Isaacowitz [11] demonstrated that familiarity influences recognition of emotions in older but not young adults. This suggests that older adults rely on additional knowledge about the person with whom they are communicating and this knowledge may help in correctly perceiving emotional facial expressions.

2.1.1.2 Possible Mechanisms

There is some evidence that differences between younger and aging adults when they view emotional faces might in part be due to "own-age bias" (attention and memory for faces of one's own age group are often superior to attention and memory for faces of another age group). In order to elucidate the mechanisms of the own-age bias in emotion perception, Ebner et al. [12] examined functional magnetic resonance imaging (fMRI) results in young and older adults during a task that included viewing a series of faces with varying emotional valence and age. Results showed greater involvement of the ventromedial prefrontal cortex, insula, and amygdala in older adults' processing of own-age faces compared with other-age faces. These results suggest greater engagement of brain regions associated with emotional processing when older adults view faces of people who are of their own age rather than younger faces. This is important to consider when interpreting findings of emotional aging studies, as most use stimuli depicting younger adults.

The changes in the brain that occur with aging that might account for these changes in the recognition of emotional faces and, especially, the negative emotions of anger, fear, and sadness are not known. Based on lesion and brain imaging studies, there are

several modular networks that appear to be critical for the naming or recognition of emotional faces. Visual perception of emotional faces appears to be in part mediated by the visual association areas, such as the fusiform gyrus, the right parietal lobe, and the amygdala [13]. Studies of patients with right hemisphere lesions have revealed that damage to the right hemisphere appears to be more likely to impair facial emotional discrimination than lesions of the left hemisphere [13]. There are also functional imaging studies in healthy participants that reveal that the right hemisphere is dominant for the recognition of facial emotional expressions [13]. Adolphs [14] performed volumetric co-registration of lesions from a large group of patients with focal brain lesions in order to map the shared location associated with facial affect recognition disorders. They found that impaired recognition of emotional facial expressions was associated with damage to the right somatosensory cortices, the right anterior supramarginal gyrus, and the right insula. Harciarek and Heilman [15] studied the ability of patients who had strokes of the anterior or posterior portions of the right hemisphere to recognize emotional faces. They found that patients with anterior or posterior lesions were impaired in facial emotional recognition but that patients with anterior right hemisphere lesions were particularly impaired at recognizing faces expressing emotions with negative valence.

The right hemisphere primarily mediates facial emotional recognition [13] and one of the major theories about changes in the brain that are associated with aging is called the right hemisphere-aging hypothesis. This hypothesis posits that with aging, there is a loss of neurons and neuronal connectivity and alterations in neurotransmitter systems. With these changes, there is a decline in functions mediated by these networks. Aging-related decline in functions that are mediated by the right hemisphere are greater than those mediated by the left hemisphere [16, 17]. The reasons for this asymmetrical decline are not entirely known. However, the loss of neurons with aging is not as great as the loss of subcortical white matter, and in the right hemisphere, there is relatively more white matter than in the left hemisphere [18, 19]. Because facial emotion recognition is dependent on the very long white matter pathways connecting visual association areas, the amygdala (located in the anterior part of the temporal lobes) and sensory-motor cortex, the recognition of facial emotions may be particularly vulnerable to aging-related degradation of white matter.

Phillips and Allen [20] demonstrated a relationship between emotional perception and moods, such as depression and anxiety. Recent work has sought to determine the effect of mood-congruency on emotion perception as a function of aging. Mood congruency is the degree of congruence between the mood of the perceiver and the affect conveyed by the perceived face. Coupland et al. [21] reported that low positive affect decreased the identification of happy faces, while negative affect increased the identification of disgust. Suzuki et al. [22] reported that aging-related decreases in negative affect were associated with similar decreases in identification of sad faces. Voelkle et al. [23] sought to determine the relationship between mood, temporal sequence, and emotion perception across the life span. Younger and older adults provided multidimensional emotion ratings of faces over ten sessions. Older adults in a positive mood were more likely to accurately perceive positive faces than when in a negative mood, but a similar pattern was not seen in younger adults. These findings illustrate the complex interplay between mood and emotion perception across the life span.

2.1.2 Comprehension of Speech Prosody

2.1.2.1 Observations

Speech prosody ("It is not what you said but how you said it") is another important means of emotional communication. With aging, there is often a decrement in hearing, and without intact hearing it may be difficult to comprehend prosody. Orbelo, Testa, and Ross [24] evaluated the ability of older and younger healthy participants without hearing impairment to produce and comprehend affective prosody. They found that the production of affective prosody, measured by variation in fundamental frequency, was unimpaired in older participants. In contrast, however, comprehension of affective prosody by older participants was impaired, particularly for tasks with reduced verbal semantic content. Demenescu, Mathiak, and Mathiak [25] replicated these findings and determined that capacity for emotion recognition of emotional faces was significantly correlated with the capacity for comprehension of affective prosody. This study provides further support for the concept that aging-related impairment in comprehension of emotional prosody cannot be entirely explained by hearing impairment.

2.1.2.2 Possible Mechanisms

Orbelo et al. [24] noted that the pattern of performance on affective prosody comprehension tasks in aging participants resembled the pattern found after right-brain damage. They suggested that aging-related loss of comprehension of affective prosody is most likely due to a processing deficit involving the right hemisphere. Alternatively, aging-related deficits in comprehension of affective prosody could be related to impairment in pitch perception. Pitch perception is important in comprehending prosody, and older people often have impairments in pitch perception. In addition, older people often have cognitive deficits. However, later research by Orbelo et al. showed that impaired comprehension of affective prosody in elderly subjects is not predicted by aging-related hearing loss or aging-related cognitive decline [26].

2.2 Emotional Expression

2.2.1 Faces

2.2.1.1 Observations

In a study of emotional facial expressivity, Pedder et al. [27] had older and younger participants view 30 positive and 30 negative pictures from the International Affective Picture System (IAPS) [28] and measured their facial responses to these emotional pictures using electromyography (EMG). These investigators reported that, when watching these pictures, the increase in facial muscle EMG activity in older adults was significantly less than in the younger participants.

2.2.1.2 Possible Mechanisms

The reduction of facial movements in response to emotional picture viewing can have many possible mechanisms. One reason could be aging-related suppression of emotional expression ("keeping a stiff upper lip"). This ability is a critical element in managing social communication and could be adaptive. Other factors, from changes in perception to aging-related sarcopenia of the facial muscles, could also account for changes in facial expressivity. One of the tests that might help to understand this change is to have older and younger participants imitate faces. If their imitation was normal, this change could not be related to sarcopenia. Unfortunately, we could not find any studies testing this hypothesis.

2.2.2 Emotional Prosody

Aging effects on emotional prosodic production have not been studied in depth, but there has been some recent work in the area. Sen, Isaacowitz, and Schirmer [29] examined the role of speaker age and listener sex in a large group of healthy participants aged 19–34 years and 60–85 years. Participants categorized verbal propositionally neutral sentences spoken by ten younger and ten older speakers with happy, neutral, sad, or angry prosody. Acoustic analyses indicated that expressions from younger and older speakers denoted the intended emotion and both groups had similar accuracy. Thus, this important aspect of emotional communication appears to be spared in normal aging.

2.3 Verbal-Alexithymia

The word "alexithymia" comes from three Greek stems: *a*, without; *lexis*, word; *thymos*, emotion. Alexithymia is the inability or reduced ability to use words (propositional language) to express emotions. There have been several studies that have suggested that, with aging, there is an increase in alexithymia. Most of these studies have used the 20-Item Toronto Alexithymia Scale (TAS-20). However, other studies have shown minimal or no impact of aging on alexithymia [30, 31].

The TAS-20 is a self-report scale comprised of 20 items. Each item is rated on a five-point Likert scale. Most studies using this scale interpret the data obtained in terms of three major subscales. One subscale assesses the ability of the person responding to the items to identify the emotional feelings and to distinguish them from the somatic sensations that accompany emotional arousal. For example, one item states, "I am often confused about what emotion I am feeling." A second subscale assesses the ability of the person to describe his or her feelings to other people. For example, one item states, "I am able to describe my feelings easily." The last subscale assesses externally oriented thinking. For example, one item states, "'Looking for hidden meanings in movies or plays distracts from their enjoyment." Therefore, it is primarily the first two subscales (do not know what I am feeling and unable to describe my feeling) that might be able to detect alexithymia. There are, however, several major problems in detecting alexithymia using the Toronto Alexithymia Scale. First, this assessment uses self-report and some patients with alexithymia also have anosognosia. Second, the assessment cannot distinguish people who are feeling or experiencing fewer emotions from those who cannot name or

verbally express their emotions. Therefore, more research is needed to develop methods to better evaluate alexithymia in a standardized manner.

Theoretically, there are two possible mechanisms that could account for true alexithymia. First, there could be a somewhat independent lexical-semantic network for storing emotional words. When this network becomes degraded, people may not be able to find the words to express their emotional feelings. However, according to this hypothesis, they should also be impaired in naming others people's emotions from faces, scenes, speech prosody, and emotional stories. On the other hand, even when they cannot name or describe the emotions, they should be able to detect the emotional valence (positive or negative), the degree to which these stimuli are arousing, and whether or not the emotion is naturally associated with approach or avoidance behavior (or neither).

Second, the right hemisphere plays a critical role in perceiving and experiencing several emotions. With damage to the corpus callosum, a person who has normal sensation in their left hand might not be able to name the objects placed in that hand or name objects viewed in the left visual field. They are unable to name these objects because their left hemisphere contains the verbal lexicon and with callosal disconnection, these sensory percepts cannot access the verbal lexicon [32]. In a similar manner, patients with callosal disconnection might also be impaired in transferring emotion percepts from the right to the left hemisphere. For example, TenHouten et al. [33] showed a 3-minute film depicting the deaths of a baby and of a boy to patients who had undergone corpus callosotomy for treatment of refractory epilepsy and matched normal control subjects. All subjects were questioned about the symbolic and emotional content of the film. These investigators performed a content analysis of the participants' spoken and written responses and found that, in comparison to normal controls, the patients with callosotomy produced fewer affect-laden words – evidence of alexithymia. With aging, there is a loss of callosal connections [34], and this might play a role in aging-related alexithymia.

Perhaps one of the best means of testing for true alexithymia would be to show pictures from the IAPS, or a similar means of eliciting emotions, while measuring autonomic responses and having the person grade valence and arousal. After viewing these pictures, the participants would verbally describe the picture and the feelings it evoked. The analysis would focus on the use of words that describe emotions. If a person had normal emotional responses but could not verbally denote the emotions they experienced, this would suggest alexithymia. Unfortunately, we could find no studies that used this type of procedure to assess aging effects on alexithymia.

3 Emotional Experience

Wundt [35] proposed that primary emotional experiences vary in three dimensions: (1) quality or valence (positive-good to negative-bad), (2) excitement or arousal (high to low), and (3) impetus to action (high to low). Heilman et al. [13] suggested that the impetus to action associated with an emotional experience could be characterized by approach to the stimulus, as can be seen with anger, or avoidance of the stimulus, as can be associated with fear or disgust.

A number of studies, using a variety of different tasks and stimuli, have sought to determine whether aging adults show evidence of changes in their experience of emotions. For example, Backs, da Silva, and Han [36] used the Self-Assessment Manikin (SAM) ratings to determine whether groups of younger and older adults had similar affective experiences to pictures from the IAPS. These investigators found age group differences. Younger adults reported pleasant-arousing pictures to be more pleasant and arousing than did the aging adults. Grühn and Scheibe also examined aging effects on response to pictures from the IAPS [37]. Unlike Backs, da Silva, and Han [36], they reported that the older participants found the positive pictures more positive than did the younger participants. The reason for this difference between results is not known. In addition, Grühn and Scheibe found that the older adults perceived negative pictures as more negative and more arousing than did the younger participants.

The intensity of the startle eye blink is modulated by arousal and emotional valence in that its magnitude is typically augmented while viewing aversive-arousing pictures (e.g., attack, threat) and suppressed while viewing pleasant-arousing pictures [38]. Feng et al. [39] found that when younger and older participants viewed positive and negative pictures from the IAPS, they had opposite reactions. The younger adults showed a potentiated startle when viewing negative pictures compared with positive pictures. Older adults exhibited a potentiated startle when

viewing positive pictures compared with negative or neutral pictures. These results are compatible with those of Grühn and Scheibe [37], who reported that the older participants found the positive pictures more positive compared with the younger participants. Le Duc et al. [40] also investigated the relationship between eye blink startle response and emotion perception in young and older adults. They found that when viewing positive images, older adults had a larger eye-blink startle response compared with the younger participants. Although the results of these studies are not in complete agreement, they suggest that older adults, when compared with younger adults, experience greater pleasure and arousal with positive stimuli.

Hillmire et al. [41] explored this aging-related "positivity effect" in an event-related potential (ERP) study. Participants were presented with photographs of emotional faces, and the ERPs elicited by the onset of angry, sad, happy, and neutral faces were recorded. These emotional expressions elicit a positive deflection in the waveforms elicited by emotional expressions relative to neutral faces early in the time course of the ERP. These waveforms, referred to as "fronto-central emotional positivity" (FcEP), are thought to reflect enhanced early processing of emotional expressions. The results of the Hillmire et al. study revealed that the young adults show an early FcEP to negative emotional expressions and older adults show an early FcEP to positive emotional expressions. These findings provide additional evidence that older and younger healthy participants differentially process positive and negative emotional stimuli and are congruent with the aging-related "positivity effect" observed in the behavioral studies discussed above.

There are several possible reasons why older healthy participants might process emotional stimuli differently from younger people. The first reason, already discussed earlier in this chapter, is that with aging, there appears to be a greater decrement in right than left hemisphere functions. There have been many studies that have suggested that, whereas the left hemisphere mediates positive emotions, the right mediates negative emotions [13]. This will be further discussed in the next section.

A second possible explanation for aging-related differences in valence detection is that, with aging, there is a particularly severe decrement in functions mediated by the frontal lobes. Neuroimaging research now enables investigators to determine functional connectivity between the regions of the brain comprising various neural networks. With aging, there is a loss of subcortical white matter connectivity. The functions of the frontal lobes are strongly dependent on white matter connectivity with the temporal and parietal lobes, as well as with the thalamus, basal ganglia, portions of the limbic system, and other structures. With aging, there is degeneration of most cerebral white matter. However, given that frontal lobe functions are so heavily dependent on white matter connectivity, aging-related white matter deterioration provides a ready explanation for aging-related impairment in frontal functions [42].

Emotions can be classified as good and bad or having a positive or negative valence. It has been posited that whereas positive evaluations produce approach behaviors, negative evaluations produce avoidance. In fact, it is reasonable to view the neural basis for approach and avoidance behavior associated with emotions as an actual component of the composite cerebral representations of emotions. Chen and Bargh had participants respond to stimuli by either pushing or pulling a lever [43]. They found that participants were faster to respond to stimuli with a negative valence when pushing the lever away (avoidance) than when pulling it toward them (approach) and were faster to respond to positive stimuli by pulling than by pushing. This pattern held even when evaluation of the stimuli was irrelevant to the participants' conscious task. Denny-Brown and Chambers [44] noted that, whereas the frontal lobes mediate disengagement and withdrawal behaviors, the temporal and parietal lobes appear to mediate approach behaviors. Since there are aging-related decrements in frontal lobe functions, there may be relative disinhibition of the temporal and parietal lobes with a relative increase in activation of the posterior temporal and parietal lobes, leading to an increase in the approach behaviors that are often associated with positive emotions. However, we are unaware of studies of aging effects on approach and avoidance in relation to emotional stimuli.

A third possible explanation for the aging-related positivity effect is aging-related degradation of the amygdala [45]. Because the amygdala is more reactive to negative than to positive emotional stimuli, aging-related degradation of the amygdala could lead to a shift favoring greater responses to positive stimuli. Support for this hypothesis comes from observations of people with amygdala lesions. Berntson et al. [46]

measured emotional arousal and judgment of valence (positive or negative) to a graded series of emotional pictures in patients with amygdala lesions and a control group with lesions sparing the amygdala. The patients with damage to the amygdala showed a complete lack of an arousal gradient across negative stimuli but displayed a typical arousal gradient with positive stimuli. These results do not seem to be attributable to the inability of the patients with amygdala injury to perceive these negative stimuli, since they accurately recognized and categorized the valence of the stimuli. Rather, they suggest that with amygdala lesions, negative stimuli are not as arousing. Aging-related degradation of the amygdalae may have the same effect. Support for this amygdala atrophy–age related positivity effect comes from a functional imaging study, which showed that older adults have less functional amygdala activation to negative stimuli than do younger participants [47].

Emotional resilience is a person's ability to adapt to stressful situations. Previous studies have suggested that low emotional resilience may correlate with increased amygdala activation. Studies have suggested that emotional resilience increases with age, and this aging-related high resilience might also be related to amygdala atrophy and/or decreased connectivity [48].

4 Aging-Related Changes in Mood

4.1 Depression

With aging, there is a lower incidence of depression than in younger adults [49]. Depression is estimated to affect as many as 10% of adults aged 55 and older [50, 51]. Throughout life, some of the factors that appear to reduce the probability of developing depression include socioeconomic success, a higher level of education, social engagement, religious or spiritual involvement, and finding meaning in life [52]. Risk factors for depression include chronic medical conditions, exposure to stressful life events, such as the loss of loved ones (e.g., spouses), social isolation, and physical and functional decline [53]. Aging adults, when compared with younger adults, might present with more of the somatic features of depression, such as sleep dysregulation, fatigue, and reduced processing speed (bradyphrenia). Aging adults are less likely to endorse alterations of mood, such as dysphoria, than are younger adults, and this appears to be particularly true of men [52, 54–56].

Differences in depressive symptomatology and etiology are often described in terms of age of onset (early or late), although there is no clear cutoff point between the two [56]. Depression that develops later in life is often associated with cerebrovascular disease characterized by white matter hyperintensities and silent brain infarctions [57]. Aging people with depression are more likely to have cognitive deficits [52, 58], suggesting a link between white matter pathology and depression. We are not aware of any data on the relationship between depression and aging-related changes in the otherwise healthy brain.

Aging adults with a depressed mood often have more weight loss and less suicidal ideation than younger people with depression [59]. Younger adults with depression are more likely to have a strong family history of mood disorders; more salient personality contributors, such as high trait neuroticism; and a higher prevalence of personality disorders [60–63].

4.2 Anxiety

Anxiety disorders affect up to 15% of elderly adults [64]. Anxiety seems to be qualitatively similar in the young and the old. Generalized anxiety disorder (GAD) is the most common anxiety diagnosis [51]. However, aging adults more often have associated somatic complaints [65, 66]. Most studies of phobic disorders report a prevalence of 1–3% in those 65 and older, with agoraphobia being the most common [64]. As with depression, we are not aware of any data on the relationship between anxiety or phobic disorders and aging-related changes in the otherwise healthy brain.

4.3 Anhedonia

4.3.1 Clinical

Anhedonia is the reduced ability to experience pleasure from activities that were previously found to be enjoyable. Anhedonia can induce diminished motivation to engage in a potentially pleasurable activity (anticipatory anhedonia) and loss of the enjoyment experienced from the activity itself (consummatory anhedonia) [67]. Anhedonia is often a key feature of depression, as the diagnosis of major depression requires the presence of either depressed mood or anhedonia [68]. However, anhedonia may occur in the absence of depression. Anhedonia can also be associated with executive dysfunction. Aging is often

associated with anhedonia: as many as one-third of community-dwelling aging adults may have elements of anhedonia [63, 69–76].

4.3.2 Possible Mechanisms

The reward system of the brain is a critical element in the mediation of enjoyment and also strongly influences engagement in activities that have been pleasurable (hedonic activities). The reward system includes many areas of the brain, including the frontal lobes, the nucleus accumbens, the ventral striatum, and the dopaminergic system [77]. The degree of hedonic impact may be related to dopamine neurotransmission from the mesolimbic dopaminergic system to the shell of the nucleus accumbens [78]. With normal aging, dopamine levels decrease approximately 10% per decade, and the anhedonia associated with aging might be related to normal aging-related changes in the dopaminergic neurotransmitter system [79, 80]; however, since the network important to hedonic tone includes other areas of the brain, such as the prefrontal cortex, it is possible that the aging-related changes in the capacity for enjoyment are related to the aging-related deterioration of other structures such as the frontal lobes.

Aging-related alterations in frontal lobe and limbic system functions (Chapter 12), as well as in dopaminergic systems (Chapter 15), have been extensively studied. However, it is not yet clear how changes in these systems might account for anhedonia. In one study, however, Thobois et al. [81] performed a randomized controlled trial of piribedil, a relatively selective D2/D3 dopamine agonist, and assessed anhedonia with the Snaith–Hamilton Pleasure Scale. They found that piribedil led to a trend toward improvement in quality of life and a reduction of anhedonia.

4.4 Apathy

The term "apathy" derives from the Latin *apatheia* (*a*, without, and *pathos*, suffering). However, the term "apathy" has subsequently come to mean without feelings or emotions.

Marin [82–84] defined three necessary components of the apathy syndrome: (1) behavioral symptoms characterized by marked reduction in self-initiated actions, decreased productivity, or a general diminution in goal-directed behaviors; (2) cognitive symptoms characterized by a marked reduction in goal-directed cognition, such as impaired elaboration of action plans and blunted cognitive inquisitiveness; and (3) emotional symptoms characterized by lack of feeling or affective responsivity and a lack of concern for oneself and others [83]. Marin's [82] view of cognitive, emotional, and behavioral subdomains of apathy has been supported by subsequent factor analytic studies. It has now been adopted in the development of provisional diagnostic criteria for use in both research and clinical settings [85].

Unfortunately, only the third component of Marin's broad definition truly corresponds to apathy, while the first two components correspond to some combination of akinesia and abulia. Apathy, as broadly defined by Marin, is observed in diseases that induce frontal-executive dysfunction, such as Parkinson's disease, Huntington's disease, vascular dementia, and head trauma. Although this apathy syndrome has been accepted by some investigators and clinicians, the conflation of apathy with akinesia and abulia is problematic and some researchers believe that Marin's third component, the emotional component, is synonymous with anhedonia [85]. Anhedonia may be observed with changes in the brain related to aging (see below), but it is also a common and often definitive symptom of depression, particularly in the aged. Many elderly patients with depression manifest anhedonia in the absence of sadness and thus may be considered as having apathy.

Although apathy, broadly defined as Marin proposed, is a common symptom in many neurological disorders, some studies have described apathy in otherwise healthy aging adults [86–88]. Brodaty et al. [89], using the Apathy Evaluation Scale, reported elevated apathy in 6% of healthy (nondemented and nondepressed) community-dwelling older adults, aged 58–85 years. In addition, over the 5-year study period, prevalence increased to as much as 15.8% and appeared to be greater in men than women. For the most part, however, this scale assesses abulia, and therefore, not surprisingly, this study found that higher apathy scores were associated with declines in activities. A recent study conducted by Kawagoe et al. [90] found that 26% of their sample of healthy older adults who reported clinically significant apathy had evidence of executive dysfunction. Resting state fMRI revealed decreased functional connectivity between the ventral striatum and frontal cortical regions. Several previous studies have also implicated frontal-basal ganglia networks in the

development of apathy, broadly defined, in both clinical and healthy older adult populations [88, 91–96].

Some studies have addressed apathy defined in the narrower sense of Marin's third component. Berntson et al. [46] studied patients with damage to their amygdala, as well as control participants, by measuring emotional arousal and judgment of valence (positive and negative) of emotional pictures. The patients with damage to the amygdala showed a complete lack of an arousal gradient across negative stimuli. Aging-related degradation of the amygdala [45] may have the same effect. Support for the hypothesis that atrophy of the amygdala may account for aging-related alteration of emotion comes from a functional imaging study that showed that older adults have less functional amygdala activation to negative stimuli than do younger participants [47].

5 Emotional Regulation

Emotional regulation is the ability to control one's own emotions. Studies of emotional regulation have, in general, highlighted a tendency for older adults to focus on positive over negative emotional information.

It is often assumed that the better a person can regulate their emotions, the better off they are in terms of their emotional well-being. Aging adults appear to be excellent regulators of their own emotions, and therefore, they typically report higher levels of emotional well-being than do younger adults [97]. For example, a study that employed self-report measures to examine emotion regulation performance and maintenance in younger and older adults found that the older group more successfully decreased negative emotional reactions to a film clip [98].

To help explain this difference between younger and older adults, Carstensen et al. [99] advanced the Socioemotional Selectivity Theory (SST). According to this theory, older adults place a higher emphasis on emotion regulation goals because of a perception that their time yet to live is limited. Consistent with this theory is the observation that the same phenomenon has been seen in younger adults with life-threatening illnesses [100]. A second theory advanced to explain the aging-related decrease in negative emotional experiences posits the existence of a "cognitive reappraisal" emotion regulation strategy. This strategy involves changing an emotional response by reinterpreting the meaning of the situation that evoked the emotion. Cognitive reappraisal has been shown to be one of the most beneficial active emotion regulation strategies; reduced use of this strategy has been associated with increased levels of anxiety and depression [101]. However, one study suggested that older individuals actually are less likely to use active regulation strategies than young or middle-aged individuals [102].

The differences in regulation of emotions by older and younger adults might have a neurological basis and might be strongly influenced by alterations in the ability to experience emotions. Successful emotion regulation with aging has been reported with decreased amygdala activation and has been found to be associated with cognitive performance, and especially measures of executive functioning [103]. These investigators had younger and aging adults perform a cognitive reappraisal task during fMRI. On each trial, participants viewed positive, negative, or neutral pictures and either naturally experienced the emotion induced by the image ("experience" condition) or attempted to detach themselves from the image ("reappraise" condition). Across both age groups, cognitive reappraisal activated the left inferior frontal gyrus and reduced amygdala activation. However, the younger participants were better able to activate this area of the prefrontal cortex, and thus this mechanism cannot explain why, with aging, people can successfully decrease negative emotional reactions to adverse stimuli. Perhaps, as discussed in Section 3, "Emotional Experience," with aging there are alterations in right hemisphere functions and changes in the limbic system, especially the amygdala, and these changes might allow healthy aging people to more easily regulate negative emotions. However, more research is needed to better understand this change with aging.

6 Conclusion

In summary, aging is associated with many changes in the brain that can influence emotional communication, emotional feelings and experiences, moods, and regulation of emotions. In this chapter, we have identified some consistent patterns of change in emotional function associated with aging and have attempted to provide plausible mechanistic accounts. However, there is still much research that is needed to better identify and clarify these changes, as well as to further understand both the mechanisms and causes of these changes. Even in the absence of disease, it is important to learn how detrimental changes associated with aging might be prevented, treated, and managed.

Acknowledgments

The authors would like to thank Dawn Bowers, Brittany Rohl, Francesca Lopez, and Bonnie Scott for their help.

References

1. Kaszniak AW, Menchola M. Behavioral neuroscience of emotion in aging. In *Behavioral Neurobiology of Aging*. Berlin: Springer; 2011, pp. 51–66.

2. Ross ED, Homan RW, Buck R. Differential hemispheric lateralization of primary and social emotions. *Neuropsychiatry, Neuropsychology, and Behavioral Neurology*. 1994;7(1):1–9.

3. Ruffman T, Henry JD, Livingstone V, Phillips LH. A meta-analytic review of emotion recognition and aging: implications for neuropsychological models of aging. *Neuroscience &*

Biobehavioral Reviews. 2008 Jan 1;32(4):863–81.

4. Sullivan S &. Ruffman T. Social understanding: how does it fare with advancing years? *British Journal of Psychology*. 2004;95:1–18.

5. Isaacowitz DM, Löckenhoff CE, Lance RD, Wright R, Sechrest L, Riedel R, et al. Age differences in recognition of emotion in lexical stimuli and facial expressions. *Psychology and Aging*. 2007;22:147–59.

6. Campbell A, Ruffman T, Murray JE, Glue P. Oxytocin improves emotion recognition for older males. *Neurobiology of Aging*. 2014 Oct 1;35(10):2246–8.

7. Sullivan S, Campbell A, Hutton SB, Ruffman T. What's good for the goose is not good for the gander: age and gender differences in scanning emotion faces. *The Journal of Gerontology: Series B*. 2017 May 1;72(3):441–7.

8. Krendl AC, Rule NO, Ambady N. Does aging impair first impression accuracy? Differentiating emotion recognition from complex social inferences. *Psychology and Aging*. 2014 Sep;29(3):482.

9. Sarabia-Cobo CM, García-Rodríguez B, Navas MJ, Ellgring H. Emotional processing in patients with mild cognitive impairment: the influence of the valence and intensity of emotional

stimuli: the valence and intensity of emotional stimuli influence emotional processing in patients with mild cognitive impairment. *Journal of the Neurological Sciences*. 2015 Oct 15;357 (1–2):222–8.

10. English T, Carstensen L. Emotional experience in the mornings and the evenings: consideration of age differences in specific emotions by time of day. *Frontiers in Psychology*. 2014 Mar 6;5:185.

11. Stanley JT, Isaacowitz DM. Caring more and knowing more reduces age-related differences in emotion perception. *Psychology and Aging*. 2015 Jun;30 (2):383.

12. Ebner NC, Johnson MR, Rieckmann A, Durbin KA, Johnson MK, Fischer H. Processing own-age vs. other-age faces: neuro-behavioral correlates and effects of emotion. *Neuroimage*. 2013 Sep 1;78:363–71.

13. Heilman KM, Blonder LX, Bowers DA, Valenstein ED. Emotional disorders associated with neurological diseases. In Heilman KM, Valenstein E, editors. *Clinical Neuropsychology*. New York: Oxford University Press; 2012, pp. 466–503.

14. Adolphs R. Recognizing emotion from facial expressions: psychological and neurological mechanisms. *Behavioral and Cognitive Neuroscience Reviews*. 2002 Mar;1(1):21–62.

15. Harciarek M, Heilman KM. The contribution of anterior and posterior regions of the right hemisphere to the recognition of emotional faces. *Journal of Clinical and Experimental Neuropsychology*. 2009 Apr;31 (3):322–30. doi: 10.1080/ 13803390802119930.

16. Albert MS, Moss MB. *Geriatric Neuropsychology*. Guilford Press; 1988.

17. Brown JW, Jaffe J. Hypothesis on cerebral dominance. *Neuropsychologia*. 1975 Jan 1;13 (1):107–10.

18. Gur RC, Packer IK, Hungerbuhler JP, Reivich M, Obrist WD, Amarnek WS, et al. Differences in the distribution of gray and white matter in human cerebral hemispheres. *Science*. 1980 Mar 14;207(4436):1226–8.

19. Pujol J, López-Sala A, Deus J, Cardoner N, Sebastián-Gallés N, Conesa G, et al. The lateral asymmetry of the human brain studied by volumetric magnetic resonance imaging. *Neuroimage*. 2002 Oct 1;17(2):670–9.

20. Phillips LH, Allen R. Adult aging and the perceived intensity of emotions in faces and stories. *Aging Clinical and Experimental Research*. 2004 Jun 1;16(3):190–9.

21. Coupland NJ, Sustrik RA, Ting P, Li D, Hartfeil M, Singh AJ, Blair RJ. Positive and negative affect differentially influence identification of facial emotions. *Depression and Anxiety*. 2004;19 (1):31–4.

22. Suzuki A, Hoshino T, Shigemasu K, Kawamura M. Decline or improvement? Age-related differences in facial expression recognition. *Biological Psychology*. 2007 Jan 1;74(1):75–84.

23. Voelkle MC, Ebner NC, Lindenberger U, Riediger M. A note on age differences in mood-congruent vs. mood-incongruent emotion processing in faces. *Frontiers in Psychology*. 2014 Jun 26;5:635.

24. Orbelo DM, Testa JA, Ross ED. Age-related impairments in comprehending affective prosody with comparison to brain-damaged subjects. *Journal of Geriatric Psychiatry and Neurology*. 2003 Mar; 16(1):44–52.

25. Demenescu LR, Mathiak KA, Mathiak K. Age- and gender-related variations of emotion recognition in pseudowords and

faces. *Experimental Aging Research*. 2014;40(2):187–207. doi: 10.1080/0361073X.2014.882210.

26. Orbelo DM, Grim MA, Talbott RE, Ross ED. Impaired comprehension of affective prosody in elderly subjects is not predicted by age-related hearing loss or age-related cognitive decline. *Journal of Geriatric Psychiatry and Neurology*. 2005 Mar;18(1):25–32.

27. Pedder DJ, Terrett G, Bailey PE, Henry JD, Ruffman T, Rendell PG. Reduced facial reactivity as a contributor to preserved emotion regulation in older adults. *Psychology and Aging*. 2016 Feb;31 (1):114–25. doi: 10.1037/ a0039985.

28. Lang PJ, Bradley MM, Cuthbert BN. International affective picture system (IAPS): technical manual and affective ratings. NIMH Center for the Study of Emotion and Attention. 1997:39–58. www2.unifesp.br/dpsicobio/adap/ instructions.pdf.

29. Sen A, Isaacowitz D, Schirmer A. Age differences in vocal emotion perception: on the role of speaker age and listener sex. *Cognition & Emotion*. 2017 Oct;24:1–16. doi: 10.1080/02699931.2017.1393399.

30. Lane RD, Sechrest L, Reidel R. Sociodemographic correlates of alexithymia. *Comprehensive Psychiatry* 1998;39:377–85.

31. Salminen JK, Saarijärvi S, Äärelä E, Toikka T, Kauhanen J. Prevalence of alexithymia and its association with sociodemographic variables in the general population of Finland. *Journal of Psychosomatic Research*. 1999 Jan 1;46(1):75–82.

32. Bogen JE. The callosal syndromes. In Heilman KM, Valenstein E, editors. *Clinical Neuropsychology*. New York: Oxford University Press; 1993, pp. 337–407.

33. TenHouten WD, Hoppe KD, Bogen JE, Walter DO. Alexithymia and the split brain.

I. Lexical-level content analysis. *Psychotherapy and Psychosomatics*. 1985;43(4):202–8.

34. Lockhart SN, DeCarli C. Structural imaging measures of brain aging. *Neuropsychology Review*. 2014 Sep;24(3):271–89. doi: 10.1007/s11065-014-9268-3.

35. Wundt W. *Grundriss der Psychologic*, 6th edn., Leipzig; 1904. Philosophische Studien.;13.

36. Backs RW, da Silva SP, Han K. A comparison of younger and older adults' self-assessment manikin ratings of affective pictures. *Experimental Aging Research*. 2005 Oct–Dec;31 (4):421–40.

37. Grühn D, Scheibe S. Age-related differences in valence and arousal ratings of pictures from the International Affective Picture System (IAPS): do ratings become more extreme with age? *Behavior Research Methods*. 2008 May;40 (2):512–21.

38. Smith JC, Bradley MM, Lang PJ. State anxiety and affective physiology: effects of sustained exposure to affective pictures. *Biological Psychology*. 2005 Jul 1;69(3):247–60.

39. Feng MC, Courtney CG, Mather M, Dawson ME, Davison GC. Age-related affective modulation of the startle eyeblink response: older adults startle most when viewing positive pictures. *Psychology and Aging*. 2011 Sep;26 (3):752–60.

40. Le Duc J, Fournier P, Hébert S. Modulation of prepulse inhibition and startle reflex by emotions: a comparison between young and older adults. *Frontiers in Aging Neuroscience*. 2016 Feb 23;8:33.

41. Hilimire MR, Mienaltowski A, Blanchard-Fields F, Corballis PM. Age-related differences in event-related potentials for early visual processing of emotional faces. *Social Cognitive and Affective Neuroscience*. 2013 Jun 13;9 (7):969–76.

42. Antonenko D, Flöel A. Healthy aging by staying selectively connected: a mini-review. *Gerontology*. 2014;60(1):3–9. doi: 10.1159/000354376.

43. Chen M., Bargh J. A. (1999). Consequences of automatic evaluation: immediate behavioral predispositions to approach or avoid the stimulus. *Pers. Soc. Psychol. Bull.* 25:215–24.

44. Denny-Brown D, Chambers RA. The parietal lobes and behavior. *Research Publications Association for Research in Nervous and Mental Disease*. 1958;36:35–117.

45. Cacioppo JT, Berntson GG, Bechara A, Tranel D, Hawkley LC. Could an aging brain contribute to subjective well-being? The value added by a social neuroscience perspective. In Todorov A, Fiske ST, Prentice DA, editors. *Social Neuroscience: Toward Understanding the Underpinnings of the Social Mind*. Oxford: Oxford University Press; 2011, 249–62.

46. Berntson GG, Bechara A, Damasio H, Tranel D, Cacioppo JT. Amygdala contribution to selective dimensions of emotion. *Social Cognitive and Affective Neuroscience*. 2007 Jun 1;2 (2):123–9.

47. Mather M, Canli T, English T, Whitfield S, Wais P, Ochsner K, et al. Amygdala responses to emotionally valenced stimuli in older and younger adults. *Psychological Science*. 2004 Apr;15 (4):259–63.

48. Leaver AM, Yang H, Siddarth P, Vlasova RM, Krause B, St Cyr N, et al. Resilience and amygdala function in older healthy and depressed adults. *Journal of Affective Disorders*. 2018 Sep;237:27–34. doi: 10.1016/j.jad.2018.04.109

49. Hasin DS, Goodwin RD, Stinson FS, Grant BF. Epidemiology of major depressive disorder: results from the National Epidemiologic Survey on Alcoholism and Related Conditions. *Archives of General Psychiatry*. 2005 Oct 1;62 (10):1097–106.

50. Lyness JM, King DA, Cox C, Yoediono Z, Caine ED. The importance of subsyndromal depression in older primary care patients: prevalence and associated functional disability. *Journal of the American Geriatrics Society*. 1999 Jun;47(6):647–52.

51. Reynolds K, Pietrzak RH, El-Gabalawy R, Mackenzie CS, Sareen J. Prevalence of psychiatric disorders in US older adults: findings from a nationally representative survey. *World Psychiatry*. 2015 Feb;14(1):74–81.

52. Fiske A, Wetherell JL, Gatz M. Depression in older adults. *Annual Review of Clinical Psychology*. 2009 Apr 27;5:363–89.

53. Bruce ML, McAvay GJ, Raue PJ, Brown EL, Meyers BS, Keohane DJ, et al. Major depression in elderly home health care patients. *American Journal of Psychiatry*. 2002 Aug 1;159(8):1367–74.

54. Gallo JJ, Anthony JC, Muthén BO. Age differences in the symptoms of depression: a latent trait analysis. *Journal of Gerontology*. 1994 Nov 1;49(6):P251–P264.

55. Gallo JJ, Rabins PV, Lyketsos CG, Tien AY, Anthony JC. Depression without sadness: functional outcomes of nondysphoric depression in later life. *Journal of the American Geriatrics Society*. 1997 May;45(5):570–8.

56. Kessler RC, Chiu WT, Demler O, Walters EE. Prevalence, severity, and comorbidity of 12-month DSM-IV disorders in the National Comorbidity Survey Replication. *Archives of General Psychiatry*. 2005 Jun 1;62(6):617–27.

57. Xekardaki A, Santos M, Hof P, Kövari E, Bouras C, Giannakopoulos P. Neuropathological substrates and structural changes in late-life depression: the impact of vascular

burden. *Acta Neuropathologica.*
2012 Oct 1;124(4):453–64.

58. Beekman AT, de Beurs E, van
Balkom AJ, Deeg DJ, van Dyck R,
van Tilburg W. Anxiety and
depression in later life: co-
occurrence and communality of
risk factors. *American Journal of
Psychiatry.* 2000 Jan 1;157
(1):89–95.

59. Janssen J, Beekman AT, Comijs
HC, Deeg DJ, Heeren TJ. Late-life
depression: the differences
between early- and late-onset
illness in a community-based
sample. *International Journal of
Geriatric Psychiatry: A Journal of
the Psychiatry of Late Life and
Allied Sciences.* 2006 Jan;21
(1):86–93.

60. Heun R, Papassotiropoulos A,
Jessen F, Maier W, Breitner JC.
A family study of Alzheimer
disease and early- and late-onset
depression in elderly patients.
Archives of General Psychiatry.
2001 Feb 1;58(2):190–6.

61. Gade A, Kristoffersen M, Kessing
LV. Neuroticism in remitted
major depression: elevated with
early onset but not late onset of
depression. *Psychopathology.*
2015;48(6):400–7.

62. Brodaty H, Luscombe G, Parker
G, Wilhelm K, Hickie I, Austin
MP, et al. Early and late onset
depression in old age: different
aetiologies, same phenomenology.
Journal of Affective Disorders.
2001 Oct 1;66(2–3):225–36.

63. Ritchie CS, Hearld KR, Gross A,
Allman R, Sawyer P, Sheppard K,
et al. Measuring symptoms in
community-dwelling older
adults: the psychometric
properties of a brief symptom
screen. *Medical Care.* 2013 Oct;51
(10):949.

64. Bryant C, Jackson H, Ames D.
The prevalence of anxiety in older
adults: methodological issues and
a review of the literature. *Journal
of Affective Disorders.* 2008 Aug
1;109(3):233–50.

65. Fuentes K, Cox B. Assessment of
anxiety in older adults: a
community-based survey and
comparison with younger adults.
Behaviour Research and Therapy.
2000 Mar 1;38(3):297–309.

66. Palmer BW, Jeste DV, Sheikh JI.
Anxiety disorders in the elderly:
DSM-IV and other barriers to
diagnosis and treatment. *Journal
of Affective Disorders.* 1997 Dec
1;46(3):183–90.

67. Treadway MT, Zald DH.
Reconsidering anhedonia in
depression: lessons from
translational neuroscience.
*Neuroscience & Biobehavioral
Reviews.* 2011 Jan 1;35(3):537–55.

68. American Psychiatric Association.
*Diagnostic and Statistical Manual
of Mental Disorders* (DSM-5).
Washington, DC: American
Psychiatric Association; 2013.

69. Lampe IK, Kahn RS, Heeren TJ.
Apathy, anhedonia, and
psychomotor retardation in
elderly psychiatric patients and
healthy elderly individuals.
*Journal of Geriatric Psychiatry and
Neurology.* 2001 Mar;14(1):11–16.

70. Quaranta D, Marra C, Gainotti G.
Post-stroke depression: main
phenomenological clusters and
their relationships with clinical
measures. *Behavioural Neurology.*
2012;25(4):303–10.

71. Andreasen NC. Negative
symptoms in schizophrenia:
definition and reliability. *Archives
of General Psychiatry.* 1982 Jul
1;39(7):784–8.

72. Chapman LJ, Chapman JP, Raulin
ML. Scales for physical and social
anhedonia. *Journal of Abnormal
Psychology.* 1976 Aug;85(4):374.

73. Fawcett J, Clark DC, Scheftner
WA, Hedeker D. Differences
between anhedonic and normally
hedonic depressive states. *The
American Journal of Psychiatry.*
1983 Aug;140(8):1027–30.

74. Snaith RP, Hamilton M, Morley S,
Humayan A, Hargreaves D,

Trigwell P. A scale for the
assessment of hedonic tone the
Snaith–Hamilton Pleasure Scale.
The British Journal of Psychiatry.
1995 Jul;167(1):99–103.

75. Gard DE, Gard MG, Kring AM,
John OP. Anticipatory and
consummatory components of the
experience of pleasure: a scale
development study. *Journal of
Research in Personality.* 2006 Dec
1;40(6):1086–102.

76. Treadway MT, Buckholtz JW,
Schwartzman AN, Lambert WE,
Zald DH. Worth the "EEfRT"?
The effort expenditure for rewards
task as an objective measure of
motivation and anhedonia. *PloS
One.* 2009 Aug 12;4(8):e6598.

77. Berridge KC, Robinson TE. What
is the role of dopamine in reward:
hedonic impact, reward learning,
or incentive salience? *Brain
Research Reviews.* 1998;28:309–69.

78. Stein DJ. Depression, anhedonia,
and psychomotor symptoms: the
role of dopaminergic
neurocircuitry. *CNS Spectrums.*
2008;13(7):561–65.

79. Mukherjee J, Christian BT,
Dunigan KA, Shi B, Narayanan
TK, Satter M, et al. Brain imaging
of 18F-fallypride in normal
volunteers: blood analysis,
distribution, test-retest studies,
and preliminary assessment of
sensitivity to aging effects on
dopamine D-2/D-3 receptors.
Synapse. 2002 Dec 1;46(3):170–88.

80. Nyberg L, Bäckman L. Cognitive
aging: a view from brain imaging.
New Frontiers in Cognitive Aging.
2004:135–60.

81. Thobois S, Lhommée E, Klinger
H, Ardouin C, Schmitt E, Bichon
A, et al. Parkinsonian apathy
responds to dopaminergic
stimulation of D2/D3 receptors
with piribedil. *Brain.* 2013
May;136(Pt 5):1568–77. doi:
10.1093/brain/awt067.

82. Marin RS. Apathy: a
neuropsychiatric syndrome. *The
Journal of Neuropsychiatry and*

Clinical Neurosciences. 1991 Summer;3(3):243–54.

83. Marin RS. Apathy: concept, syndrome, neural mechanisms, and treatment. *Seminars in Clinical Neuropsychiatry* 1996 Oct;1(4):304–14.

84. Marin RS, Wilkosz PA. Disorders of diminished motivation. *The Journal of Head Trauma Rehabilitation.* 2005 Jul 1;20 (4):377–88.

85. Starkstein SE, Leentjens AF. The nosological position of apathy in clinical practice. *Journal of Neurology, Neurosurgery & Psychiatry.* 2008 Oct;79 (10):1088–92.

86. Cummings JL, Benson DF. Psychological dysfunction accompanying subcortical dementias. *Annual Review of Medicine.* 1988 Feb;39(1):53–61.

87. Stuss DT, Van Reekum R, Murphy KJ. Differentiation of states and causes of apathy. In Borod JC, editor. *Series in Affective Science: The Neuropsychology of Emotion.* New York: Oxford University Press; 2012, pp. 340–63.

88. Levy R, Dubois B. Apathy and the functional anatomy of the prefrontal cortex–basal ganglia circuits. *Cerebral Cortex.* 2005 Oct 5;16(7):916–28.

89. Brodaty H, Altendorf A, Withall A, Sachdev P. Do people become more apathetic as they grow older? A longitudinal study in healthy individuals. *International Psychogeriatrics.* 2010 May;22 (3):426–36.

90. Kawagoe T, Onoda K, Yamaguchi S. Apathy and executive function

in healthy elderly – resting state fMRI study. *Frontiers in Aging Neuroscience.* 2017 May 9;9:124.

91. Alexopoulos GS, Hoptman MJ, Yuen G, Kanellopoulos D, Seirup JK, Lim KO, et al. Functional connectivity in apathy of late-life depression: a preliminary study. *Journal of Affective Disorders.* 2013 Jul 1;149 (1–3):398–405.

92. Cardinal RN, Parkinson JA, Hall J, Everitt BJ. Emotion and motivation: the role of the amygdala, ventral striatum, and prefrontal cortex. *Neuroscience & Biobehavioral Reviews.* 2002 May 1;26(3):321–52.

93. Carriere N, Besson P, Dujardin K, Duhamel A, Defebvre L, Delmaire C, et al. Apathy in Parkinson's disease is associated with nucleus accumbens atrophy: a magnetic resonance imaging shape analysis. *Movement Disorders.* 2014 Jun;29 (7):897–903.

94. Bonnelle V, Manohar S, Behrens T, Husain M. Individual differences in premotor brain systems underlie behavioral apathy. *Cerebral Cortex.* 2015 Nov 12;26(2):807–19.

95. Levy R. Apathy: a pathology of goal-directed behaviour. A new concept of the clinic and pathophysiology of apathy. *Revue neurologique.* 2012 Aug 1;168(8–9):585–97.

96. Murayama K, Matsumoto M, Izuma K, Matsumoto K. Neural basis of the undermining effect of monetary reward on intrinsic motivation. *Proceedings of the National Academy of Sciences.* 2010 Dec 7;107(49):20911–16.

97. Cacioppo JT, Hawkley LC, Kalil A, Hughes ME, Waite L, Thisted RA. Happiness and the invisible threads of social connection. In Eid M, Larsen RJ, editors. *The Science of Subjective Well-Being.* New York: Guilford Press; 2008, pp. 195–219.

98. Scheibe S, Blanchard-Fields F. Effects of regulating emotions on cognitive performance: what is costly for young adults is not so costly for older adults. *Psychology and Aging.* 2009 Mar;24(1):217.

99. Carstensen LL, Isaacowitz DM, Charles ST. Taking time seriously: a theory of socioemotional selectivity. *American Psychologist.* 1999 Mar;54(3):165.

100. Carstensen LL, Fredrickson BL. Influence of HIV status and age on cognitive representations of others. *Health Psychology.* 1998 Nov;17(6):494.

101. Garnefski N, Kraaij V, Spinhoven P. Negative life events, cognitive emotion regulation and emotional problems. *Personality and Individual Differences.* 2001 Jun 1;30(8):1311–27.

102. Brummer L, Stopa L, Bucks R. The influence of age on emotion regulation strategies and psychological distress. *Behavioural and Cognitive Psychotherapy.* 2014 Nov;42 (6):668–81.

103. Winecoff A, LaBar KS, Madden DJ, Cabeza R, Huettel SA. Cognitive and neural contributors to emotion regulation in aging. *Social Cognitive and Affective Neuroscience.* 2010 Apr 12;6 (2):165–76.

Aging and Attention

Ian H. Robertson and Paul M. Dockree

1 Introduction

Attention is the ability to *select,* within and between sensory modalities, the stimuli that will be further processed and those that will not, including stimuli of which we are aware but are deemed unimportant (e.g., listening to a person speaking while ignoring the flickering screen of a television in the background). The networks that mediate attention also provide the ability to *switch* between one stream of information (e.g., reading a newspaper) and another (e.g., an airport announcement), as well as to switch between top-down (intentionally allocated) and bottom-up (stimulus-induced) attention. Vigilance is the ability to *sustain* attention to a particular stream of information in the absence of novelty, emotion-arousing qualities, or perceived difficulty in responding [1]. Different forms of attention may require use of different networks and even different neuromodulators and neurotransmitters. For example, Posner has suggested that different forms of attention might be more strongly linked to different neurotransmitter systems, for example, selection to the acetylcholine system, switching to the dopamine system, and sustaining attention to the norepinephrine system [2].

With aging, there are changes in these attentional networks and in the allocation of attention that may be particularly important as they may adversely influence work, activities of daily living, and social interactions. Since aging is associated with a gradual degradation of cholinergic, dopaminergic, and noradrenergic function [3–5], it is not surprising to find widespread attentional changes associated with aging. With these changes in neurotransmitters, as well as other aging-related changes, such as white matter connectivity, there is no clear consensus about the brain mechanisms accounting for aging-related changes in attention.

The precise pathological-functional relationships that can and have been defined with lesion studies of younger adults cannot be fully used to understand the alterations of attention in aging individuals. For example, spatial orientation paradigms of the type developed by Posner have enabled us to understand how strokes in specific locations affect the allocation of spatial attention [1, 2]. Aging-related deficits in spatial orientation have been demonstrated, but a recent review concludes that these deficits are probably mediated by a number of factors and cannot be confidently attributed to a specific defect in orienting mechanisms [6]. An electrophysiological study of aging supports this conclusion, finding no evidence of aging-related ERP changes associated with orienting and alerting systems but definite evidence of ERP changes consistent with alteration of executive control [7].

In a recent review [6] of meta-analyses of aging, executive control, and attention, aging-related deficits were found. For example, there were aging-related changes in dual-task performance and global task-switching but not with local task switching or selective attention. This finding was recently confirmed in an fMRI BOLD study [8].

While deficits in inhibitory processes have been observed with aging, resulting in top-down suppression deficits that impair working memory [9], the generality of this finding was placed in doubt by a recent review. It revealed that aging-related inhibitory deficits in selective attention appear to be sensory modality–dependent, such that older adults are disproportionately affected when visual distraction accompanies an auditory task but not vice versa. Also, aging-related inhibitory deficits, in this review, were not apparent in the spatial domain, and, furthermore, it was not clear that the deficits observed were a result of a failure of enhancement of the target stimuli rather than a failure of top-down inhibition of the distractor stimuli.

Elucidating the possible mechanistic relationships between attention and aging poses a number of methodological challenges. First, attention almost always is measured in ways that involve motor, perceptual, memory, emotional, and other systems in the brain. Given the aging-related changes in these systems (see Chapters 5, 7, 9 and 11), it can be challenging to separate out attention-specific deficits from impairments related either to these other systems or to their interactions with higher level attention control systems.

Second, processes described as "attention" interact with frontal executive functions (Chapter 12) involving inhibitory and strategic processes controlling cognition. Even quite simple attention tasks can have a strong strategic component [10]. Executive dysfunction characterized by inconsistently applied, and possibly compensatory, top-down executive control can result in apparent impairments in basic attention processes.

Third, many if not most attention tasks require rapid processing. Slowing of information processing can masquerade as an attentional deficit [11]. A number of processes that slow with aging can impact attention, including error processing [12], decision-making [13] and working memory [14].

An important study by Backman, Nyberg, and colleagues exemplifies the challenge of delineating specific cognitive losses in older people. Compared with younger participants, healthy older adults showed a failure to modulate frontoparietal activity in relation to cognitive load in a spatial working memory task. However, when a PET measure of dopamine D1 binding potential was covaried statistically, the aging-related differences in fMRI BOLD signal were either eliminated or greatly attenuated [3]. This finding raises the possibility that apparent aging-related cognitive dysfunction, including impairments in attentional processes, may actually reflect aging-related changes in underlying systems, for example, neurotransmitter functions.

The delineation of aging-related attention deficits may be complicated by the evolution of strategies to *compensate* for changes in brain chemistry, structure, and function. These include adopting a more conservative criterion before responding in order to minimize errors [15], slowing responses to alter speed-error trade-offs [16], and engaging in more effortful, controlled processing for some tasks [17], while relying more on automatic processes for others (see Chapter 12).

For all the above reasons, we will not attempt in this chapter to characterize further the specific – and possibly elusive – attention deficits shown by older people in the context of the multiple and complex confounds that render the measurement of attention

difficult in this group. Excellent reviews of this area do exist (e.g., [18]), which we will not summarize here, except to say that on most measures of attention, aging-related deficits do appear to vary considerably, with one important exception: sustained attention.

Sustained attention is less consistently impaired when comparing younger and older adults than other aspects of attention, such as selection and switching [19–24]. Two large cross-sectional studies across the life span [25, 26] suggest that sustained attention ability follows a unique trajectory with a plateau in performance in middle adulthood before later decline in older adulthood. This mid-life maturation of sustained attention may, in part, explain why differences between older and younger adults are not always detected. A meta-analysis of a large number of fMRI studies has shown that sustained attention processes strongly localize to the right frontoparietal cortex [27]. Furthermore, sustained attention is preferentially modulated by the noradrenalin/norepinephrine neurotransmitter system [28], which in turn plays a central role in cognitive reserve [4, 29, 30].

This chapter will focus on the possible role of a number of attention-related processes in the complex dynamics of the aging brain as it reorganizes to maintain function. It will focus on the potential role of a right hemisphere network in enabling older people to maintain adequate attention to their environment as a multitude of biological changes take place in their brains. Kenneth Heilman and his colleagues were pioneers in identifying a right hemisphere role in the maintenance of basic arousal processes in the brain, and a recent review has indeed suggested that aging is associated with a rightward shift in visuospatial attention [31]. Adequate arousal provides the essential underpinning for all types of attention. It is therefore fitting that this chapter in this volume should take this particular perspective on attention and aging.

2 Cognitive Reserve

Many individuals who have shown no symptoms of dementia while alive are found to have evidence of brain pathology on postmortem examination. Most of these cases are distinguished by higher education, a history of mental stimulation, above-average intelligence, and rich social networks [32, 33]. This phenomenon of preserved intellect in the face of pathology defining a dementing process has been attributed to the acquired flexibility, resilience, and efficiency of brain networks [34, 35]. It is usually termed "cognitive reserve." It has been defined in a way that incorporates the closely linked concepts of brain reserve [32] and brain maintenance [36]:

> Cognitive reserve is the thinking capacity and adaptation of the mechanisms that protect and maintain optimal cognition in functioning across multiple contexts and in the face of multiple pathologies and stressors. (IFA Global Think Tank on Ageing Cognitive Reserve, 2017)

Robertson, one of the current authors [29], has proposed that noradrenaline may be of particular importance in mediating the capacity of the brain to maintain cognitive functioning in the face of a number of age-related biological changes. Subsequent studies have given support to this norepinephrine hypothesis [4, 30, 37]. Briefly, each of the components of cognitive reserve, including education level, intelligence, social engagement, and mental stimulation, has a specific link to the noradrenaline system. For example, fluid intelligence is highly correlated with baseline pupil diameter across a range of socioeconomic and racial groups [38], and pupillary function indexes noradrenaline activity [39]. Over a lifetime, people high in cognitive reserve experience many millions of brief infusions of noradrenaline consequent to their high level of mental stimulation. Furthermore, noradrenaline is a neuromodulator that promotes optimal coordination of neural firing within and between neural networks [40], as well as enhancing synaptogenesis [41] and neurogenesis [42]. It also reduces inflammation as well as the toxicity and aggregation of amyloid plaques in the brain [43]. The locus coeruleus (LC) is activated by cognitive and physical functions that (1) are arousing and effortful; (2) are interesting, novel, and productive of excitement; (3) require sustained attention [27]; and (4) involve self-awareness and self-monitoring. Resultant increases in brain norepinephrine can protect against some aging-related changes of the brain. A right hemisphere frontoparietal cortical network appears to play an important role in all four of these processes [44] and appears to be important in making compensatory changes in the aging brain.

3 The Special Role of Attention in Aging

Compensatory processes in the aging brain engage neuroplastic mechanisms that, in turn, are strongly dependent on the ability to sustain attention to

stimuli. Although learning mechanisms are central to the instantiation of compensatory changes in the brain, sustained attention is a key precondition for effective learning [42]. In this way, sustained attention serves as a gateway to neuroplasticity [45]. Normal learning processes, such as those that underpin recovery and rehabilitation, depend on neuroplasticity, which in turn requires attention to the relevant stimulus-response elements of the to-be-learned behavior; without this attention, plastic reorganization does not occur [46]. We have supportive evidence in humans showing, for example, that recovery of left-hand motor function after right hemisphere stroke is specifically predicated on sustained attention capacity [45]. Painstaking motor rehearsal demands plasticity-affording, sustained attention over time to routine, even boring, repetitions. To the extent that attention falls away, motor rehearsal will result in few, if any, neuroplastic changes. The same principle applies to cognitive and sensory domains. Arousal is a prerequisite for optimal attention [47] and novelty is a major driver of arousal [48]. The ability to monitor one's behavior and errors is critical for learning and compensation [49] and such self-awareness is also heavily dependent on adequate arousal [50].

The behaviors commonly associated with senescence include routine rather than novelty, familiar tasks rather than challenging, low arousal rather than high arousal, and undemanding mental activity that is less dependent on sustained attention. This highly predictable, unchallenging, low-tempo, unforced way of life also reduces the requirements for self-monitoring because so little is unpredictable; mistakes or difficulties that would normally trigger self-monitoring, and hence self-awareness, are limited.

The contributors to cognitive reserve that mitigate the effects of normal and abnormal aging include education, intelligence, mental challenge, and dense social networks, all of which foster the antithesis of senescence – namely, novelty over routine, sustained versus drifting attention, higher rather than lower arousal, and more rather than less self-awareness.

There is, however, a major problem with this crucial compensatory network for the aging brain. The same frontoparietal regions of the brain that mediate those attentional-arousal functions important for developing cognitive reserve are also the areas of the brain that appear to be the most vulnerable to the effects of aging. A number of studies report reduced brain volume [51, 52] and lowered metabolism [53, 54] in these regions, as well as functional changes characterized by a reduced leftward bias for spatial attention-related processing with aging [55–59]. Two aging-related changes appear to assail these right hemispheric frontoparietal networks. The first is a change in structure caused by a number of as yet poorly understood processes. Neuroimaging studies of functional and structural connectivity have demonstrated aging-related changes and structural degeneration in most parts of the hemispheric white matter. However, the greatest deterioration appears to occur in the frontal networks, which are very dependent on white matter connectivity.

With aging, there is loss of noradrenergic cells in the locus coeruleus. Of all the brain stem nuclei, the locus coeruleus is the only one for which cell density predicts rate of cognitive decline in humans [37]. Norepinephrine concentrations are higher in the right hemisphere [60], and, as mentioned above, senescence is associated with an asymmetrical deterioration of right hemisphere networks.

4 Sustained Attention

An unparalleled investigation of the life-span trajectories in a large sample of 10,430 people has revealed unique aging-related changes in sustained attention that are distinguishable from other facets of cognition [25]. Fortenbaugh et al. [25] derived measures of response time variability and accuracy from performance on the gradual-onset continuous performance test (gradCPT). Participants are required to respond to the more frequent (90%) photographs of city scenes and withhold their responses to rare (10%) mountain scenes. A novel aspect of the test is a gradual transition from one scene to the next, and, as such, performance is more dependent on endogenous processes and less influenced by sudden exogenous onsets and offsets typical of punctate stimuli. Performance on this task revealed a pattern of aging-related incremental improvement in participants' ability to sustain attention peaking at 43 years of age and declining thereafter (see Figure 10.1). As the authors note, this sets sustained attention apart from cognitive functions linked to fluid intelligence, such as information processing speed and working memory, which decline from the mid-20s onward [61], and functions linked to crystallized intelligence, such as the accumulation of knowledge and experience, which show no decrement until after the mid-60s [62].

This unique mid-life advantage in sustained attention may be attributable to the pattern of maturation

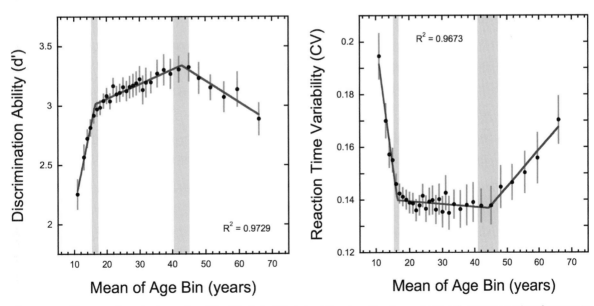

Figure 10.1 Measures of sustained attention ability (discriminability index (d') and reaction time variability), illustrating a peak performance in mid-life followed by decline. Error bars show 95% confidence intervals. Modified from Fortenbaugh FC, DeGutis J, Germine L, Wilmer JB, Grosso M, Russo K, et al. Sustained attention across the life span in a sample of 10,000: dissociating ability and strategy. *Psychol Sci.* 2015;26(9):1497–510.

and degeneration of white matter over the human life span. MRI studies suggest that mean diffusivity and myelin content (measured by the R1 (1/T1) sequence) reach their maximum at ~40 years of age and decline thereafter [63], mirroring the sustained attention performance patterns reported by Fortenbaugh et al. [25]. Peak sustained attention in mid-life may also, in part, reflect accruing practice in engagement of this cognitive mechanism over time with the multiple responsibilities of family, work, and community placing unique demands on middle-aged adults [64]. It is clear from alertness training protocols in the laboratory that sustained attention can be augmented by practice at any age [65]. However, given the degeneration of white matter fascicles destined for the prefrontal cortices and the related decline in frontal functions that begins in middle age, it is unclear as to whether the dominant role of the right prefrontal cortex (PFC) for sustained attention can still be exploited and upregulated in older adults to ameliorate deficits in this capacity.

Our research group has investigated whether the aging-related decline of sustained visual attention relatable to right hemispheric dysfunction could be improved with noninvasive brain stimulation. Specifically, we have examined whether behavioral markers and associated electrophysiological signatures of sustained attention in older adults can be normalized by increasing excitability of the right lateral PFC with anodal transcranial direct current stimulation (tDCS). In one experiment [66], low performing older adults ($n = 26$) were selected based on their percentile scores (<50%) on the Sustained Attention to Response Test

(SART) (normative data from the Irish Longitudinal Study of Ageing [67]). Their performance was then measured under both real tDCS and sham tDCS during two versions of the SART, one with fixed and one with random stimulus presentation [68, 69]. During the fixed presentation, nine numbers are presented repeatedly in a fixed order. Participants are required to respond to each number with the exception of the number 3 (no-go trial). This version is more sensitive to sustained attention failures because its monotonous regularity leads to distraction and task disengagement. During the random SART, stimuli are presented in an unpredictable order and are more likely to elicit errors that reflect a failure of response inhibition. Using both the *fixed* and *random* tests, we have provided evidence that the two types of action error they elicit are physiologically dissociable despite being behaviorally indistinguishable from each other (i.e., the same unintended response) [70]. During tDCS, we found that right PFC stimulation reduced the number of errors in older adults during the *fixed* SART but not the *random* SART, suggesting a selective improvement of processes linked to sustained attention but not response inhibition (see Figure 10.2).

Electrophysiological data collected during tDCS helped explain a possible mechanism underlying this improvement. Two event-related potential (ERP) components during the fixed SART were affected by tDCS within the first 200 milliseconds of stimulus processing, providing insight into the mechanisms of tDCS-related improvement. A greater amplitude of the *P2f component* was measured over prefrontal

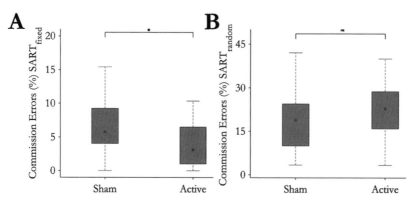

Figure 10.2 The effect of right PFC tDCS during fixed and random SART conditions. Anodal stimulation over the right prefrontal cortex reduced commission errors during the fixed SART (A) and but not during the random SART (B). Modified from Brosnan MB, Arvaneh M, Harty S, Maguire T, O'Connell RG, Robertson IH, Dockree PM. Prefrontal modulation of the sustained attention network in ageing, a tDCS-EEG co-registration approach. *J Cogn Neurosci.* 2018;13:1–16.

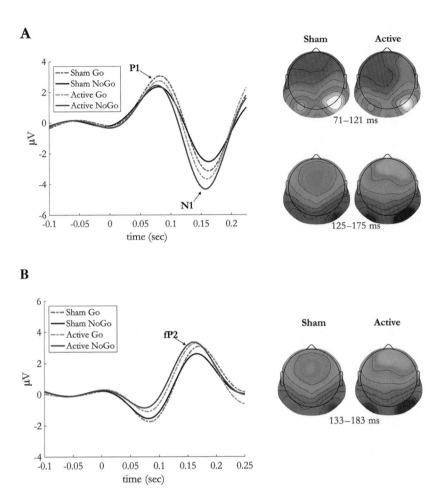

Figure 10.3 The effects of anodal tDCS on the selection negativity amplitude (A) and on the frontal P2 (P2f) amplitude (B) during the fixed SART. ERP plots illustrating the effect of stimulation by trial type (left) and scalp plots (right) showing the topography of the components of interest (P1: 71–121 milliseconds; N1: 125–175 milliseconds; P2f: 133–183 milliseconds) during active and sham stimulation (for go and no-go trials). Modified from Brosnan MB, Arvaneh M, Harty S, Maguire T, O'Connell RG, Robertson IH, Dockree PM. Prefrontal modulation of the sustained attention network in ageing, a tDCS-EEG co-registration approach. *J Cogn Neurosci.* 2018;13:1–16.

regions, suggesting greater top-down recruitment of attentional resources across the task. In addition, there was evidence of an enhanced *selection negativity* effect over parieto-occipital regions, specifically on no-go trials, suggesting that greater sensory amplification of goal-relevant features was induced by right PFC stimulation (see Figure 10.3). By contrast, tDCS did not change any of the task-relevant ERP signals elicited during the *random* SART, including the frontal P3 marker of response inhibition. These electrophysiological effects support the hypothesis that neuromodulation of the right PFC can potentiate a functional network in which top-down prefrontal inputs can increase stimulus-evoked signaling in visual regions, supporting task performance. More generally, the findings suggest that a potential for plasticity exists within this right-lateralized network in low-performing older adults, and interventions that target the right PFC, in particular, hold promise for promoting long-lasting changes in sustained attention function. Since the lateral PFC has been identified as a highly interconnected regional hub [71], upregulation of its function might mitigate the impact of aging-related neural decline. Indeed, tDCS using the same right lateral PFC stimulation parameters (current strength, anode/cathode electrode placement) also increases error awareness in older adults [72]. This may reflect enhanced sustained attention capacity [73], a potentially important means of offsetting the detrimental effects of aging on the ability to monitor one's errors [74].

5 Error Awareness

Failures to detect everyday cognitive errors are often related to aging-related inattention and distraction. These failures might prevent the growing realization with aging one has limitations that necessitate a change of strategy. Laboratory paradigms that capture error awareness may therefore provide an assay of this key monitoring function. We have found that older adults are aware of 25% fewer errors than younger adults during a go/no-go response inhibition task in which participants were trained to signal their "awareness" by making a response on the subsequent trial to the error [74]. This aging-related deficit in error awareness was present even when sensory and motor response times were controlled, thereby parsing out the influence of aging-related reduction in processing speed. It is modifiable by right PFC stimulation [72]. A deficit in awareness of errors is also associated with cognitive difficulties in daily life, derived from reports of daily attentional and memory functioning [74]. A common approach for measuring self-awareness is to make a comparison between an individual's report and that of a significant other or informant [75]. A discrepancy between the two reports provides an indirect measure of an impairment in self-awareness. Harty et al. [73] found that older adults who underreported attentional failures and memory problems in daily life (compared with informant reports) were also less aware of errors in the laboratory.

The existence of an aging-related deficit in error awareness initially appears at odds with a more commonly observed phenomenon: older adults are typically more cautious, adopting a conservative response strategy to minimize error. Fortenbaugh and colleagues [25], in their life-span study of attentional processes (cited above), parsed sustained attention into two underlying components ("ability" and "strategy") using exploratory factor analysis. Although "ability" declined from age 43 onward, "strategy," which was characterized by slower reaction times and reduced willingness to respond in the case of uncertainty, exhibited a monotonic increase across the life span. One might hypothesize that a conservative response strategy that increases with age would support error awareness. However, new unpublished data from our group [76] suggest that strategic slowing improves task accuracy but hinders error awareness in older adults. In a simplified version of the error awareness task used by Harty et al. [73], participants were required to respond to colored stimuli but withhold their response when the stimulus that appeared was either blue in color or a repeat of the previous colored stimulus. Following a response inhibition error, participants were instructed to signal their awareness with a second button press. An interaction was apparent in which older adults demonstrated lower levels of error awareness than younger adults but achieved higher levels of overall task accuracy compared with their younger counterparts (Figure 10.4).

These findings suggest that older and younger adults show a reverse relationship between response selection and error monitoring. Older adults appear to favor a cautious response strategy that improves response selection accuracy, even as they appear to be less aware of errors, possibly reflecting poor monitoring and momentary lapses of attention. Longer RTs on error trials were associated with higher overall levels of unawareness in older adults, suggesting that their cautious strategy not only reduced error but also appeared to reduce error awareness. By contrast, the faster responses of the younger adults were associated with a greater speed/accuracy trade-off, yielding more errors of response selection and inhibition. However, the errors associated with their speeded responses appear to be more likely to capture their attention.

To further elucidate the differences between the older and younger adults in error-processing mechanisms, we examined the well-known error-related ERP component – the error positivity (Pe) component – that has previously been shown to vary in amplitude as a function of awareness [77]. Understanding the temporal dynamics of the Pe has the potential to elucidate the impact of aging on error awareness. It may be useful to consider error awareness as a metacognitive decision process whereby evidence for an erroneous response is accumulated until a decision threshold is reached [78, 79]. The temporal dynamics of the Pe provide a useful measure to track this process [80]. First, the build-up rate of the signal (calculated as the slope of a straight line 100 milliseconds prior to the Pe peak latency [Figure 10.5]) reflects the rate at which evidence is accumulated by this metacognitive decision process. Second, the peak signal amplitude represents the decision threshold, and third, the peak latency marks the

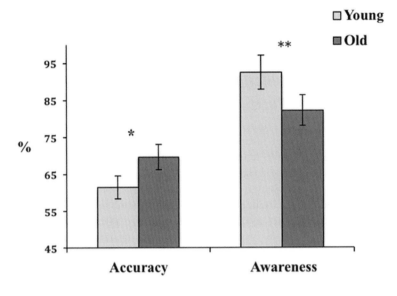

□ **Young**

■ **Old**

Figure 10.4 Mean percentage task accuracy and error awareness scores in younger and older adults during a response inhibition error awareness task. ** p < 0.001; * p < 0.05.

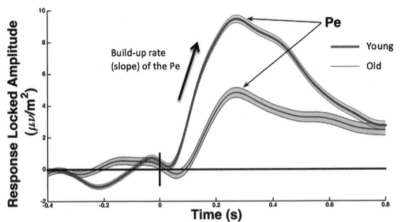

Figure 10.5 Error positivity (Pe). Older adults exhibited a reduced build-up rate and reduced Pe mean amplitude compared with younger adults. Waveform is the average for erroneous responses to which participants subsequently signaled their awareness with a button press (i.e., aware errors only). A clear age group difference in signal build-up rate (slope) and the mean peak amplitude of the Pe is apparent.

point at which conscious awareness would be most likely to emerge. We found that older adults exhibited a reduced signal build-up rate and attenuated amplitude of the Pe component compared with young adults (see Figure 10.5). This implies that poor error awareness in older adults may be explained by less efficient accumulation of evidence and ultimately diminished strength of evidence informing conscious awareness of the error.

Recent evidence suggests that medial frontal (MF) delta/theta (2–7 Hz) activity may also be a useful measure of error processing. Increased spectral activity within this band is associated with a higher build-up rate of the Pe and higher levels of error awareness [81]. Harty and colleagues [82] have demonstrated that, conversely, an aging-related reduction in MF

delta/theta accompanies a lower build-up rate of the Pe and a reduced level of error detection in older adults. Diminished top-down signaling from prefrontal cortex, reflected by reduced mid-frontal theta activity [83], may compromise the accumulation of evidence necessary for conscious awareness.

Error awareness paradigms provide a powerful tool in the investigation of specific mechanisms of self-monitoring that are critical in daily life. The evidence presented so far has demonstrated the deterioration of these neurocognitive mechanisms in older adults. However, there is cause for optimism: autonomic nervous system reactivity, which is responsive to alertness training [69, 84], has recently been shown to covary with error awareness in young adults [85]. Richard Ridderinkhof's group at the University of

Amsterdam assessed functional connectivity in young healthy participants during performance of a challenging and error-prone task. In addition, they measured pupil diameter, which has been shown to covary with BOLD activity in the human locus coeruleus [86] and with spiking activity in an LC single unit recording study with monkeys [87]. Thus, pupillary diameter is a tractable marker of the arousal and autonomic functioning of the locus coeruleus–noradrenergic (LC/NA) system. Ridderinkhof and colleagues found that changes in pupil diameter were associated with changes in brain connectivity between the anterior insular cortices (AIC), task-related networks, and regions of the default mode network during states of error awareness. During aware errors, connectivity increased between the AIC and task-related networks, indicating greater capacity for performance monitoring. In the same time frame, connectivity decreased between the AIC and the default mode network, suggesting a suspension of task-irrelevant processing. Increased pupil diameter was associated with both these patterns of increased and decreased connectivity with the AIC, suggesting that autonomic arousal was involved in these shifts between cortical networks. Unaware errors were linked to both insufficient autonomic arousal (indexed by smaller pupil diameter) and the absence of right AIC activation.

These findings support the conjecture that impaired error-monitoring in older adults might, in part, be explained by diminished autonomic arousal reactivity that fails to support shifts in the functional connectivity of cortical networks centered on the right AIC. Noradrenergic drugs, which amplify the effects of LC activity, have been shown to exert remote changes in frontoparietal connectivity during human attention [88]. There is the potential for modulation of LC/NA function (by means of pharmacological or nonpharmacological approaches such as alertness training) to increase interregional cortical connectivity centered on the AIC to rebalance cortical networks in support of error awareness in the aging brain.

6 Conclusions

The focus of this chapter was on the potential role of a predominantly right hemisphere network in allowing aging people to maintain adequate attention to their environment as a multitude of biological changes take place in their brains. The complexity of the findings on aging-related attentional changes is in part due to

the fact that certain right hemisphere–dominant processes may be both more vulnerable to aging *and* more important in mediating the compensatory dynamics associated with cognitive reserve, in particular, arousal, sustained attention, novelty processing, and self-monitoring.

Self-reported cognitive reserve assessed with the CR Index questionnaire [89] is strongly correlated with faster perceptual processing in the right hemisphere compared with the left, as assessed by hemifield asymmetries in visual attention to stimuli presented in the right and left hemifield [90]. The research by Ridderinkhof's group suggests that the right anterior insula may play a pivotal role in processes underlying error-monitoring and error-correcting and that noradrenergic activity may be an important modulator of these processes. These processes appear to incorporate critical adjustments by the aging brain to aging-related biological changes – particularly in the brain's neurotransmitter systems.

A full understanding of the nature of aging-related attention changes is not possible without taking into account the pervasive alterations in brain connectivity and in neurotransmitters, such as noradrenaline and dopamine. Such "low level" alterations may explain much of the variance in apparent old–young differences in "higher" attentional functions, as for example shown by the near-elimination of aging-related differences in fMRI working memory activations when striatal dopamine activity is covaried [3].

These neurotransmitter systems, however, are themselves plastic and their responsivity varies with the behavioral and environmental patterns of older people. For example, dopamine receptor density varies in relation to perceived social status [91]. The result of this complex of dynamically changing and interacting multilevel processes is that a characterization of the attentional deficits associated with aging may not be the most fruitful scientific quest. Rather, the study of the nature of the dynamic adjustments made by the aging brain in relation to its environment and self-perceptions may be more useful because it leads to the possibility of leveraging such dynamics in the service of enhanced cognitive aging.

One indicator of the value of this approach can be seen in the only published study showing the potential to prevent dementia over a 10-year period [92] through a training program that focused on speed of processing and visuo-spatial function, both strongly right hemisphere–dominant processes [93].

References

1. Posner MI, Petersen SE. The attention system of the human brain. *Annual Review of Neuroscience.* 1990;13:25–42.

2. Posner MI, Rothbart MK. Research on attention networks as a model for the integration of psychological science. *Annual Review of Psychology.* 2007;58:1–23.

3. Backman L, Karlsson S, Fischer H, Karlsson P, Brehmer Y, Rieckmann A, et al. Dopamine D1 receptors and age differences in brain activation during working memory. *Neurobiology of Aging.* 2011;32(10):1849–56.

4. Mather M, Harley CW. The locus coeruleus: essential for maintaining cognitive function and the aging brain. *Trends in Cognitive Sciences.* 2016;20 (3):214–26.

5. Rolls ET, Deco G. Stochastic cortical neurodynamics underlying the memory and cognitive changes in aging. *Neurobiology of Learning and Memory.* 2015;118:150–61.

6. Erel H, Levy DA. Orienting of visual attention in aging. *Neuroscience & Biobehavioral Reviews.* 2016;69:357–80.

7. Williams RS, Biel AL, Wegier P, Lapp LK, Dyson BJ, Spaniol J. Age differences in the Attention Network Test: evidence from behavior and event-related potentials. *Brain and Cognition.* 2016;102:65–79.

8. Nashiro K, Qin S, O'Connell MA, Basak C. Age-related differences in BOLD modulation to cognitive control costs in a multitasking paradigm: global switch, local switch, and compatibility-switch costs. *NeuroImage.* 2018;172:146–61.

9. Gazzaley A, Clapp W, Kelley J, McEvoy K, Knight RT, D'Esposito M. Age-related top-down suppression deficit in the early stages of cortical visual memory processing. *Proceedings of the National Academy of Sciences.* 2008;105(35):13122–6.

10. Ollman R. Choice reaction time and the problem of distinguishing task effects from strategy effects. *Attention and Performance VI.* 1977:99–113.

11. Salthouse TA. Aging and measures of processing speed. *Biological Psychology.* 2000;54 (1–3):35–54.

12. O'Connell RG, Dockree PM, Robertson IH, Bellgrove MA, Foxe JJ, Kelly SP. Uncovering the neural signature of lapsing attention: electrophysiological signals predict errors up to 20 s before they occur. *Journal of Neuroscience.* 2009;29 (26):8604–11.

13. O'Connell RG, Dockree PM, Kelly SP. A supramodal accumulation-to-bound signal that determines perceptual decisions in humans. *Nature Neuroscience.* 2012;15 (12):1729.

14. Arnsten AFT. Catecholamine modulation of prefrontal cortical cognitive function. *Trends in Cognitive Sciences.* 1998;2:436–47.

15. Ratcliff R, Thapar A, McKoon G. The effects of aging on reaction time in a signal detection task. *Psychology and Aging.* 2001;16 (2):323.

16. Ram N, Rabbitt P, Stollery B, Nesselroade JR. Cognitive performance inconsistency: intraindividual change and variability. *Psychology and Aging.* 2005;20(4):623.

17. Alain C, McDonald KL, Ostroff JM, Schneider B. Aging: a switch from automatic to controlled processing of sounds? *Psychology and Aging.* 2004;19(1):125.

18. Verhaeghen P, Cerella J. Aging, executive control, and attention: a review of meta-analyses. *Neuroscience & Biobehavioral Reviews.* 2002;26(7):849–57.

19. Berardi A, Parasuraman R, Haxby JV. Overall vigilance and sustained attention decrements in healthy aging. *Experimental Aging Research.* 2001;27(1):19–39.

20. Jackson JD, Balota DA. Mind-wandering in younger and older adults: converging evidence from the sustained attention to response task and reading for comprehension. *Psychology and Aging.* 2012;27(1):106.

21. Staub B, Doignon-Camus N, Després O, Bonnefond A. Sustained attention in the elderly: what do we know and what does it tell us about cognitive aging? *Ageing Research Reviews.* 2013;12 (2):459–68.

22. Carriere JS, Cheyne JA, Solman GJ, Smilek D. Age trends for failures of sustained attention. *Psychology and Aging.* 2010;25 (3):569.

23. Giambra LM. Sustained attention and aging: overcoming the decrement? *Experimental Aging Research.* 1997;23(2):145–61.

24. Giambra LM, Quilter RE. Sustained attention in adulthood: a unique, large-sample, longitudinal and multicohort analysis using the Mackworth Clock-Test. *Psychology and Aging.* 1988;3(1):75.

25. Fortenbaugh FC, DeGutis J, Germine L, Wilmer JB, Grosso M, Russo K, et al. Sustained attention across the life span in a sample of 10,000: dissociating ability and strategy. *Psychol Sci.* 2015;26 (9):1497–510.

26. McAvinue LP, Habekost T, Johnson KA, Kyllingsbaek S, Vangkilde S, Bundesen C, et al. Sustained attention, attentional selectivity, and attentional capacity across the lifespan. *Attention, Perception, & Psychophysics.* 2012;74 (8):1570–82.

27. Singh-Curry V, Husain M. The functional role of the inferior

parietal lobe in the dorsal and ventral stream dichotomy. *Neuropsychologia.* 2009;47:1434–48.

28. Robertson I. A right hemisphere role in cognitive reserve. *Neurobiology of Aging.* 2014;35:1375–85

29. Robertson IH. A noradrenergic theory of cognitive reserve: implications for Alzheimer's disease. *Neurobiology of Aging.* 2013;34:298–308.

30. Clewett DV, Lee T-H, Greening S, Ponzio A, Margalit E, Mather M. Neuromelanin marks the spot: identifying a locus coeruleus biomarker of cognitive reserve in healthy aging. *Neurobiology of Aging.* 2016;37:117–26.

31. Benwell CSY, Thut G, Grant A, Harvey M. A rightward shift in the visuospatial attention vector with healthy aging. *Frontiers in Aging Neuroscience.* 2014;6.

32. Valenzuela MJ, Sachdev P. Brain reserve and dementia: a systematic review. *Psychological Medicine.* 2006;36(4):441–54.

33. Barulli D, Stern Y. Efficiency, capacity, compensation, maintenance, plasticity: emerging concepts in cognitive reserve. *Trends in Cognitive Sciences.* 2013;17(10):502–9.

34. *Cognitive Aging: Progress in Understanding and Opportunities for Action.* Blazer DG, Yaffe K, Liverman CT, editors. Washington, DC: National Academies Press; 2015.

35. Stern Y. What is cognitive reserve? Theory and research application of the reserve concept. *Journal of the International Neuropsychological Society.* 2002;8 (3):448–60.

36. Nyberg L, Lövdén M, Riklund K, Lindenberger U, Bäckman L. Memory aging and brain maintenance. *Trends in Cognitive Sciences.* 2012;16(5):292–305.

37. Wilson RS, Nag S, Boyle PA, Hizel LP, Yu L, Buchman AS, et al. Neural reserve, neuronal density in the locus ceruleus, and cognitive decline. *Neurology.* 2013;80:1202–8.

38. Tsukahara JS, Harrison TL, Engle RW. The relationship between baseline pupil size and intelligence. *Cognitive Psychology.* 2016;91:109–23.

39. Murphy P, O'Connell R, O'Sullivan M, Robertson I, Balsters J. Pupil diameter covaries with BOLD activity in human locus coeruleus. *Human Brain Mapping.* 2014;35:4140–54.

40. Sara SJ. The locus coeruleus and noradrenergic modulation of cognition. *Nature Reviews Neuroscience.* 2009;10:211–23.

41. Parnavelas JG, Blue ME. The role of the noradrenergic system on the formation of synapses in the visual cortex of the rat. *Developmental Brain Research.* 1982;3(1):140–4.

42. Jhaveri DJ, Mackay EW, Hamlin AS, Marathe SV, Nandam LS, Vaidya VA, et al. Norepinephrine directly activates adult hippocampal precursors via β3-adrenergic receptors. *Journal of Neuroscience.* 2010;30 (7):2795–806.

43. Heneka MT, Nadrigny F, Regen T, Martinez-Hernandez A, Dumitrescu-Ozimek L, Terwel D, et al. Locus ceruleus controls Alzheimer's disease pathology by modulating microglial functions through norepinephrine. *Proceedings of the National Academy of Sciences.* 2010;107 (13):6058–63.

44. Robertson IH. A right hemisphere role in cognitive reserve. *Neurobiology of Aging.* 2014;35 (6):1375–85.

45. Robertson I, Ridgeway V, Greenfield E, Parr A. Motor recovery after stroke depends on intact sustained attention: a two-year follow-up study. *Neuropsychology.* 1997;11:290–5.

46. Recanzone Ga, Schreiner C, Merzenich MM. Plasticity in the frequency representation of primary auditory cortex following discrimination training in adult owl monkeys. *The Journal of Neuroscience.* 1993;13(1):87–103.

47. Maki B, McIlroy W. Influence of arousal and attention on the control of postural sway. *Journal of Vestibular Research.* 1996;6 (1):53–9.

48. Vankov A, Hervé-Minvielle A, Sara SJ. Response to novelty and its rapid habituation in locus coeruleus neurons of the freely exploring rat. *European Journal of Neuroscience.* 1995;7 (6):1180–7.

49. Wessel JR. Error awareness and the error-related negativity: evaluating the first decade of evidence. *Frontiers in Human Neuroscience.* 2012;6:88.

50. Graf H, Abler B, Freudenmann R, Beschoner P, Schaeffeler E, Spitzer M, et al. Neural correlates of error monitoring modulated by atomoxetine in healthy volunteers. *Biological Psychiatry.* 2011;69:890–7.

51. Brickman AM, Zimmerman ME, Paul RH, Grieve SM, Tate DF, Cohen RA, et al. Regional white matter and neuropsychological functioning across the adult lifespan. *Biological Psychiatry.* 2006;60(5):444–53.

52. Nyberg L, Salami A, Andersson M, Eriksson J, Kalpouzos G, Kauppi K, et al. Longitudinal evidence for diminished frontal cortex function in aging. *Proc Natl Acad Sci U S A.* 2010;107 (52):22682–6.

53. Lu H, Xu F, Rodrigue KM, Kennedy KM, Cheng Y, Flicker B, et al. Alterations in cerebral metabolic rate and blood supply across the adult lifespan. *Cereb Cortex.* 2011;21(6):1426–34.

54. Small GW, Ercoli LM, Silverman DH, Huang SC, Komo S, Bookheimer SY, et al. Cerebral metabolic and cognitive decline in persons at genetic risk for Alzheimer's disease. *Proc Natl Acad Sci U S A.* 2000;97 (11):6037–42.

55. Benwell CS, Thut G, Grant A, Harvey M. A rightward shift in the visuospatial attention vector with healthy aging. *Front Aging Neurosci.* 2014;6:113.

56. Brown JW, Jaffe J. Hypothesis on cerebral dominance. *Neuropsychologia.* 1975;13 (1):107–10.

57. Cherry BJ, Hellige JB. Hemispheric asymmetries in vigilance and cerebral arousal mechanisms in younger and older adults. *Neuropsychology.* 1999;13 (1):111–20.

58. Clark LE, Knowles JB. Age differences in dichotic listening performance. *Journal of Gerontology.* 1973;28(2):173–8.

59. Learmonth G, Benwell CSY, Thut G, Harvey M. Age-related reduction of hemispheric lateralisation for spatial attention: an EEG study. *Neuroimage.* 2017;153:139–51.

60. Oke A, Keller R, Mefford I, Adams R. Lateralization of norepinephrine in human thalamus. *Science.* 1978;200:1411–13.

61. Hartshorne JK, Germine LT. When does cognitive functioning peak? The asynchronous rise and fall of different cognitive abilities across the life span. *Psychol Sci.* 2015;26(4):433–43.

62. Kaufman AS, Horn JL. Age changes on tests of fluid and crystallized ability for women and men on the Kaufman Adolescent and Adult Intelligence Test (KAIT) at ages 17–94 years. *Arch Clin Neuropsychol.* 1996;11(2):97–121.

63. Yeatman JD, Wandell BA, Mezer AA. Lifespan maturation and degeneration of human brain white matter. *Nat Commun.* 2014;5:4932.

64. Lachman ME, Teshale S, Agrigoroaei S. Midlife as a pivotal period in the life course: balancing growth and decline at the crossroads of youth and old age. *International Journal of Behavioral Development.* 2015;39 (1):20–31.

65. Van Vleet TM, DeGutis JM, Merzenich MM, Simpson GV, Zomet A, Dabit S. Targeting alertness to improve cognition in older adults: a preliminary report of benefits in executive function and skill acquisition. *Cortex.* 2016;82:100–18.

66. Brosnan MB, Arvaneh M, Harty S, Maguire T, O'Connell RG, Robertson IH, Dockree PM. Prefrontal modulation of the sustained attention network in ageing, a tDCS-EEG co-registration approach. *J Cogn Neurosci.* 2018;13:1–16.

67. O'Halloran AM, Finucane C, Savva GM, Robertson IH, Kenny RA. Sustained attention and frailty in the older adult population. *Journals of Gerontology Series B: Psychological Sciences and Social Sciences.* 2014;69(2):147–56.

68. Dockree PM, Kelly SP, Robertson IH, Reilly RB, Foxe JJ. Neurophysiological markers of alert responding during goal-directed behavior: a high-density electrical mapping study. *Neuroimage.* 2005;27(3):587–601.

69. O'Connell RG, Bellgrove MA, Dockree PM, Lau A, Fitzgerald M, Robertson IH. Self-Alert Training: volitional modulation of autonomic arousal improves sustained attention. *Neuropsychologia.* 2008;46 (5):1379–90.

70. O'Connell RG, Dockree PM, Bellgrove MA, Turin A, Ward S, Foxe JJ, et al. Two types of action error: electrophysiological evidence for separable inhibitory and sustained attention neural mechanisms producing error on go/no-go tasks. *J Cogn Neurosci.* 2009;21(1):93–104.

71. Buckner RL, Sepulcre J, Talukdar T, Krienen FM, Liu H, Hedden T, et al. Cortical hubs revealed by intrinsic functional connectivity: mapping, assessment of stability, and relation to Alzheimer's disease. *J Neurosci.* 2009;29 (6):1860–73.

72. Harty S, Robertson IH, Miniussi C, Sheehy OC, Devine CA, McCreery S, et al. Transcranial direct current stimulation over right dorsolateral prefrontal cortex enhances error awareness in older age. *J Neurosci.* 2014;34 (10):3646–52.

73. McAvinue L, O'Keeffe F, McMackin D, Robertson IH. Impaired sustained attention and error awareness in traumatic brain injury: implications for insight. *Neuropsychol Rehabil.* 2005;15(5):569–87.

74. Harty S, O'Connell RG, Hester R, Robertson IH. Older adults have diminished awareness of errors in the laboratory and daily life. *Psychol Aging.* 2013;28 (4):1032–41.

75. Fleming JM, Strong J, Ashton R. Self-awareness of deficits in adults with traumatic brain injury: how best to measure? *Brain Injury.* 1996;10(1):1–15.

76. Lacey E. Behavioural and electrophysiological aspects of error processing in healthy ageing and Alzheimer's disease. PhD diss., Trinity College Dublin; 2018.

77. O'Connell RG, Dockree PM, Bellgrove MA, Kelly SP, Hester R, Garavan H, et al. The role of cingulate cortex in the detection of errors with and without awareness: a high-density electrical mapping study. *European Journal of Neuroscience.* 2007;25(8):2571–9.

78. Steinhauser M, Yeung N. Error awareness as evidence accumulation: effects of speed-accuracy trade-off on error signaling. *Frontiers in Human Neuroscience*. 2012;6:240.

79. Yeung N, Summerfield C. Metacognition in human decision-making: confidence and error monitoring. *Philosophical Transactions of the Royal Society B: Biological Sciences*. 2012;367 (1594):1310–21.

80. Murphy PR, Robertson IH, Allen D, Hester R, O'Connell RG. An electrophysiological signal that precisely tracks the emergence of error awareness. *Frontiers in Human Neuroscience*. 2012;6:65.

81. Murphy PR, Robertson IH, Harty S, O'Connell RG. Neural evidence accumulation persists after choice to inform metacognitive judgments. *Elife*. 2015;4.

82. Harty S, Murphy PR, Robertson IH, O'Connell RG. Parsing the neural signatures of reduced error detection in older age. *Neuroimage*. 2017;161:43–55.

83. Cavanagh JF, Frank MJ. Frontal theta as a mechanism for cognitive control. *Trends in Cognitive Science*. 2014;18(8):414–21.

84. Braun N, Debener S, Solle A, Kranczioch C, Hildebrandt H. Biofeedback-based self-alert training reduces alpha activity and stabilizes accuracy in the Sustained Attention to Response Task. *Journal of Clinical and Experimental Neuropsychology*. 2015;37(1):16–26.

85. Harsay HA, Cohen MX, Spaan M, Weeda WD, Nieuwenhuis S, Ridderinkhof KR. Error blindness and motivational significance: shifts in networks centering on anterior insula co-vary with error awareness and pupil dilation. *Behavioural Brain Research*. 2018 Dec 14;355:24–35.

86. Murphy PR, O'Connell RG, O'Sullivan M, Robertson IH, Balsters JH. Pupil diameter covaries with BOLD activity in human locus coeruleus. *Human Brain Mapping*. 2014;35 (8):4140–54.

87. Joshi S, Li Y, Kalwani RM, Gold JI. Relationships between pupil diameter and neuronal activity in the locus coeruleus, colliculi, and cingulate cortex. *Neuron*. 2016;89 (1):221–34.

88. Coull JT, Buchel C, Friston KJ, Frith CD. Noradrenergically mediated plasticity in a human attentional neuronal network. *Neuroimage*. 1999;10(6):705–15.

89. Nucci M, Mapelli D, Mondini S. Cognitive Reserve Index questionnaire (CRIq): a new instrument for measuring cognitive reserve. *Aging Clinical and Experimental Research*. 2012;24(3):218–26.

90. Brosnan MB, Demaria G, Petersen A, Dockree PM, Robertson IH, Wiegand I. Plasticity of the right-lateralized cognitive reserve network in ageing. *Cerebral Cortex*. 2018;28:1749–59.

91. Martinez D, Orlowska D, Narendran R, Slifstein M, Liu F, Kumar D, et al. Dopamine type 2/3 receptor availability in the striatum and social status in human volunteers. *Biological Psychiatry*. 2010;67(3):275–8.

92. Edwards JD, Xu H, Clark DO, Guey LT, Ross LA, Unverzagt FW. Speed of processing training results in lower risk of dementia. *Alzheimer's & Dementia: Translational Research & Clinical Interventions*. 2017;3(4):603–11.

93. Coslett HB, Bowers D, Heilman KM. Reduction in cerebral activation after right hemisphere stroke. *Neurology*. 1987;37:957–62.

Chapter 11

Changes in Motor Programming with Aging

Kenneth M. Heilman

1 Introduction

The human motor system includes many structures in the brain, such as the motor cortex and corticospinal system, the premotor cortex, basal ganglia, and cerebellum. These networks, together with the motor units (e.g., spinal anterior horn cells, motor nerves, and muscles) can mediate an almost infinite number of movements. Thus, to successfully interact with our environment, with others, and with ourselves, this wonderful motor system requires movement-action programs. With aging, there are changes of the motor units. The muscles get smaller and transmission of neural impulses slows. In addition, the ratio of motor nerve to muscle fiber changes so that each motor nerve activates more muscle fibers. The primary purpose of this chapter, however, is to review the changes that occur in the motor programs with aging. There are two major types of motor programs, action-intentional and motor-praxic. The motor-praxic programs provide the corticospinal system and motor units with the information needed to know about *how* to make skilled, purposeful movements. The action-intentional programs provide the corticospinal system with information about *when* to move. Studies of patients with brain injury have shown that there are several forms of impairment in the "how" networks causing different forms of programming impairments called apraxias. There are also several forms of "when" impairments, called action-intentional disorders. In this chapter, we will discuss the networks that mediate the praxis and action-intention functions and how these functions might be altered with aging.

2 Praxis Programming and Aging

When interacting with the environment or self, there are several "hows" of the arms and hands that need to be programmed, including (1) how to posture the hand and arm, (2) how to move the joint or joints

to make the correct movements, (3) how fast to move each of the joints, (4) how much force to use, (5) how to sequence a series of actions to complete the goal of these actions, and (6) how to coordinate the use of the right and left hands.

The human's hands are very deft and can make such precise and rapid movements that an outside observer may have difficulty seeing these movements. The human hands and fingers can also make independent but coordinated finger movements.

Older people often have local structural changes of their joints, muscle, tendons, and bones. These changes can influence older people's ability to perform skilled purposeful movements. When assessing praxis, such as hand and finger deftness, it is important to take these disorders into consideration. However, even in the absence of structural changes, older people often exhibit a decline in their ability to perform purposeful skilled movements [1, 2].

Studies of patients with neurological diseases suggest that there are independent networks responsible for hand and finger deftness, as well as spatial and speed programming. Impairment of hand and finger deftness, as well as the ability to make independent and coordinated finger movements, was termed limb-kinetic apraxia by Liepmann in1920 [3]. Impairment of the ability to perform correct upper limb postures and joint movements is called ideomotor apraxia [3]. Whereas many of the diseases that cause apraxia, such as stroke, Parkinson's disease, and Alzheimer's disease, occur in older people, the goal of this chapter is to discuss how normal aging might influence these "how" action skills.

2.1 Hand and Finger Deftness and Dexterity

2.1.1 Speed

One of the mostly commonly reported changes in motor activities with aging is a slowing of movements [4].

Slowing has been shown with pointing, grasping, and reaching movements [5, 6]. The express pathway for initiating movement is the corticospinal system. The nerve cells in the sensorimotor cortex send their axons directly down to the spinal cord and the corticospinal neurons directly excite the lower motor neurons responsible for action initiation. Good and coworkers [7] performed a voxel-based morphometric study of the gray matter of 465 heathy human brains and found that one of the major areas that reveals a loss of gray matter with aging was the sensorimotor cortex.

Reaching, grasping, and pointing movements do require sensory feedback (they are closed loop), and therefore, with slowing of movements, it may be unclear if the slowing is caused by slowness of the action or other factors such as impairment of motor programming, sensory perception, or feedback. In contrast to these closed-loop movements, open-loop movements, such as finger tapping, require little sensory feedback or planning. Ruff and Parker [8] studied finger tapping in older and younger men and woman. They found that with aging there was no slowing of the men's finger tapping, but the women's tapping speed did show some slowing.

There are often warning stimuli in the environment that may prepare a person to make open-loop movements. Van Gerven, Hurks, and Adam [9] have demonstrated that when older people are provided with a valid warning stimulus, this stimulus does reduce the time it takes them to respond (reaction time) but not as much as in younger people. Sometimes the warning stimulus provides incorrect information about the required action. These investigators also examined the cost of invalid cues. They found out that invalid cues slowed the reaction times of older participants more than the reaction times of the younger participants. In addition, studies have revealed that, when initiating a movement, healthy older people are more likely to engage their antagonist muscles and may even activate these muscles before they activate agonist muscles [10].

Yordanova and coworkers studied processing speed in older and younger healthy participants [11]. They found significant age-related slowing of responses in a choice-reaction time task. Analysis of event-related potentials (ERPs) suggested that this slowing did not originate from the early processing of the stimulus or processing of response selection. Instead, it was produced by slower activation of the contralateral motor cortex. These authors concluded that aging is accompanied by a functional dysregulation of motor cortex excitability during sensorimotor processing, with this deficit becoming progressively more evident with greater task complexity.

The supplementary motor area (SMA) typically activates before the motor cortex and provides the motor cortex with firing instructions. Hoffstaedter and co-investigators, using voxel-based morphometry and whole-brain resting-state functional connectivity data, reported that, with aging, there was a reduction of connectivity of the SMA with the motor cortex and that the slower activation pattern, in part, might be related to this reduction in functional connectivity [12].

Koppelmans and coworkers [13] examined cerebellar gray and white matter volume as a function of aging and motor performance. These investigators found that there was a relationship between the loss of white matter of the right cerebellum and right-hand tapping speed.

Ross and coinvestigators [14] reported that in older people who are without Parkinson's disease, there is a decrease in the neuron density in the substantia nigra (SN). Therefore, it is also possible that the slowing associated with aging might be related to a loss of these dopaminergic neurons.

2.1.2 Accuracy

As discussed above, with aging, people commonly develop motor slowing (bradykinesia). Although this slowing with aging may be entirely related to degradation of the cerebral, basal ganglia, or cerebellar networks important in motor programming, in general older people are more averse to risk than younger people. Therefore, it is possible that, at least in part, slowing may be a learned procedure for enhancing the accuracy and/or precision of movements. Lamb and coinvestigators [15] tested the ability of healthy younger and older adults to use a pen to alternately mark a card centered directly in front of them and each of a number of circles distributed across a more distally placed page. Performance was timed and participants were instructed to complete the task as quickly as possible, while not sacrificing accuracy for speed. The circle sizes and hand used varied by trial. They found that the older adults performed the task more slowly for all target circles. As the circles decreased in size, the older adults performed the task still more slowly compared with the younger participants. However, the younger participants exhibited a greater decline in accuracy. Thus, it appears that during this aiming task, healthy older adults were less likely than younger adults to sacrifice accuracy for speed, and, at least in part, older peoples' slowing might be a learned adaptive strategy.

When reaching for a target, there are two phases, an initial phase, in which there is a rapid open-loop movement, and then a closed-loop "homing-in" phase. It has been reported that older healthy people slow down their primary movement and therefore undershoot the target of the movement more than do younger people [16]. In the second, closed-loop, homing-in phase, older people take more time to complete the closed-loop, feedback-based adjustments. Although this movement strategy results in overall longer movement times, the older people can spend relatively more time on homing-in and have greater accuracy as shown in the study by Lamb and coworkers [15].

What is not known from this study is what would happen if we used an experimental paradigm that required the older participant to perform at a more rapid speed. Would their accuracy decline more than in the younger participants? In addition, if we used a metronome to slow the younger participants' actions, would they be as accurate as the older participants or even more accurate? Similarly, if we used a metronome in an attempt to speed the older participants' actions, could we get them to move as rapidly as the younger participants and, if they could perform as rapidly, would their accuracy remain better than the younger participants' or would their performance degrade more than that of the younger participants? These questions are unanswered and remain to be tested.

When performing reaching-aiming movements, both visual and proprioceptive perception are important for locating the target and providing knowledge about the position of the upper limb. Wright, Adamo, and Brown [17] have reported that with aging, there is a decline in the detection of passive wrist movements, suggesting that there may be an age-related decline in proprioception. However, in the study of Lamb et al. [15], the older subjects were more accurate than the younger subjects and this difference cannot be fully explained by a proprioceptive deficit or a decline in visual acuity. However, it is possible that with faster movements, there may be a decline in proprioceptive or visual perception and this needs to be further investigated.

Van Halewyck and coinvestigators [18] compared the aiming performance of physically active and sedentary older adults with that of younger adults and found that it was only the sedentary older adults who exhibited slower aiming-reaching movements, suggesting that the adage "use it or lose it" may also be correct for reaching-aiming movements.

In the study paradigm used above by Lamb et al. [15], the participants did not have to carefully program the distance needed for an accurate movement because the board that contained the target circles limited their distance. However, when someone is going to pick up a glass of water from a table, they have to compute not only the egocentric horizontal and vertical angles that the arm and hand must be moved but also the distance the hand has to move. The paradigm used by Lamb et al. did not enable examination of distance accuracy.

2.1.3 Independent and Coordinated Hand–Finger Movements

Deftness and dexterity depend not only on speed and accuracy but also on the ability to perform independent but coordinated finger–hand–arm movements. There are two tests of this form of dexterity/deftness that are often used clinically and experimentally: the grooved pegboard test and the coin rotation test [19]. There are many forms of the grooved pegboard test sold by different companies. In general, the test employs a board with multiple holes that are circular except for a little groove located at a particular position (e.g., 1 o'clock, 9 o'clock, 2 o'clock, etc.). The pegs are also circular but each has a little ridge that fits into the groove. All the pegs are initially found in a basin in the board that is close to the subject. The subject is instructed to place all the pegs in the holes as rapidly as possible. Performing this test requires that the participant lift up just one of the pegs at a time, and the pincher grasp requires finger deftness. The arm moves the hand to the hole, which requires accuracy of arm extension, and finally, to get the peg into the hole, the participant has to rotate the peg so that the irregularity in the peg is aligned with the irregularity in the hole. The score is the time it takes to complete this task. As expected, healthy participants perform better with their preferred hand and woman do better than men. There is also slowing with aging. In a study by Ruff and Parker [8], whereas with aging there was little slowing of finger tapping, both men and woman had slowing of the grooved pegboard test performance. This dissociation suggests that this slowing is not related to bradykinesia but rather to differences in finger precision and accuracy. However, with these closed-loop movements, accuracy and precision depend on sensory feedback, especially touch, and studies have revealed that with aging there is a degradation of touch perception [20]. Therefore, it is unclear if the slowing in grooved pegboard test performance is related to a motor programming deficit, a sensory-perceptual disorder, or both. Another test of hand–finger deftness/dexterity is the coin rotation test [19]. In this test, a nickel is given to the participant, who is asked to rotate this nickel as rapidly as possible between their thumb, index, and middle finger. Although there are several means of scoring this test, most studies employ either the number of 180-degree rotations made in 10 seconds or the time required to make twenty 180-degree rotations. Unfortunately, we could find no studies that examined performance as a function of age; however, one study did reveal that performance on the grooved pegboard test and the coin rotation test were strongly correlated [21].

To learn whether in people who are right handed, it is the left hemisphere that helps to program deft movements for both hands, Heilman, Meador, and Loring [22] studied patients who were undergoing hemispheric anesthesia (the Wada test) to determine if there was a laterality difference in deftness of the hand that was on the same side as the hemisphere (ipsilateral) that was anesthetized. Hanna-Pladdy and her colleagues [19], using the coin rotation task, assessed the hand ipsilateral to the hemisphere that was injured by a stroke. Both studies reported that people with a right-hand preference who have left hemispheric dysfunction are more likely to have a loss of deftness of their left ipsilesional hand than are people who have right hemisphere dysfunction. These findings suggest that for right-handed people, their left hemisphere plays a particularly important role in programming deft movements of both hands.

Evidence that this programming information is transferred from the left to the right hemisphere by means of the corpus callosum comes from a study by Acosta, Bennett, and Heilman [23]. They reported a right-handed man who developed memory impairment and, on brain imaging, was found to have a septum pellucidum cyst that was causing mild dilatation of the occipital and temporal horns of the lateral ventricles. After this cyst was removed surgically, he

had postoperative imaging that revealed a lesion of the middle portion of his corpus callosum. Following surgery, he had a limb-kinetic apraxia of his left but not right hand. The finding that this man with a callosal disconnection exhibited limb-kinetic apraxia of his left hand suggests that the corpus callosum is critical in allowing the left hemisphere's motor areas to enable the right hemisphere's motor system to program deft movements of the left hand.

Mitrushina and coworkers [24] tested a large group of healthy older people using the grooved pegboard, a tapping test, and the pin test. The pin test required participants to place pins into small holes. Although somewhat similar to the grooved pegboard test, according to these investigators, the pin test requires greater finger movement accuracy. They found that when performing the pin test, superiority of performance of the right-hand relative to that of the left increased with aging. This increase in superiority of the right hand with aging on this highly demanding task supports the hypothesis that with aging, there is a reduction in callosal functioning. An alternative hypothesis is that with aging there is a greater decrement of right than left hemisphere functioning [25].

If there were a decrement of right hemisphere functions with aging, then a similar finding would be expected with finger tapping. However, aging-related hand performance asymmetry with tapping was not as great as with the pin test. This finding provides support for the callosal deficit hypothesis over the right hemisphere decrement hypothesis. In addition, Reuter-Lorenz and Stanczak [26] performed a reaction time task that required the interhemispheric transfer of information (i.e., reaction times with the left hand to visual stimuli presented to the right visual hemifield and vice versa) and compared this performance with intrahemispheric reaction times (i.e., reaction times of the left hand to stimuli presented to the left visual hemifield). They found that the older participants had greater slowing with the task requiring interhemispheric communication.

Anatomic studies of the corpus callosum have revealed that with normal aging there is atrophy of the corpus callosum with anterior portions showing greater atrophy than posterior portions [27]. The corpus callosum is not only important for transferring motor programming information from the dominant left hemisphere to the motor areas of the right hemisphere, but it is also critical in allowing the two hands to work together. There have been reports that older healthy adults are relatively impaired at performing bimanual tasks, especially when the two hands are moving out of phase with each other [28, 29]. The performance of such tasks requires interhemispheric interactions. Fling et al. [29] used structural magnetic resonance and diffusion tensor imaging to investigate age-related changes in the relationships between callosal macrostructure, microstructure, and motor performance on bimanual tasks. They found that when compared with the younger participants, the older adults' anterior corpus callosum was smaller and there was poorer white matter integrity in the callosal mid-body.

The mechanism accounting for the reduced ability of older adults to perform bimanual tasks when the two hands are out of phase may be different from the mechanism underlying the impairment in placing pins in a small hole with the left hand. Interhemispheric communication via the corpus callosum can be either facilitatory or inhibitory. In the performance of bimanual tasks, there appears to be motor programming information that is transmitted via the corpus callosum from the left to the right hemisphere. However, in order to perform bilateral movements that are out of phase, interhemispheric inhibition is necessary and the interhemispheric connections between primary motor and premotor cortices, such as the presupplementary and supplementary premotor areas, and convexity premotor cortex appear to be important for interhemispheric inhibition [30, 31].

2.2 Force

The control of force exerted by the fingers is a critical element in handling and using objects, tools, and implements. In most studies, investigators use a grasp, lift, and hold paradigm. If the force of the grasp is too great, fragile objects may be damaged or even crushed. In addition, with the use of a greater force than needed, there may be problems with manipulation of the object that is being held. In contrast, if the force is too small, the object may be dropped or the person making these movements might not be able to make the desired alterations of movement.

There are several stages in the process of exerting requisite forces in lifting, holding, and using objects. First, there is an anticipatory stage in which we approach the object that we are going to hold. In this stage, based on viewing the object and stored

knowledge about the weight and texture of this object, we estimate the force that will be needed. An incorrect estimate can lead to a poor result. For example, if served what appears to be a glass mug of beer, if the mug is made of plastic and thus is much lighter than anticipated, there is a chance of applying too much lifting force and tossing the beer in the air. The force of the grip on the object also, in part, depends on the texture of the surface. Since this glass of beer is cold and the bar serving it is hot and humid, there may be condensed water on the surface of the mug, which would make it slippery. Therefore, one might use a stronger grasp to prevent the mug from slipping.

Diermayr, McIsaac, and Gordon [32] reviewed the literature on grip force control in the elderly. They found that with aging there was a decrement in control of the forces exerted by the fingers. In addition, during the use of more proximal muscles like those used to rotate the arm at the elbow, as is done when performing tasks such as using a screwdriver to drive a screw into a wall, older people exhibit unsteadiness in their control of force. These findings suggest a more generalized aging-related impairment in force control. However, the mechanism underlying this change in force control has not been determined. It is possible that these impairments in force might be related to impaired feedback or impaired programming. Unfortunately, it is not fully known which brain areas are specifically involved in the precision grip task; however, several studies have suggested an important role of the premotor cortex, the basal ganglia, and the thalamus [33].

2.3 Motor Learning

When growing up in the streets of Brooklyn I learned to play many sports. Although I was never a great athlete, my ability to play almost all sports was respectable. Even when my brother Fred brought me to the mountains of Vermont, I was able to learn to ski pretty well. When I finished my neurology residency training in Boston and came to Gainesville, I learned that Gainesville had many golf courses and the cost of playing was very reasonable. Even the University of Florida, where I was worked, had a wonderful golf course. In addition, many of my coworkers and friends played golf. I therefore decided to learn to play golf. I thought golf should be easy to learn because, unlike other sports, the ball that I had to hit was not moving.

I purchased some golf clubs and decided that I should first go to a golf range and just hit some balls. I rapidly learned that I was wrong! Golf is not easy to learn. I have practiced, taken lessons, and I have now been playing golf for more than two decades, but I am still a terrible golfer and rarely break a score of 100. Being a neurologist who performs neurobehavioral research and being a terrible golfer, I wanted to learn why I had trouble improving my game. When I learned to play other sports in Brooklyn, I was young. I did not start to play golf until I was in my fifties. I therefore thought that this disability might be related to aging.

William Thorpe [34] studied birds' ability to learn their songs. He found that young chaffinches, after hearing adult chaffinches sing, were able to produce these songs when they matured. In contrast, if these young birds were not able to hear these mature birds sing, when they matured they were unable to produce these songs. This indicated that they had to hear the songs to learn how to produce them. Another group of these birds was allowed to hear the songs only after they matured. They too could not learn the songs. These observations suggest an age of acquisition effect.

Bottjer and Johnson [35] castrated chaffinches at an early age. When young, the birds did not hear adult birds sing their song, but, when they were older and they did hear these songs, they were able to learn them. This finding suggested that the apparent age of acquisition effect observed by Thorpe was strongly influenced by testosterone.

Age of acquisition effects on motor learning, apparently modulated by hormonal environment, have also been observed in humans. For example, children who did not speak English in the country in which they were born and who immigrated to America before puberty, after being here for a few years or even months, rarely have any accent when they speak English. In contrast, those who come to America later in their lives, even after living in America for decades, almost invariably still have a foreign accent [36]. The reason for their persistent accent is that they have not entirely learned how to correctly move their articulatory apparatus to precisely reproduce the phonetics of the new language.

After my trouble learning to play golf, I found that this aging-related change in motor learning is not restricted to speech. There is some evidence that learning to play a sport at an early age may allow a person to play that sport better than when they attempt to learn this sport at a later age. In regard to golf, Tiger Wood's father started to teach him when he was just 10 months old. Many other famous golfers also started to play at an early age. For example, Jack Nicklaus started playing golf before he was 10. Arnold Palmer began playing when he was 4 years old and Ben Hogan was 9 years old when he started. It would have been interesting if they, as well as other great golfers, had identical twins and the great golfer's twin sibling did not start playing golf until a later age. This would allow us to separate the effects of genetics and early learning, thereby allowing us to learn if age of learning a new motor skill makes this difference.

The changes in the brain that alter motor learning with puberty and adolescence remain to be fully discovered; however, while probably unrelated to these changes with puberty, there is also a decrease in motor learning that occurs in older age. The learning of new motor skills (procedural memory) is achieved by brain networks that are different from the networks that mediate other forms of memory such as working memory or episodic memory. An example of this dissociation comes from studies of the famous patient HM.

Scoville and Milner [37] first described HM. After having both of his hippocampi removed to control his epilepsy, he had a permanent severe deficit in the formation of new episodic memories. Lesions in many other portions of the Papez circuit (fornix, mammilo-thalamic track, anterior thalamus, retrosplenial cortex) can also cause deficits of episodic memory formation. However, Corkin [38] reported that HM was able to learn new motor skills, such as rotatory pursuit. When performing this task, HM had to keep a metal wand on a metal disk located on a revolving wheel. With repeated testing, the amount of disk contact time HM maintained increased; however, he could not recall previously performing this task and had to be given instruction each day.

Unfortunately, the networks that allow people to learn new motor skills – procedural memories – are not entirely known. There is, however, some evidence that a frontal lobe–basal ganglia (striatum) network plays an important role. The striatum receives dopaminergic input from the substantia nigra and the frontal lobes receive dopaminergic input from the mesencephalic tegmentum. Patients with Parkinson's disease have a 70–80% loss of their dopaminergic cells in their midbrain and these cells provide the basal ganglia with dopamine, a critical neurotransmitter for the function of the basal ganglia. Many studies have revealed that patients with Parkinson's disease are impaired in learning new motor skills [39, 40].

In another study Rodrigue, Kennedy, and Raz [41] studied older adults' ability to perform mirror drawing and found that the older adults required more training to reach asymptote. Analyses of individual learning curves indicated that the effects of age on mirror-tracing speed were greater at longitudinal follow-up than at baseline, with older adults requiring more training to reach asymptote. Kennedy and Raz [42] also examined how participants' ability to learn mirror drawing was related to brain atrophy. They found it was the lateral frontal cortex volume that best correlated with the decline in procedural memory acquisition.

The frontal cortex is strongly connected with the basal ganglia, and the functions mediated by the frontal lobes appear to be the most dependent on long white matter connections. Bennett and coinvestigators [43] studied the relationship between white matter connectivity and procedural learning. They found that with aging there was a reduction of procedural learning and that these changes were related to a loss of connectivity between the dorsolateral frontal lobe and the neostriatum.

3 Action-Intentional Programs and Aging

In addition to knowing "how" to interact with objects in the environment, with other people, and with themselves, people also need to know "when" to act. There are four major "whens." They include when to initiate an action, when to persist at an action or series of actions, when not to act, and when to stop acting. Knowing "when" depends on action-intentional programs that can activate the motor cortex, as well as those that inhibit or deactivate the motor cortex. As in the brain, executives of corporations have to decide not only on a plan of action but also on when their workers need to initiate, persist, and stop activities. The functions mediated by the frontal lobes are often called "executive functions" (see Chapter 12). Thus, "when" disorders could be called executive-motor dysfunction. Impairments in these action-intentional programs, like impairments in the praxis programs, can cause severe disability.

3.1 Action Initiation Impairments

There are several types of deficits in the ability to initiate actions. An inability to initiate actions is called "akinesia," and a delay in the initiation of actions is called "hypokinesia." These impairments may involve all movements made by the body, or specific parts of the body such as an arm (limb akinesia). They may be directional, leftward or rightward, upward or downward – directional akinesia and directional hypokinesia. For example, patients with a large right hemispheric stroke may deviate their eyes toward the right. Although this is called a "gaze palsy," this is an example of an ocular directional akinesia. There is also a hemispatial akinesia: patients fail to move or have a reduced ability to make movement in one-half of egocentric (body-centered) space. Finally, akinesia and hypokinesia might also be primarily for self-initiated actions and not for actions that are in response to stimuli. This disorder is called "akinesia paradoxica."

Most of these forms of akinesia are seen in patients who have neurological diseases such as stroke and Parkinson's disease; however, the major difference in action initiation between healthy older and younger people is hypokinesia, with older people having longer response times. For example, Woods and coworkers [44] reported that simple reaction time latencies, which include both the latency for detection of the go stimulus and the time to produce the response, increase significantly with aging (0.55 ms/year). These investigators computed stimulus detection time by subtracting movement initiation time, measured by finger tapping test, from the stimulus reaction times. They found that the stimulus detection time averaged about 131 milliseconds and that the detection time was unaffected by the participant's age. Therefore, the increase in reaction time latencies with aging appear to be primarily due to slowed motor output.

The reason for this slowing of reactions or response times is not entirely understood. There is age-related slowing in nerve conduction velocity as well as slowed muscle contraction [45]. However, Serbruyns and coworkers [46] demonstrated that slowing with aging is related to alterations in subcortical myelin, as measured by magnetization transfer ratio. In addition, as mentioned above in the accuracy section, the slowing with aging might, at least in part, be a learned procedure for enhancing the accuracy and/or precision of movements [15].

Howes and Boller [47] studied patients with unilateral hemispheric lesions. In their population of participants, lesions of the right hemisphere were not larger than those of the left; however, when they tested reaction times of these participants' ipsilateral hands, they found that the patients with right hemisphere lesions had slower reaction times than those with left hemisphere lesions. Heilman and Van den Abell [48] wanted to determine whether the right hemisphere is dominant for motor activation (physiologic readiness to response). Twenty-four healthy participants were tested for their reaction times in response to light stimuli given in central vision. However, these participants were intermittently and randomly presented lateralized warning stimuli preceding the imperative stimulus. The effect of warning stimuli projected to the right hemisphere in reducing reaction times of the right hand was greater than the effect of warning stimuli projected to the left hemisphere in reducing left hand reaction times. These results support the hypothesis that the right hemisphere plays a dominant role in activating the motor system. It is thus possible that aging-related increases in reaction time are related to a shift in the balance of hemispheric function. Hurtz and coworkers [49] studied the cortical thickness of normal elderly people and found that overall there was a greater loss of gray matter in the right than left hemisphere. They found that the greatest changes were in the sensory-motor cortex and in the supplementary motor areas. Of course, with studies of cortical thickness, one must always ask whether observed changes are primary or related to altered use of the cortex in question.

Krehbiel, Kang, and Cauraugh [50] identified 27 studies that reported bimanual movement performance measured as a function of age. They found that when performing bimanual tasks, older participants displayed reduced accuracy and longer execution time compared with the younger participants. In addition, Leinen and coinvestigators [51] had participants perform tasks that required the hands to perform contrasting movements and found that the older people had a strong tendency to produce mirror movements.

Whereas there are several possible causes of this decrement in performing bimanual movements, studies of the corpus callosum have revealed that with aging there is a loss of callosal connectivity [29].

There is also a decrease in interhemispheric motor inhibition, and it may be the age-related loss of this interhemispheric inhibition that accounts for the slowing in bimanual tasks [52].

3.2 Impersistence

One of the most common tests of impersistence was initially described by C. Miller Fisher and subsequently studied by Kertesz and his coworkers [53], who asked patients to close their eyes, keep their mouth open, and protrude their tongue for 20 seconds. They found that inability to maintain all three postures for the full 20 seconds was associated with lesions of the right hemisphere, particularly the right frontal lobe. However, review of the literature did not reveal any studies that reported motor impersistence as a function of healthy aging.

3.3 Perseveration

Sandson and Albert [54] described two major types of motor perseveration. Patients with *recurrent* perseveration inappropriately repeat a previous response to a subsequent stimulus, and patients with *continuous* perseveration have an abnormal prolongation of the same activity or inappropriately continue the same activity. One of the most commonly used tests is the rampart test, in which the participant is asked to draw a series of continuous alternating squares and triangles or to write in script a series of Ms and Ns (mnmnmnmn). Another test involves asking the patient to draw a series of triple loops; people who perseverate tend to make more than three loops.

There have not been many studies that have examined motor perseveration as a function of aging; however, Suchy and coinvestigators [55] had older and younger patients perform the Push-Turn-Taptap task. This task requires participants to perform motor sequences that become progressively more complex across the four blocks of the task. It is designed to assess the speed and accuracy of action planning, action learning, and motor control. These investigators found that the older participants often made perseverative errors. They also performed functional MR, which revealed anomalies involving frontal-subcortical circuits.

Many of our purposeful actions are based on cognitive decisions. One of the most sensitive and commonly used tests for cognitive perseveration is the Wisconsin Card Sorting Test, and studies have revealed that with aging there is an increase in perseverative errors [56]. These investigators also found that this increase in cognitive perseverative errors was associated with a decrease in regional cortical volumes in the prefrontal cortex. Further support for the postulate that aging is associated with an increase in motor perseveration comes from a study by Niermeyer, Suchy, and Ziemnik [57]. In this study, older and younger healthy participants' executive functions were assessed using the Delis-Kaplan Executive Function System. These investigators also assessed motor sequencing using the Push-Turn-Tap-tap task and demonstrated that older participants' motor sequencing performance is more reliant on executive functioning and more susceptible to complexity than that of younger adults.

3.4 Defective Response Inhibition

People with defective response inhibition make incorrect motor responses that appear to be induced by the perception of a stimulus. For example, Luria described two tasks used to assess defective response inhibition. In one task, participants are asked to raise two fingers when the examiner raises one finger and vice versa. When the participant raises the same number of fingers as the examiner, it is a form of echopraxia and echopraxia is a form of defective response inhibition. In another test, the examiner instructs the patient to raise one finger when the examiner raises two fingers and not to raise any fingers when the examiner raises one finger. Patients with defective response inhibition will raise one finger when the examiner raises one or two fingers.

Another means of assessing defective response inhibition is the go/no-go test. Rey-Mermet and Gade [58] selected 176 studies in which young and older adults were tested on tasks employing commonly used measures of response inhibition. They reported that for most tasks the results speak against an inhibition deficit associated with older age; however, they did find that older participants have an inhibition impairment on the stop-signal and go/no-go tasks. For example, in the go/no-go task, participants are instructed to press a key as rapidly as possible when a certain letter appears on the screen, but not to press when any other letter appears. Whereas the "go" letter frequently appears on the screen, another (no-go) letter will infrequently appear. Older participants are

more likely to press the key to these "no go" letters than are younger participants.

Whereas Luria's tests and the go/no-go test described above examine response inhibition to visual stimuli, Shoraka and coworkers [59] assessed older versus younger participants with the tactile crossed response task. In this test, the seated subject is asked to place their hands on their lap, palms down, and when touched on their left hand, to lift their right hand off their lap as rapidly as possible, and when touched on their right hand, to lift their left hand off their lap as rapidly as possible. These investigators found that the older healthy participants made more errors than did the younger participants. Unlike Luria's tests, this tactile crossed response test is strongly dependent on interhemispheric communication. With aging, in addition to degradation of frontal lobe functions, there appears to be alteration in cerebral myelin, particularly in the corpus callosum, as reflected in reduced magnetization transfer ratio [46]. Therefore, it is not entirely clear whether the aging-related deficit in crossed response inhibition is related to an aging-related deficit in frontal executive functions, impaired callosal interhemispheric communication, or a combination.

3.5 Pathophysiology of Age-Related Decline in Action-Intentional (When) Functions

Defects in response inhibition could be considered a form of inappropriate approach behavior. Denny-Brown (personal communication) noted that all animals from the simplest to the most complex have two major forms of behavior: approach and avoidance. Denny-Brown and Chambers [60] noted that ablation of monkeys' parietal lobes induces avoidance reactions to stimuli. These monkeys even avoided foods that, before this ablation, attracted them. Touching these animals with parietal lesions could also cause a very vigorous withdrawal. In contrast to the withdrawal seen with parietal lesions, frontal lesions are associated with inappropriate approach behaviors, including a grasp reflex of the hand when the palm is touched, as well as sucking and rooting reflexes when the lips or cheek are touched. In addition, patients with frontal lesions can demonstrate magnetic apraxia [61]. Patients with magnetic apraxia reach for objects that they see but for which they have no need. Lhermitte [62] described "utilization behavior." Patients with frontal lesions will often pick up and use objects that they see when there is no reason to use these objects. For example, if there are a pen and notebook on a table, the patient with utilization behavior from frontal dysfunction will often pick up the pen, open the notebook, and write in it, even if this behavior is inappropriate to the circumstances. Whereas all these abnormal approach behaviors are associated with frontal lobe dysfunction, the lesion that causes this dysfunction is not always located in the frontal lobes, and frontal dysfunction, such as utilization behavior, can be caused by lesions in structures that interact with the frontal lobe cortex [63]. Although with normal aging an increase of abnormal behaviors such as a grasp reflex, magnetic apraxia, and utilization behavior has not been reported, defective response inhibition can be considered a form of inappropriate approach behavior, and it is primarily deficits in the frontal subcortical networks that cause defective response inhibition and the other action-intentional disorders discussed above.

3.5.1 Hemispheric-Right-Left Asymmetries

As mentioned, for people who are right handed, disorders of the "how" systems, such as ideomotor apraxia (IMA), are almost always associated with left hemisphere dysfunction. Action-intentional disorders are often caused by disorders that injure both hemispheres, but when they are caused by unilateral hemispheric dysfunction, they are most likely to be due to injury to the right hemisphere. For example, the action-intentional disorders that have been reported to occur with right frontal injury include limb akinesia [64], directional akinesia [65], perseveration [54], and motor impersistence [53]. In a study testing reaction time of the ipsilesional hand in patients with an infarction of one cerebral hemisphere, patients with right hemisphere infarctions exhibited greater slowing than did patients with left hemisphere infarctions, even when the hemispheric lesions were matched for size [47]. Furthermore, many of the action-intentional defects induced by right hemisphere dysfunction may not be limited to the left arm, the left hemispace, or movements in a leftward direction, but can involve both sides of the body. In addition, patients with a right hemispheric infarction are more likely to develop apathy and abulia [66]. Apathetic-abulic patients are less active and patients with less activity are more likely to

develop decubiti as well as pulmonary emboli from thrombophlebitis.

Hemispheric specialization permits parallel processing. Therefore, when the left hemisphere is programming "how" information, the right can be programming "when" information. The anatomic and physiological basis for the right hemisphere's dominance in mediating intentional activity is not entirely known. However, intentional processing appears to be an executive function and when executives decide to have their employees produce a product, they often base this decision on the need for this product. There are three systems that are important in detecting our needs: (1) portions of the limbic system, such as the amygdala, that are critical for the mediation of externally activated emotions, such fear and anger; (2) the hypothalamus, which monitors our body's internal milieu and induces drives to maintain homeostasis; and (3) semantic-declarative memory (knowledge) networks, which store the knowledge of how to satisfy our current needs as well as what actions should be taken so that future needs can be satisfied. One of the major connections between the limbic system and the cerebral cortex is via the subgenual anterior cingulate gyrus (Brodmann's area 25). The subgenual anterior cingulate gyrus is connected to all the major subcortical components of the limbic system, including the amygdala, the periaqueductal gray, nucleus accumbens, the nucleus of the solitary tract, the dorsal motor nucleus of the vagus, and the intermediate zone of the spinal cord (site of preganglionic autonomic neurons) [67]. Area 25 is in turn heavily connected with ventromedial orbitofrontal cortex and with pregenual anterior cingulate cortex (Brodmann's area 32) [68], an area implicated in intentional gating of action plans [69]. Injury to the bilateral anterior medial hemispheres, typically caused by extreme vasospasm in the wake of anterior communicating aneurysm rupture, involves the anterior cingulate gyri (infra-, pre-, and supragenual), SMA, and pre-SMA. This injury is associated with a profound action-intentional disorder called "akinetic mutism." Patients with this disorder do not initiate speech or actions. The relative contributions of damage to each of the regions damaged by this injury is unknown. However, injury to or degeneration of the ventral portion of right anterior cingulate cortex might be particularly important because this region provides motivational information to frontal neocortical areas. The right anterior cingulate gyrus appears to play a dominant role in action-intentional programming [70].

The cingulate gyrus also projects to the inferior parietal lobe, and the inferior parietal lobe, by means of the superior longitudinal fasciculus, connects with the lateral frontal lobes. This network, as well as many other sensory association areas, might be important in providing the frontal lobes with the knowledge about "when" actions as needed. As will be described below, getting all this information to the frontal lobe executive system is highly dependent on neuronal connectivity, and with aging there is a loss of this connectivity, especially in the right hemisphere.

3.5.2 Intrahemispheric Networks

Studies of patients with focal injuries, such as stroke and degenerative diseases, suggest that there are two major frontal lobe "when" networks. Patients with injury to the medial portions of the frontal lobes appear to primarily have impairments in the initiation of endogenously evoked actions. Although patients with these injuries often have problems with self-initiation, they are often better able to respond to external stimuli. In contrast, patients with injury to the lateral frontal cortex are more likely to reveal impairments in exogenously evoked actions.

As mentioned, the initiation of actions, the persistence of actions until a task is completed, and the termination of actions when the task is completed or the actions are unsuccessful are dependent on the normal functioning of the frontal executive network. The proper functioning of this frontal executive network is dependent on information this network receives from cognitive-semantic networks that store declarative memories (knowledge), and these declarative-knowledge networks are primarily located in the temporal and parietal association cortices.

Other than input from the olfactory system, the frontal lobes have no direct sensory input from the external world; they receive information about the external world from posterior sensory association areas. These posterior cortical sensory association areas are primarily connected to the frontal lobes by the superior longitudinal fasciculus. The superior longitudinal fasciculus includes SLF-I, which connects the superior parietal cortex to the supplementary motor area and the adjacent medial frontal cortex; SLF-II, which connects the inferior parietal lobule with the dorsal premotor area and adjacent prefrontal cortex; and SLF-III, which connects the supramarginal gyrus

to the ventral premotor cortex. The temporal lobes also contain sensory association areas, which connect to the frontal lobes by means of the uncinate and arcuate fasciculi. These intrahemispheric connections are important for providing the frontal lobes with knowledge about the environment, knowledge about past experiences, and knowledge about the behaviors that were successful and unsuccessful.

The basal ganglia are also a critical element of the action-intentional network. Different areas of the frontal lobes have specific connections with the basal ganglia, including the caudate and putamen. The striatum projects to the internal portion of the globus pallidus, as well as the pars reticularis of the substantia nigra, and the globus pallidus projects to specific thalamic nuclei that in turn project back to the frontal lobes. Physiological as well as clinical studies have revealed that these frontal, basal ganglia, thalamic reentrant circuits are critical for the function of the "when" motor action-intentional network. Therefore, the many diseases that are associated with basal ganglia dysfunction may be associated with impairments of the action-intentional system.

Since the frontal lobes are so dependent on input from other portions of the brain, the normal function of this portion of the action-intentional network is highly dependent on the integrity of white matter tracts that connect these subcortical and cortical areas with the frontal lobes. Therefore, with aging and the associated deterioration of the white matter pathways, such as the superior longitudinal fasciculi, the anterior limb of the internal capsule, and the anterior corona radiata, there is often a decrement of action-intentional functions.

4 Management and Treatment

As mentioned, Van Halewyck and coworkers [18] compared the aiming-reaching performance of physically active and sedentary older adults with that of younger adults. These investigators found that it was only the sedentary older adults who had the slower aiming-reaching movements. Although not fully studied, physical and cognitive exercises might be the best means of preventing and treating the changes in "how" and "when" motor programming discussed above.

Unfortunately, there have not been many studies that have systematically investigated possible medications that might treat the motor changes associated with aging. However, when possible, the first step should always be prevention. Since many of the changes associated with aging are related to the alterations of white matter connectivity and small vessel disease is often the cause of deep white matter injury, it is critical that hypertension be diagnosed and treated as early as possible. However, even in the absence of hypertension, with aging there may be decreased perfusion of blood into the small arteries that feed the subcortical white matter as a result of cerebral arteriolosclerosis [71]. There are several agents that might be helpful, such as ergoloid mesylates (Hydergine), which is a cerebrovasodilator, and pentoxifylline (Trental), which reduces the viscosity of blood. These medications might be helpful by increasing the blood flow to the white matter; however, these medications have not been studied for preventing and treating the white matter changes associated with aging and are thus are not approved for this use.

Patients with multiple sclerosis often suffer with fatigue, and their fatigue, as well as the fatigue associated with Parkinson's disease, is often successfully treated with amantadine. This medication was initially used to treat patients with influenza, and the mechanisms by which it helps fatigue in these patients is not known. In addition, this medication has not been used with healthy older people to learn if can also help them with early fatigue. However, even in the absence of the signs of Parkinson's disease with aging, there is a loss of dopaminergic neurons, and many of the alterations of the motor system that occur with aging in some respects mirror the signs of Parkinson's disease. Thus, trials using dopamine agonists may be worthwhile.

References

1. Desrosiers J, Hébert R, Bravo G, Rochette A. Age-related changes in upper extremity performance of elderly people: a longitudinal study. *Exp Gerontol.* 1999 Jun;34 (3):393–405.

2. Ranganathan VK, Siemionow V, Sahgal V, Yue GH. Effects of aging on hand function. *J Am Geriatr Soc.* 2001 Nov;49(11):1478–84.

3. Liepmann, H. Apraxia. *Ergbn Ges Med.* 1920, 1:516–43.

4. Jiménez-Jiménez FJ, Calleja M, Alonso-Navarro H, Rubio L, Navacerrada F, Pilo-de-la-Fuente B, Plaza-Nieto JF, Arroyo-Solera M, García-Ruiz PJ, García-Martín E, Agúndez JA. Influence of age and gender in motor performance in healthy subjects. *J Neurol Sci.* 2011 Mar 15;302(1–2):72–80. doi: 10.1016/j.jns.2010.11.021.

5. Seidler RD, Bernard JA, Burutolu TB, Fling BW, Gordon MT, Gwin JT, Kwak Y, Lipps DB. Motor control and aging: links to age-related brain structural, functional, and biochemical effects. *Neurosci Biobehav Rev.* 2010 Apr;34(5):721–33. doi: 10.1016/j.neubiorev.2009.10.005.

6. Carmeli E, Patish H, Coleman R. The aging hand. *J Gerontol A Biol Sci Med Sci.* 2003 Feb;58 (2):146–52.

7. Good CD, Johnsrude IS, Ashburner J, Henson RN, Friston KJ, Frackowiak RS. A voxel-based morphometric study of ageing in 465 normal adult human brains. *Neuroimage.* 2001 Jul;14(1 Pt 1):21–36.

8. Ruff RM, Parker SB. Gender- and age-specific changes in motor speed and eye-hand coordination in adults: normative values for the Finger Tapping and Grooved Pegboard Tests. *Percept Mot Skills.* 1993 Jun;76(3 Pt 2):1219–30.

9. Van Gerven PWM, Hurks PPM, Adam JJ. Both facilitatory and inhibitory impairments underlie age-related differences of proactive cognitive control across the adult lifespan *Acta Psychol (Amst).* 2017 Sep;179:78–88. doi: 10.1016/j.actpsy.2017.07.005. n;76 (3 Pt 2):1219–30.

10. Arnold P, Vantieghem S, Gorus E, Lauwers E, Fierens Y, Pool-Goudzwaard A, Bautmans I. Age-related differences in muscle recruitment and reaction-time performance. *Exp Gerontol.* 2015

Oct;70:125–30. doi: 10.1016/j. exger.2015.08.005.

11. Yordanova J, Kolev V, Hohnsbein J, Falkenstein M. Sensorimotor slowing with ageing is mediated by a functional dysregulation of motor-generation processes: evidence from high-resolution event-related potentials. *Brain.* 2004 Feb;127(Pt 2):351–62.

12. Hoffstaedter F, Grefkes C, Roski C, Caspers S, Zilles K, Eickhoff SB. Age-related decrease of functional connectivity additional to gray matter atrophy in a network for movement initiation. *Brain Struct Funct.* 2015 Mar;220 (2):999–1012. doi: 10.1007/ s00429-013-0696-2.

13. Koppelmans V, Hirsiger S, Mérillat S, Jäncke L, Seidler RD. Cerebellar gray and white matter volume and their relation with age and manual motor performance in healthy older adults. *Hum Brain Mapp.* 2015 Jun;36 (6):2352–63. doi: 10.1002/ hbm.22775.

14. Ross GW, Petrovitch H, Abbott RD, Nelson J, Markesbery W, Davis D, Hardman J, Launer L, Masaki K, Tanner CM, White LR. Parkinsonian signs and substantia

nigra neuron density in decendents elders without PD. *Ann Neurol.* 2004 Oct;56(4):532–9.

15. Lamb DG, Correa LN, Seider TR, Mosquera DM, Rodriguez JA Jr, Salazar L, Schwartz ZJ, Cohen RA, Falchook AD, Heilman KM. The aging brain: movement speed and spatial control. *Brain Cogn.* 2016 Nov;109:105–11. doi: 10.1016/j.bandc.2016.07.009.

16. Poston B, Van Gemmert AW, Barduson B, Stelmach GE. Movement structure in young and elderly adults during goal-directed movements of the left and right arm. *Brain Cogn.* 2009 Feb;69 (1):30–8. doi: 10.1016/j.bandc.2008.05.002.

17. Wright ML, Adamo DE, Brown SH. Age-related declines in the detection of passive wrist movement. *Neurosci Lett.* 2011 Aug 15;500(2):108–12. doi: 10.1016/j.neulet.2011.06.015.

18. Van Halewyck F, Lavrysen A, Levin O, Elliott D, Helsen WF. The impact of age and physical activity level on manual aiming performance. *J Aging Phys Act.* 2015 Apr;23(2):169–79. doi: 10.1123/japa.2013-0104.

19. Hanna-Pladdy B, Mendoza JE, Apostolos GT, Heilman KM. Lateralised motor control: hemispheric damage and the loss of deftness. *J Neurol Neurosurg Psychiatry.* 2002 Nov;73(5):574–7.

20. Thornbury JM, Mistretta CM. Tactile sensitivity as a function of age. *J Gerontol.* 1981 Jan;36 (1):34–9.

21. Hill BD, Barkemeyer CA, Jones GN, Santa Maria MP, Minor KS, Browndyke JN. Validation of the coin rotation test: a simple, inexpensive, and convenient screening tool for impaired psychomotor processing speed. *Neurologist.* 2010 Jul;16 (4):249–53. doi: 10.1097/NRL.0b013e3181b1d5b0.

22. Heilman KM, Meador KJ, Loring DW. Hemispheric asymmetries of

limb-kinetic apraxia: a loss of deftness. *Neurology.* 2000 Aug 22;55(4):523–6.

23. Acosta LM, Bennett JA, Heilman KM. Callosal disconnection and limb-kinetic apraxia. *Neurocase.* 2014;20(6):599–605.

24. Mitrushina M, Fogel T, D'Elia L, Uchiyama C, Satz P. Performance on motor tasks as an indication of increased behavioral asymmetry with advancing age. *Neuropsychologia.* 1995 Mar;33 (3):359–64.

25. Dolcos F, Rice HJ, Cabeza R. Hemispheric asymmetry and aging: right hemisphere decline or asymmetry reduction. *Neurosci Biobehav Rev.* 2002 Nov;26 (7):819–25.

26. Reuter-Lorenz PA, Stanczak L. Differential effects of aging on the functions of the corpus callosum. *Dev Neuropsychol.* 2000;18 (1):113–37.

27. Hou J, Pakkenberg B. Age-related degeneration of corpus callosum in the 90+ years measured with stereology. *Neurobiol Aging.* 2012 May;33(5):1009.e1–9. doi: 10.1016/j.neurobiolaging.20.

28. Bangert AS, Reuter-Lorenz PA, Walsh CM, Schachter AB, Seidler RD. Bimanual coordination and aging: neurobehavioral implications. *Neuropsychologia.* 2010;48:1165–70.

29. Fling BW, Walsh CM, Bangert AS, Reuter-Lorenz PA, Welsh RC, Seidler RD. Differential callosal contributions to bimanual control in young and older adults. *J Cogn Neurosci.* 2011 Sep;23(9):2171–85. doi: 10.1162/jocn.2010.21600.

30. Ni Z, Gunraj C, Nelson AJ, Yeh IJ, Castillo G, Hoque T, Chen R. Two phases of interhemispheric inhibition between motor related cortical areas and the primary motor cortex in human. *Percept Mot Skills.* 1993 Jun;76(3 Pt 2):1219–30.

31. Grefkes C, Eickhoff SB, Nowak DA, Dafotakis M, Fink GR

Dynamic intra- and interhemispheric interactions during unilateral and bilateral hand movements assessed with fMRI and DCM. *Neuroimage.* 2008 Jul 15;41(4):1382–94. doi: 10.1016/j.neuroimage.2008.03.048.

32. Diermayr G, McIsaac TL, Gordon AM. Finger force coordination underlying object manipulation in the elderly – a mini-review. *Gerontology.* 2011;57(3):217–27. doi: 10.1159/000295921.

33. Ameli M, Dafotakis M, Fink GR, Nowak DA. Predictive force programming in the grip-lift task: the role of memory links between arbitrary cues and object weight. *Neuropsychologia.* 2008;46 (9):2383–8. doi: 10.1016/j.neuropsychologia.2008.03.011.

34. Thorpe WH. The learning of song patterns with especial references to the song of the chaffinch, *Fringilla coelebs. Ibis* 1958;100:535–70.

35. Bottjer SW, Johnson F. Circuits, hormones, and learning: vocal behavior in songbirds. *J Neurobiol.* 1997 Nov;33 (5):602–18. Review.

36. Asher JJ, Garcia RC. The optimal age to learn a foreign language. *Modern Language Journal.* 1969;53:334–41.

37. Scoville WB, Milner B. Loss of recent memory after bilateral hippocampal lesions. *J Neurol Neurosurg Psychiatry.* 1957;20:11–21.

38. Corkin S. Acquisition of motor skill after bilateral medial temporal-lobe excision. *Neuropsychologia.* 1968;6:255–65.

39. Saint-Cyr JA, Taylor AE, Lang AE. Procedural learning and neostriatal dysfunction in man. *Brain.* 1988 Aug;111 (Pt 4):941–59.

40. Harrington DL, Haaland KY, Yeo RA, Marder E. Procedural memory in Parkinson's disease: impaired motor but not

visuoperceptual learning. *J Clin Exp Neuropsychol*. 1990 Mar;12(2):323–39.

41. Rodrigue KM, Kennedy KM, Raz N. Aging and longitudinal change in perceptual-motor skill acquisition in healthy adults. *J Gerontol B Psychol Sci Soc Sci*. 2005 Jul;60(4):P174–P181.

42. Kennedy KM, Raz N. Age, sex and regional brain volumes predict perceptual-motor skill acquisition. *Cortex*. 2005 Aug; 41(4):560–9.

43. Bennett IJ, Madden DJ, Vaidya CJ, Howard JH Jr, Howard DV. White matter integrity correlates of implicit sequence learning in healthy aging. *Neurobiol Aging*. 2011 Dec;32(12):2317.e1–12. doi: 10.1016/j.neurobiolaging.2010.03.017.

44. Woods DL, Wyma JM, Yund EW, Herron TJ, Reed B. Factors influencing the latency of simple reaction time. *Front Hum Neurosci*. 2015; 23;9:193. doi: 10.3389/fnhum.2015.00193.9: 131.

45. Lewis RD, Brown JM. Influence of muscle activation dynamics on reaction time in the elderly. *Eur J Appl Physiol Occup Physiol*. 1994;69(4):344–9.

46. Serbruyns L, Leunissen I, van Ruitenbeek P, Pauwels L, Caeyenberghs K, Solesio-Jofre E, Geurts M, Cuypers K, Meesen RL, Sunaert S, Leemans A, Swinnen SP. Alterations in brain white matter contributing to age-related slowing of task switching performance. *Brain Mapp*. 2016 Nov;37(11):4084–98. doi: 10.1002/hbm.23297.

47. Howes D, Boller F. Evidence for focal impairment from lesions of the right hemisphere. *Brain*. 1975;98:317–32.

48. Heilman KM, Van Den Abell T. Right hemispheric dominance for mediating cerebral activation. *Neuropsychologia*. 1979;17(3–4):315–21.

49. Hurtz S, Woo E, Kebets V, Green AE, Zoumalan C, Wang B, Ringman JM, Thompson PM, Apostolova LG. Age effects on cortical thickness in cognitively normal elderly individuals. *Dement Geriatr Cogn Dis Extra*. 2014 Jul 1;4(2):221–7. doi: 10.1159/000362872.

50. Krehbiel LM, Kang N, Cauraugh JH. Age-related differences in bimanual movements: a systematic review and meta-analysis. *Exp Gerontol*. 2017 Nov;98:199–206. doi: 10.1016/j.exger.2017.09.001.

51. Leinen P, Vieluf S, Kennedy D, Aschersleben G, Shea CH, Panzer S. Life span changes: performing a continuous 1:2 bimanual coordination task. *Hum Mov Sci*. 2016 Apr;46:209–20. doi: 10.1016/j.humov.2016.01.004.

52. Langan J, Peltier SJ, Bo J, Fling BW, Welsh RC, Seidler RD. Functional implications of age differences in motor system connectivity. *Front Syst Neurosci*. 2010 Jun 7;4:17. doi: 10.3389/fnsys.2010.00017.

53. Kertesz A, Nicholson I, Cancelliere A, Kassa K, Black SE. Motor impersistence: a right-hemisphere syndrome. *Neurology*. 1985 May;35(5):662–6.

54. Sandson J, Albert ML. Perseveration in behavioral neurology. *Neurology*. 1987 Nov;37(11):1736–41.

55. Suchy Y, Lee JN, Marchand WR. Aberrant cortico-subcortical functional connectivity among women with poor motor control: toward uncovering the substrate of hyperkinetic perseveration. *Neuropsychologia*. 2013 Sep;51(11):2130–41.

56. Head D, Kennedy KM, Rodrigue KM, Raz N. Age differences in perseveration: cognitive and neuroanatomical mediators of performance on the Wisconsin Card Sorting Test. *Neuropsychologia*. 2009 Mar;47(4):1200–3. doi: 016/j.neuropsychologia.2009.01.003.

57. Niermeyer MA, Suchy Y, Ziemnik RE. Motor sequencing in older adulthood: relationships with executive functioning and effects of complexity. *Clin Neuropsychol*. 2017 Apr;31(3):598–618. doi: 10.1080/13854046.2016.1257071.

58. Rey-Mermet A, Gade M. Inhibition in aging: what is preserved? what declines? a meta-analysis. *Psychon Bull Rev*. 2017 Oct 10. doi: 10.3758/s13423-017-1384-7.

59. Shoraka AR, Otzel DM, M Zilli E, Finney GR, Doty L, Falchook AD, Heilman KM. Effects of aging on action-intentional programming. *Neuropsychol Dev Cogn B Aging Neuropsychol Cogn*. 2018 Mar;25(2):244–58. doi: 10.1080/13825585.2017.1287854.

60. Denny-Brown D, Chambers RA. The parietal lobe and behaviour. *Res Publ Assoc Res Nerv Ment Dis*. 1958; 36:35–117.

61. Denny-Brown D. The nature of apraxia. *J Nerv Ment Dis*. 1958;126:9–32.

62. Lhermitte F. "Utilization behaviour" and its relation to lesions of the frontal lobes. *Brain*. 1983;106:237–55.

63. Eslinger PJ, Warner GC, Grattan LM, Easton JD. "Frontal lobe" utilization behavior associated with paramedian thalamic infarction. *Neurology*. 1991 Mar;41(3):450–2.

64. Coslett HB, Bowers D, Heilman KM. Reduction in cerebral activation after right hemisphere stroke. *Neurology*. 1987 Jun;37(6):957–62.

65. Heilman KM, Bowers D, Coslett HB, Whelan H, Watson RT. Directional hypokinesia: prolonged reaction times for leftward movements in patients with right hemisphere lesions and neglect. *Neurology*. 1985 Jun;35(6):855–9.

66. Brodaty H, Sachdev PS, Withall A, Altendorf A, Valenzuela MJ, Lorentz L Frequency and clinical,

neuropsychological and neuroimaging correlates of apathy following stroke – the Sydney Stroke Study. *Psychol Med.* 2005 Dec;35(12):1707–16.

67. Devinsky O, Morrell MJ, Vogt BA. Contributions of anterior cingulate cortex to behaviour. *Brain.* 1995;118: 279–306.

68. Joyce MKP, Barbas H. Cortical connections position primate area 25 as a keystone for interoception, emotion, and memory. *Journal of Neuroscience.* 2018; 38:1677–98.

69. Nadeau SE, McCoy KJM, Crucian GP, Greer RA, Rossi F, Bowers D, et al. Cerebral blood flow changes in depressed patients after treatment with repetitive transcranial magnetic stimulation. Evidence of individual variability. *Neuropsychiatry, Neuropsychol Behav Neurol.* 2002;15:159–75.

70. Yan H, Zuo XN, Wang D, Wang J, Zhu C, Milham MP, Zhang D, Zang Y. Hemispheric asymmetry in cognitive division of anterior cingulate cortex: a resting-state functional connectivity study. *Neuroimage.* 2009 Oct 1;47(4):1579–89. doi: 10.1016/j. neuroimage.2009.05.080.71.

71. Kryscio RJ, Abner EL, Nelson PT, Benbnett D, Schneider J, Yu L, et al. The effect of vascular neuropathology on late-life cognition: results from the SMART Project. *J Prev Alzheimers Dis.* 2016 3:85–91.

Chapter 12

Alterations in Executive Functions with Aging

Donald T. Stuss and Fergus I. M. Craik

1 Introduction

Adult aging is often associated with declining efficiency of executive functions (EFs), and these changes have, in turn, been attributed to aging-related changes in the frontal lobes and in frontal systems. However, questions have been raised about the nature, validity, and specificity of these relationships. What is the operational definition of EF or, in specific studies, what operational definition was used? What measures are used to assess EF, and what is the relationship of these measures to the operational definitions? What is the relationship of these constructs to neuroanatomy? Finally, how are neural networks to be considered within this brain–behavior relationship?

Our review is structured as follows. The first section highlights studies of cognitive aging, that is, experimental, theoretically motivated approaches to understanding aging-related changes in cognitive functioning. The next section emphasizes research in aging and EF from a neuropsychological standpoint with a spotlight on studies using putative tests of EF and/or frontal lobe functioning. A review of studies of EF in association with structural and/or functional imaging indices follows. In the last section, we attempt to integrate these concepts, not to postulate a new theory but to suggest a way forward in addressing the questions that have been raised.

This review is selective rather than exhaustive. The focus is on normal or healthy aging and does not address issues involving alterations in EF that occur with mild cognitive impairment and the different forms of dementia.

1.1 Operational Definitions

Executive functions have been defined as "those capacities that enable a person to engage successfully in independent, purposive, self-serving behavior" ([1], p. 42); Lezak [1] identifies initiation, planning, purposive action, self-monitoring, self-regulation, and

volition as specific executive functions. Other frequently discussed EFs include working memory, inhibition, monitoring, and flexibility (set shifting). Deficits in these functions have been most commonly observed after frontal lobe damage. Over time, the terms "executive dysfunction" and "frontal lobe dysfunction" became virtually synonymous, and recently the term EF has been broadened even more. Patients with frontal lobe dysfunction often have pathology involving many regions of their frontal lobes, and even extending elsewhere. They exhibit a variety of deficits in domains other than cognition, such as affective and behavioral function, as well as changes in personality. In aggregate, these deficits may affect instrumental and activities of daily living. Terms such as "frontal lobe syndrome" and "dysexecutive syndrome" have been used to encompass all these deficits. In a word, the term "EF" often means different things to different researchers and clinicians.

In this review, we use the term "EF" as used in the original papers. However, we foreshadow Section 5, on "Integration," by indicating that there are often problems with the way the term "EF" is currently used. First, the incorporation of affective, behavioral, and personality changes overextends the cognitive definition proposed by Lezak, resulting in muddying of the term's operational definition. It is therefore important to consider whether a more precise definition of EF can be found. Second, the frontal lobes are very large (estimated at 25–33% of the entire cortex) with more than 15 Brodmann areas, each with architectonic specificity and many having specific connectivity with nonfrontal regions. Anatomical distinctions imply potential functional specificity. Third, functions such as working memory have been shown to involve brain regions other than frontal lobes. There are two potential implications: (1) certain functions may be mediated by multiple brain regions – a neural network; and (2) the strict localization of at least some definitions of EF is not possible at the present time.

2 Cognitive Aging Studies

It is generally agreed that many cognitive functions decline in efficiency in the course of adult aging, although it is also the case that some functions decline more than others [2, 3]. The abilities that decline include speed of processing, working memory, and episodic memory, whereas those that hold up well with age include world knowledge and vocabulary level [2]. Well-maintained functions appear to involve information and actions that have been thoroughly learned and are used on a regular basis, whereas the functions that decline with aging typically involve novel processes and procedures, often of a complex nature. This difference is captured by the theory of fluid and crystallized intelligence, which contrasts the ability to solve new problems with abilities that draw on well-learned knowledge and procedures. A complementary distinction has been made between representations and control, where *representations* are the set of crystallized schemas that are the basis for memory and knowledge of the world, and *control* is the set of fluid operations that enable intentional processing and adaptive cognitive performance. Representations are generally well maintained into older adulthood, whereas control (fluid intelligence) tends to peak in early adulthood and decline thereafter [4].

Cognitive control is not a monolithic entity but is itself composed of various processes and procedures – executive processes – which may change with age in different ways. Over the last 25 years or so, researchers and theorists have emphasized different aspects of EF as being the primary component responsible for aging-related decline in cognitive functioning and have also speculated as to how these aspects may be related to the frontal lobes and other brain regions. One such analysis was carried out by Verhaeghen and Cerella [5], who reviewed a set of existing meta-analyses and found no clear evidence for aging-related deficits in selective attention or in the specific costs (diminishing processing speed) related to local task switching. However, they did find evidence for deficits in dual-task performance and in global task-switching. Reimers and Maylor [6] also found aging-related deficits in global but not local processing. They conducted an online study of more than 5,000 participants aged 10–66 years. They had their participants perform speeded face categorization based on gender (G) or emotion (E) in single task blocks (either

all G decisions or all E decisions) or switching blocks, in which G and E decisions alternated (GGEEGGEE ...). General (global) switching cost, defined by the difference in performance time between a switching block and a single task block, decreased to the age of about 17 and then increased almost linearly from age 18 on. In contrast, specific (local) switching cost, defined by the difference in performance time between EG or GE sequences and GG or EE sequences *within* a switching block, remained remarkably stable across the entire age range. Verhaeghen and Cerella [5] also found evidence for aging-related increments in dual-task costs (the time associated with performing two tasks concurrently relative to the time to perform the tasks individually). They concluded that one major problem associated with cognitive aging is difficulty in simultaneously maintaining two distinctive task sets, where "set" implies preparedness to carry out some activity in a rapid and efficient manner.

One influential analysis of executive functions was published by Miyake and coworkers [7]. They measured the performance of 137 college students on a selection of commonly used EF tasks and then used factor analysis to identify three latent variables – mental set shifting, information updating and monitoring, and inhibition of prepotent responses – that contributed differentially to performance of the individual tasks. These three latent variables correlated moderately strongly with each other. There are two possible conclusions from this observation: (1) "pure" EFs do not exist; and (2) the EF tests used in the factor analysis engaged many different processes, and even the EFs in each test may not be the same; that is, a task or test is not a process. As Jacoby [8] pointed out some years ago, cognitive tasks and abilities are rarely "process-pure" but, rather, draw on several underlying processes and presumably on several different brain regions.

Many publications have explored adult age differences in the three EFs identified by Miyake et al. [7]. With regard to set switching, it is generally agreed that aging-related deficits are found in global but not local switching [5]. A slightly different approach was taken by Zelazo, Craik, and Booth [9], who measured perseverative errors – responses that would have been correct by the prior rule – in a set-switching task. In a life-span study, they found that the proportions of such errors declined from 10% in children aged 8–9 years to 4% in young adults, but rose again to 10% in adults aged 65–74 years. Similar results were reported by Cepeda, Kramer, and Gonzalez de Sather [10] with the additional findings that older participants took longer to disengage from the current task set than younger adults, but that the older group also benefited more than their younger counterparts from continued practice. All in all, it seems clear that mental flexibility, as measured by set-switching tasks, declines in the course of healthy aging.

The notion that inhibitory processes are less effective in older adults is a dominant one in studies of cognitive aging. Many of the relevant ideas and associated empirical studies stem from the work of Hasher, Zacks, and their colleagues. They have proposed that cognitive control involves both excitatory and inhibitory processes, the former to enhance task-relevant information (e.g., by focusing attention on crucial stimuli and appropriate responses) and the latter to suppress task-irrelevant information (e.g., by not attending to interfering stimuli and resisting misleading response tendencies). In their view, excitatory processes are largely spared in older adults, but inhibitory processes are impaired, thereby reducing cognitive control and precision of information processing [11]. In another influential article, Hasher and Zacks [12] proposed impairments of working memory functioning in older adults involving three domains: *access*, *deletion*, and *restraint*, with "access" referring to the selection and retention of relevant information in working memory, "deletion" referring to the efficient deletion of unwanted information, and "restraint" referring to the ability to override "prepotent" automatic response tendencies that are potentially disruptive to current task performance. An example of restraint or inhibition is given by the Stroop effect (see below) in which participants are instructed to name the color of the print (e.g., blue) and not to read the written color word (e.g., "red"). Thus, the participant must inhibit the overlearned tendency to say "red" when shown the word "red," when the correct response is "blue" – the color in which the stimulus word is printed. Another more striking clinical example of the inability to restrain "automatic" or overlearned responses is the phenomenon of "utilization behavior" described by Lhermitte [13], in which patients with frontal lobe damage inappropriately carry out actions strongly associated with objects placed in front of them.

There are a number of effects of these aging-related processing inefficiencies: older adults are more susceptible to interference and distraction by irrelevant stimuli; more likely to maintain no-longer-relevant information in working memory, thereby reducing the capacity to process new information; and less able to inhibit "default" responses that are not appropriate to the current situation. Information in working memory is in conscious awareness and, as such, is critical to comprehension, learning, and decision-making. The inhibition of automatic or prepotent responses is one of the major functions of working memory as this enables the person to respond appropriately to changing environmental demands. The efficiency of this function has been measured by performance on the Stroop task. Older adults typically take longer to inhibit word reading than their younger counterparts, as shown by West and Alain [14], supporting the notion that inhibitory processes decline with age. On the other hand, the results of a meta-analysis by Verhaeghen and De Meersman [15] suggest that the age sensitivity of the Stroop effect may be attributable to general slowing.

Updating is the third executive function identified by Miyake et al. [7]. Relevant tasks include ones in which response-relevant information is constantly changing so that "goal maintenance" information in working memory must be constantly updated [16]. Aging-related deficits in updating tasks were reported by De Beni and Palladino [17]. One commonly used measure of updating is the n-back task. There are various versions of this task, but the simplest version is one in which the participant is given a long string of letters and must detect repetitions of the same letter exactly n-back in the series, where n is typically 1, 2, or 3. For example, in a three-back task the string J G R F A **R** A X P B Q **P** X S has two targets, **R** and **P**; the letters A and X are also repeated, but not three back in the series. Older adults are typically slower and make more errors on this task [18].

The constructs of working memory and executive processes are often difficult to compare across different studies, as researchers have their own perspective on their nature and relationships. Working memory was originally conceived by Baddeley and Hitch [19] as a temporary buffer storage system in which the information "held in mind" could be processed and manipulated by executive functions, but in recent years the emphasis has shifted to the notion of working memory as the major center for cognitive control – thereby embodying the various executive processes discussed by Miyake et al. [7] and others. The label "working memory" in cognitive psychology has thus largely become an umbrella term to encompass a variety of related functions concerned with temporary storage and control operations. By this broad definition, working memory involves at least two types of control functions, those associated with the selective engagement of specific posterior networks and those associated with the inhibition of networks that are inappropriate for current circumstances.

Measures of working memory include complex span procedures, such as digit span backward, in which participants must both hold information in mind and manipulate that information or process additional information, as well as set-switching and *n*-back tasks. By all these measures, working memory performance declines with age, and, as illustrated by Salthouse [20], the decline starts when people are in their 20s. Another such task is the alpha span test. In this test, participants are given a short sequence of words and their task is to rearrange the words mentally and say them back in correct alphabetic order. It was found that performance on this task peaks when participants are in their 20s and then declines monotonically with increasing age [21]. The EFs involved in such complex span tasks include updating and the mental skills of coordination and management, whose decline with age was discussed and illustrated by Mayr and Kliegl [22]. Complex span tasks should be distinguished from "simple span" tasks in which participants repeat back a sequence of digits or words in the same order as they were presented (i.e., without the need for manipulation or transformation). Aging-related performance decrements on such simple span tasks are comparatively slight [23], perhaps because performance involves the relatively automatic "articulatory loop" described by Baddeley and Hitch [19]. These findings make the point that the clinical use of simple memory span tests to "assess memory" does not even yield a valid measure of short-term memory. Rather, memory span measures largely reflect the capacity of the articulatory loop. There are two final points to be made about working memory. First, there is a growing consensus that working memory operations depend on both frontal [24, 25] and posterior brain networks [26]. Frontal networks are concerned with control aspects, whereas posterior networks reflect the specific content of the material being held and actively processed. The second point is that the construct of

working memory has much in common with the construct of fluid intelligence; both decline with age and overlap in ways discussed by Salthouse [20].

Two further bodies of work are central to the topic of aging-related differences in cognitive control: those of Jacoby and his colleagues [27, 28] and those of Braver, Barch, and their colleagues [29, 30]. Jacoby [8] proposed two dissociable processes involved in recognition memory: familiarity and recollection. Of the two, recollection involves memory for the context of initial occurrence and is controlled, conscious, and deliberate, whereas familiarity is typically context free, driven by the perceptual input, and is largely cost free in terms of processing resources. In line with other work on aging and executive processes, the controlled process of recollection declines with age but the automatic process does not, with the consequence that older adults are impaired in their recollection of specific episodes, thereby allowing familiarity, past experience, and habit to play a more dominant (and sometimes misleading) role in recognition memory [27, 28]. The conclusion that recollection declines with age but familiarity does not receives further support from the results of a study by Koen and Yonelinas [31] in which they found converging evidence from several different methods of estimating these measures. Koen and Yonelinas [32] presented evidence that the hippocampus is critical for recollection, whereas familiarity is dependent on the integrity of the perirhinal cortex.

The second approach to studying the effects of aging on executive functions was proposed by Braver, Barch, and their colleagues [29, 30]. They suggested that a common feature of many executive control tasks is that they rely on internal representations of task-appropriate sets or goals. This thought led to the formulation of their *goal maintenance account* of working memory, in which they postulate that maintenance of current task goals in working memory reflects activation in lateral prefrontal cortex, modulated by the neurotransmitter dopamine. The active maintenance of the goal influences the flow of processes in other brain regions that are concerned with perception, the selection of appropriate actions, and memory retrieval. Braver and colleagues propose that aging-related declines in the functions of lateral PFC and dopamine result in an impairment in the older adult's ability to maintain goal information over time [29, 30] (see also Chapters 11, 13, and 14). An excellent comprehensive account of the effects of aging on goal maintenance is provided by Braver and West [16].

To return to more general topics, a number of big-picture ideas have been advanced in the last few decades to capture fundamental reasons for aging-related declines in cognitive performance. These include general slowing [33], reflecting the undeniable evidence that reaction times (RTs) are slower and response latencies are greater in older than in younger adults. It is less clear how a decline in processing speed could account for the equally undeniable aging-related declines in working memory perform-ance, although Salthouse [34] has suggested that the limit on the number of distinct ideas that can be kept active in working memory may be set by the rate at which information can be processed.

A second general idea is that inhibitory processes become less effective with increasing age [12]. A persuasive case for such effects has been made by Hasher, Zacks, and their colleagues. They suggest that older adults are less able than younger adults to sup-press the processing and retrieval of items designated as to be forgotten. Specifically, in comparison with younger adults, older adults produced more "to be forgotten" word intrusions on an immediate recall test.

A third idea is that processing resources decline with age, presumably reflecting underlying biological changes, and that this decline in attentional capacity or even "mental energy" results in aging-related impairments in cognitive control and in memory encoding and retrieval processes [35]. One experi-mental finding in favor of the reduced processing resources account is that when attention is divided by having participants perform two cognitive tasks simultaneously, younger adults' performance quanti-tatively resembles that of older adults working under undivided attention [36].

A final theoretical account emphasizes the increasing difficulty experienced by older adults in the "self-initiation" of such higher mental activities as memory retrieval and complex decision-making [37, 38]. Craik's further suggestion was that retrieval and other complex processes depend substantially on input from the external environment, such that internally generated self-initiation and support pro-vided by the external environment are complemen-tary and act in concert to yield effective performance. This notion is illustrated in Figure 12.1, which shows a set of common laboratory memory tasks arranged from top to bottom in terms of increasing

environmental support and therefore declining need for processing resources and cognitive control. Free recall and time-based prospective memory have high resource requirements and high need for cognitive control and are typically associated with large aging-related decrements. These decrements imply that older adults require more support from the external context for many higher cognitive activities. By the same token, they will benefit disproportionately from external support and aging-related deficits will decline when such support is provided [35, 37, 38]. In the final section of this chapter, we suggest that self-initiated activities are linked to energization functions mediated by the superior medial regions of the frontal lobes.

2.1 Summary

Cognitive changes with aging appear to be grouped into two major categories. First, there is slowed pro-cessing speed, and second, there are impairments in executive or control processes such as inhibition, set shifting, monitoring, and working memory. Many of these aging-related problems have been attributed to a decline in "attentional resources" and to difficulties with "self-initiation" of cognitive processes, which in turn may reflect fundamental aging-related decreases in processing speed and decreased effectiveness of executive processes.

3 Neuropsychological Studies of Aging and Executive Functions

Neuropsychological studies differ from cognitive aging approaches because of their greater focus on the rela-tionship of function to brain organization and func-tional localization. Thus, in this section we will discuss some of the more widely used classic neuropsycho-logical tests of EF. There is, however, an obvious over-lap, particularly in an emphasis on processing speed.

3.1 Processing Speed/Reaction Time

Diminishing processing speed "may deserve special status in the context of cognitive aging" ([39, p. 246; see also [33]) as it accounts for 70–80% of age-related variance in other cognitive variables. Controlling for the impact of processing speed on other variables might help to dissociate the roles of different control processes. Although some conclude that older indi-viduals are slower in both simple and more complex

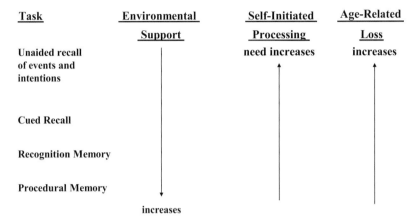

Age-related memory loss a function of:

1. **PERSON** unable to execute controlled processing

   (self-initiated activity; frontal inefficiency)

2. **TASK** requires self-initiated processing

3. **ENVIRONMENT** fails to compensate (via cues, context)

Task	Environmental Support	Self-Initiated Processing	Age-Related Loss
		need increases	increases
Unaided recall of events and intentions			
Cued Recall			
Recognition Memory			
Procedural Memory			
	increases		

Figure 12.1 The leftmost column shows memory tasks arranged from top to bottom in terms of increasing environmental support and decreasing need for self-initiated processing. The topmost tasks are those (such as free recall and some types of prospective memory) that require most self-initiated activity, and therefore show the greatest age-related losses. Speculatively, the ability to perform self-initiated activities depends on the integrity of frontal lobe circuits (see text).

reaction time (RT) tasks [40], others propose that task demands interact with processing speed. For example, simple RT is quite constant until age 50 before showing aging effects, while four-choice RT slows throughout the entire adult age range [41]. This suggests that there may be more than one factor influencing the slowing of processing speed with aging. Godefroy and colleagues [42] pursued this by examining the effect of divided attention on various simple RT measures, as well as the effect of age on perceptual, motor, decision, and attentional processes. They concluded that the slowing cannot be due solely to deficits in working memory and higher-order processes but that there is also basic perceptual-motor slowing. They also suggested that the alterations of these different functions may become relevant at different ages (e.g., attentional decline after age 60); that is, there are different phases of aging, depending on what is being measured.

A perhaps more interesting consideration is not processing speed per se but intra-individual variability (IIV), the changes in stability of performance of an individual. In general, the performance of older adults is more variable [43–46]. IIV decreases with age until the third decade of life, at which point it begins to increase [41], even controlling for speed of response [47]. Hultsch, MacDonald, and Dixon [44] compared a younger witih an older group and then

retested these groups every 3 years (older participants) or every 6 years on four tests, all of which required speeded response: simple RT, choice RT, lexical decision, and semantic decision. Other measures included perceptual speed, working memory, episodic memory, and crystallized abilities. They measured both group variability (between persons or inter-individual) and intra-individual variability (both across tasks and over time). All measures of variability were larger in the older than the younger group, even when speed was controlled.

There are at least three reasons why IIV is a particularly interesting dependent variable. First, IIV has been reported in studies of patients with focal frontal pathology, and the underlying mechanisms of IIV vary depending on the location of the lesion [48, 49]. These data therefore suggest that different mechanisms might be affecting performance. Second, IIV can be measured in tasks other than RT, such as word-list learning [50] and verbal fluency [51]. Third, one can use feedback to reduce IIV in older adults, particularly in those with higher education [52].

3.2 The Classic Neuropsychological Tests

Neuropsychologists have commonly used certain measures of EF to study the effects of age on performance – for example, the Wisconsin Card Sorting Test

(WCST), Stroop, Hayling Sentence Completion, and Trail Making Test (TMT) – because they were designed to measure the classic EFs such as inhibition, planning, monitoring, and disengagement with switching. WCST performance does deteriorate with aging. One study indicated that as early as age 50, there was evidence of more overall errors, perseverative errors, and fewer categories achieved [53]. A meta-analysis of these studies demonstrated a large aging effect size in WCST performance, particularly in the number of perseverative errors [54]. Deterioration was most severe for the oldest group, aged 80–90. Education influenced performance, especially in people with fewer than 12 years of education. Different mechanisms have been offered to explain the deterioration in WCST performance with aging. These include reduced processing speed affecting the use of feedback [55], impairment in updating working memory [56], and impaired set-shifting [57]. Some have suggested a combination of impaired processes affecting performance on the WCST. For example, Gamboz and colleagues [58] concluded that faulty inhibition, working memory, and global (but not local) switching were relevant. Ashendorf and McCaffrey [59] asked younger and older participants to verbalize their response strategy when placing each card; their results suggested that in the older participants, there was poor set-shifting and set maintenance.

The Stroop test is very commonly used in studies of aging, as the different conditions (e.g., word reading, color naming, and word–font color interference) provide the possibility of isolating specific processes. There have also been variations in the presentation. Research studying the effects of aging on the Stroop test, in particular, the interference condition, demonstrates larger Stroop effects in healthy older adults compared with younger ones (e.g., [60, 61]). Different reasons for the deterioration have been suggested, including aging-related slowing rather than impairment of a specific cognitive process [33, 62, 63]. A role for other variables above and beyond aging has also been proposed: general health and biological life events that impact performance, sex differences (no effect or superior performance by women), and lesser education in the older groups [61–63].

Some authors have attempted to dissociate processes by manipulating presentation of the Stroop. For example, Ludwig and colleagues [64] compared blocked presentation (only one type of stimulus is presented repeatedly and the expected response does

not change; e.g., read the words, name the colors, interference condition) with item-by-item presentation (all three types of stimuli are presented randomly and the response required is based on the nature of the stimulus). Their results suggested that there was an aging effect with the blocked but not with the item-by-item presentation. Bélanger et al. [65] used a similar approach but it yielded somewhat different results. They presented pure blocks of incongruent items and mixed blocks of congruent (75%) and incongruent. The pure blocks allowed the study of other strategies that do not call on inhibitory mechanisms, since maintenance of the task goal then becomes paramount and the ability to resist interference is not a factor. Thus, according to these authors, this approach provided a more detailed insight into potentially different EF changes with aging, which may be dependent on task context: aging increased vulnerability to interference and also (but only partially) impaired goal-maintenance capabilities. Section 5, on "Integration," suggests possible reasons for these results.

The Trail Making Test (TMT) consists of two parts, A and B. Trail Making Test A consists of 25 circles numbered from 1 to 25 distributed over a sheet of paper. The participant is instructed to draw lines to connect the numbers as quickly as possible but not to sacrifice accuracy for speed and to avoid lifting the writing instrument (pen or pencil). In Part B, the circles are alternatively numbered (1–13) or lettered (A to L). The participant is requested to draw lines connecting these circles by alternating between the numbers and letters (e.g., 1-A-2-B-3-C). Many proposals have been offered for cognitive processes that are engaged in both parts of the test and processes that differ in the two parts. For example, both tasks require making fast and accurate movements between former targets and new targets; working memory to recall the next target; and allocation of global attention to find the target circle on the paper as well as to encode where future targets are located. Part B makes greater demands on working memory and requires the alternative shifting of attention between two different stimulus categories, numbers and letters.

Research results have been somewhat conflicting. Lindsey and Coppinger [66] partialed out performance on Part A and other simple capabilities, such as visual search, from Part B, and found that performance on Part B was no longer correlated with age, although Part A performance was related to age. Salthouse and Fristoe [67], on the other hand, demonstrated that the slowing with age on the TMT occurred on both Parts A and B, although it was greater in Part A.

These results illustrate an important question regarding the mechanisms underlying cognitive aging, previously noted: Is the problem just slowing of basic processing speed [66], is slowing greater with more complex cognitive tasks because they demand additional EF processes, is slowing greater with more complex cognitive tasks because they demand more effort independent of EF, or is it a combination of these factors? The weight of evidence in the neuropsychological studies reviewed above favors the concept that slowing with aging is caused primarily by reduced processing speed with the caveat that this reduction may reflect some combination of basic perceptual-motor slowing and slowing of specific higher-order cognitive processes.

Some studies have used multiple measures of EF. Wecker and colleagues [68] studied subtests of the Delis-Kaplan Executive Function battery. They concluded that there are aging effects on certain EFs that are best revealed when component parts are considered. This finding suggested possible aging-related differences between various types of EF that should be borne in mind when considering the effects of aging on EF. Other studies used different tests. An investigation of 938 participants who were between 20 and 89 years of age, using simple and choice RT, as well as card-sorting and the Golden version of the Stroop, revealed that there were aging-related declines in performance on all tests, with processing speed accounting for much of the variance in the Stroop and WCST results [69]. However, there was an effect of age even after controlling for speed, which they interpreted as "possibly different inhibitory control processes." Lin and colleagues [70], studying a different ethnic population (Chinese), also argued for multiple processes. They used a group of different EF tests, such as the Hayling Sentence Completion Test, Modified Six Elements Task, counting, and classics such as the WCST and Stroop. Comparison of old (60–70) and old-old (> 70) adults indicated that the older participants were worse on the WCST and Modified Six Elements Test but exhibited some decline in performance on the other tasks. Since the tests were selected as examples of different processes, they concluded that some EF processes, such as allocation of attention,

planning, and initiation, were more affected than other processes.

3.3 Summary

The majority of aging studies of processing speed and those using different neuropsychological tests of executive function have concluded that there is a decline in performance in the course of normal healthy aging. Slowed processing speed has been a very common finding, and often this impairment has been suggested as the major reason for deterioration in performance on other tests, such as the WCST. However, there has been a lack of clarity on the reasons for slowed responses, and there appears to be an effect of type of test used and/or method of test administration. One problem in the research has been the inconsistent or imprecise definition of EF. This issue has been addressed by some by attempting to separate underlying cognitive mechanisms affecting performance. This effort led to a proposal that there are EF changes with aging that are independent of speed of processing. Not all agree on the types of EF processes that are impaired, but there is general agreement that "possible differences between various types of executive functions require further study" [68]. This research has been hampered by a lack of an agreed-on model of EF or frontal lobe functioning and imprecise operational definitions of EF. We will return to this theme in the last section.

4 Brain–Behavior Approaches to Understand Cognitive Aging

With more readily available structural-anatomical and functional imaging, there has been a growth in research evaluating brain–behavior relationships associated with aging. As with behavioral studies, the imaging studies discussed here focus largely on tests of EF.

4.1 Structural Imaging Measures of Brain Aging

Studies of cortical changes have noted thinning associated with aging in prefrontal areas and relative sparing of temporal/parahippocampal regions [71] (see also Chapter 4). Analysis of T1 structural MRI scans in more than 100 nondemented individuals ranging in age from 19 to 93 revealed that cortical thickness began to diminish as early as middle age [72]. Thinning was widespread but was most prominent in the prefrontal area with relative sparing of temporal/parahippocampal regions. These authors also noted that their results did not support the idea that cortical atrophy proceeds in reverse of the order of maturational development, although this concept may still be relevant for myelin deterioration.

While gray matter changes in studies comparing middle-aged and senior individuals do not correlate with simple RT [73], Head et al. [74] found that more perseverative errors on the WCST were specifically associated with a lower prefrontal cortical volume. Bettcher and colleagues [75] administered a series of EF tests to 202 healthy older adults. Above and beyond the ever-present slowing in processing speed, the performance on the EF tests could be explained by a two-factor model – shifting/inhibition and updating working memory. They did not find a specific relationship between prefrontal anatomic parameters and EF. They concluded that a broad network of frontal and posterior regions was necessary for performance on "frontal lobe" tests and that changes of the corpus callosum and cingulate gyri might better predict EF after accounting for global gray matter atrophy.

These and other findings were put into context in two major reviews. Lockhart and DeCarli [76] reviewed the brain-aging research using structural MRI, including regional volume, cortical thickness, and white matter (WM) integrity. They concluded that there were "highly consistent age-related differences in brain structure, particularly frontal lobe *and* [emphasis added; see first paragraph in this section] medial temporal regions that are also accompanied by age-related differences in frontal and medial temporal lobe mediated cognitive abilities" (p. 1). They also suggested that the integrity of the corpus callosum might affect performance. Yuan and Raz [77] noted in their review that the reports addressing the frontal/aging hypothesis were inconsistent. In this review, which included about 4,000 articles on aging and EF, they found only 52 acceptable articles out of the 231 that were related to aging and brain structure. This list was further narrowed to 33 studies after excluding studies that found a relationship between EF and prefrontal structure size only after controlling for other variables such as education and age, the latter in essence affecting the ability to show an aging effect. Effect size depended on the type of EF task, with prefrontal cortex volume correlating more strongly with the WCST performance than with digit span backward, TMT performance, or verbal fluency. There was also some indication of specific anatomic-behavioral relationships, with larger effect sizes associated with differences in lateral and medial but not orbital prefrontal regions. Finally, "bigger was better" – better EF performance was observed with greater prefrontal volume and cortical thickness.

4.2 White Matter Tracts/Pathways

Executive functions rely on coordinated processing between the frontal lobes and anatomically distributed cortical and subcortical regions of the brain. Researchers began to look specifically at the relationship of EF to WM pathways connecting with the frontal lobes because studies of aging monkeys demonstrated that, with aging, there were WM changes. Therefore, cortical disconnection might contribute to the decline of EF observed with aging, even in the absence of disease. In human studies, diffusion tensor imaging (DTI) is well suited for studying cortical disconnection as these noninvasive studies provide information about the structural integrity of the connections between neural networks and particularly the frontal regions [78] (see also [74]). DTI measures the degree to which water molecules are free to diffuse in particular directions. For example, water can diffuse relatively freely along the axis of axons but has limited ability to diffuse in directions perpendicular to this axis. DTI studies of aging humans have shown that there is typically deterioration of WM marked by less diffusion along axons and greater diffusion across axons, most clearly in the frontal lobes but also in parietal and temporal regions [78–81]. These observations led to a growing linkage of EF performance to the integrity and connectivity of neural networks.

Examining speed of processing in relation to WM changes, Yang, Bender, and Raz [82] found that in healthy normal elderly adults with normal-appearing white matter (NAWM), there was evidence of more WM changes in the anterior than posterior regions. There was, however, no relation of NAWM diffusion properties to RT measures. IIV may be a more sensitive measure. IIV is related to WMH [83, 84], WM volume [85, 86], and DTI measures [87]. The relationship between IIV and brain measures is apparently stronger for the frontal regions.

Other investigators have examined the relation of WM integrity, defined by DTI, to performance on specific neuropsychological tests, particularly of EF, but also other functions such as memory. While older individuals who had low EF scores had frontal WM abnormalities, those with memory problems showed more medial temporal lobe WM deterioration [81]. Kennedy and Raz [88] used DTI in 52 adults aged 19–81 to examine WM integrity and its relation to tests of processing speed, inhibition, working memory, task switching, and episodic memory. The association between WM changes and alterations in cognitive function varied with task: changes in WM in frontal regions were associated with poorer working memory and processing speed; changes in posterior regions with deficient inhibition and task switching; and changes in medial-temporal regions with poorer episodic memory. They concluded: "Because longitudinal studies show that posterior association regions, e.g., inferior parietal lobule, are just as sensitive to aging as prefrontal regions . . ., and because executive functions indeed depend on both prefrontal and posterior parietal cortices, the term 'associative regional aging' may be more appropriate than the 'frontal aging' hypothesis" (p. 924). Hirziger and colleagues [81] assessed 200 healthy individuals older than 64 years who had normal MMSE scores. The TMT and Stroop were used to measure inhibition, task-switching, and processing speed. Although degradation in WM integrity was greatest within the frontal regions, the associations between task performance and anatomical change suggested the importance of other regions, including parietal and temporal lobes.

4.3 Functional Imaging Studies of EF and Aging

Functional imaging studies assessing the effects of aging provide another perspective beyond structural brain changes by recording alterations in brain activation, particularly in response to task demands. There are several salient observations. First, activation in functional imaging tasks varies from no aging-related differences to decreased as well as increased activation in specific regions of prefrontal cortex [89–91]. Second, functional imaging studies indicate that many brain regions respond to task demands, not just frontal (although frontal engagement is often most prominent), supporting the importance of studying the contribution of different regions within networks (e.g., [92]). Third, rather than general aging-related changes, there appear to be process- and region-specific activations, emphasizing the importance of

understanding what tasks are used and what processes are required to complete the tasks [93, 94].

Perhaps most importantly, functional imaging studies have led to hypotheses about the meaning of the activations. Both under- and overactivation, depending on task demands, may be observed with aging [95]. The mechanism of overactivation was analyzed by dividing older individuals into high and low performers on tests of EF and memory functions [80]. The overactivation was task and region dependent, with low-performing older adults showing greater synaptic activity in the frontal lobes than higher-performing older adults. The authors concluded that less wiring requires more firing, an explanation for over-recruitment with age. This paper has important implications for understanding mechanisms with its emphasis on dissociating processes engaged by complex tasks.

Systematic reviews, however, have elaborated on different possible mechanisms. Maillet and Rajah [90] reviewed functional imaging papers that included measures of gray matter volume in prefrontal or medial temporal regions and concluded that there may be multiple mechanisms underlying the differences in activation, the type of mechanism being dependent on brain integrity and task demands. Spreng and colleagues [91] completed a meta-analysis of functional neuroimaging studies in four specific cognitive domains (perception, memory encoding, memory retrieval, and EF) and concluded that aging-related decrements involved multiple brain regions, including the prefrontal areas, other frontal regions such as the frontal eye fields, parietal areas, ventral occipital lobes, and the postcentral gyrus. They called this a "task-positive network." Older adults exhibited greater activity in this network, particularly in frontal regions, suggesting greater allocation of frontal control processes to enable function at the same level as younger adults (see also [96]). There was again some suggestion of frontal control process specificity, with different frontal regions in the network associated with different behavioral outcomes in older adults. Turner and Spreng [97] proposed a dual account: deficient lateral PFC modulation of the frontoparietal network and reduced suppression of the default mode network as tasks increase in difficulty. They argue that the two processes co-occur and that older adults tend to rely to a greater extent on more posteriorly stored representations to complete tasks.

4.4 Hemispheric Asymmetries

Robertson [98] summarized evidence of the importance of the right lateral and inferior parietal lobe in maintaining performance on many tasks, but also noted that this was only one of several possible regions affected with aging. On psychometric tests, spatial scores decline with aging more than verbal scores, a finding that has been interpreted by some to suggest a greater aging-related decline in right hemisphere function. Several imaging studies appear to demonstrate differential right frontal and parietal changes with aging. In a PET study of healthy younger participants exploring mechanisms, sustained attention for object selection was associated with activation of the right frontal and parietal regions that declined over time unless there was a requirement to respond selectively to target objects [93]. Thus, aging-associated changes in right fronto-parietal engagement could reflect either changes in mechanisms underlying sustained attention, mechanisms underlying object selection, or their interaction.

Context helps interpretation of these data. Most of the studies that have demonstrated hemispheric asymmetries suggestive of alteration of right hemisphere processes with aging have used tests that are more sensitive to right hemisphere functioning. For example, Vallesi and colleagues [99] determined, in an fMRI study, that aging differentially impacts brain processes occurring in the fore period of RT tasks, processes that have been particularly linked to right lateral frontal regions in lesion and imaging studies. That is, the right hemisphere asymmetry was task and process specific (see also [93]). Nebes and colleagues [100] directly tested the right hemisphere deterioration with aging hypothesis using tachistoscopic and dichotic presentation of visual and auditory information. Their conclusion was that there was no evidence for selective right hemisphere deterioration with aging.

Rajah and D'Esposito [101] performed a qualitative meta-analytic review of all the functional magnetic resonance imaging and positron emission tomography studies of the effects of aging on working and episodic memory to determine if any region-specific changes have been observed. They found that with normal aging, distinct PFC regions exhibit different patterns of functional change. Normal aging may be related to deficits in function in right dorsal and anterior PFC, but as a result of these changes, functional compensation in left dorsal and anterior PFC might occur.

In other words, it is important to understand task demands and network interactions when analyzing brain–behavior relations associated with aging. If one analyzes the types of tasks that seem to support the right hemisphere decrement hypothesis, many if not all of them involve maintaining and sustaining performance, and there is growing evidence of right frontal specificity for mediating persistence and monitoring of performance [102] (see Section 5.1, on "Specificity of Frontal Lobe Functions," and also Chapter 11). There is a final argument for caution: anatomical studies do not suggest specific right frontal deterioration [103].

4.5 Brain and Cognitive Resilience

The study of cognitive changes associated with aging, particularly of EF, is complicated by the general concept of brain and cognitive reserve, or resilience. Cognitive reserve [104] may be defined broadly as the ability to maintain cognitive performance at a level better than brain integrity might predict. Several factors have been implicated in cognitive reserve, including education [52, 61], bilingualism [105], musical training, social interactions, differential recruitment of brain networks, and alternative cognitive strategies. The specific mechanisms accounting for cognitive reserve remain unclear, since aging individuals often have other a priori qualities, such as being more enterprising and more persistent.

Although the details about biological reserve have been known for years, more recently, the differences in brain structure are being recognized as an important consideration for understanding the changes associated with aging. The interaction of biological development and brain functional maintenance with cognitive reserve requires further study. The brain, particularly the prefrontal regions, is sensitive to vascular changes, especially those due to cerebrovascular disease [76, 106]. Although common, cerebrovascular disease is often clinically silent among older individuals [107, 108]. These brain structural changes may be seen as early as mid-life [76]. Hypertension is common with aging and often leads to atherosclerosis and small vessel disease [109] with associated damage to long white matter connections. As mentioned above, frontal lobe function is highly dependent on frontal connectivity with posterior association cortices, as well as the thalamus and caudate. Reduced EF efficiency has been associated with vascular risk factors [106, 110]. Increased blood pressure is associated with reduced processing speed and impaired performance on EF tasks, the latter even when covaried for speed (e.g., [110]). Nyberg and colleagues [111] argued for a broader concept of brain maintenance: better performance is associated with less structural brain damage, a principle that stands independently of aging and that is important for all processes, not just EF.

4.6 Summary

Structural imaging studies have shown brain changes (typically deterioration) associated with aging, measured in terms of either cortical thickness or WM integrity. There is evidence that distinct EF processes are implicated, as well as specific brain location–behavior associations. There is, however, lack of unanimity in the definition of EF processes and which ones are altered with aging. Although aging changes are not confined to frontal regions, they are often more prominent in these regions; nevertheless, there is an increasing emphasis on the importance of networks, especially with the advent of functional imaging. Network analysis has led to efforts to dissociate cognitive processes (both EF and those that are more domain specific) required for performance of complex tasks to understand the mechanisms underlying aging-related changes in brain function. Not understanding task process/brain region dissociations may lead to erroneous conclusions about changes with aging; this may be one reason for the hypothesis of hemispheric asymmetry with aging.

5 Integration

In the introductory Section 1, we emphasized that the study of alterations in executive functions with aging was likely confounded by unclear and inconsistent operational definitions, of both EFs and anatomical specificity. In our review of the literature, this lack of clarity was evident. Although there were multiple suggestions of the possibility of subtypes of EF processes, the definitions and results were inconsistent. Because of this, associations with specific brain regions were also inconsistent. In this section, we highlight our current understanding of the functions of the frontal lobes based on multiple studies of the deficits reported in patients with a focal lesion and

supported by functional imaging research. The results of these studies will be used as a means for developing an approach to the study the alterations of "executive functions" associated with aging.

5.1 Specificity of Frontal Lobe Functions

The Experimental Approach: Focal lesion research is considered a critical element in defining specific EF/brain relations because lesion research with an anatomically limited single lesion can best elucidate a functional-anatomic relationship [112].

The Theoretical Basis, Starting with Attention: We first assumed that the generic supervisory attentional system could be divided into separable processes [112]. Second, there was a need for more precise operational definitions of specific EF processes operating within the tasks that assess EF. These postulates had two implications: performance on most EF tests requires multiple processes and the use of an "EF" *task* does not automatically indicate a unique process. Third, there is a commonly held belief that frontal lobe control processes are required only in complex or novel situations. This was tested by starting with very simple tasks. It was possible that separation of processes was hampered by too many processes occurring simultaneously. Commonly used neuropsychological tests such as verbal fluency, WCST, Stroop, and TMT were also evaluated (see [113] for a review). Finally, analyses of tasks strongly suggested that a specific set of frontal attentional control processes could be hypothesized to explain functioning on any given EF test.

Viewed through the theory of a supervisory attentional system, and informed by discrete lesion analyses, three frontal lobe control processes could explain performance on all of the classic tasks listed above: (1) energization, the activation or driving of a behavior (initiation and maintenance of a selected action or target in active attention); (2) planning; and (3) a function that subsumes monitoring quality of performance and staying on task. These processes are not only operationally distinct, but also mediated by anatomically separate nodes in a network. Only two of these control processes were considered to fit a definition of EF.

We consider the first a frontal lobe control process but not an EF in the classical use of the term. The superior medial frontal lobe plus the anterior pre- and supra-genual cingulate gyrus appear to mediate energization, the activation or driving of a behavior (initiation and maintenance of a selected action or target in active attention). The term "energization" was selected since the terms activation, drive, and effort have come to have multiple meanings. Extensive damage to this region results in abulia, severe apathy, or even akinetic mutism. If damage is less extensive, patients are nevertheless slow to initiate and sustain mental processes. Since this energization function is important for all processes, impairment in initiating and sustaining any behavior, when present, is observed in many tests, including language tests such as verbal fluency. The energization deficit is best isolated anatomically and functionally with cognitively simple but speed-demanding reaction time tests [114], since demands posed by more complex tasks require additional processes associated with more activation.

The generic definitions of EF usually include terms such as planning, monitoring, task switching, and inhibition. Our results indicate that the other two processes required in many attentional/EF tasks fit this definition: (1) planning and (2) a function that subsumes monitoring quality of performance and staying on task, each linked to a hemisphere-specific anatomic substrate [102, 114–117]. Both are related to lateral prefrontal regions, with hemispheric asymmetry. Deficits in planning, including impaired selection of a goal (task setting), deciding sub-steps to achieve that goal, and establishing a criterion to respond, tend to occur with left lateral frontal lobe damage, particularly ventrolateral. The right lateral frontal area, on the other hand, appears to be important in monitoring quality of performance (e.g., were errors made?) or the occurrence of stimuli over time (staying on task). Finer distinctions are likely possible within these regions. These two domains of function can be conceptually grouped under the broader term "executive" function, since they can be considered to fit the true definition of "executive": planning, organizing, and monitoring to control and constrain lower-level, more automatic, domain-specific functions. Although we limit the term "executive functions" to those related to the lateral frontal regions, the most important conclusion is that there are anatomically separable and functionally distinct processes associated with the frontal lobes that should not be grouped under one umbrella term.

The differentiation of frontal lobe functions that led to the identification of three processes required

for attentional tasks has been empirically validated. Importantly, the results have been consistent across different groups of patients with focal frontal lesions and across task modalities (e.g., memory, language, RT – see [113, 118] for reviews). There is anatomical support in that both the EF (lateral frontal cortex) and energization (ACG/superior medial frontal) processes map onto two of the three prefrontal frontal-subcortical networks documented by Alexander, deLong, and Strick [119].

The value of these results is illustrated in analyses of two favorite classes of EF tasks, those probing inhibition and switching (often used in cognitive aging research). In the original theoretical proposal of Stuss and colleagues [112], inhibition was proposed as a possible independent process. However, subsequent studies did not confirm this particular hypothesis. Performance on inhibitory tasks such as the Stroop was most parsimoniously explained by the more basic processes of energization, monitoring, and planning (findings that were partially implied in the aging research by Ludwig et al. [64] and Bélanger and colleagues [65]). Two factors were important in revealing these distinctions: specific brain–behavior relations and context of test administration. The effects of these factors were evident in both lesion and functional imaging [120] research, with different Stroop paradigms, and in different patient groups and healthy controls. For example, if the Stroop interference condition was presented in a blocked format, impairment was associated with pathology in the ACG/superior medial frontal areas, and in the healthy controls, with activation in these same regions [121]. In participants with ACG/superior medial frontal pathology, the waxing and waning of correct responses suggested difficulty in maintenance (energization of the target) of the goal over time. If the task was presented in unblocked manner, lesions of the left ventro-lateral region produced an increased number of incorrect responses to distractors, indicating a problem in planning and establishing a set to respond correctly [122]. Shallice and colleagues demonstrated similar dissociations and similar processes operating in task-switching paradigms [102].

That is, inhibition and switching are not processes – they are broad descriptive terms for the demands of the task. Each test requires multiple operations related to the separable attentional processes as well as to non-frontal functions. Factor analysis of such tests will not yield individual brain-related processes.

Moving beyond Attention – Lessons from Neuro-anatomy: Neuroanatomy provides the basis for two other possible functions, beyond attention, associated with the frontal regions. Anatomical connectivity, specifically the prefrontal/subcortical circuitry identified by Alexander et al. [119], isolates a third prefrontal node in orbitofrontal/ventral medial regions, important for behavioral and emotional self-regulation (see [118] for a review). Developmental anatomy supports a distinction between two major moieties: cognition and memory (archicortical-hippocampal) and social and emotional (paleo-olfactory) [123]. In the frontal regions, then, this would be reflected by a distinction between the lateral/EF functions and ventral/orbitofrontal social emotional functions.

More recent research indicates that metacognition/theory of mind (thinking about thinking) is associated with more polar frontal regions, that is, Brodmann's area 10, the brain region latest to develop phylogenetically and ontogenetically. This region has a more integrative function.

Implications: There are multiple important implications of this frontal lobe lesion research. The first relates to operational definitions. There is no single frontal system; the frontal lobes and EF are not synonymous; and the frontal lobes have different control functions, some related to activation/energization, others to EF, others to emotional regulation, and still others to a more meta-cognitive/integrative ability. Frontal lobe functions can be divided into four distinct categories, each related to a different frontal region, an organization that is compatible with brain development and brain connectivity [118]. All four categories (i.e., energization, executive functions (planning and monitoring), emotional regulation, and metacognition) can be considered domain-general control functions related to specific frontal brain regions that interact with non-frontal domain-specific functions over time in response to contextual demands.

Although lesion research has identified separable frontal nodes, these are parts of complex networks. Alterations of task demands have demonstrated the roles that the frontal control component plays and when. Depending on the task demand or context, one or more of the anatomically distinct frontal regions may be recruited. Complex tasks may require the use of multiple regions and networks, making dissociations difficult, and simple tasks may be better suited to studying the functions of specific networks. Networks may work top-down or bottom-up, again depending on environmental context and task requirements, demonstrating the specific functions mediated by different regions of the frontal lobes [124]. This is evident in all functions, including language [125], where complex goal-directed communications, such as narratives, require not only basic language operations but also the functions of the frontal lobes, such as planning, sequencing, monitoring, and inhibiting responses.

5.2 Application to EF Changes with Aging

We suggest that this scheme for understanding frontal lobe functions [118] also provides a framework for the interpretation of current findings and for the development of future studies of aging-related changes in executive functions. Several of the ideas presented in the previous section have been expressed in studies of aging, although not specifically within the frontal framework. From a general methodological view, several of the functional imaging studies reported above used differences in context to start dissociating processes. There has also been a growing consensus in many aging studies that a task does not represent a process (e.g., [8, 59]). Instead of using more generic terms such as task switching or inhibition, using the framework discussed above might help to decipher which fundamental processing defects account for deficient performance on a given task. We used this approach in a direct comparison of older adults with younger adults with focal lesions [126]. Performance on specific measures of control processes involving memory was comparable between older individuals with intact brains and younger adults with focal lesions.

For a fuller understanding of executive functions, the specific roles of different neuroanatomical and functional networks should be considered. For example, in cortico-cortical networks, the lateral frontal regions are more related to strategic control aspects (with possible functional specificity as outlined above), and postcentral regions reflect the domain-specific content of information being held and actively processed. These considerations can also be viewed in cognitive terms of control versus automatic and recollection versus familiarity. This concept also appears compatible with the proposals of Macpherson and colleagues [25] regarding a dorsolateral theory of normal aging. These investigators subdivided the frontal lobes into the dorsolateral and ventromedial regions and assessed aging effects on performance of three tasks of executive function and working memory particularly dependent on dorsolateral prefrontal function and three tasks of emotion and social decision-making particularly dependent on ventromedial prefrontal function. They found aging-related differences in performance on all the tasks that were dependent on dorsolateral prefrontal dysfunction. In contrast, aging-related differences were not found on the majority of the tasks dependent on ventromedial prefrontal dysfunction. The results support a specific dorsolateral prefrontal theory of cognitive changes with age, rather than a global decline in frontal-lobe function.

Perhaps the most interesting comparison comes in the consideration of changes in processing speed. With aging, there are likely some basic perceptuomotor changes stemming from slowing of neuronal processes [42]. Beyond this, however, the interaction of slowing and task demands suggests the effect of deficient activation/energization, since a hallmark of inefficient medial frontal functioning is slowing related to task demands. Eyler and colleagues [96], in a review of functional imaging studies of aging effects, noted that better cognitive performance is often related to more brain responsiveness in many association cortices. However, this association was not universal, and was seen mainly in the frontal cortex. This suggests that good performance is supported by greater activation of the frontal cortex, and this increased frontal activation might be in response to a decline in non-frontal regions [127].

In the 1980s Craik and colleagues introduced the concept that an aging-related deficit in self-initiated processing might be a contributor to declining cognitive efficiency. Deficits in self-initiation have been linked to lesions of the anterior cingulate gyrus and superior medial frontal cortex, regions of the brain that have been posited to be critical to energization. Thus, Craik's proposal suggests that aging-related deficits in cognitive efficiency, particularly observable as task demands increase, could be related to aging-related deterioration in dorsomedial frontal and anterior cingulate function, an idea that finds support in several imaging studies (e.g., [95, 128]). As noted previously, the reduced ability of older adults to self-initiate control processes implies that they require more support from external context for many higher cognitive activities, but also that they will benefit disproportionately when such support is available [35, 37, 38]. This idea of impaired energization is also adaptable to the concept of reserve in that, if either cognitive or brain reserve is depleted, more effort (activation, energization) would be required.

6 Summary

This review suggests that the study of "EF" changes with aging would be better served by understanding the specific processes, defined above, that are related to domain-general (i.e., frontally mediated) control functions, differentiating these from changes in domain-specific functions (e.g., familiarity in memory, i.e., posteriorly mediated). In addition, it appears important to examine the role of context and task demands in relation to the need for increased effort (energization), and to relate these more detailed approaches to either structural or functional imaging changes.

References

1. Lezak MD. *Neuropsychological assessment*, 3rd ed. New York: Oxford University Press; 1995.

2. Park DC, Reuter-Lorenz P. The adaptive brain: Aging and neurocognitive scaffolding. *Annu Rev Psychol* 2009;60: 173–96.

3. Zacks RT, Hasher, L, Li, KZH. Human memory. In: Craik FIM, Salthouse TA, editors. *The handbook of aging and cognition*. Mahwah, NJ: Lawrence Erlbaum; 2000, pp. 293–357.

4. Craik FIM, Bialystok E. Cognition through the lifespan: Mechanisms of change. *Trends Cogn Sci* 2006;10: 131–8.

5. Verhaeghen P, Cerella J. Aging, executive control, and attention, a review of meta-analyses. *Neurosci Biobehav Rev* 2002;26: 849–57.

6. Reimers S, Maylor EA. Task switching across the life span: Effects of age on general and specific switch costs. *Dev Psychol* 2005;41: 661–71.

7. Miyake A, Friedman NP, Emerson MJ, Witzki AH, Howerter A, Wager TD. The unity and diversity of executive functions and their contributions to complex "frontal lobe" tasks: A latent variable analysis. *Cogn Psychol* 2000;41: 49–100.

8. Jacoby LL. A process dissociation framework: Separating automatic from intentional uses of

memory. *J Mem Lang* 1991;30: 513–41.

9. Zelazo PD, Craik FIM, Booth L. Executive function across the life span. *Acta Psychol* 2004;115: 167–83.

10. Cepeda NJ, Kramer AF, Gonzalez De Sather JC. Changes in executive control across the life span: Examination of task-switching performance. *Dev Psychol* 2001;37: 715–30.

11. Hasher L, Zacks RT, May CP. Inhibitory control, circadian arousal, and age. In: Gopher D, Koriat A, editors. *Attention and performance*, vol. 17. Cambridge, MA: MIT Press; 1999, pp. 653–75.

12. Hasher L, Zacks RT. Working memory, comprehension, and aging: A review and a new view. In: Bower GH, editor. *The psychology of learning and motivation*, vol. 22. San Diego, CA: Academic Press; 1988, pp. 193–225.

13. Lhermitte F. Human autonomy and the frontal lobes. 2. Patient behavior in complex and social situations – The environmental dependency syndrome. *Ann Neurol* 1986;19: 335–43.

14. West R, Alain C. Age-related decline in inhibitory control contributes to the increased Stroop effect observed in older adults. *Psychophysiol* 2000;37: 179–89.

15. Verhaeghen P, De Meersman L. Aging and the Stroop effect: A meta-analysis. *Psychol Aging* 1998;13: 120–6.

16. Braver TS, West R. Working memory, executive control, and aging. In: Craik FIM, Salthouse TA, editors. *The handbook of aging and cognition*, 3rd ed. New York: Psychology Press; 2008, pp. 311–72.

17. De Beni R, Palladino P. Decline in working memory updating through ageing: Intrusion error analyses. *Memory* 2004;12: 75–89.

18. Salthouse TA, Atkinson TM, Berish DE. Executive functioning as a potential mediator of age-related cognitive decline in normal adults. *J Exp Psychol General* 2003;132: 566–94.

19. Baddeley AD, Hitch G. Working memory. In: Bower GH, editor. *The psychology of learning and motivation*, vol. 8. New York: Academic Press; 1974, pp. 47–89.

20. Salthouse TA. Individual differences in working memory and aging. In: Logie RH, Morris RG, editors. *Working memory and ageing*. New York: Psychology Press; 2015, pp. 1–20.

21. Craik FIM, Bialystok E, Gillingham S, Stuss DT. Alpha Span: A measure of working memory. *Can J Exp Psychol* 2018 Sep;72(3): 141–52.

22. Mayr U, Kliegl R. Sequential and coordinative complexity: Age-based processing limitations in figural transformations. *J Exp Psychol Learn Mem Cogn* 1993;19:1297–320.

23. Craik FIM. Age differences in human memory. In: Birren JE, Schaie KW, editors. *Handbook of the psychology of aging*. New York: Van Nostrand Reinhold; 1977, pp. 384–420.

24. Braver TS, Cohen JD. Working memory, cognitive control, and the prefrontal cortex: Computational and empirical studies. *Cog Processing* 2001;2: 25–55.

25. Macpherson SE, Phillips LH, Della Sala S. Age, executive function and social decision making: A dorsolateral prefrontal theory of cognitive aging. *Psychol Aging* 2002;17: 598–609.

26. D'Esposito M, Postle BR. The cognitive neuroscience of working memory. *Ann Rev Psychol* 2015;66:115–42.

27. Jennings JM, Jacoby LL. Automatic versus intentional uses of memory: Aging, attention, and

control. *Psychol Aging* 1993;8: 283–93.

28. Hay JF, Jacoby LL. Separating habit and recollection in young and older adults: Effects of elaborative processing and distinctiveness. *Psychol Aging* 1999;14: 122–34.

29. Braver TS, Barch DM. A theory of cognitive control, aging cognition, and neuromodulation. *Neurosci Biobehav Rev* 2002;26: 809–17.

30. Braver TS, Barch DM, Keys BA, Carter CS, Cohen JD, Kaye JA, et al. Context processing in older adults: Evidence for a theory relating cognitive control to neurobiology in healthy aging. *J Exp Psychol Gen* 2001;130: 746–63.

31. Koen JD, Yonelinas AP. Recollection, not familiarity, decreases in healthy aging: Converging evidence from four estimation methods. *Memory* 2016;24: 75–88.

32. Koen JD, Yonelinas AP. The effects of healthy aging, amnestic MCI and Alzheimer's disease on recollection and familiarity: A meta-analytic review. *Neuropsychol Rev* 2014;24: 332–54.

33. Salthouse TA. The processing-speed theory of adult age differences in cognition. *Psychol Rev* 1996;103: 403–28.

34. Salthouse TA. Influence of processing speed on adult age differences in working memory. *Acta Psychol* 1992;79: 155–70.

35. Craik FIM, Byrd M. Aging and cognitive deficits: The role of attentional resources. In: Craik FIM, Trehub SE, editors. *Aging and cognitive processes*. New York: Plenum Press; 1982, pp. 191–211.

36. Anderson ND, Craik FIM, Naveh-Benjamin M. The attentional demands of encoding and retrieval in younger and older adults: I. Evidence from divided

attention costs. *Psychol Aging* 1998;13: 405–23.

37. Craik FIM. On the transfer of information from temporary to permanent memory. *Philos Trans R Soc Lond B* 1983;302: 341–59.

38. Craik FIM. A functional account of age differences in memory. In: Klix F, Hagendorf H, editors. *Human memory and cognitive capabilities.* Amsterdam: North-Holland; 1986, pp. 409–22.

39. Verhaeghen P, Salthouse TA. Meta-analyses of age–cognition relations in adulthood: Estimates of linear and non-linear age effects and structural models. *Psychol Bull* 1997;122: 231–49.

40. Waugh NC, Vyas S. Expectancy and choice reaction time in early and late adulthood. *Exp Aging Res* 1980;6: 563–7.

41. Der G, Deary IJ. Age and sex differences in reaction time in adulthood: Results from the United Kingdom Health and Lifestyle Survey. *Psychol Aging* 2006;21: 62–73.

42. Godefroy O, Roussel M, Despretz P, Quaglino V, Boucart M. Age-related slowing: Perceptuomotor, decision, or attention decline? *Exp Aging Res* 2010;36: 169–89.

43. Bielak AA, Cherbuin N, Bunce D, Anstey KJ. Intraindividual variability is a fundamental phenomenon of aging: Evidence from an 8-year longitudinal study across young, middle, and older adulthood. *Dev Psychol* 2014;50: 143–51.

44. Hultsch DF, MacDonald SWS, Dixon RA. Variability in reaction time performance of younger and older adults. *J Gerontol Psychol Sci* 2002;57B: P101–P115.

45. Shammi P, Bosman E, Stuss DT. Aging and variability in performance. *Aging Neuropsychol Cogn* 1998;5: 1–13.

46. West R, Murphy KJ, Armilio ML, Craik FIM, Stuss DT. Lapses of intention and performance variability reveal age related increases in fluctuations of executive control. *Brain Cogn* 2002;49: 402–19.

47. Dykiert D, Der G, Starr JM, Deary IJ. Age differences in intra-individual variability in simple and choice reaction time: Systematic review and meta-analysis. *PLoS ONE* 2012;7(10): e45759.

48. Stuss DT, Pogue J, Buckle L, Bondar J. Characterization of stability of performance in patients with traumatic brain injury: Variability and consistency on reaction time tests. *Neuropsychol* 1994;8: 316–24.

49. Stuss DT, Murphy KJ, Binns MA, Alexander MP. Staying on the job: The frontal lobes control individual performance variability. *Brain* 2003;126: 2363–80.

50. Murphy KJ, West R, Armilio ML, Craik FIM, Stuss DT. Word list learning performance in younger and older adults: Intra-individual performance variability and false memory. *Aging Neuropsychol Cogn* 2007;14: 70–94.

51. Iskandar S, Murphy J, Baird AD, West R, Armilio J, Craik FIM, et al. Interacting effects of age and time of day on verbal fluency performance and intraindividual variability. *Aging Neuropsychol Cogn* 2016;23: 1–17.

52. Garrett DD, MacDonald SWS, Craik FIM. Intraindividual reaction time variability is malleable: Feedback- and education-related reductions in variability with age. *Front Hum Neurosci* 2012;6: article 101, 1–10.

53. Axelrod BN, Henry RR. Age-related performance on the Wisconsin card sorting, similarities, and controlled oral word association tests. *Clin Neuropsychol* 1992;6: 16–26.

54. Rhodes MG. Age-related differences in performance on the Wisconsin Card Sorting Test: A meta-analytic review. *Psychol Aging* 2004;19: 482–94.

55. Fristoe, NM, Salthouse TA, Woodard JL. Examination of age-related deficits on the Wisconsin Card Sorting Test. *Neuropsychol* 1997;11: 428–36.

56. Hartman M, Bolton E, Fehnel, SE. Accounting for age differences on the Wisconsin Card Sorting Test: Decreased working memory, not inflexibility. *Psychol Aging* 2001;16: 385–99.

57. Ridderinkhof KR, Span MM, van der Molen MW. Perseverative behavior and adaptive control in older adults: Performance monitoring, rule induction, and set shifting. *Brain Cogn* 2002;49: 382–401.

58. Gamboz N, Borella E, Brandimonte MA. The role of switching, inhibition and working memory in older adults' performance in the Wisconsin Card Sorting Test. *Aging Neuropsychol Cogn* 2009;16: 260–84.

59. Ashendorf L, McCaffrey RJ. Exploring age-related decline on the Wisconsin Card Sorting Test. *Clin Neuropsychol* 2008;22: 262–72.

60. Belleville S, Rouleau N, Van der Linden M. Use of the Hayling task to measure inhibition of prepotent responses in normal aging and Alzheimer's disease. *Brain Cogn* 2006;62: 113–19.

61. Houx PJ, Holles J, Vreeling FW. Stroop interference: Aging effects assessed with the Stroop Color-Word test. *Exp Aging Res* 1993;19: 209–24.

62. Uttl B, Graf P. Color-Word Stroop test performance across the adult life span. *J Clin Exp Neuropsychol* 1997;19: 405–20.

63. Van der Elst W, Van Boxten MPJ, Van Breukelen GJP, Jolles J. The Stroop Color-Word Test. Influence of age, sex, and education; and normative data for

a large sample across the adult age range. *Assessment* 2006;13: 62–79.

64. Ludwig C, Borella E, Tettamanti M, de Ribaupierre A. Adult age differences in the Color Stroop Test: A comparison between an item-by-item and a blocked version. *Arch Gerontol Geriatr* 2010;51: 135–42.

65. Bélanger S, Belleville S, Gauthier S. Inhibition impairments in Alzheimer's disease, mild cognitive impairment and health aging: Effect of congruency proportion in a Stroop task. *Neuropsychologia* 2010;48: 581–90.

66. Lindsey BA, Coppinger NW. Age-related deficits in sample capabilities and their consequences for Trail Making performance. *J Clin Psychol* 1969;25: 156–9.

67. Salthouse TA, Fristoe NM. A process analysis of adult age effects on a computer-administered trail making test. *Neuropsychology* 1995;9: 518–28.

68. Wecker NS, Kramer JH, Wisniewski A, Delis DC, Kaplan E. Age effects on executive ability. *Neuropsychology* 2000;14: 409–14.

69. Bugg JM, DeLosh EL, Davalos DB, Davis HP. Age differences in Stroop interference: Contributions of general slowing and task-specific deficits. *Aging Neuropsychol Cogn* 2007;14: 155–67.

70. Lin H, Chan RCK, Zheng L, Yang JT, Wang Y. Executive functioning in healthy elderly Chinese people. *Arch Clin Neuropsychol* 2007;22: 501–11.

71. Raz N, Gunning FM, Head D, Dupuis JH, McQuain J, Briggs SD, et al. Selective aging of the human cerebral cortex observed *in vivo*: Differential vulnerability of the prefrontal gray matter. *Cereb Cortex* 1997;7: 268–82.

72. Salat DH, Buckner RL, Snyder AZ, Greve DN, Desikan RSR, Busa E,

et al. Thinning of the cerebral cortex in aging. *Cereb Cortex* 2004;14: 721–30.

73. Haier RJ, Jung RE, Yeo RA, Head K, Alkire MT. Structural brain variation, age, and response time. *Cogn Affect Behav Neurosci* 2005;5: 246–51.

74. Head D, Kennedy, KM, Rodrigue KM, Raz N. Age differences in perseveration: Cognitive and neuroanatomical mediators of performance on the Wisconsin Card Sorting Test. *Neuropsychologia* 2009;47: 1200–3.

75. Bettcher BM, Mungas D, Patel N, Elofson J, Dutt S, Wynn M, et al. Neuroanatomical substrates of executive functions: Beyond prefrontal structures. *Neuropsychologia* 2016;85: 100–9.

76. Lockhart SN, DeCarli C. Structural imaging measures of brain aging. *Neuropsychol Rev* 2014;24: 271–89.

77. Yuan P, Raz N. Prefrontal cortex and executive functions in healthy adults: A meta-analysis of structural neuroimaging studies. *Neurosci Biobehav Rev* 2014;42: 180–92.

78. Makris N, Papadimitriou GM, van der Kouwe A, Kennedy DN, Hodge SM, Dale AM, et al. Frontal connections and cognitive changes in normal aging rhesus monkeys: A DTI study. *Neurobiol Aging* 2007;28: 1556–67.

79. Brickman AM, Schupf N, Manly JJ, Stern Y, Luchsinger JA, Provenzano FA, et al. APOE epsilon4 and risk for Alzheimer's disease: Do regionally distributed white matter hyperintensities play a role? *Alzheimers Dement* 2014;10: 619–29.

80. Daselaar SM, Iyengar V, Davis SW, Eklund K, Hayes SM, Cabeza RE. Less wiring, more firing: Low-performing older adults compensate for impaired white matter with greater neural

activity. *Cereb Cortex* 2015;25: 983–90.

81. Hirsiger S, Koppelmans V, Merillat S, Erdin C, Narkhede A, Brickman AM, et al. Executive functions in healthy older adults are differentially related to macro- and microstructural white matter characteristics of the cerebral lobes. *Front Aging Neurosci* 2017 Nov 30;9:373. doi: 10.3389/fnagi.2017.00373. eCollection 2017.

82. Yang Y, Bender AR, Raz N. Age related differences in reaction time components and diffusion properties of normal-appearing white matter in healthy adults. *Neuropsychologia* 2015;66: 246–58.

83. Bunce D, Anstey KJ, Cherbuin N, Burns R, Christensen H, Wen W, et al. Cognitive deficits are associated with frontal and temporal lobe white matter lesions in middle-aged adults living in the community. *PLoS ONE* 2010;5 (10). http://dx.doi.org/10.1371/journal.pone.0013567.

84. Haynes BI, Bunce D, Kochan NA, Wen W, Brodaty H, Sachdev PS. Associations between reaction time measures and white matter hyperintensities in very old age. *Neuropsychologia* 2017;96: 249–55.

85. Jackson JD, Balota DA, Duchek JM, Head D., White matter integrity and reaction time intraindividual variability in healthy aging and early-stage Alzheimer disease. *Neuropsychologia* 2012;50: 357–66.

86. Lovden M, Schmiedek F, Kennedy KM, Rodrigue KM, Lindenberger U, Raz N. Does variability in cognitive performance correlate with frontal brain volume? *Neuroimage* 2013;64: 209–15.

87. Deary IJ, Bastin ME, Pattie A, Clayden JD, Whalley LJ, Starr JM, et al. White matter integrity and

cognition in childhood and old age. *Neurology* 2006;66: 505–12.

88. Kennedy KM, Raz N. Aging white matter and cognition: Differential effects of regional variations in diffusion properties on memory, executive functions, and speed. *Neuropsychologia* 2009;47: 916–27.

89. Dennis NA, Cabeza, R. Neuroimaging of healthy cognitive aging. In: Craik FIM, Salthouse TA, editors. *Handbook of aging and cognition*, 3rd ed. Mahwah, NJ: Erlbaum; 2008, pp. 1–54.

90. Maillet D, Rajah MN. Association between prefrontal activity and volume change in prefrontal and medial temporal lobes in aging and dementia: A review. *Ageing Res Rev* 2013;12: 479–89.

91. Spreng RN, Wojtowicz M, Grady CL. Reliable differences in brain activity between young and old adults: A quantitative meta-analysis across multiple cognitive domains. *Neurosci Biobehav Rev* 2010;34: 1178–94.

92. Langenecker SA, Nielson KA, Rao SM. fMRI of health older adults during Stroop interference. *NeuroImage* 2004;21: 192–200.

93. Coull JT, Frackowiak RSJ, Frith, CD. Monitoring for target objects: Activation of right frontal and parietal cortices with increasing time on task. *Neuropsychologia* 1998;36: 1325–34.

94. Goh JO, Beason-Held LL, An Y, Kraut MA, Resnick SM. Frontal function and executive processing in older adults: Process and region specific age-related longitudinal functional changes. *NeuroImage* 2013;69: 43–50.

95. Kalpouzos G, Persson J, Nyberg L. Local brain atrophy accounts for functional activity differences in normal aging. *Neurobiol Aging* 2012;33: 62.e1–623c13.

96. Eyler LT, Sherzai A, Kaup AR, Jeste DV. A review of functional brain imaging correlates of successful cognitive aging. *Biol Psychiatry* 2011;70: 115–22.

97. Turner GR, Spreng RN. Prefrontal engagement and reduced default network suppression co-occur and are dynamically coupled in older adults: The default-executive coupling hypothesis of aging. *J Cogn Neurosci* 2015;27: 2462–76.

98. Robertson IH. A right hemisphere role in cognitive reserve. *Neurobiol Aging* 2014;35: 1375–85.

99. Vallesi A, McIntosh AR, Stuss DT. Temporal preparation in aging: A functional MRI study. *Neuropsychologia* 2009;47: 2876–81.

100. Nebes RD, Madden DJ, Berg WD. The effect of age on hemispheric asymmetry in visual and auditory identification. *Exp Aging Res* 1983;9: 87–91.

101. Rajah MN, D'Esposito M. Region-specific changes in prefrontal function with age: A review of PET and fMRI studies on working and episodic memory. *Brain* 2005;128: 1964–83.

102. Shallice T, Stuss DT, Picton TW, Alexander MP, Gillingham S. Multiple effects of prefrontal lesions on task-switching. *Philos Trans R Soc Lond B Biol Sci.* 2008;1: 1–12.

103. Raz N, Gunning-Dixon F, Head D, Rodrigue KM, Williamson A, Acker JD. Aging, sexual dimorphism, and hemispheric asymmetry of the cerebral cortex: Replicability of regional differences in volume. *Neurobiol Aging* 2004;25: 377–96.

104. Stern Y. What is cognitive reserve? Theory and research application of the reserve concept. *J Int Neuropsychol Soc* 2002;8: 448–60.

105. Bialystok E, Craik FIM, Luk G. Bilingualism: Consequences for mind and brain. *Trends Cogn Sci* 2012;16: 240–50.

106. Raz N, Rodrigue, KM, Acker JD. Hypertension and the brain: Vulnerability of the prefrontal regions and executive functions. *Behav Neurosci* 2003;117: 1169–80.

107. Brickman AM, Schupf N, Manly JJ, Luchsinger JA, Andrews H, Tang MX, et al. Brain morphology in older African Americans, Caribbean Hispanics, and whites from northern Manhattan. *Arch Neurol* 2008;65: 1053–61.

108. DeCarli C, Massaro J, Harvey D, Hald J, Tullberg M, Au R, et al. Measures of brain morphology and infarction in the Framingham heart study: Establishing what is normal. *Neurobiol Aging* 2005;26: 491–510.

109. Vasan RS, Beiser A, Seshadri S, Larson MG, Kannel WB, D'Agostino RB, et al. Residual lifetime risk for developing hypertension in middle-aged women and men: The Framingham Heart Study. *JAMA* 2002;287: 1003–10.

110. Bucur B, Madden DJ. Effects of adult age and blood pressure on executive function and speed of processing. *Exp Aging Res* 2010;36: 153–68.

111. Nyberg L, Lövdén M, Riklund K, Lindenberger U, Bäckman L. Memory aging and brain maintenance. *Trends Cogn Sci* 2012;16: 292–305.

112. Stuss DT, Shallice T, Alexander MP, Picton TW. A multidisciplinary approach to anterior attentional functions. *Ann N Y Acad Sci* 1995;769: 191–212.

113. Stuss DT, Alexander MP. Is there a dysexecutive syndrome? *Philos Trans R Soc Lond B Biol Sci* 2007;362: 901–15.

114. Alexander MP, Stuss DT, Shallice T, Picton TW, Gillingham S. Impaired concentration due to frontal lobe damage from two distinct lesion sites. *Neurology* 2005;65: 572–9.

115. Picton TW, Stuss DT, Shallice T, Alexander MP, Gillingham S. Keeping time: Effects of focal frontal lesions. *Neuropsychologia* 2006;44: 1195–209.

116. Stuss DT, Binns MA, Murphy KJ, Alexander MP. Dissociations within the anterior attentional system: Effects of task complexity and irrelevant information on reaction time speed and accuracy. *Neuropsychology* 2002;16: 500–13.

117. Stuss DT, Alexander MP, Shallice T, Picton TW, Binns MA, MacDonald R, et al. Multiple frontal systems controlling response speed. *Neuropsychologia* 2005;43: 396–417.

118. Stuss DT. Functions of the frontal lobes: Relation to executive functions. *J Int Neuropsychol Soc* 2011;17: 1–7.

119. Alexander GE, Delong MR, Strick PI. Parallel organization of functionally segregated circuits linking basal ganglia and cortex. *Ann Rev Neurosci* 1986;9: 357–81.

120. Floden D, Vallesi A, Stuss DT. Task context and frontal lobe activation in the Stroop task. *J Cogn Neurosci* 2011;23: 867–79.

121. Stuss DT, Floden D, Alexander MP, Levine B, Katz D. Stroop performance in focal lesion patients: Dissociation of processes and frontal lobe lesion location. *Neuropsychologia* 2001;39: 771–86.

122. Alexander MP, Stuss DT, Picton T, Shallice T, Gillingham S. Regional frontal injuries cause distinct impairments in cognitive control. *Neurology* 2007;68: 1515–23.

123. Pandya DN, Barnes CL. Architecture and connections of the frontal lobe. In: Perecman E, editor. *The frontal lobes revisited.* New York: IRBN Press; 1987, pp. 41–72.

124. Stuss DT. Frontal lobes and attention: Processes and networks, fractionation and integration. *J Int Neuropsychol Soc* 2006;12: 261–71.

125. Alexander MP. Impairments of procedures for implementing complex language are due to disruption of frontal attention processes. *J Int Neuropsychol Soc* 2006;12: 236–47.

126. Stuss DT, Craik FIM, Sayer L, Franchi D, Alexander MP. Comparison of older people and patients with frontal lobe lesions: Evidence from word list learning. *Psychol Aging* 1996;11: 387–95.

127. Persson J, Nyberg L, Lind J, Larsson A, Nillson LG, Ingvar M, et al. Structure–function correlates of cognitive decline in aging. *Cereb Cortex* 2006;16: 907–15.

128. Buchsbaum BR, Greer S, Chang WL, Berman KF. Meta-analysis of neuroimaging studies of the Wisconsin card-sorting task and component processes. *Hum Brain Mapp* 2005;25: 35–45.

Chapter 13

Brain Aging and Creativity

Ira S. Fischler and Kenneth M. Heilman

1 Introduction

One of the greatest of human gifts is our creative ability. Not only does scientific and artistic creativity help to improve our quality of life, but creativity often provides great joys to the person performing creatively and those who read, view, and listen to creative works. As Dietrich and Kanso state, "to study creative ideas, and how and where they arise in the brain, is to approach a defining element of what makes us human" ([1], p. 822).

Like many other mental functions, creativity might change with aging. The goal of this chapter is to review the brain functions important in creativity, the nature of age-related changes in creative ability, and the possible brain mechanisms that may account for these changes. Finally, we will consider recent work on how creative potential might be maintained, or even enhanced, as we age.

1.1 Definition of Creativity

Many dictionaries primarily define "creativity" as the ability to make new and original things. While originality is certainly a critical element of creativity, others have suggested that these original items must also be "useful" or appropriate in context. Bronowski added what we regard as a critical element when he defined creativity as finding unity in what appears to be diversity [2]. This concept of finding unity in what appears to be diversity appears to apply for both works of art such as painting, music, and literature, as well as for science. For example, great novels may have tens of thousands of sentences and dozens of themes, and great musical works have a large variety of motifs, melodies, and rhythms; however, in all these creative works the creative person is able to develop a "thread that unites." Similarly, some of the greatest theories of modern physics, such as Einstein's theories of relativity and Copernicus's heliocentric model of the solar system,

although based on myriad mathematical expressions that are difficult for most people to understand, have a unity at their apex that can be expressed simply and elegantly. For this reason, we have defined creativity as the development and systematic expression of novel orderly relationships [3, 4].

1.2 Alterations of Creativity with Aging

Given the apparent decline with age in some of the core cognitive functions that we might argue are critical for creative thinking (such as speed of cognition, efficiency of long-term memory retrieval, working memory capacity, attentional control, and inhibition, to name a few), we might expect to see systematic declines in creative productivity and quality with aging. In his studies of notable creative achievement across a variety of fields, Simonton has provided evidence that there are indeed age-related changes in creative productivity, often peaking between the ages of 30 and 50 and subsequently declining [5, 6]. On the other hand, the same author reported that the quality of creative productions by influential psychologists (quantified as the percentage of publications receiving at least one citation) remained constant over their later years [6].

There are also many anecdotal examples of highly creative individuals in diverse fields who maintained the quality of their creative production well into their later years. Titian and Monet painted "masterpieces" well into their 80s and Doris Lessing only stopped writing at age 84 – complaining she had recently lost her creative edge [7].

It has also been widely argued that the "peak years" and rate of decline in creativity with aging may vary widely across disciplines [8]. Lehman wrote that whereas poets and mathematicians typically reach their creative peaks at a relatively early age, philosophers and novelists develop their peak of creativity at a later age [9]. Lehman also argued that scientists do their highest quality work before the age of 40. However, Cole found that age had only a minor impact on scientific performance [10].

With the increased interest in "positive psychology" in aging research, some have argued that at least for some creative domains, normal aging may result not in a decline but an enhancement of creative potential. There may be neurological, behavioral, and social reasons for these improvements. For example, a decline in frontal inhibitory control could "release" more posterior temporal and parietal areas from routine or conventional patterns of thought. Since the importance of both specific neurological structures and interactions, and core cognitive mechanisms, will certainly vary across different kinds of creative domains, we might expect to see wide variation in creative abilities that change with age.

2 Stages of Creativity

The "classic" model of creativity offered by Helmholtz (as cited, e.g., by Eysenck [11]) and later Wallas [12] proposed that there are four major stages in the creative process: *preparation, incubation, illumination,* and *verification. Preparation* involves acquiring the skills and knowledge that will allow that person to develop creative ideas, as well as the means to test these ideas and develop creative products. "Distal" preparation for one's career in a domain must be accompanied, of course, by more "proximal" preparation, whereby the knowledge and skills needed to generate a particular new creative product need to be acquired.

Incubation. Anecdotally, creative people often report being confronted with a problem that they could not resolve; this initial conscious attempt at problem-solving is followed by a period during which there appears to not be any conscious thought about this problem. Subsequently, the person seems to spontaneously become aware of a solution. There have been several studies in which "unconscious" thought about a problem appeared to help the person make a better decision or generate a creative solution to a problem [13]. However, it has been difficult to empirically distinguish a process of active but unconscious problem-solving from a more passive "release from interference" and shifts in mental set over time (but see [14]).

There have also been several studies suggesting that sleep also may benefit creativity, and this

enhancement might be considered as evidence for incubation. Drago and colleagues, for example, reported that there were positive correlations between Stage 1 of NREM sleep and some measures of creativity, such as the variety of alternative uses for objects generated. In addition, these investigators noted a relationship between Stage 4 of NREM sleep and performance on laboratory tests of creativity. They also found that there was a negative correlation between REM sleep and such tests [15].

When a person cannot at first resolve a problem but later suddenly becomes aware of the solution, it is often referred to as a moment of "illumination," also called an "aha" or a "Eureka" experience. But the realization that a solution is in hand may often result not from any subconscious incubation but from a series of conscious steps during periods of exceptional effort. In any case, since illumination is the end stage of the incubation process, instead of discussing incubation and illumination as independent stages, in this chapter we will combine these aspects of the creative process and call this stage "creative innovation."

Verification: Whereas scientists do have to perform experiments in order to test their hypothesis, other innovators, such as novelists and poets, composers, visual artists, and choreographers, do not have to verify theories but rather produce works of art, music, poems, books, and so on. Therefore, in this chapter we call this last and critical stage of creativity "verification-production." Although critical, the processes used for verification-production are necessarily specific to the type or domain of creativity, and, therefore, they will not be further discussed in this chapter.

3 Neuropsychology of Creative Innovation

3.1 Divergent Thinking

Since one of the major features of creativity is novelty, the creative person needs to develop ideas and hypotheses that are different from those that have previously been proposed or accepted. This process, which has been called *divergent thinking*, was first described as an important mechanism in creativity by William James [16]. In most empirical work done on creativity over the past century, in fact, "creative ability" has commonly been operationalized through some test of divergent thinking.

There are two major steps in divergent thinking: the first is *disengagement* from current beliefs, solutions, thoughts, ideas, and products. The second step is the *generation* of alternative beliefs, solutions thoughts, ideas, and products. These are different cognitive processes that might be mediated by different neurocognitive networks. We begin our review of the neuropsychology of creativity by considering the potential role of the frontal lobes in the ability to disengage from current modes of thinking.

3.1.1 Disengagement and the Frontal Lobes

Denny-Brown and Chambers noted that with frontal lesions, monkeys and humans had abnormal approach behaviors, such as the grasp reflex and magnetic apraxia. They posited that all animals, including humans, have two basic forms of behavior: they can approach or they can avoid [17]. With evolution, humans have developed an almost infinite number of different motor and cognitive behaviors, but many of these motor behaviors, like the grasp reflex, magnetic apraxia, and the rooting and sucking reflexes, are still basically approach behaviors, while others, such as spatial neglect, have elements of avoidance. Based on these clinical and experimental observations, Denny-Brown and Chambers proposed that whereas the frontal lobes are the part of the brain important in disengagement and avoidance, the posterior temporal and parietal lobes are important for mediating approach behaviors.

Clinically, failure to disengage manifests as perseveration. One test for perseveration is the "ramparts test," whereby the patient is asked to draw a series of figures across a page where each square is followed by a triangle and each triangle is followed by a square. Patients with perseveration will often draw two or more triangles or two or more squares. Luria demonstrated similar "motor perseveration," called echopraxia, using simple motor tasks such as the "two finger–one finger task" (in which the examiner tells the patient "when you see me put up one finger you are to put up two fingers" and vice versa). Patients with frontal lobe injury tend to imitate the behavior of the examiner and will put up the same number of fingers as the examiner [18].

Berg developed the Wisconsin Card Sorting Test to assess patients for cognitive perseveration [19]. In this test, participants are given a series of cards, each depicting one or more items of the same shape. The shapes come in four different colors and there can be a different number of shapes on any given card. The participant is asked to place each card below one of four different targets: one solid red circle, two solid green triangles, three solid blue squares, and four solid yellow crosses. No card will perfectly match any target, forcing the participant to decide whether to match for shape, color, or number. However, the participant is given no explicit instructions: the examiner merely indicates whether a placement was correct or incorrect. At apparently random intervals, the sorting principle changes (e.g., from shape to color). The participant's "working hypothesis" (e.g., shape) will soon result in a sorting error. Feedback about an error should result in a change in the sorting strategy. The normal participant performing this test will switch their strategy based on these responses of the examiner, but some patients do not. Milner found that patients with intractable epilepsy who had frontal lobe foci and who were treated with frontal lobectomies were particularly impaired on the Wisconsin Card Sorting Test. Many of these patients successfully developed the initial sorting strategy, but after the change in the sorting principle, when the examiner told them that their sort was wrong, these patients often did not alter their strategy [20]. These observations support the hypothesis that the frontal lobes are critical for the ability to disengage from a specific strategy and develop alternative solutions.

Functional imaging can provide converging evidence for the localization of function based on lesion studies. Studies of regional blood flow in normal participants who are performing the Wisconsin Card Sorting Test or performing divergent-thinking creativity tests, similar to those described by Guilford [21] and Torrance [22], have revealed that the prefrontal lobes were specifically more active during performance of these tests than during control tasks that did not require divergent thinking. In addition, the amount of increased activation of the frontal lobes when performing the Wisconsin Card Sorting Test correlated with the participant's performance [23].

3.1.2 Idea Generation and the Frontal Lobes

One of the most commonly used tests for divergent thinking that stresses the production of novel ideas is the Alternative Uses Test, first described by Guilford [21]. When performing this test, participants are given the name of an object, such as a brick, and are asked to describe alternative uses of this object. The more unusual the use, relative to normative responses, the greater the "originality" score. For example, if a participant provides responses such as, "You build houses, walls, and fireplaces," they would receive a low score. In contrast, if the participant provides responses such as "You can take this brick with you to the bath and when you get out you can use it to rub off the calluses on your feet," the participant would get a high score. When Carlsson and colleagues performed functional imaging on participants who were providing alternative uses of bricks, the participants who provided highly original responses had greater frontal lobe activation than those who were less creative [24].

3.1.3 Distributed Networks for Creativity

Although studies of patients with frontal lobe lesions and functional imaging studies provide evidence that the prefrontal lobes are important for disengagement and divergent thinking, the means by which the frontal lobes accomplish these functions are not fully known. The frontal lobes have strong connections (longitudinal fasciculi) with the polymodal and sensory association areas of the temporal and inferior parietal lobes [25]. These sensory association and polymodal areas appear to store sensory and semantic-conceptual information. Whereas the representational networks that store the most common uses of objects (such as bricks for building) are perhaps the easiest to activate, success in this task appears to be dependent on activating the semantic-conceptual and sensory association networks that have been previously only weakly activated or not activated at all. Activation of these remote networks might be important in developing the alternative solutions so important in divergent thinking.

Benedek and colleagues had participants generate alternative uses, then self-sort their responses into "old" (previously known or thought of) and "new" ideas [26]. Functional imaging during this generation task showed that, overall, the generation task was associated with increased activation in left prefrontal and right medial temporal lobes. "New" ideas, however, tended to be produced later than "old" ones in each test (confirming Marbe's law that less common associative responses are also produced more slowly – and indicating the time-course of disengagement?). But the new ideas were associated with stronger activity in the left inferior parietal cortex. The responses rated as more "creative" (in originality and appropriateness) were associated with greater activity in the

orbital inferior frontal gyrus – taken by the authors as a sign of attentional control in disengaging from the "dominant but uncreative" responses.

3.2 Cerebral Connectivity, Creativity, and Insight

Although disengagement and divergent thinking are critical initial elements of the creative process, it is associative and convergent thinking that allows the creative person to find "the thread that unites." Since Paul Broca demonstrated that it is lesions of the left hemisphere that produce impairments of language [27], there have been myriad studies showing that the right and left hemispheres store different forms of knowledge and mediate different forms of cognitive activity.

In many popular accounts, the right hemisphere has been described as "the creative hemisphere." There is certainly evidence for asymmetry of function between left and right hemispheres for a number of processes that might be important for creative cognition, including visuospatial skills, allocation and scope of attention, processing of melody, and non-verbal emotional communication. But many forms of creativity should require that the creative person use the skills and knowledge mediated by both hemispheres. In order to integrate these skills and knowledge, the creative person requires interhemispheric communication. Therefore, a critical part of creative innovation – the understanding, development, and expression of orderly relationships – requires communication between these modules.

3.2.1 Interhemispheric Communication

Interhemispheric communication is primarily mediated by the corpus callosum. Early support for the postulate that interhemispheric callosal communication is important for creativity came from a study by Lewis [28]. Alfred Binet, the French psychologist who developed the first intelligence test, had initially used the Rorschach ink-blot test as a means of assessing creativity. Lewis administered the Rorschach test to eight patients before and after they had undergone sectioning of the corpus callosum to help with their intractable epilepsy. Lewis reported that the corpus callosum disconnection "tended to destroy creativity" as measured by this test. Although intriguing, it may be that this finding resulted more from the inability of the "verbal" left hemisphere to fully describe what the right hemisphere saw in these visually based projective test images than from the inability to generate and integrate creative responses through interhemispheric connections. It would be worthwhile to replicate Lewis's work using a variety of tests of creativity that range in the degree of verbal versus visuospatial demands.

Since Lewis's work, there has been little direct study of hemispheric connectivity and its role in creativity. The most intuitive hypothesis would be that greater connectivity should lead to better integration and evaluation of creative ideas. Bogen and Bogen, however, have argued that decreased callosal connectivity enhances hemispheric specialization. This independence benefits the incubation of ideas that are critical for the divergent-thinking component of creativity [29] and it is the momentary inhibition of this hemispheric independence that accounts for the illumination that is part of the innovative stage of creativity. Moore and colleagues reported some evidence that provided support of this hypothesis [30], showing a significant negative correlation between corpus callosum volume and performance on a frequently used test of creativity, the Torrance Tests of Creative Thinking [22]. Subsequently, Takeuchi and colleagues performed diffusion tensor imaging to determine the relationship between white matter connectivity and creativity [31]. In contrast to Moore and colleagues, they found that there was a significant positive relationship between creativity, as measured by the divergent thinking test, and fractional anisotropy in the body of the corpus callosum and several other regions, including the prefrontal lobes, the bilateral temporoparietal junction, and the right inferior parietal lobule. These findings provide further support for the concept that connectivity is a critical element of creativity.

3.2.2 Intrahemispheric Communication

Even within each hemisphere, there are different areas of the cerebral cortex that have different neuronal architectures, store different forms of knowledge, and instantiate different forms of cognitive activity. In addition to the axons that form the corpus callosum and carry information between the cortex of the right and left hemispheres, there are axons that carry information between cortical regions within the same hemisphere. We posit that it is widespread intrahemispheric as well as interhemispheric connectivity that allows creative people to

"thread together" representations and ideas that are critical for convergent and associative thinking.

Connectivity and Connectionist Models: Connectionist and parallel-distributed processing (PDP) models propose that it is the strength and pattern of connections between neurons that allow our brains to store information. In these models, a large set of neuronal units that are connectively linked in a network defines and instantiates a domain of knowledge. Simulation studies have shown how a large number of concepts can be represented, accessed, and modified within a domain, and there has been some theoretical work exploring how connectionist models might make sense of creative abilities and processes (e.g., [32]).

There are two different ways that connectionist networks could be recruited for creative innovation, corresponding to so-called top-down and bottom-up processing. One of the most important medical innovations was the discovery of antibiotics. When Fleming left the windows open in his laboratory and mold flew into his lab and landed on bacterial cultures, he noticed that it killed the bacteria. This is an example of how environmental stimulation can lead to activation of selected neuronal units in a new context, and thereby lead to the generation of the patterns of activation that instantiate novel concepts. However, the human brain has the capacity for top-down intentional activation, mediated by frontal executive networks. The activation of selected units in a cognitive network may produce novel *patterns* of activation and lead to the development of novel concepts. For example, for Picasso, the mental image of the handlebars over a bicycle seat led to his famous "bicycle" sculpture of the *Bull's Head*.

Creative innovation might also involve the co-activation of neuronal networks that are substantially different in content and architecture. This would allow a person to escape the constraints of existing (learned) models in a particular knowledge domain. The activation and manipulation of concepts in a network of a completely different architecture would allow the investigator or artist to ask novel "what if" questions. We might expect such "remote" co-activation to be particularly dependent on long-axon white matter tracts across different cerebral regions.

Mednick suggested that highly creative people might have different patterns of connectivity than less creative people such that connectivity in their semantic-conceptual networks to the most common associations may be relatively weaker, and their connectivity with more "remote" networks may be stronger [33]. Therefore, highly creative people may readily activate more remote and highly distributed networks. Partial support for the postulate that creative innovation is related to the recruitment of more highly distributed networks comes from electroencephalographic (EEG) studies of normal subjects that found, during creative thought, an increase of anatomically distributed coherence of EEG oscillations [34–36].

Creative innovation might also be achieved by using networks representing knowledge in one domain to help organize a different domain that may share some attributes. This "structural concept mapping" is the basis of the sort of analogical reasoning that is important to several forms of creative thinking [37, 38]. For example, Albert Einstein often began his creative process with visual-spatial representations of ideas, and subsequently translated these concepts into mathematical terms. The architecture of the networks supporting these visual representations permitted him the manipulative freedom to escape from conventional formulations, and provided the basis for creative innovation.

4 Changes in Creativity with Aging

As we noted earlier, with aging there appears to be a decrease of creativity [5, 6, 8, 39]. However, throughout history there have been many older people who were exceptionally creative. For example, at the age of 85, Giuseppe Verdi wrote *Falstaff*, one of the greatest operas. Karl Gauss made notable contributions to theoretical mathematics throughout his older age, and revised his theory of algebra at 71. At the age of 78, Benjamin Franklin invented the bifocal lens. Frank Lloyd Wright completed the design of the Guggenheim Museum in New York when he was 92 years old. However, these examples appear to be exceptions. The reason for the general decline of creativity with aging is not fully known, and is likely multifactorial. In the following sections, we will explore some of the possible reasons for this decline.

4.1 Aging, Creativity, and Intelligence

For many years, the relationship between human creativity and human intelligence has generated a large body of theory, research, and controversy [40]. Some of the controversy comes from the diverse

means by which each concept has been operationalized and measured. Most agree that creativity and intelligence are neither wholly independent nor identical, and much of the controversy has related to the means by which, and the degree to which, they are related. Guilford and Christensen, for example, proposed that creativity was a subset of intelligence, and they attempted to develop psychometric tests that could measure creativity as part of a battery of tests to measure human intelligence [41].

Although there are many definitions of intelligence, most psychologists and educators consider intelligence, in broad terms at least, as a measure of a person's ability to acquire and apply knowledge. Whereas intelligence and creativity are distinct concepts, to be creative a person does need the ability to acquire, and to apply, the knowledge required in their domain of creativity [4]. Given the documented aging-related decline in certain forms of intelligence, we might ask to what extent any declines in creative abilities might be linked to changes in intelligence.

Guilford's Alternative Uses Test remains the most commonly used test to measure divergent thinking specifically and creative ability in general [21]. As noted earlier, this test measures participants' ability to develop novel uses of common objects, such as a brick, during a fixed time interval. Guilford found that students with low IQ consistently performed poorly on these tests, but among those participants with higher IQ scores, there was no correlation between IQ and performance on the Alternative Uses test.

Another approach to examine the relationship between creativity and intelligence has been to study highly creative people's intelligence. Consistent with Guilford's results, Barron and Harrington found only a weak relationship between notable architects' creativity and their IQ. Barron and Harrington concluded that whereas in those people with a lower IQ (i.e., IQ lower than approximately 120) the IQ does predict creativity, with higher IQs there is not a strong relationship between the IQ score and creativity [42]. These results suggest that intelligence may be a necessary but not a sufficient condition for creativity.

These results, however, may be limited by the "kind" of intelligence being measured. Catell proposed that there are two distinct forms of intelligence [43], "crystallized" and "fluid." Crystallized intelligence is primarily stored memories, such as knowing that Paris is in France or having a large vocabulary. In contrast, fluid intelligence is more related to problem-solving. For example, Raven's Progressive Matrices is a nonverbal test that measures associative and convergent reasoning. The participant is shown a series of cards, each of which has a series of figures, and the participant must select the figure that would make a series complete. Tests such as the Raven's are regarded as nonverbal tests of fluid intelligence. Whereas acquiring crystallized knowledge is important in the preparation stage of creativity, it is fluid intelligence that seems critical for creative innovation and convergent thought. Tests such as Raven's Progressive Matrices may thus be a more appropriate method to assess peoples' abilities "to find the thread that unites."

In support of this view, several recent studies that have examined the relationship between fluid intelligence and frontal-executive functions and creativity have found a strong relationship between some measures of creativity and fluid intelligence. Silvia, for example, using a composite latent-variable measure of fluid intelligence, found it to be strongly predictive of divergent thinking as measured by performance on Guilford's Alternative Uses Test [44].

Lee and Therriault also used latent-variable measures for fluid intelligence and found it was significantly predictive of both divergent thinking, as measured by several tests, including the Torrance Tests, and associative-convergent thinking, as measured by Mednick's Remote Associates Test [45]. Mednick's Remote Associates Test [33] provides participants with a series of three words and the participant has to find a fourth word that is associated with these three words. This test, unlike the Alternative Uses Test, is a measure of convergent thinking. The relationship between fluid intelligence and creativity was strongest when modeled through the mediating variable of "associative fluency," as measured by three different word-production tasks. In our lab, we have found that a composite intelligence variable, with both crystallized (vocabulary) and fluid (matrix reasoning) components, was predictive of self-reported creative behavior. This relationship was mediated wholly by performance on the associative reasoning Remote Associates test rather than a divergent thinking variable (as measured by the Alternative Uses Test) [46].

With aging, there is often a decrease in what is termed performance IQ on tests such as the Wechsler Adult Intelligence Scale (WAIS). Several of the tests on this portion of the IQ test require fluid intelligence. Even when the older participants are tested without time constraints, they do less well on the performance IQ of the WAIS than do younger subjects [47]. In contrast, with aging there is often an improvement in some of the tests for crystallized intelligence such as vocabulary. Together, these results suggest that with aging there is an increase in crystallized intelligence, but a decrease of fluid intelligence [48].

4.2 Creativity and the Aging Brain

Presumably, these declines in fluid intelligence and decreasing creative innovation are mediated by changes in the brain with age. As people get older there is a greater possibility that they may develop a disease of the brain, such as stroke or Alzheimer's disease, and these diseases can certainly adversely influence creativity. However, degenerative dementia is not always associated with a reduction of creativity. For example, with aging some people get a degenerative disorder called primary progressive aphasia, and in one form of this disorder, called semantic dementia, there have been reports of the emergence of visual and musical creativity. It is hypothesized that loss of left anterior frontotemporal function facilitates activity of the right posterior hemispheric structures, leading to de novo creativity observed in visual artistic representation [49].

Even in the absence of diseases such as stroke and Alzheimer's disease, there are of course many normal age-related biological changes of the brain (see Chapter 2). With aging the brain decreases in both size and weight. This reduction starts about the age of 50 and is progressive; however, anatomical studies of the aging brain in people who did not have a disease of the brain have revealed that the loss of neurons from the age of 20 to 90 years is minimal, only about 10% [50]. Although there is only a small percentage of neurons lost with aging, many of the neurons that are lost are located in brain areas that might be critical to creativity, including the frontal lobes as well as the inferior parietal lobes, along with portions of the temporal lobe neocortex.

4.3 Connectivity and the Aging Brain

Aging-related changes in connectivity may be more important to loss of creativity than loss of neurons. With aging, there is often a substantial decrease in dendritic branching or arborization, such that these neurons are less connected, or less efficiently connected, with other neurons. Finding the thread that unites often requires co-activation and communication between areas of the brain that are distant from one another. These intrahemispheric and interhemispheric connections are formed by axons that for the most part travel in the subcortical white matter. With aging, the loss of gray matter (primarily composed of neurons and their dendritic processes) is much less severe than the loss of white matter (primarily composed of myelinated axons), and most of the brain volume and brain weight that is lost with aging is primarily related to loss of white matter [51]. In addition, the total myelinated fiber length of axons decreases with aging [50]. Furthermore, the areas of the brain that show the greatest white matter loss with aging are those that myelinate the latest – the frontal lobes, which are still myelinating when people are in their early 20s. In addition, the corpus callosum is primarily composed of myelinated neurons that travel from one hemisphere to the other. With aging, there is also a thinning of the corpus callosum [52] as well as evidence of a decrease in interhemisphere communication mediated by the corpus callosum [53]. Thus, it is possible that the decrease in interhemispheric as well as intrahemispheric connectivity with aging might be directly related to the loss of creative potential.

The claim that creative potential may be closely related to connectivity and communication efficiency among brain regions points to the importance of using the increasingly precise tools available for mapping that connectivity in the study of creativity, and the effects of aging on creativity. To date, there has been little such work. For example, we know of no studies using recently developed "coherence" measures in the EEG to explore changes in connectivity between specific brain regions and how they may be associated with changes in creativity with aging. Similarly, although several studies mentioned previously have shown that white matter integrity (as measured by diffusion tensor imaging) is correlated with creative performance, none of those studies had age as a factor.

In the past several years, in the face of the inconsistent results of studies attempting to "localize" creative innovation skill in general terms [1, 54], there has been a blossoming of research on the neuroscience of creativity from a more connectionist, distributed brain-systems perspective [55, 56]. Much of this work has focused on the interplay between two broadly conceived neural networks. The so-called default-mode network (DMN) is comprised of the medial orbital-frontal and posterior cingulate cortex and precuneus, medial prefrontal cortex, anterior cingulate, and midline and inferior parietal regions. It shows greater activity during rest and "internally driven" tasks. In contrast, the central executive network (CEN) – comprising the dorsolateral prefrontal cortex, anterior cingulate gyrus, and anterior lateral inferior parietal cortex – shows greater activity with externally driven tasks requiring attention and high information-processing demands [57]. Summarizing this growing body of research, Beaty and colleagues [56] suggest that tasks involving generation of innovative ideas or thoughts may be dominated by DMN activity, while tasks (or stages of tasks) involving the evaluation of those generated ideas may show greater "coupling" and co-activation of the two networks.

We have studied a small sample of older individuals ($n = 18$) for such an association, examining correlations between fractional anisotropy (FA) measures of white matter integrity in selected neural fiber tracts and these participants' performance on a battery of common creativity tests [58]. To date, none of these anatomic-functional correlations has reached significance; however, the correlations between the frontoparietal tract measures and creativity have approached significance. This is likely due to the very small sample size, and we hope to replicate the study with a much larger sample and with a variety of measures of connectivity, including volumetric measures of white matter as well as dynamic measures of interregional communication as afforded by the EEG. A recent study by Takeuchi and colleagues found that an advanced version of voxel-based morphometry (VBM) revealed a significant correlation between white matter volume and performance in a divergent-thinking test, at least among female subjects, but FA scores of the same regions did not show this relationship [59].

4.4 The Aging Frontal Lobes

As mentioned, creative innovation requires disengagement from previously used ideas, concepts, strategies, and products with the development of new ones. Ridderinkhof and colleagues tested a population of healthy participants with the Wisconsin Card Sorting Test. These investigators found that the older participants were more likely to get stuck in set than were the younger subjects [60]. In our own study comparing younger and older individuals on an extensive battery of both performance and self-report measures of "creative cognition," we found that the biggest decline in performance with age was on the Wisconsin Card Sorting Test, with older participants showing almost four times the number of perseverative errors observed with younger participants [58]. These results suggested that the older subjects' reduced performance on this test was not related to an inability to initially identify the rule for sorting, but, rather, their reduced ability to disengage from a previously successful strategy.

Loss of neurons in the frontal lobes and loss of connectivity between the frontal lobes and subcortical structures (e.g., medial dorsal thalamus, the basal ganglia, the basal forebrain, the ventral tegmental area, and the hypothalamus) and posterior neocortical association cortices in the temporal, parietal, and occipital lobes impairs frontal-executive functions. To learn the lobes of the brain that undergo the greatest functional deterioration, Mittenberg and colleagues studied older and younger participants using neuropsychological tests designed to assess the functions of the frontal, parietal, and temporal lobes, and found that it was primarily a decrease of frontal lobe function that was associated with aging [61]. The finding that frontal-executive functions decrease with aging more than functions mediated by other parts of the brain is consistent with frontal lobe function being highly dependent on white matter connectivity and the loss in white matter connectivity with aging.

Whereas a loss of white matter connectivity and neurons within the frontal and prefrontal regions with aging may account for older people's propensity to get "stuck in set" or have "cognitive rigidity," another possibility for the decrement associated with aging may be related to changes in neurotransmitters, especially dopamine. Using functional imaging (PET), Volkow and colleagues reported that with aging a decrease of dopamine is associated with a decrease of frontal lobe activation [62]. The cells that produce dopamine are found in the midbrain and project to both the basal ganglia and frontal cortex. The mesocortical pathway transmits dopamine from the ventral tegmental area of the midbrain to the frontal cortex. Takeuchi and colleagues used voxel-based morphometry to identify the gray matter correlates of individual creativity as measured by a divergent thinking test. They reported positive correlations between regional gray matter volume in the ventral tegmental area and divergent thinking, suggesting to these authors that dopaminergic activation

of the frontal lobes was an important factor in divergent thinking [63]. It was not clear, however, if there was adequate correction for family-wise error rate, and the major source of activation in the midbrain was periaqueductal gray, so their results should be taken with caution.

This interpretation is clouded, however, by the fact that the Alternative Uses Test may depend on acquired knowledge and experience, as well as divergent thinking. We tested 30 older and 30 younger subjects using the Alternative Uses Test and unexpectedly found that the older subjects performed *better* than the younger subjects [64]. To help explain this finding, we posited that perhaps the older subjects had more experiences with these objects than did the younger subjects. We have since replicated this finding [58], showing that older participants generated more distinct uses (9.4) than did younger participants (7.6), and provided far more elaborations to their responses (4.9 vs. 1.8).

4.5 Risks and Rewards: The Aging Gambler

In 1610, Galileo made observations with his new telescope that supported the heliocentric theory of Nicolaus Copernicus. The Roman Inquisition tried Galileo and found that he promoted heresy. He was sentenced to indefinite imprisonment and kept under house arrest until he died. Clearly, creative achievement sometimes come at great risk. Finally, in 1992, Pope John Paul II wrote, "Thanks to his intuition as a brilliant physicist and by relying on different arguments, Galileo, who practically invented the experimental method, understood why only the sun could function as the centre of the world, as it was then known, that is to say, as a planetary system."

In a 2013 interview for Art Works Blog, filmmaker George Lucas said, "If you're creating things, you're doing things that have a high potential for failure, especially if you're doing things that haven't been done before." Since there is a high probability of failure, creative innovation is a risky behavior and failure often has a cost and can even be painful. Yet visual artists, composers, authors, scientists, and many people from other professions are strongly motivated to produce creative works. When successful, the production of creative work can provide the creator a great sense of reward.

In 1954 James Olds and Peter Milner inserted electrodes into the septal region of the brain of rats [65]. When these rats pressed a lever, they received electrical stimulation to the region of the septum and adjacent nucleus accumbens. This stimulation was so rewarding to these rats that they would repeatedly press this lever to receive this electrical stimulation, with some rats pressing the lever up to 2,000 times per hour. Subsequent research has revealed that the ventral tegmental area of the midbrain sends dopaminergic neurons to the nucleus accumbens. A person receives the joy-pleasure of reward when these neurons that innervate the nucleus accumbens release dopamine. The nucleus accumbens is part of network that includes the ventral striatum and is highly connected with the ventral medial frontal lobes, as well as the cingulate gyrus.

Several studies have found that older individuals are less likely to engage in risky behaviors than younger people. For example, Rutledge and colleagues studied a large population of older and younger participants in which the participants could choose between safe and risky options. These investigators found that the number of risky options chosen in trials with greater potential gains decreased gradually with aging [66]. Deakin and colleagues examined risk-taking in a large cohort of adults using a computer-based gambling test and also found risk-taking decreased with age. Aging was also associated with longer deliberation times [67]. Rutledge and colleagues proposed that it was an age-related decline in dopamine that may be responsible for the observed decrease in risk-taking. However, it is also possible that dopamine serves only to define the operational neurophysiological state of target neurons. In this view, the decline in risk-taking behavior is related to alterations in frontal function that may be independent of dopamine.

For the most part, motivational and "cognitive style" factors have received little attention in the study of creativity, though this may be changing [68]. The one personality factor that has been the focus of most work on creativity and cognitive style is what is called "openness to experience," which on face would seem closely linked to willingness to take risks. Sharp and colleagues recently reported that higher openness to experience was positively associated with performance on a range of cognitive tests among older individuals [69]. We would predict that declines in risk-taking with aging would be particularly associated with declines in performance on tasks requiring innovative thinking, but we know of no study that directly tested this hypothesis.

4.6 Right Hemisphere Deterioration with Aging

Another possible reason for any decrease in creativity with aging is that the right hemisphere mediates functions that appear to deteriorate more than those mediated by the left hemisphere [70]. When older and younger healthy participants took the WAIS, it was found that with aging there is greater deterioration of performance IQ than there is of verbal IQ. Whereas visual-spatial tasks such as block construction are part of the performance IQ, language tests such as vocabulary are part of the verbal IQ. Investigators have found that the right hemisphere appears to be dominant for mediating visual-spatial functions and the left hemisphere is dominant for mediating language functions. One interpretation of this observation is that this age-related decrease of visual-spatial abilities may be related to a decrement of right hemispheric function.

There are many other visual-spatial functions that have been shown to deteriorate with aging, even when using untimed tests [71]. For example, there is a test in which the participants are shown incomplete drawings of objects and the person taking the test is required to recognize and name the object. When performing this test, older subjects have more trouble recognizing these objects than do the younger participants [72]. Recognition of an object with incomplete information is a form of convergent thinking and "insight" often accompanied by a sudden "aha" moment, suggesting an important link to later stages of innovative thought, especially in the visual-spatial domain.

The right hemisphere also appears to be more important in mediating global than local attention and perception [73]. The Navon figure is a large figure made up of smaller figures, for example, many smaller letter Ts arranged to make a large letter A. When younger people view the Navon figure, they more often see the global configuration first (e.g., the letter A) and then the smaller letters (e.g., T). Older participants often report the small letter first. To see the "thread that unites" often requires global processing.

The reason that, with aging, there appears to be a decrement of right hemisphere functions is not fully known. Gur and colleagues studied the ratio of gray to white matter in the left versus right hemisphere. They found that there is relatively more white matter relative to gray matter in the right than left hemisphere

[74]. The white matter contains axons that connect different areas of the brain with other areas that are some distance from each other. Therefore, this asymmetry of white matter suggests that the left hemisphere primarily transfers information within or between contiguous regions and the right hemisphere transfers intrahemispheric information across regions that are greater distances apart. Since the functions performed by the right hemisphere may be more dependent on long myelinated axons and with aging there is a greater loss of white than gray matter, the right hemisphere should be more adversely affected by aging than the left hemisphere. Thus, the decrease of creativity with aging might be primarily related to a decrease of right hemisphere functions.

4.7 Aging Brain, Conceptual Relationships, and Depth of Processing

Objects can be related to each other by virtue of shared features and/or functional relationships (i.e., associative relationships), or they may be related because they are linked to an abstract concept. For example, when the participants are shown three objects such as a rifle, a bow, and an arrow and then are asked to group the two objects that are most closely related, there are two possible responses. A person could select a bow and arrow based on their functional relationship, or a bow and rifle because these two objects can be related by a more abstract concept (e.g., weapons that emit projectiles; hunting; war). Denney asked participants to group objects and found that elderly people are more likely than younger subjects to group these objects on the basis of functional relationships than by abstract conceptual relationships [75].

The means by which the brain develops these associative and abstract relationships is not known with certainty. Grouping by associative relationships can be done based on the "mere contiguity" of sensory (iconic) memories. For example, a person might be able to image a bow together with an arrow easier than they could image a bow together with a rifle, because a bow and arrow are more often seen together than a rifle with a bow. Grouping at a semantic-conceptual level is arguably more abstract (i.e., less dependent on sensory associations) than grouping on an associative level. In order to group at the semantic-conceptual level, a person must "draw away" (Latin *abstractus*) from the sensory-iconic level of

processing. Determining associative relationships could thus be performed within a "local" sensory modality, but determining conceptual relationships often depends on the activation of widely distributed networks. Also, there is evidence that abstract conceptualization is particularly supported by frontal lobe function. For example, it is relatively spared in patients with semantic dementia, which is, for much of its course, a temporal lobe disorder [76, 77].

Studies of the "priming" or speeding of simple decisions about words have shown that both abstract, semantic/conceptual relations (e.g., prince-boy) and functional associative relations (e.g., horse-doctor) can facilitate lexical (word-nonword) decisions [78]. Badham and colleagues found that older and younger subjects benefited equally from conceptual (what they termed "integrative") relations and functional associative relations in a lexical decision task, as well as in a simple paired-associate task [79]. In contrast, much research on "levels of processing" in more complex episodic memory tasks suggests that aging brings a decline in depth of processing. For example, Simon found the effectiveness of semantic contextual cues to be diminished in older subjects, while that of phonemic cues was unchanged [80]. Together, these results may indicate that although the networks representing conceptual and associative connections may remain largely intact, the ability to access and make use of the two kinds of knowledge may change differentially with aging.

4.8 Interventions to Conserve Creative Potential in Aging

4.8.1 Cosmetic Neuropharmacology?

It is possible that the age-related decline in creativity is, to some degree, sensitive to pharmaceutical interventions (see also Chapters 15 and 17). In the section on risk and rewards, we mentioned that creativity often requires the creative person to take risks. We also mentioned that the ventral tegmental area of the midbrain sends dopaminergic neurons to the nucleus accumbens and a person receives the pleasure of reward when these neurons release dopamine in the nucleus accumbens. Several studies have found that with aging there is a reduction in riskier behaviors, although the extent of change varies across domains [81]. Rutledge and colleagues suggested that this reduction might be related to the aging-related decline in dopamine [66]. If this hypothesis is correct, then pharmacologically enhancing dopaminergic function could reverse this decline.

Patients with Parkinson's disease have a great reduction of neurons that produce dopamine. When treated with dopamine agonists, patients with PD did increase their creativity [82]. There have been no treatment studies of the influence of dopamine agonists on older people without Parkinson's disease, but with healthy aging there is a reduction of dopamine, so it is possible that dopaminergic medications could increase older peoples' creativity.

Oxytocin is a neurohormone that often decreases with age [83]. De Dreu and colleagues reported in a placebo-controlled trial that the administration of intranasal oxytocin increased global processing as assessed by recognition of "global" versus "local" targets in Navon figures, and improved divergent thinking [84], as evaluated by performance on the Alternative Uses Test. In addition, oxytocin led to improvement in tests of convergent creative thinking.

4.8.2 Cognitive-Behavioral Interventions, Aging, and Creativity

There is increasing interest in both physical interventions and behavioral interventions that might sustain or enhance cognitive abilities as we age. One intriguing example was reported by Chapman and colleagues [85]. They compared the effects of physical training (PT) with those of a "cognitive-reasoning training" (CT) program conducted over 12 weeks in older (aged 56–75) subjects. The outcome measure was performance on a novel "innovative thinking" task and its association with regional cerebral blood flow and resting DMN and CEN functional connectivity. The cognitive training consisted of their SMART (Strategic Memory Advanced Reasoning Training) course [86], which focuses on metacognitive skills of "strategic attention" (filtering task-relevant from irrelevant information), "integrated reasoning" (abstracting key aspects or goals in a task), and "innovation" (updating ideas and perspectives, and looking for ways to improve everyday task performance).

Before, during, and after training, subjects were given a "multiple interpretations measures" (MIM) task, in which one of three short passages about an unknown historical person's life experiences is read, and subjects are asked to generate "as many high-level interpretations" as they can that may be inferred from the passage. The task is designed to be a more ecologically valid version of the Alternative Uses Test. MIM scores are the number of "high-quality" (essentially, more thematic and abstract) responses to a given passage, so both productivity and quality of responses are measured.

In contrast to either the PT group or a wait-list control group, the CT group showed sustained improvement in response generation scores from the pretest to later tests. Analyses of resting-state MRI data obtained after the end of training differentiated the CT group from the other groups in several ways. First, there was greater cerebral blood flow in medial orbital-frontal cortex and posterior cingulate cortex – purported components of the DMN – for SMART training versus the other conditions. This suggested to these authors that training produced a more "prepared" DMN for the generative aspects of the MIM task.

Within-group correlations between high-quality MIM scores and the functional connectivity measures were significant only for the CT group. The correlation was *negative* for the DMN network, but *positive* for the CEN network. These results seem consistent with the role of the CEN during the evaluative phase in producing "high-quality" responses. It would be interesting to differentiate the sheer number of responses from their quality; we would predict that the former would show a positive correlation with DMN connectivity.

These kinds of findings show the promise and potential of training interventions to maintain and enhance creative abilities through changes in the brain systems that mediate creative cognition. Our hope is that it is not so much "use it or lose it," but "use it and thrive."

5 Conclusions

Although creativity is one of the most important of human attributes, studies of creativity are still limited when compared with studies of memory and language. It has been repeatedly reported that with aging there is a decrease in creativity; however, the type of changes with aging and the underlying brain mechanisms that could account for this aging-related decrement have not been fully studied. Therefore, there is a great need for research that will allow us to further understand the brain mechanisms that allow humans to be creative, as well as how these functions can be developed and nurtured, and, with aging maintained or even enhanced. There also is a great need for clinicians to learn how the different functions critical for creativity may be tested. Finally, we need to learn more about the adverse influence of diseases and aging on creativity and how these too can be ameliorated.

References

1. Dietrich A, Kanso R. A review of EEG, ERP, and neuroimaging studies of creativity and insight. *Psychol Bull* 2010; **136**: 822–48.

2. Bronowski J. *Science and Human Values*. New York: Harper and Row, 1972.

3. Heilman KM, Nadeau SE, Beversdorf DO. Creative innovation: Possible brain mechanisms. *Neurocase* 2003; **9**: 369–79.

4. Heilman KM. *Creativity and the Brain*. New York: Psychology Press, 2005.

5. Simonton DK. Quality, quantity and age: The careers of 10 distinguished psychologists. *Int J Aging Hum Dev* 1985; **21**: 241–54.

6. Simonton DK. *Greatness: Who Makes History and Why?* New York: Guilford Press, 1994.

7. Cohen GD. *The Creative Age: Awakening Human Potential in the Second Half of Life*. New York: Avon, 2000.

8. Abra J. Changes in creativity with age: Data, explanations, and further predictions. *Int J Aging Hum Dev* 1989; **28**: 105–26.

9. Lehman HC. *Age and Achievement*. Princeton, NJ: Princeton University Press, 1953.

10. Cole S. Age and scientific performance. *Amer J Sociol* 1979; **84**: 958–77.

11. Eysenck HJ. *Genius: The Natural History of Creativity*. Cambridge: Cambridge University Press, 1995.

12. Wallas G. *The Art of Thought*. New York: Harcourt Brace, 1926.

13. Sio UN, Ormerod TC. Does incubation enhance problem solving? A meta-analytic review. *Psychol Bull* 2009; **135**: 94–120.

14. Ritter SM, Dijksterhuis A. Creativity – The unconscious foundations of the incubation period. *Front Hum Neurosci* 2014; **8**: Article ID 215.

15. Drago V, Foster PS, Heilman KM, et al. Cyclic alternating pattern in sleep and its relationship to creativity. *Sleep Med* 2011; **12**: 361–6.

16. James W. *The Principles of Psychology*. New York: Holt, 1890.

17. Denny-Brown D, Chambers RA. The parietal lobe and behavior. *Res Publ – Assoc Res Nerv Mental Dis* 1958; **36**: 35–117.

18. Luria AR. Frontal lobe syndrome. In: Vinkin PJ, Bruyn GW, eds. *Handbook of Clinical Neurology*, vol. 2. Amsterdam: North Holland, 1969, 725–57.

19. Berg EA. A simple objective technique for measuring flexibility in thinking. *J Gen Psychol* 1948; **39**: 15–22.

20. Milner B. Behavioural effects of frontal-lobe lesions in man. *Trends Neurosci* 1984; **7**: 403–7.

21. Guilford JP. Creativity: Yesterday, today and tomorrow. *J Creative Behav* 1967, **1**: 3–14.

22. Torrance EP. *Torrance Tests of Creative Thinking*. Bensenville, IL: Scholastic Testing Service, 1974.

23. Weinberger DR, Berman KF, Zec RF. Physiologic dysfunction of dorsolateral prefrontal cortex in schizophrenia: I. Regional cerebral blood flow evidence. *Arch Gen Psychiatr* 1986; **43**: 114–24.

24. Carlsson I, Wendt PE, Risberg J. On the neurobiology of creativity: Differences in frontal activity between high and low creative subjects. *Neuropsychologia* 2000; **38**: 873–85.

25. Pandya DN, Barnes CL. Architecture and connections of the frontal lobe. In: Perecman E, ed. *The Frontal Lobes Revisited*. New York: IRBN Press, 1987, 41–72.

26. Benedek M, Jauk E, Fink A., et al. To create or to recall? Neural mechanisms underlying the generation of creative new ideas. *Neuroimage* 2014; **88**: 125–33.

27. Broca P. Localisation des functions cerebrales siege du language articule. *Bull Société d'Anthropol* 1863; **4**: 200–8.

28. Lewis RT. Organic signs, creativity, and personality characteristics of patients following cerebral commissurotomy. *Clin Neuropsychol* 1979; **1**: 29–33.

29. Bogen JE, Bogen GM. Creativity and the corpus callosum. *Psychiatr Clin* 1988; **11**: 293–301.

30. Moore DW, Bhadelia RA, Billings RL, et al. Hemispheric connectivity and the visual–spatial divergent-thinking component of creativity. *Brain Cognit* 2009; **70**: 267–72.

31. Takeuchi H, Taki Y, Sassa Y, et al. White matter structures associated with creativity: Evidence from diffusion tensor imaging. *Neuroimage* 2010; **51**: 11–18.

32. Martindale C. Creativity and connectionism. In: Smith SE, Ward TB, Fink RA, eds. *The Creative Cognition Approach*. Cambridge, MA: MIT Press, 1995, 249–68.

33. Mednick SA. The associative basis of the creative process. *Psychol Rev* 1962; **69**: 220–32.

34. Petsche H. Approaches to verbal, visual and musical creativity by EEG coherence analysis. *Int J Psychophys* 1996; **24**: 145–59.

35. Jausovec N, Jausovec K. Differences in resting EEG related

to ability. *Brain Topogr* 2000; **12**: 229–40.

36. Kounios J, Fleck JI, Green DL, et al. The origins of insight in the resting brain. *Neuropsychologia* 2008; **46**: 281–91.

37. Gentner D, Bowdle B. Metaphor as structure-mapping. In: Gibbs RW Jr., ed. *The Cambridge Handbook of Metaphor and Thought*. New York: Cambridge University Press, 2008, 109–28.

38. Glucksberg S. How metaphors create categories – quickly. In Gibbs RW Jr., ed. *The Cambridge Handbook of Metaphor and Thought*. New York: Cambridge University Press, 2008, 67–83.

39. Lindauer MS. *Aging, Creativity and Art*. New York: Plenum, 2003.

40. Sternberg RJ, O'Hara LA. Creativity and intelligence. In: Sternberg RJ, ed. *The Cambridge Handbook of Creativity*. New York: Cambridge University Press, 1999, 251–72.

41. Guilford JP, Christensen PW. The one-way relationship between creative potential and IQ. *J Creative Behav* 1973; **7**: 247–52.

42. Barron F, Harrington DM. Creativity, intelligence and personality. *Annu Rev Psychol* 1981; **32**: 439–76.

43. Catell RB. The theory of fluid and crystallized intelligence: A critical experiment. *J Educ Psychol* 1963; **54**: 1–22.

44. Silvia PJ. Another look at creativity and intelligence: Exploring higher-order models and probable confounds. *Pers Indiv Differ* 2008; **44**: 1012–21.

45. Lee CS, Therriault DJ. The cognitive underpinnings of creative thought: A latent variable analysis exploring the roles of intelligence and working memory in three creative thinking processes. *Intelligence* 2013; **41**: 306–20.

46. Lee CS, Therriault DJ, Fischler IS, et al. The role of intelligence in

creative thinking processes and behavior. Paper presented at the meeting of the American Psychological Association, Orlando, FL, 2012 Aug 2–5.

47. Storandt M. Age, ability level, and method of administering and scoring the WAIS. *J Gerontol* 1977; **32**: 175–8.

48. Ryan JJ, Sattler JM, Lopez SJ. Age effects on Wechsler Adult Intelligence Scale-III subtests. *Arch Clin Neuropsychol* 2000; **15**: 311–17.

49. Miller ZA, Miller BL. Artistic creativity and dementia. *Prog Brain Res* 2013; **204**: 99–112.

50. Pakkenberg B, Pelvig D, Marner L, et al. Aging and the human neocortex. *Exp Gerontol* 2003; **38**: 95–9.

51. Tang Y, Whitman GT, Lopez I, Baloh RW. Brain volume changes on longitudinal magnetic resonance imaging in normal older people. *J Neuroimaging* 2001; **11**: 393–400.

52. Hopper KD, Patel S, Cann TS, et al. The relationship of age, gender, handedness, and sidedness to the size of the corpus callosum. *Acad Radiol* 1994; **1**: 243–8.

53. Reuter-Lorenz PA, Stanczak L. Differential effects of aging on the functions of the corpus callosum. *Dev Neuropsychol* 2000; **18**: 113–37.

54. Sawyer K. The cognitive neuroscience of creativity: A critical review. *Creativ Res J* 2011; **23**: 137–54.

55. Jung RE, Vartanian O, eds. *The Cambridge Handbook of the Neuroscience of Creativity*. New York: Cambridge University Press, 2018.

56. Beaty RE, Benedek M, Silvia PJ, Schacter DL. Creative cognition and brain network dynamics. *Trends Cognit Neurosci* 2016; **20**: 87–95.

57. Bressler SL, Menon, V. Large-scale brain networks in cognition:

Emerging methods and principles. *Trends Cognit Neurosci* 2010; **14**: 277–90.

58. Fischler IS, Heilman KM, Williamson J. Creative cognition in younger and older participants. Paper presented at the meeting of the Center for Neuropsychological Studies, University of Florida, Gainesville, 2015 May 15.

59. Takeuchi H, Taki Y, Nouchi R, et al. Creative females have larger white matter structures: Evidence from a large sample study. *Hum Brain Mapp* 2017; **38**: 414–30.

60. Ridderinkhof KR, Span MM, van der Molen MW. Perseverative behavior and adaptive control in older adults: Performance monitoring, rule induction, and set shifting. *Brain Cognit* 2002; **49**: 382–401.

61. Mittenberg W, Seidenberg M, O'Leary DS, DiGiulio DV. Changes in cerebral functioning associated with normal aging. *J Clin Exp Neuropsychol* 1989; **11**: 918–32.

62. Volkow ND, Logan J, Fowler JS, et al. Association between age-related decline in brain dopamine activity and impairment in frontal and cingulate metabolism. *Am J Psychiatry* 2000; **157**: 75–80.

63. Takeuchi H, Taki Y, Sassa Y, et al. Regional gray matter volume of dopamine rich system associate with creativity: Evidence from voxel-based morphology. *Neuroimage* 2010; **51**: 578–85.

64. Leon SA, Altmann L, Abrams, L, et al. Divergent task performance in older adults: Declarative memory or creative potential? *Creativ Res J* 2014; **26**: 21–9.

65. Olds J, Milner P. Positive reinforcement produced by electrical stimulation of septal area and other regions of rat brain. *J Comp Physiol Psychol* 1954; **47**: 419–27.

66. Rutledge RB, Smittenaar P, Zeidman P, et al. Risk taking for potential reward decreases across

the lifespan. *Curr Biol* 2016; **26**: 1634–9.

67. Deakin J, Aitken M, Robbins T, Sahakian BJ. Risk taking during decision-making in normal volunteers changes with age. *J Int Neuropsychol Soc* 2004; **10**: 590–8.

68. Sternberg RJ. A triangular theory of creativity. *Psychol Aesth Creativ Arts* 2018; **12**: 50–67.

69. Sharp, ES, Reynolds, CA, Pedersen NL, Gatz M. Cognitive engagement and cognitive aging: Is openness protective? *Psychol Aging* 2010; **25**: 60–73.

70. Dolcos F, Rice HJ, Cabeza R. Hemispheric asymmetry and aging: Right hemisphere decline or asymmetry reduction? *Neurosci Biobehav Rev* 2002; **26**: 819–25.

71. Koss E, Haxby JV, DeCarli C, et al. Patterns of performance preservation and loss in healthy aging. *Dev Neuropsychol* 1991; **7**: 99–113.

72. Read DE. Age-related changes in performance on a visual-closure task. *J Clin Exp Neuropsychol* 1988; **10**: 451–66.

73. Fink GR, Marshall JC, Halligan PW, et al. Hemispheric specialization for global and local processing: The effect of stimulus category. *Proc Biol Sci* 1997; **264**: 487–94.

74. Gur RC, Packer IK, Hungerbuhler JP, et al. Differences in the distribution of gray and white matter in human cerebral hemispheres. *Science* 1980; **207**: 1226–8.

75. Denney NW. Classification criteria in middle and old age. *Dev Psychol* 1974; **10**: 901–6.

76. Breedin S, Saffran EM, Coslett HB. Reversal of the concreteness effect in a patient with semantic dementia. *Cognitive Neuropsychology* 1994; **11**: 617–60.

77. Nadeau SE. *The Neural Architecture of Grammar.* Cambridge, MA: MIT Press, 2012.

78. Fischler I. Semantic facilitation without association in a lexical decision task. *Mem Cognit* 1977; **5**: 335–9.

79. Badham SP, Estes Z, Maylor EA. Integrative and semantic relations equally alleviate age-related associative memory. *Psychol Aging* 2012; **27**: 141–52.

80. Simon E. Depth and elaboration of processing in relation to age. *J Exp Psychol Hum Learn Mem* 1979; **5**: 115–24.

81. Bonem, EM, Ellsworth, PC, Gonzalez, R. Age differences in risk: Perceptions, intentions and domains. *J Behav Dec Making* 2015; **28**: 317–30.

82. Faust-Socher A, Kenett YN, Cohen OS, et al. Enhanced creative thinking under dopaminergic therapy in Parkinson disease. *Ann Neurol* 2014; **75**: 935–42.

83. Huffmeijer R, IJzendoorn MH, Bakermans-Kranenburg MJ. Aging and oxytocin: A call for extending human oxytocin research to aging populations – A mini-review. *Gerontology* 2013; **59**: 32–59.

84. De Dreu KW, Baas M, Roskes M, et al. Oxytonergic circuitry sustains and enables creative cognition in humans. *Soc Cogn Affect Neur* 2014; **9**: 1159–65.

85. Chapman SB, Spence JS, Aslan S, Keebler MW. Enhancing innovation and underlying neural mechanisms via cognitive training in healthy older adults. *Front Aging Neurosci* 2017; **9**: Article ID 314.

86. Chapman SB, Mudar RA. Enhancement of cognitive and neural functions through complex reasoning training: Evidence from clinical and normal populations. *Front Sys Neurosci* 2014; **8**: Article ID 69.

Attractor Network Dynamics, Transmitters, and Memory and Cognitive Changes in Aging

Edmund T. Rolls

1 Introduction

This chapter starts with a concise overview of attractor networks that are implemented in the cerebral cortex by excitatory connections between pyramidal cells, and that implement processes such as short-term memory, episodic memory, attention, and decision-making. Then, the means by which the decline of some neurotransmitters that occurs with aging influence the stability of these attractor networks are described, with this analysis having implications for treatment.

An *attractor* network is a group of neurons with excitatory interconnections that can settle into a stable pattern of firing [1–4] (see Chapter 8 for a simple conceptual introduction to attractor networks). This chapter explains how attractor networks in the cerebral cortex are important for long-term memory, short-term (working) memory, attention, and decision-making, with a fuller description as well as demonstration programs that run in Matlab or Octave provided [1]. The chapter then describes how the random firing of neurons can influence the stability of these networks by introducing stochastic noise, and how these effects are involved in probabilistic decision-making and are also implicated in some disorders of cortical function, such as poor short-term memory and attention that occur with during normal aging [5]. Each memory pattern stored in an attractor network through associative synaptic modification consists of a subset of the neurons firing. These patterns could correspond to short-term memories, long-term memories, perceptual representations, or thoughts.

2 Attractor Networks

2.1 Attractor Network Architecture, and the Storage of Memories

2.1.1 Architecture and Memory Storage

The architecture of an attractor or autoassociation network is shown in Figure 14.1. External inputs e_i

activate the neurons in the network, and produce firing y_i, where i refers to the ith neuron. The neurons are connected by recurrent collateral synapses w_{ij}, where j refers to the jth synapse on a neuron. By these synapses, an input pattern on e_i is associated with itself, and thus the network is referred to as an autoassociation network [6–8]. Because there is positive feedback via the recurrent collateral excitatory synaptic connections, the network can sustain persistent firing. These synaptic connections are assumed to build up by an associative (Hebbian) learning mechanism [9] (according to which, the more two neurons are simultaneously active, the stronger the neural connection becomes). The associative learning rule for the change in the synaptic weight is as shown in Eqn. (1):

$$\delta w_{ij} = k \cdot y_i \cdot y_j \tag{1}$$

where k is a constant, y_i is the activation of the dendrite (the postsynaptic term), y_j is the presynaptic firing rate, and δw_{ij} is the synaptic weight. The inhibitory interneurons are not shown. The inhibitory interneurons receive inputs from the pyramidal cells and make negative feedback connections onto the pyramidal cells to control their activity.

In order for biologically plausible autoassociative networks to store information efficiently, heterosynaptic long-term depression (LTD) (as well as long-term potentiation) is required [1, 8, 10]. This type of LTD helps to remove the correlations between the training patterns that arise when the neurons have positive-only firing rates. The effect of the LTD can be to enable the effect of the mean presynaptic firing rate to be subtracted from the training patterns [1, 8, 10].

2.1.2 Memory Recall

During recall, the external input e_i is applied and produces output firing, operating through the non-linear activation function described below. The firing is fed back by the recurrent collateral axons shown in

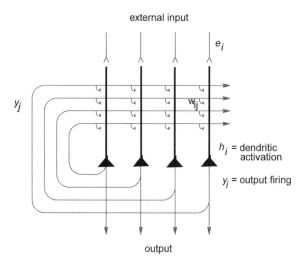

external input

e_i

y_j

w_{ij}

h_i = dendritic activation

y_i = output firing

output

Figure 14.1 The architecture of an autoassociative or attractor neural network (see text).

Figure 14.1 to produce activation of each output neuron through the modified synapses on each output neuron. The activation h_i produced by the recurrent collateral effect on the ith neuron is the sum of the activations produced in proportion to the firing rate of each axon y_j operating through each modified synapse w_{ij}, that is,

$$h_i = \Sigma_j y_j w_{ij} \tag{2}$$

where Σ_j indicates that the sum is over the C input axons to each neuron, indexed by j. This is a dot or inner product computation between the input firing vector y_j ($j = 1, C$) and the synaptic weight vector w_{ij} ($j = 1, C$) on neuron i. It is because this is a vector similarity operation, closely related to a correlation between the input vector and the synaptic weight vector, that many of the properties of attractor networks arise, including completion of a memory when only a partial retrieval cue is applied (often referred to as content addressable memory) [1]. The output firing y_i is a nonlinear function of the activation produced by the recurrent collateral effect (internal recall) and by the external input e_i:

$$y_i = f(h_i + e_i) \tag{3}$$

The activation function should be nonlinear, and may be, for example, binary threshold, linear threshold, sigmoid, and so on. The threshold at which the activation function operates is set in part by the effect of the inhibitory neurons in the network (not shown in Figure 14.1). The threshold prevents the positive

feedback inherent in the operation of attractor networks from leading to runaway neuronal firing. It also allows optimal retrieval of a memory without interference from other memories stored in the synaptic weights [1, 3].

The recall state (which could be used to implement short-term memory, or memory recall) in an attractor network can be thought of as a local minimum in an energy landscape [2], where the energy would be defined as:

$$E = -\frac{1}{2} \sum_{i,j} w_{ij} (y_i - \langle y \rangle) (y_j - \langle y \rangle) \tag{4}$$

where y_i is the firing of neuron i, and $\langle y \rangle$ indicates the average firing rate. The intuition here is that, if both y_i and y_j are above their average rates and are exciting each other through a strong synapse, then the firing will tend to be stable and maintained, resulting in a low energy state that is stable. Although this energy analysis applies formally only with a fully connected network with symmetric synaptic strengths between neurons (which would be produced by an associative learning rule), it has been shown that the same general properties apply if the connectivity is diluted and becomes asymmetric [7, 8, 11–13].

Autoassociation attractor systems have two types of stable fixed points: a spontaneous state with a low firing rate, and one or more persistent states with high firing rates in which the neurons keep firing (Figure 14.2). Each one of the high firing rate attractor states can implement a different memory. When the system is moved to a position in the space by an external retrieval cue stimulus, it will move to the closest stable attractor state. The area in the space within which the system will move to a stable attractor state is called its basin of attraction. This is the process involved in completion of a whole memory from a partial retrieval cue.

2.2 Properties of Attractor Networks
2.2.1 Completion

An important and useful property of these attractor networks is that they complete an incomplete input vector, allowing recall of a whole memory from a small fraction of it. The memory recalled in response to a fragment is that stored in the memory that is closest in pattern similarity (as measured by the dot product, or correlation). Because the recall is iterative and progressive, the recall can be perfect.

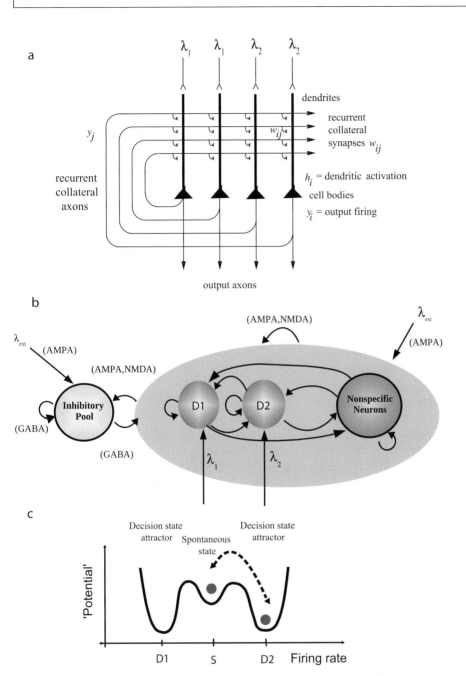

Figure 14.2 (a) Attractor or autoassociation network architecture for decision-making. The evidence for decision 1 is applied via the λ_1 inputs, and for decision 2 via the λ_2 inputs. The synaptic weights *wij* have been associatively modified during training in the presence of λ_1 and at a different time of λ_2. When λ_1 and λ_2 are applied, each attractor competes through the inhibitory interneurons (not shown) until one wins the competition and the network falls into one of the high firing rate attractors that represents the decision. The noise in the network caused by the random spiking of the neurons means that on some trials, for given inputs, the neurons in the decision 1 attractor are more likely to win, and on other trials the neurons in the decision 2 attractor are more likely to win. This makes the decision-making probabilistic, for, as shown in (c), the noise influences when the system will jump out of the spontaneous firing stable (low-energy) state S, and whether it jumps into the high firing state for decision 1 or decision 2 (D). (b) The architecture of the integrate-and-fire network used to model vibrotactile decision-making (see text).

2.2.2 Short-Term Memory

An autoassociation or attractor memory not only is useful as a long-term memory, in, for example, the memory for particular past episodes (see below), but can also be used as a short-term (working) memory, in which iterative processing around the recurrent collateral loop keeps a representation or series of representations active until another input cue is received or the task is completed. This is often used by the brain and is a prototypical property of cerebral neocortex [1].

2.2.3 Graceful Degradation or Fault Tolerance

If the synaptic weight vector $\mathbf{w}_i$ on each neuron has synapses missing (e.g., during development) or loses synapses (e.g., with brain damage or aging), then the activation h_i will still be reasonable, because h_i is the dot product (correlation) of the input firing rate vector and the weight vector. The same argument applies if whole input axons are lost. If an output neuron is lost, then the network cannot itself compensate for this, but the next network in the brain is likely to be able to generalize or complete if its input vector has some elements missing, as would be the case if some output neurons of a preceding autoassociation network were damaged. These processes constitute graceful degradation.

2.2.4 Storage Capacity, and the Sparseness of the Representation

Hopfield, using the approach of statistical mechanics, showed that, in a fully connected attractor network with fully distributed binary representations (e.g., for any one pattern, half the neurons are in the high firing state of 1, and the other half are in the low firing state of 0 or -1), the number of stable attractor states, corresponding to the number of memories that can be successfully retrieved, is approximately $0.14C$, where C is the number of connections on each neuron from the recurrent collateral connections [2–4].

We (Treves and Rolls) have performed quantitative analyses of the storage and retrieval processes in attractor networks [1, 7, 8, 11, 12]. We have extended previous formal models of autoassociative memory (see [3]) by analyzing a network either with graded response units (so as to represent more realistically the continuously variable rates at which neurons fire) or with incomplete connectivity [8, 11]. We have found that, in general, the maximum number, p_{max},

of firing patterns that can be (individually) retrieved is proportional to the number C^{RC} of (associatively) modifiable recurrent collateral synapses per neuron, by a factor that increases roughly with the inverse of the sparseness, a, of the neuronal representation (see below for definition of sparseness).[1]

The outcome of these analyses is that the number of memories that can be stored in a cortical attractor network is proportional to the number of synapses per neuron and that, with the sparsenesses of the representations present in the cerebral cortex, the number of memories is on the order of the number of synapses per neuron. Thus, if a typical pyramidal neuron in the cerebral cortex has 10,000 synapses devoted to the recurrent collateral connections, then such a local network in a small part of the neocortex, perhaps 2 millimeters in radius, could play a role in storing on the order of 10,000 memories [1]. Some details follow.

The neuronal population sparseness a of the representation can be measured by extending the binary notion of the proportion of neurons that are firing to any one stimulus or event as

$$a = \left(\sum_{i=1,n} r_i/N \right)^2 / \sum_{i=1,n} \left(r_i^2/N \right) \quad (5)$$

where r_i is the firing rate of the ith neuron in the set of N neurons. The sparseness ranges from $1/N$, when only one of the neurons responds to a particular stimulus (a local or grandmother cell representation), to a value of 1.0, attained when all the neurons are responding to a given stimulus. Approximately,

$$p_{max} \cong \frac{C^{RC}}{a \ln (1/a)} k \quad (6)$$

where k is a factor that depends weakly on the detailed structure of the rate distribution, on the connectivity pattern, and so on, but is roughly in the order of 0.2–0.3 [8]. For example, for $C^{RC} = 12,000$ (the number of recurrent collateral synapses on a hippocampal CA3 neuron in the rat [14]) and $a = 0.02$, p_{max} is calculated to be approximately 36,000. This analysis emphasizes the utility of having a sparse representation in the

---

[1] Each memory representation is precisely defined in the theory: it is a set of firing rates of the population of neurons (which represent a memory) that can be stored and later retrieved, with retrieval being possible from a fraction of the originally stored set of neuronal firing rates.

hippocampus, for this enables many different memories to be stored [1, 15, 16]. These quantitative analyses have been confirmed numerically [1, 13, 17].

2.2.5 The Dynamics of the Recurrent Attractor Network – Fast Recall

The analysis of the capacity of a recurrent network described above considered steady state conditions of the firing rates of the neurons. The question arises of how quickly the recurrent network would settle into its final state. If these settling processes took on the order of hundreds of milliseconds, they would be much too slow to contribute usefully to cortical activity, whether in the hippocampus or the neocortex [1, 18–20].

It has been shown that if the neurons are treated not as McCulloch–Pitts neurons, which are simply "updated" at each iteration or cycle of time steps (and assume the active state if the threshold is exceeded), but instead are analyzed and modeled as "integrate-and-fire" neurons in real continuous time, then the network can effectively "relax" into its recall state very rapidly, in one or two time constants of the synapses [1, 7, 21, 22]. This corresponds to perhaps 20 milliseconds in the brain. One factor in this rapid dynamics of autoassociative networks with brain-like integrate-and-fire membranes and synaptic properties is that, with some spontaneous activity, some of the neurons in the network are close to firing threshold already before the recall cue is applied, and hence some of the neurons are very quickly pushed by the recall cue into firing. Thus, information starts to be exchanged very rapidly (within 1–2 milliseconds of brain time) through the modified synapses by the neurons in the network. The progressive exchange of information, starting early on within what would otherwise be thought of as an iteration period (of perhaps 20 milliseconds, corresponding to a neuronal firing rate of 50 spikes per second), is the mechanism accounting for rapid recall in an autoassociative neuronal network made biologically realistic in this way. Further analysis of the fast dynamics of these networks, if they are implemented in a biologically plausible way with integrate-and-fire neurons, is provided in appendix A5 of Rolls and Treves [7], and elsewhere [1, 20–22].

2.3 Attractor Networks for Short-Term Memory

Pyramidal neurons in the cerebral cortex have a relatively high density of excitatory connections to each other within a local area of 1–3 millimeters [1, 23–25]. These local recurrent collateral excitatory connections provide a positive-feedback mechanism (which is kept under control by GABA inhibitory interneurons) that enables a set of neurons to maintain their activity for many seconds to implement a short-term memory [26]. Each memory is formed by the set of the neurons in the local cortical network that were coactive when the memory was formed, resulting in strengthened excitatory connections between that set of neurons through the process of long-term potentiation, which is a property of these recurrent collateral connections.

Attractor networks appear to operate in many cortical areas, including the prefrontal cortex, an area that is important in attention and short-term memory, as shown, for example, by firing in the delay period of a short-term memory task [1, 27–32]. Short-term memory is the ability to hold information online during a short time period [32].

It has been proposed that, whereas it is a property of all cortical areas that they have an ability to maintain neuronal activity by the attractor properties implemented by the recurrent collateral connections, the prefrontal cortex has a special role in short-term memory because it can act as an offline store as follows [1]. First, we note that a perceptual brain area, such as the inferior temporal cortex, must respond to every new incoming set of objects in the world so that we can see them, and this is inconsistent with maintaining their firing in an attractor state that represents an object or objects seen seconds ago. For this reason, for a short-term memory to be maintained during periods in which new stimuli are to be perceived, there must be separate networks for the perceptual and short-term memory functions, and indeed two coupled networks, one in the inferior temporal visual cortex for perceptual functions, and another in the prefrontal cortex for maintaining the short-term memory, for example, when intervening stimuli are being shown, provide a precise model of the interaction of perceptual and short-term memory systems [33, 34]. This model shows how a prefrontal cortex attractor (autoassociation) network could be triggered by a sample visual stimulus represented in the inferior temporal visual cortex in a delayed match to sample task, and could keep this attractor active during a memory interval in which intervening stimuli are shown. Then, when the sample stimulus reappears in the task as a match stimulus, the inferior temporal cortex module shows a large response to the match stimulus because it is activated by both the visual incoming match stimulus and the consistent back-projected memory of the sample stimulus still being represented in the prefrontal cortex memory module. The prefrontal attractor can be stimulated into activity by the first stimulus when it is inactive, but once in its high firing rate attractor state, it is relatively stable because of the internal positive feedback, and is not likely to be disturbed by further incoming stimuli. The internal recurrent connections must be stronger than the feedforward and feedback connections between the two cortical areas for this to work [1, 33, 34].

This computational model makes it clear that in order for ongoing perception to occur unhindered, implemented by posterior cortex (parietal and temporal lobe) networks, there must be a separate set of modules that is capable of maintaining a representation over intervening stimuli. This is the fundamental understanding offered for the evolution and functions of the dorsolateral prefrontal cortex, and it is this ability to provide multiple separate short-term attractor memories that provides, I suggest, the basis for its functions in planning [1].

The impairments of attention induced by prefrontal cortex damage may be accounted for in large part by an impairment in the ability to stably hold the object of attention in the short-term memory systems in the prefrontal cortex [1, 27, 35].

2.4 Stability of Attractor States

Using an integrate-and-fire approach, the individual neurons, synapses, and ion channels that comprise an attractor network can be simulated, and when a threshold is reached, the cell fires [1]. The firing times of the neurons can be approximately like those of neurons in the brain, approximately Poisson distributed; that is, the firing time is approximately random for a given mean rate. The random firing times of neurons are one source of noise in the attractor network and can influence the stability of the network [1, 36–39]. The attractor dynamics can be pictured as energy landscapes in which basins of attraction correspond to valleys and the attractor states to fixed points at the bottom of the valleys. The stability of an attractor is characterized by the average time in which the system stays in the basin of attraction under the influence of noise, which provokes

transitions to other attractor states. Noise results from the interplay between the Poissonian character of the spikes and the finite-size effect due to the limited numbers of neurons in the network. Two factors determine the stability. First, if the attractors are shallow (as in the left compared with the right valley in Figure 14.2c), less force is needed to move to a neighboring valley. *If the firing rates of the neurons are low, this reduces the depth of the basins of attraction by reducing the positive feedback between the set of neurons in the attractor. This is a key concept in understanding the effects of aging on memory, attention, and cognition, and a key foundation for many of the hypotheses about the effects of normal aging that are considered later in this chapter.* Second, a high level of noise increases the likelihood that the system will jump over an energy boundary from one state to another. We envision that the brain, as a dynamical system, has characteristics of such an attractor system, replete with statistical fluctuations.

This type of model can then be applied to the prefrontal cortex and used to link these low-level neuronal properties to the cognitive functions such as short-term memories that result from the interactions between thousands of neurons in the whole network. In order to maintain a short-term memory, these interactions have to remain stable, and several factors influence the stability of such a short-term memory attractor state with noise inherent in its operation.

First, the stable states of the network are the "low energy" states in which one set of the neurons, connected by strengthened recurrent collateral synapses, and representing one memory, is activated (see Figure 14.2). The higher the firing rates of this set of neurons, the stronger will be the negative feedback inhibition by the GABA inhibitory interneurons to the other excitatory (pyramidal) neurons in the network. This will keep the short-term memory state stable and will prevent distracting inputs to the other, inhibited neurons in the network from taking over [40]. Any factor that reduces the currents through the NMDA receptor channels (NMDARs) on the pyramidal cells (or via AMPA receptors) would decrease the firing rates of the set of activated neurons and tend to make the network more distractible [41–43].

Second, the strong synaptic connections implemented by the recurrent collateral synapses between the excitatory neurons in the network (e.g., the pyramidal cells in the prefrontal cortex) also tend to promote stability by enhancing the firing of the neurons that are active for a short-term memory [44]. This helps to keep the energy low in the Hopfield equation (see Eqn. 4), and thus to make it difficult to jump from one energy minimum over a barrier to a different energy minimum that represents a different memory.

Third, the operation of the network is inherently noisy and probabilistic, owing to the random spiking of the individual neurons in the network and the finite size of the network [45–49]. The random spiking will sometimes (i.e., probabilistically) be large in neurons that are not among those in the currently active set representing the short-term memory in mind; this chance effect, perhaps in the presence of a distracting stimulus, might make the network jump over an energy barrier between the memory states into what becomes a different short-term memory, resulting in distraction. In a different scenario, the same type of stochastic noise could make the network jump from a spontaneous state of firing, in which there is no item in short-term memory, to an active state in which one of the short-term memories becomes active. The effects of noise operating in this way would be more evident if the firing rates were low (resulting in a low energy barrier over which to jump) or if the GABA inhibition was reduced, which would make the spontaneous firing state less stable. GABA interneurons normally inhibit the neurons that are not in the active set that represent a memory, but hypofunction of the NMDARs on GABA interneurons could diminish this inhibition.

Fourth, the stability of the attractor state is enhanced by the long time constants (around 100 milliseconds) of the NMDARs in the network [50–53]. The contribution of these long time constants (long in relation to those of the alpha-amino-3-hydroxy-5-methyl-4-isoxazole propionate (AMPA) excitatory receptors, which are on the order of 5–10 milliseconds) is to smooth out in time the statistical fluctuations that are caused by the random spiking of populations of neurons in the network, and thus to make the network more stable and less likely to jump to a different state. The different state might represent a different short-term memory, or the noise might return the active state back to the spontaneous level of firing, producing failure of the short-term memory and failure to maintain attention. Further, once a neuron is strongly depolarized, the voltage dependence of the NMDARs may tend to promote further

firing [50]. If the NMDARs were less efficacious, the short-term memory network would be less stable because the effective time constant of the whole network would be reduced, owing to the greater relative contribution of the short time constant AMPA receptors to the effects implemented through the recurrent collateral excitatory connections between the pyramidal cells [51, 52, 54].

2.5 Attractor Network Stability and Psychiatric Disorders

It is hypothesized that some of the cognitive symptoms of schizophrenia, including poor short-term memory and attention, can be related to a reduced depth in the basins of attraction of the attractor networks in the prefrontal cortex that implement these functions [42, 43, 55]. The reduced depth of the basins of attraction may be related to hypoglutamatergia [56, 57] and/or changes in dopaminergic function, which act partly by influencing glutamatergic function [1, 43, 58–61]. The negative and positive symptoms of schizophrenia may be related to similar underlying changes, but expressed in different parts of the brain, such as the orbitofrontal and anterior cingulate cortex, as well as the temporal lobes [1, 42, 43, 55].

Obsessive-compulsive disorder has been linked to overstability in cortical attractor networks involved in short-term memory, attention, and action selection. It is hypothesized, at least in part, to be induced by hyperglutamatergia [1, 44].

In depression, the theory is being developed that the lateral orbitofrontal cortex, which is involved in detecting when rewards are smaller than expected, has a non-reward attractor that is overactive, resulting in persistent negative ruminating thoughts, hence sadness [62–66].

2.6 Attractor Networks, Noise, and Decision-making

A biologically plausible model, motivated and constrained by neurophysiological data, has been formulated to establish an explicit link between probabilistic decision-making and the way in which the noisy (i.e., stochastic) firing of neurons influences which attractor state (representing a decision) is reached when there are two or more competing inputs or sources of evidence to the attractor network [1, 38,

39, 48, 67–71]. The way in which these decision-making attractor network models operate is as follows. The model is an attractor network set up to have two (or more) possible high firing rate attractor states, one for each of the two (or more) decisions, as illustrated in Figure 14.2b. The evidence for each decision (1 vs. 2, etc.) biases each of the two attractors via the external inputs λ_1 and λ_2. The attractors are supported by strengthened synaptic connections in the recurrent collateral synapses between the (e.g., cortical pyramidal) neurons activated when λ_1 is applied, or when λ_2 is applied. (This is an associative or Hebbian process set up during a learning stage by a process like long-term potentiation.) When inputs λ_1 and λ_2 are applied, there is positive feedback via the recurrent collateral synaptic connections and competition is implemented through the inhibitory inter-neurons so that there can be only one winner. The network starts in a low spontaneous state of firing. When λ_1 and λ_2 are applied, there is competition between the two attractors, each of which is pushed toward a high firing rate state, and eventually, depending on the relative strength of the two inputs and the noise in the network caused by the random firing times of the neurons, one of the attractors will win the competition, and it will reach a high firing rate state. The firing of the neurons in the other attractor will be inhibited, resulting in a low firing rate. Because this is a nonlinear positive feedback system, the final firing rates are in what is effectively a binary decision state of high firing rate or low firing rate and do not reflect the exact relative values of the two inputs, λ_1 and λ_2, once the decision is reached. The noise in the network, caused by the random spiking of the neurons, is important to the operation of the network because it enables the network to jump out of a stable spontaneous rate of firing to a high firing rate and to do so probabilistically, depending on whether, on a particular trial, there is relatively more random firing in the neurons of one attractor than the other. This can be understood in terms of energy landscapes, where each attractor (the spontaneous state, and the two high firing rate attractors) is a low energy basin, and the spiking noise helps the system to jump over an energy barrier into another energy minimum, as illustrated in Figure 14.2c. If λ_1 and λ_2 are equal, then the decision that is taken is random and probabilistic, with the noise in each attractor determining which decision is taken on a particular trial. If one of the inputs is larger than the other, then the decision is biased toward it, but is still probabilistic. Because this is an attractor network, it has short-term memory properties implemented by the recurrent collaterals, which tend to promote a state once it is started. These help it to maintain the firing once it has reached the decision state, enabling a suitable action to be implemented even if this takes some time.

It might be posited that, if the depth of the basins of attraction is impaired with normal aging by one of more of the mechanisms described below, then this impairment might have an effect on decision-making systems of this type in the brain. It is possible in these circumstances that decisions might become noisier, that is, less closely related to the decision variables; slower; and not maintained as well in the short term. Planning related to the decision would not be maintained as persistently as with unreduced depths of the basins of attraction. This is an idea that arises from considering this type of decision-making system, and it would be of interest to further explore this proposal.

2.7 Hippocampal versus Neocortical Attractor Networks

The neocortical networks have local recurrent collateral connections between the pyramidal cells that achieve a high density only for a few millimeters across the cortex. It is hypothesized that this organization enables the neocortex to have many local attractor networks, each concerned with a different type of processing, short-term memory, long-term memory, and decision-making [1]. This is important, for recall that the capacity of an attractor network is set to first order by the number of connections onto a neuron from other neurons in the network. If there were widespread recurrent collateral connections in the neocortex so that the whole neocortex operated as a single attractor, the total memory capacity of the neocortex would be only that of a single attractor network (on the order of thousands of memories), a possibility that has been ruled out [1, 72]. There are great advantages in having large numbers of local but weakly coupled neocortical attractor networks. Some have been described above and many more are described by Rolls [1, 73].

It has been suggested, however, that one network in the brain, the hippocampal CA3 network, does operate as a *single* attractor network [1, 7, 15, 16, 74–83] (see related approaches, not emphasizing the relative importance of a single attractor network (or CA3 [84]), including [85–88])). Part of the anatomical basis for this single attractor network is that the recurrent collateral connections between the CA3 neurons are very widespread and have a chance of contacting any other CA3 neuron in the network [14, 89, 90]. The underlying theory is that the widespread connectivity in this network allows any one set of active neurons, perhaps representing one part of an episodic memory, to have a fair chance of making modifiable synaptic contacts with any other set of CA3 neurons, perhaps representing another part of an episodic memory. (An episodic memory is a memory of a single event or episode, such as where one ate dinner, with whom one ate, what was eaten, and what was discussed.) This widespread connectivity providing for a single attractor network means that any one part of an episodic memory can be associated with other components of events in the episodic memory. (This is what I mean by calling this an arbitrary memory, in that any arbitrary set of events can be associated with any other.) This functionality would be impossible in the neocortex, as the connections are local. Thus, this is a special contribution that the hippocampus can make when encoding an event in episodic memory [1, 81, 91, 92]. Any reduction of the firing rates of neurons in this CA3 network and the hippocampal system in general, which might occur with normal aging, would be expected to impair episodic memory by reducing the depths of the basins of attraction of hippocampal memory-related networks.

3 Attractor Networks, Transmitters, and Normal Aging

3.1 Introduction

As described above, cognitive symptoms such as poor short-term (working) memory and a decrement in top-down attention could arise from reduced depth in the basins of attraction of prefrontal and other cortical networks, as well as the effects of noise [1, 5, 39]. The hypothesis is that the reduced depth in the basins of attraction would make short-term memory unstable, so that sometimes the continuing firing of neurons that implement short-term memory would cease, and the system, under the influence of noise, would fall back out of the short-term memory state into spontaneous firing. Top-down attention requires

an intact short-term memory to hold the object of attention in mind. This is the source of the top-down attentional bias that influences competition from other networks that are receiving incoming signals. Therefore, disruption of short-term memory is also predicted to impair the stability of attention, as well as many other cognitive and executive functions that depend on the stability of short-term memory.

In this section I consider the hypothesis that the impairments in short-term memory and attention that are commonly associated with normal aging occur because the stochasticity of the dynamics is increased. This increase is caused by a reduced depth in the basins of attraction of cortical attractor networks involved in short-term memory and attention. Reduced short-term memory and impaired attention are commonly associated with aging, as are impairments in episodic memory [93]. Short-term memory and top-down attention are related to the operation of the dorsolateral prefrontal cortex [94, 95] using attractor networks that also provide the source of the top-down bias for attention [1]. Episodic memory utilizes attractor networks in the hippocampus [1, 16]. First, we examine some of the neurobiological changes that occur during normal aging and formulate hypotheses about how they might alter the depth of the basins of attraction of the attractor networks in the brain involved in short-term memory, attention, and episodic memory. Then we test these hypotheses by integrate-and-fire simulations with stochastic dynamics (caused by the almost Poisson nature of the spike trains of the neurons) in order to investigate how these neurobiological changes may influence the performance of these memory and attention systems. This leads to a discussion of ways in which some of the effects found might be ameliorated by different types of treatment.

Given that there is much knowledge about the neurobiology of normal aging [96, 97], an aim of the present approach is to provide a mechanistic, computational neuroscientific, stochastic neurodynamics framework for analysis of how the operation of cortical memory circuits involved in short-term memory, attention, and episodic memory, are altered by these changes [5]. This in turn has implications for how to ameliorate the changes in the operation of cortical networks during normal aging.

Neurodynamical hypotheses about the effects of the neurobiology of aging on attractor network functions in memory, attention, and cognition are developed next.

3.2 NMDA Receptor Hypofunction

One change associated with aging is a decrease in the functions of the NMDA receptors [98]. This change would act to reduce the depth of the basins of attraction, both by reducing the firing rate of the neurons in the active attractor and by decreasing the strength of the potentiated synaptic connections that support each attractor as the currents passing through these potentiated synapses decrease. If the NMDA receptor–activated channel conductances are reduced, then the depth of the basins of attraction will be reduced because the firing rates decline as a result of reduced excitatory inputs to the neurons, and because the synaptic coupling weights are effectively reduced because the synapses can pass only reduced currents.

I, therefore, hypothesize that with normal aging, *short-term memory and attention* will be impaired because the basins of attraction of the prefrontal cortex attractor networks mediating these functions [95, 99] and of other postcentral cortex areas that send inputs to the prefrontal cortex will have reduced depth and will therefore be less stable. This loss of stability will result in an increased proportion of trials on which the short-term memory will not be maintained [1, 5, 73]. Similarly, I hypothesize that with aging, *episodic memory* will be impaired because the basins of attraction of the hippocampal attractor networks mediating these functions [1] will have a reduced depth and will therefore be less stable, resulting in an increased proportion of trials on which the episodic memory will not be correctly recalled and actively maintained for the short period when it is used. Reduced functionality of AMPA receptors might also contribute, though NMDA receptors are of especial interest because of their long time constants.

3.3 Dopamine

D1 receptor blockade in the prefrontal cortex can impair short-term memory [100, 101]. Part of the reason for this may be that D1 receptor blockade can decrease NMDA receptor–activated ion channel conductances [40, 58]. Thus part of the role of dopamine in the prefrontal cortex in short-term memory can be accounted for by a decreased depth in the basins of attraction of prefrontal attractor networks [43]. The decreased depth would be due to both the decreased firing rate of the neurons and the reduced efficacy of the modified synapses as their channels

would be open less (see Eqn. 4). Dopaminergic innervation of the prefrontal cortex may decline with aging [102]. The decrease in dopamine could contribute to the reduced short-term memory and attention associated with aging, just as in Parkinson's disease, in which there are also be dopamine-related cognitive impairments.

During development, short-term memory and related executive functions implemented in the dorsolateral prefrontal cortex only mature when dopamine becomes functional in this cortical region [103]. These effects may also be related to an effect of dopamine acting, for example, via NMDA receptors [104] to increase neuronal firing rates and thus the stability of short-term memory attractor networks.

Tests of the neurodynamical hypothesis that reductions in dopamine in the prefrontal cortex in normal aging could, by reducing NMDA receptor–activated synaptic conductances, impair short-term memory and related attentional and executive functions are described in Section 3.7.1, "NMDA Receptor Hypofunction and Reduced Synaptic Strength."

3.4 Norepinephrine, cAMP, and HCN Channels

Norepinephrine (noradrenaline), acting on alpha2A-adrenoceptors, can strengthen working memory implemented in recurrent attractor neural networks in the dorsolateral prefrontal cortex by inhibiting cyclic adenosine monophosphate (cAMP) [105]. cAMP closes hyperpolarization-activated cyclic nucleotide-gated (HCN) channels (see also Chapter 3). The HCN channels on the distal dendrites allow K^+ (and Na^+) to pass through, generating an h current that shunts the effects of synaptic inputs [106], including inputs from the recurrent collateral connections. Thus, noradrenaline, by reducing shunting inhibition of the synaptic inputs, strengthens the attractor network, that is, maintains it more stably for more prolonged periods. Part of the evidence comes from iontophoresis of agents that influence these cAMP-activated HCN channels on single neurons in the macaque dorsolateral prefrontal cortex [105].

Noradrenaline reaches the cortex from the locus coeruleus, and a reduction in noradrenaline in aging and mild cognitive impairment [107], together with a loss of alpha2A adrenoceptors in the aged prefrontal cortex [108] and decreased excitation of noradrenergic neurons [109], would thus tend to impair short-term memory. The effect is modeled in the simulations described below, which involve decreasing the synaptic input associated with the recurrent collaterals by reducing the NMDA synaptic conductance. The effect is to reduce the firing rates of the excitatory (pyramidal) cells in the simulation and thus to make the short-term memory less stable by reducing the depth of the basins of attraction. The simulation described below in fact predicts the changes in the firing rates that have been found experimentally [105].

Although this may or may not be due only to changes in the noradrenergic system with aging, the loss of persistent firing is related to increased cAMP-K+ channel signaling [110] arising from a loss of phosphodiesterase-4A (PDE4A) [111]. The loss of PDE4A leads to hyperphosphorylation of tau and vulnerability to degeneration, an effect that is most relevant to Alzheimer's disease.

3.5 Impaired Synaptic Modification

Another factor that may contribute to the memory and cognitive changes associated with aging is that long-lasting associative synaptic modification, as assessed by long-term potentiation (LTP), is more difficult to achieve in older animals and decays more quickly [96] (see Chapter 3). This would tend to weaken the synaptic strengths that support an attractor, and this weakening could progress over time, thus directly reducing the depth of the attractor basins. This would impact episodic memory, the memory for particular past episodes, such as where one was at breakfast on a particular day, who was present, and what was eaten [1, 16, 83]. The reduction of synaptic strengths over time could also affect short-term memory, which requires that the synapses supporting a short-term memory attractor be modified in the first place using LTP, before the attractor is used [112].

In view of these changes, boosting glutamatergic transmission is being explored as a means of enhancing cognition and minimizing its decline in aging. Several classes of AMPA receptor potentiators have been described in the last decade. These molecules bind to allosteric sites on AMPA receptors, slow desensitization, and thereby enhance signaling through the receptors. Some AMPA receptor potentiating agents have been explored in rodent models [113]. These treatments might increase the depth of the basins of attraction.

Another factor is that Ca^{2+}-dependent processes affect Ca^{2+} signaling pathways and impair synaptic function in an aging-dependent manner, consistent with the Ca^{2+} hypothesis of brain aging and dementia [98] (see Chapter 3). In particular, an increase in Ca^{2+} conductance can occur in aged neurons. CA1 pyramidal cells in the aged hippocampus have an increased density of L-type Ca^{2+} channels that might lead to disruptions in Ca^{2+} homeostasis, contributing to the plasticity deficits that occur during aging [114].

My neurodynamical hypothesis is that with aging, impaired synaptic modification during learning and/or poorer maintenance of synaptic modifications after learning could impair episodic memory, short-term memory, and related attentional and executive functions. I test this below by analyzing the effects on the stochastic dynamics of attractor networks of reducing NMDA receptor–activated synaptic conductances to simulate the effect of less strong synapses.

3.6 Cholinergic Function
3.6.1 Cerebral Cortical Acetylcholine and Aging

Another change with aging is a reduction in cortical acetylcholine. Acetylcholine in the neocortex has its origin largely in the cholinergic neurons in the basal magnocellular forebrain nuclei of Meynert [115]. The correlation of clinical dementia ratings with the reductions in a number of cortical cholinergic markers such as choline acetyltransferase, muscarinic and nicotinic acetylcholine receptor binding, and levels of acetylcholine suggested an association between cholinergic hypofunction and cognitive deficits. This led to the formulation of the cholinergic hypothesis of memory dysfunction in senescence and in Alzheimer's disease [97]. In this section I generate hypotheses about how this reduction in acetylcholine in aging may influence the stochastic dynamics of attractor networks involved in short-term memory and thereby degrade cognitive functions that depend on short-term memory such as attention. For top-down attention, the subject to which attention is being allocated must be maintained in a short-term memory [73].

The cells in the basal magnocellular forebrain nuclei of Meynert lie just lateral to the lateral hypothalamus in the substantia innominata and extend forward through the preoptic area into the diagonal band of Broca [115]. The majority of these cells, but not all, are cholinergic [116], and they project directly to the cerebral cortex [115]. They provide the major cholinergic input to the cerebral cortex. If they are lesioned, the cortex is depleted of acetylcholine [115]. Loss of these cells does occur in Alzheimer's disease, and there is consequently a reduction in cortical acetylcholine in this disease [97, 115]. This loss of cortical and hippocampal acetylcholine may contribute to episodic memory impairment as well as other cognitive impairments in patients with Alzheimer's disease; however, the cognitive impairment caused by a loss of these basal forebrain cholinergic neurons may not be either the earliest factor or the major factor in the pathogenesis of the cognitive impairments associated with Alzheimer's disease. In monkeys, it has been shown that damage to basal forebrain cholinergic neurons can also impair attention and short-term memory [116]. There are only limited numbers of these cholinergic basal forebrain neurons (on the order of thousands). Given that there is a relative paucity of these neurons, it is not likely that they are directly storing learned information because the number of different patterns that could be represented and stored is so small (the number of different patterns that could be stored is dependent in a leading way on the number of input connections to each neuron in a pattern associator [1]). With the projections of these few neurons distributed throughout the cerebral cortex, the memory capacity of the whole system would be impractically small. Instead, these neurons could modulate storage in the cortex of information derived from what provides the numerical majority of input to cortical neurons, the glutamatergic terminals of other cortical neurons. This modulation may operate by setting thresholds for cortical cells to the appropriate value, or by more directly influencing the cascade of processes involved in long-term potentiation [117]. There is indeed evidence that acetylcholine is necessary for cortical synaptic modifiability, as shown by studies in which depletion of acetylcholine and noradrenaline impaired cortical LTP/synaptic modifiability [118]. However, age-related damage to the basal forebrain cholinergic neurons is also likely, and with a reduction of cholinergic input, cortical neurons become much more sluggish in their responses and show much more firing rate adaptation [119, 120].The question then arises of whether the basal forebrain cholinergic neurons tonically release acetylcholine, or whether they release it particularly in response to some external influence. To examine this, recordings have been made from basal forebrain neurons, at least some of which project to the cortex [71], and some of which will have been the cholinergic neurons just described. It has been found that some of these neurons respond to visual stimuli associated with rewards, such as food [121–125], or with punishment [126]; that others respond to novel visual stimuli [127]; and that others respond to a range of visual stimuli. For example, in one set of recordings, one group of these neurons (1.5%) responded to novel visual stimuli while monkeys performed recognition or visual discrimination tasks [127]. A complementary group of neurons, located more anteriorly, responded to familiar visual stimuli in the same tasks [127, 128]. A third group of neurons (5.7%) responded to positively reinforcing visual stimuli in visual discrimination and recognition memory tasks [124, 125]. In addition, a considerable proportion of these neurons (21.8%) responded to any visual stimuli shown in the tasks, and some (13.1%) responded to the tone cue that preceded the presentation of the visual stimuli in the task, alerting the monkey to the impending visual stimuli [127]. These neurons did not respond to touch to the leg that induced arousal, so their responses did not simply reflect arousal. Neurons in this region receive inputs from the amygdala [115, 129] and orbitofrontal cortex, and it is probably via the amygdala (and orbitofrontal cortex) that the information described above reaches and activates the basal forebrain neurons. Neurons with similar response properties have been found in the amygdala, and the amygdala appears to be involved in decoding visual stimuli that are associated with reinforcers or are novel [71].

3.6.2 Acetylcholine Reduction and Impaired Synaptic Modification and Modulation

Based on this neurobiological evidence, it is therefore suggested that the normal physiological function of these basal forebrain neurons is to send a general activation signal to the cortex when certain classes of environmental stimuli occur [71]. These environmental stimuli are often the stimuli to which a behavioral response is appropriate or required, such as positively or negatively reinforcing visual stimuli or novel visual stimuli. The effect of the firing of these neurons on the cortex is excitatory and, in this way, produces activation. This cortical activation may produce arousal and may thus facilitate concentration and attention, which are both impaired in

Alzheimer's disease. The reduced arousal and concentration may contribute to the memory disorders; however, the acetylcholine released from these basal magnocellular neurons may be more directly involved in memory formation (encoding). Bear and Singer [118] showed that long-term potentiation, used as an indicator of the synaptic modification that underlies learning, requires the presence in the cortex of acetylcholine as well as noradrenaline. In a similar way, acetylcholine in the hippocampus makes it more likely that LTP will occur, probably through activation of an inositol phosphate second messenger cascade [117]. In the hippocampus and prefrontal cortex, acetylcholine may simultaneously decrease transmission in recurrent collateral excitatory connections, and this may have the beneficial effect of reducing the effects of memories already stored in the recurrent collaterals so that they do not excessively influence the neuronal firing when new memories must be stored [130]. The adaptive value of the cortical strobe provided by the basal forebrain magnocellular neurons may thus be that it facilitates memory storage, especially when significant (e.g., reinforcing) environmental stimuli are detected. This means that memory storage is likely to be conserved (new memories are less likely to be laid down) when significant environmental stimuli are not present.

It is therefore hypothesized that one way in which impaired cholinergic neuron function is likely to impair memory is by reducing the depth of the basins of attraction of hippocampal and cortical networks. Alteration of synapses that are needed for the hippocampal encoding of episodic memory and the neocortical maintenance of short-term memory is reduced. This makes both the recall of long-term episodic memories and the maintenance of short-term memory less reliable in the face of stochastic noise. This hypothesis is tested in the simulations described below by analyzing the effects on the stochastic dynamics of attractor networks by reducing NMDA receptor–activated synaptic conductances to simulate the effect of reduced synaptic connectivity.

In addition to this effect of acetylcholine on LTP, acetylcholine can act via a nicotinic receptor to enhance thalamocortical transmission [131]. At least in early cortical processing stages, this would be expected to increase cortical neuronal responses to stimuli and thereby increase attention to stimuli as well as the likelihood that the effects of the stimuli would lead to information storage. A reduction in acetylcholine in aging would thus be predicted, when acting by this mechanism, to decrease attention to and short-term memory of environmental stimuli.

In addition to these effects of acetylcholine, the neurotransmitter can also act via a nicotinic receptor to increase the firing of cortical GABA inhibitory neurons [132]. A reduction of acetylcholine in aging would thereby be expected to produce an increase in the firing of cortical excitatory neurons, and this might partially compensate for some of the other effects of reduced acetylcholine, which tend to impair the operation of short-term memory systems. This is investigated in the simulations described below and elsewhere [5].

Some of these effects of acetylcholine on the operation of cortical systems involved in attention have been investigated in a cortical model of visual processing in early cortical visual areas [133]. We investigated the effects of reductions of acetylcholine on the operation, stability, and stochasticity of cortical memory and short-term memory systems in aging in an integrate-and-fire model of these memory processes [5].

3.6.3 Acetylcholine Reduction and Spike Frequency Adaptation

Another property of cortical neurons is that they tend to adapt with repeated input [119, 120]. However, this adaptation is most marked in brain slices in which there is no acetylcholine. One effect of acetylcholine is to reduce this adaptation [134]. It appears that the afterhyperpolarization (AHP) that follows the generation of a spike in a neuron is primarily mediated by two calcium-activated potassium currents, I_{AHP} and the sI_{AHP} [135, 136], which are activated by calcium influx during action potentials. The I_{AHP} current is mediated by small conductance calcium-activated potassium (SK) channels and its time course primarily follows cytosolic calcium, rising rapidly after action potentials and decaying with a time constant of 50 to several hundred milliseconds [136]. In contrast, the kinetics of the sI_{AHP} are slower, exhibiting a distinct rising phase and decaying with a time constant of 1–2 seconds [135]. A variety of neuromodulators, including acetylcholine (ACh) (acting via muscarinic receptors), as well as noradrenaline and glutamate (acting via G-protein-coupled receptors), suppress the sI_{AHP} and thus reduce spike-frequency adaptation.

When recordings are made from single neurons operating in physiological conditions in the awake behaving monkey, peristimulus time histograms of inferior temporal cortex neuronal responses to visual stimuli show only limited adaptation. There is typically an onset of the neuronal response at 80–100 milliseconds after the stimulus, followed within 50 milliseconds by the highest firing rate. There is afterward some reduction in the firing rate, but the firing rate is still typically more than half-maximal 500 milliseconds later [1, 137]. Thus, under normal physiological conditions, firing rate adaptation can occur but it is not large, even when cells are responding at a high rate (at, e.g., 100 spikes per second) to a visual stimulus. One of the factors that keeps the response relatively maintained may, however, be the presence of acetylcholine. Its depletion in aging and some disease states [97] could lead to less sustained neuronal responses (i.e., more adaptation), and this may contribute to the symptoms found with aging. In particular, if acetylcholine is low, the resultant reduced firing rates that may occur as a function of time would gradually, over a few hundred milliseconds, reduce the depth of the basin of attraction and thus destabilize short-term memory when noise is present, as shown in Eqn. 4. Such changes would thereby impair short-term memory and top-down attention.

The effects of this adaptation can be studied by including a time-varying intrinsic (potassium-like) conductance in the cell membrane [1, 21]. This can be done by specifying that this conductance, which if open tends to shunt the membrane and thus to prevent firing, opens by a fixed amount with the potential excursion associated with each spike, and then relaxes exponentially to its closed state. In this manner, sustained firing driven by a constant input current occurs at lower rates after the first few spikes. If the relevant parameters are set appropriately, this firing pattern is similar to the behavior observed in vitro of many pyramidal cells.

It is hypothesized that this spike frequency adaptation will reduce the depth of the basins of attraction of attractor networks involved in memory, including short-term memory, and will make the memory less reliable from trial to trial, and less robust against the effects of spiking-related and other noise. This hypothesis is tested as described below and elsewhere [5] with an implementation of the spike-frequency adaptation mechanism using Ca^{2+} activated K^+ hyperpolarizing currents [5, 138].

3.7 Integrate-and-Fire Attractor Network Simulation Results

3.7.1 NMDA Receptor Hypofunction and Reduced Synaptic Strength

The effect of reduction in the NMDA receptor–activated channel conductances on the short-term memory performance of a simulated integrate-and-fire attractor network are shown in Figure 14.3 [5]. The network had two main populations of neurons, similar to what is shown in Figure 14.2. Population S1 was activated at time = 1–3 seconds, and then tested to see whether it reliably maintained the high firing rate in a short-term memory attractor state when the memory cue was removed at time = 3 seconds, as illustrated in Figure 14.4. This reduction simulates the effect of reduction in synaptic strength, or in the amount of glutamate released per action potential, or in the conductance of the NMDA receptor channel. It was found that a rather small reduction in synaptic strength (caused, e.g., by less efficacious LTP), or in the NMDA receptor channel conductance of 5%, causes a major reduction in the percentage of trials on which the short-term memory is maintained (Figure 14.3). The reduction also makes the spontaneous firing rate state just a little more stable. The reason that the reduction of NMDA conductance decreases the persistence of the short-term memory is that the firing rates become reduced, as illustrated in Figure 14.4, for the condition in which NMDA conductance is reduced by 5% [5]. This reduction of the firing rate decreases the depth of the basin of attraction of the short-term memory population of neurons (the "S1 pool"), and this in turn makes the short-term memory state more susceptible to the effects of the noise due to the almost Poisson firing times of the neurons, as explained elsewhere [1, 39].

The reduction in firing rate is also relevant to any effects produced in a particular neuronal population and, for example, can be reflected in hypoemotionality due to reduced firing in emotion-related states elicited by reward and nonreward in the orbitofrontal and anterior cingulate cortex [62, 71].

3.7.2 Effects of Spike Frequency Adaptation Mediated by a Reduction in Acetylcholine

Figure 14.4 also shows the effects of increasing AHP conductance (gAHP) to simulate the effects of

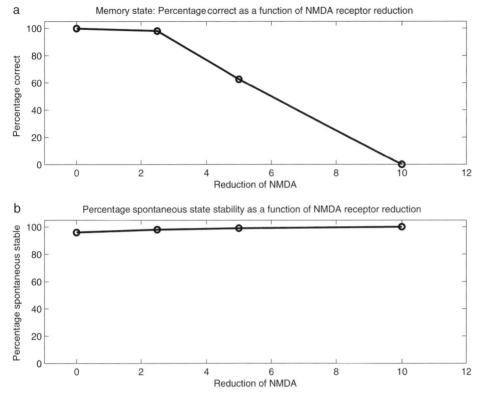

a

Memory state: Percentage correct as a function of NMDA receptor reduction

b

Percentage spontaneous state stability as a function of NMDA receptor reduction

Figure 14.3 Effects of reductions of NMDA receptor conductance on short-term memory in the integrate-and-fire network. (a) The effects of different reductions of NMDA receptor conductance on the percentage of short-term memory trials that show correct short-term memory at the end of a 2-s delay period. The criterion for correct short-term memory was a firing rate in the cued pool of neurons S1 that was > 10 spikes per second higher at the end of the delay period than for the uncued pool of neurons S2. (b) The percentage of trials on which the spontaneous firing rate state was stable (with a firing rate of < 10 spikes per second) at the end of the 1-s spontaneous firing rate period (before a short-term memory cue was applied to pool S1) as a function of the reduction of NMDA receptor conductance. Each data point is based on 1,000 trials [5]. From Rolls, E.T., and G. Deco, Stochastic cortical neurodynamics underlying the memory and cognitive changes in aging. *Neurobiology of Learning and Memory*, 2015. 118: 150–161

different reductions of acetylcholine in normal aging. It is shown that when the network was in the attractor state, the firing rate was reduced. This in turn markedly reduced the persistence of short-term memory [5]. The decrease in firing rates decreases the depth of the basin of attraction and makes it more probable that the system will be knocked out of its high firing rate state by the noise related to the Poisson nature of the spike times. Superimposed on this reduction of the firing rates produced by the Ca^{2+}-mediated after-spike hyperpolarization, the gradual reduction in the firing rate, in the period of 1.0–1.5 seconds, demonstrates firing rate adaptation, which has a similar time course to that recorded in single neurons in the inferior temporal visual cortex of the awake behaving macaque [137]. Also of interest is that after the cue is removed from pool S1 at time = 3 seconds, the neurons decrease their firing rates for several hundred

milliseconds, while the spike frequency adaptation recovers. During this post-cue period of reduced firing, the spike frequency adaptation mechanism makes the network especially vulnerable to being knocked out of the attractor by the spiking-dependent noise in the system.

It is thus predicted that enhancing cholinergic function is one treatment that may help to minimize the reduction in the short-term memory performance of attractor networks, involved in short-term memory and attention, that may occur in aging.

3.7.3 Reducing GABA Function When NMDA Receptor Functionality Is Reduced

The results in Figure 14.3 show that when NMDA functionality, glutamate transmission, or excitatory synaptic strength are reduced, short-term memory is impaired. This impairment appears to be related to

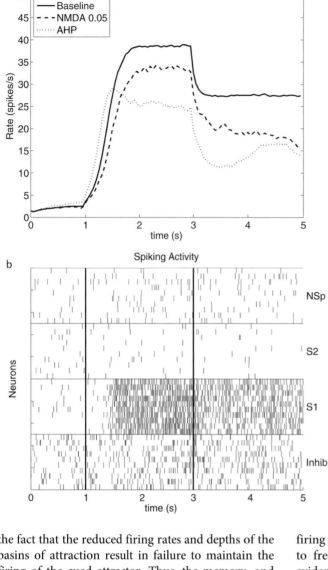

a

Figure 14.4 (a) Effects of reductions of NMDA receptor conductance (by 5%; NMDA 0.05) and of spike frequency adaptation (gAHP) on the firing rates of neurons in the short-term memory integrate-and-fire network. The baseline condition is with no reduction of NMDA conductances and no spike frequency adaptation. Time course: 0–1 second is spontaneous activity; 1–3 seconds is when the short-term memory cue is applied to neuron pool S1; 3–5 seconds is the period after the cue is removed and the short-term memory should be maintained by the firing rates of pool S1, which is what are shown. The firing rates are shown purely for correct trials for pool S1, that is, when the spontaneous firing state was stable and when the firing rate remained high in pool S1 (i.e., greater than 10 spikes per second more than in pool S2) until the end of the trial. The gAHP conductance was 40 nS for the AHP condition, and 0 for the other conditions. (b) Rastergrams showing the spiking activity of 10 randomly selected neurons in each pool on a typical trial for the baseline condition of no reduction in NMDA and no spike-frequency adaptation. S1, S2: the two specific pools. NSp: the nonspecific pool. Inhib: the pool of inhibitory neurons. From Rolls, E.T., and G. Deco, Stochastic cortical neurodynamics underlying the memory and cognitive changes in aging. *Neurobiology of Learning and Memory*, 2015. 118: 150–161

the fact that the reduced firing rates and depths of the basins of attraction result in failure to maintain the firing of the cued attractor. Thus, the memory, and any attentional effect maintained by it, is frequently lost. Would a reduction of inhibitory transmission mediated by GABA reduction alleviate this problem, by allowing the firing rates to remain high in a cued attractor after the cue is removed? It was shown that a reduction by 10% in the GABA synaptic conductance can at least partially help the memory to be maintained [5]. However, the effects of the reduction of GABA to help maintain a cued high firing rate attractor short-term memory state comes at a cost. It was found that the reduced inhibition produced by a 10% reduction in GABA causes the spontaneous

firing rate state (i.e., before the recall cue is applied) to frequently become unstable. The instability was evident in that, even when no recall cue was applied, the network would sometimes jump from the spontaneous firing rate state to a high firing rate state, provoked by the spiking-related noise in the system. Thus, simply reducing the inhibition in the system to compensate for the decreased excitatory synaptic transmission in aging may not be a useful approach to treatment. This is because of the risk that the spontaneous firing rate state, when no stimuli are applied, will become unstable, such that the network jumps into a state of high firing. This reduced inhibition could increase the risk of disorders such as hallucinations or epilepsy.

3.8 Implications

The reduced depth in the basins of attraction that the different neurobiological mechanisms produce in relation to normal aging could have a number of effects that are relevant to the cognitive changes in aging:

First, the stability of short-term memory networks would be impaired, and it might be difficult to hold items in short-term memory for a long period, as the noise might more easily push the network out of its shallow attractor.

Second, top-down attention would be impaired, in two ways. First, the short-term memory network holding the object of attention in mind would be less stable, so that the source of the top-down bias for the biased competition in other cortical areas might disappear. Second, even when the short-term memory for attention is still in its persistent attractor state, it would be less effective as a source of the top-down bias because the firing rates would be lower, as shown in Figure 14.4.

Third, the recall of information from episodic memory systems, such as object-place memory [1], would be impaired. This would arise because the positive feedback from the recurrent collateral synapses that helps the system to fall into a basin of attraction, representing in this case the recalled memory, would be less effective. The network would be more noisy overall, and in particular, the attractor state would not be maintained for the several seconds necessary for the recalled memory to be used.

Fourth, any reduction of the firing rate of the pyramidal cells caused by NMDA receptor hypofunction would itself be likely to impair new learning involving LTP.

In addition, if the NMDA receptor hypofunction were expressed not only in the prefrontal cortex, where it would affect short-term memory, and in the temporal lobes, where it would affect episodic memory [1], but also in the orbitofrontal cortex, then we would predict some reduction in emotion and motivation with aging, as these functions rely on the orbitofrontal cortex [63, 71], where there would be a reduction in firing rate due to the NMDA receptor hypofunction.

Although a decrease of GABA efficacy may help to maintain a network in an attractor state when NMDA receptor–mediated effects are reduced, this comes at the cost of reducing the stability of the spontaneous firing state when no cues are applied [5]. The effect of instability in the spontaneous firing rate state when no stimuli are applied is that the network enters one of its high firing rate attractor states even without any external input. This would increase the risk, for example, of hallucinations or epilepsy. Thus, reducing inhibition is likely to be an unsafe way, in terms of stochastic neurodynamics, to treat the short-term memory and attentional problems in aging. Instead, a better approach would be to use treatments that would increase the excitatory glutamatergic transmission in cortical networks. This might (after careful and full testing) involve effects such as that of glycine in upwardly modulating the NMDA receptor [139]; agents such as AMPAkines that increase transmission through effects on the AMPA glutamatergic receptors [139]; agents that mimic dopaminergic or cholinergic effects; or other types of stimulants, including perhaps caffeine. Indeed, one of the advantages of the stochastic neurodynamics approach is that it allows combinations of such approaches to be tested, allowing exploration of approaches where any one agent is in low concentration to minimize any side effects. Part of the interest of this stochastic dynamics approach to aging is that it provides a way to test treatments and combinations of pharmacological treatments that may together help to minimize the cognitive symptoms and signs of aging. The approach facilitates the investigation of drug combinations that may together be effective in doses lower than when only one drug is given. Further, this approach may lead to predictions for effective treatments that need not necessarily restore the particular change in the brain that caused the symptoms, but may engage alternative routes to restore the stability of the dynamics. For example, nicotine (self-administered by gum or patch) might increase the firing rates of neurons in some of the relevant brain systems, and this might ameliorate some of the symptoms. Consistent with this proposal, nicotinic stimulation may improve cognition and neural functioning and may also elevate mood in depression [140, 141], both of which are predicted from the effects described here of acetylcholine on the stability of memory networks in the prefrontal cortex and hippocampus, as well as on the firing rates of neurons in areas such as the orbitofrontal and anterior cingulate cortex involved in emotion and mood.

In the context of normal aging, if the depth of the basins of attraction is impaired by one of more of the mechanisms described above, then this might have an effect on decision-making systems of the type illustrated in Figure 14.2. In these circumstances, decisions might become noisier, that is, less closely related to the decision variables; slower; and they might not be maintained well in the short term. Planning related to the decision would not necessarily be maintained as persistently as with unreduced depths of the basins of attraction. This is an idea that arises from considering this type of decision-making system, and it would be of interest to explore this proposal further.

Finally, although the research described here has focused on attentional and short-term memory changes in normal aging, the results are also relevant to the preclinical changes in Alzheimer's disease, in which synaptic transmission and plasticity in NMDA receptors may be reduced because of effects related to soluble Aβ oligomers [142].

References

1. Rolls, E.T., *Cerebral Cortex: Principles of Operation.* Oxford: Oxford University Press, 2016.

2. Hopfield, J.J., Neural networks and physical systems with emergent collective computational abilities. *Proceedings of the National Academy of Science USA*, 1982. **79**: 2554–2558.

3. Amit, D.J., *Modeling Brain Function.* Cambridge: Cambridge University Press, 1989.

4. Hertz, J., A. Krogh, and R.G. Palmer, *An Introduction to the Theory of Neural Computation.* Wokingham: Addison-Wesley, 1991.

5. Rolls, E.T., and G. Deco, Stochastic cortical neurodynamics underlying the memory and cognitive changes in aging. *Neurobiology of Learning and Memory*, 2015. **118**: 150–161.

6. Kohonen, T., E. Oja, and P. Lehtio, *Storage and processing of information in distributed memory systems*, in *Parallel Models of Associative Memory*, G.E. Hinton and J.A. Anderson, editors. Hillsdale, NJ: Lawrence Erlbaum, 1981, pp. 129–167.

7. Rolls, E.T., and A. Treves, *Neural Networks and Brain Function.* Oxford: Oxford University Press, 1998.

8. Treves, A., and E.T. Rolls, What determines the capacity of autoassociative memories in the brain? *Network*, 1991. **2**: 371–397.

9. Hebb, D.O., *The Organization of Behavior: A Neuropsychological Theory.* New York: Wiley, 1949.

10. Rolls, E.T., and A. Treves, The relative advantages of sparse versus distributed encoding for associative neuronal networks in the brain. *Network*, 1990. **1**: 407–421.

11. Treves, A., Graded-response neurons and information encodings in autoassociative memories. *Physical Review A*, 1990. **42**: 2418–2430.

12. Treves, A., and E.T. Rolls, Computational constraints suggest the need for two distinct input systems to the hippocampal CA3 network. *Hippocampus*, 1992. **2**: 189–199.

13. Rolls, E.T., et al., Simulation studies of the CA3 hippocampal subfield modelled as an attractor neural network. *Neural Networks*, 1997. **10**: 1559–1569.

14. Amaral, D.G., N. Ishizuka, and B. Claiborne, Neurons, numbers and the hippocampal network. *Progress in Brain Research*, 1990. **83**: 1–11.

15. Treves, A., and E.T. Rolls, A computational analysis of the role of the hippocampus in memory. *Hippocampus*, 1994. **4**: 374–391.

16. Kesner, R.P., and E.T. Rolls, A computational theory of hippocampal function, and tests of the theory: new developments. *Neuroscience and Biobehavioral Reviews*, 2015. **48**: 92–147.

17. Rolls, E.T., Advantages of dilution in the connectivity of attractor networks in the brain. *Biologically Inspired Cognitive Architectures*, 2012. **1**: 44–54.

18. Rolls, E.T., Neurophysiological mechanisms underlying face processing within and beyond the temporal cortical visual areas. *Philosophical Transactions of the Royal Society of London B*, 1992. **335**: 11–21.

19. Rolls, E.T., Consciousness absent and present: a neurophysiological exploration. *Progress in Brain Research*, 2003. **144**: 95–106.

20. Panzeri, S., et al., Speed of feedforward and recurrent processing in multilayer networks of integrate-and-fire neurons. *Network*, 2001. **12**(4): 423–440.

21. Treves, A., Mean-field analysis of neuronal spike dynamics. *Network*, 1993. **4**: 259–284.

22. Battaglia, F.P., and A. Treves, Stable and rapid recurrent processing in realistic autoassociative memories. *Neural Computation*, 1998. **10**: 431–450.

23. Braitenberg, V., and A. Schütz, *Anatomy of the Cortex.* Berlin: Springer-Verlag, 1991.

24. Abeles, M., *Corticonics: Neural Circuits of the Cerebral Cortex.* New York: Cambridge University Press, 1991.

25. Rolls, E.T., and W.P.C. Mills, Computations in the deep vs superficial layers of the cerebral cortex. *Neurobiology of Learning and Memory*, 2017. **145**: 205–221.

26. Goldman-Rakic, P.S., Cellular basis of working memory. *Neuron*, 1995. **14**: 477–485.

27. Goldman-Rakic, P.S., The prefrontal landscape: implications of functional architecture for understanding human mentation and the central executive. *Philosophical Transactions of the Royal Society B*, 1996. **351**: 1445–1453.

28. Fuster, J.M., Executive frontal functions. *Experimental Brain Research*, 2000. **133**(1): 66–70.

29. Fuster, J.M., and G.E. Alexander, Neuron activity related to short-term memory. *Science*, 1971. **173**: 652–654.

30. Kubota, K., and H. Niki, Prefrontal cortical unit activity and delayed alternation performance in monkeys. *Journal of Neurophysiology*, 1971. **34**(3): 337–347.

31. Funahashi, S., C.J. Bruce, and P.S. Goldman-Rakic, Mnemonic coding of visual space in monkey dorsolateral prefrontal cortex. *Journal of Neurophysiology*, 1989. **61**: 331–349.

32. Fuster, J.M., *The Prefrontal Cortex*. 4th ed. London: Academic Press, 2008.

33. Renart, A., N. Parga, and E.T. Rolls, *A recurrent model of the interaction between the prefrontal cortex and inferior temporal cortex in delay memory tasks*, in *Advances in Neural Information Processing Systems*, S.A. Solla, T.K. Leen, and K.-R. Mueller, editors. Cambridge, MA: MIT Press, 2000, pp. 171–177.

34. Renart, A., et al., A model of the IT-PF network in object working memory which includes balanced persistent activity and tuned inhibition. *Neurocomputing*, 2001. **38–40**: 1525–1531.

35. Goldman-Rakic, P.S., and H.-C. Leung, *Functional architecture of the dorsolateral prefrontal cortex in monkeys and humans*, in *Principles of Frontal Lobe Function*, D.T. Stuss and R.T. Knight, editors. New York: Oxford University Press, 2002, pp. 85–95.

36. Tuckwell, H., *Introduction to Theoretical Neurobiology*. Cambridge: Cambridge University Press, 1988.

37. Jackson, B.S., Including long-range dependence in integrate-and-fire models of the high interspike-interval variability of cortical neurons. *Neural Computation*, 2004. **16**(10): 2125–2195.

38. Deco, G., E.T. Rolls, and R. Romo, Stochastic dynamics as a principle of brain function. *Progress in Neurobiology*, 2009. **88**: 1–16.

39. Rolls, E.T. and G. Deco, *The Noisy Brain: Stochastic Dynamics as a Principle of Brain Function*. Oxford: Oxford University Press, 2010.

40. Brunel, N., and X.J. Wang, Effects of neuromodulation in a cortical network model of object working memory dominated by recurrent inhibition. *Journal of Computational Neuroscience*, 2001. **11**: 63–85.

41. Durstewitz, D., J.K. Seamans, and T.J. Sejnowski, Neurocomputational models of working memory. *Nature Neuroscience*, 2000. **3 Suppl**: 1184–1191.

42. Loh, M., E.T. Rolls, and G. Deco, A dynamical systems hypothesis of schizophrenia. *PLoS Computational Biology*, 2007. **3** (11): e228. doi:10.1371/journal. pcbi.0030228.

43. Rolls, E.T., et al., Computational models of schizophrenia and dopamine modulation in the prefrontal cortex. *Nature Reviews Neuroscience*, 2008. **9**: 696–709.

44. Rolls, E.T., M. Loh, and G. Deco, An attractor hypothesis of obsessive-compulsive disorder. *European Journal of Neuroscience*, 2008. **28**: 782–793.

45. Brunel, N., and V. Hakim, Fast global oscillations in networks of integrate-and-fire neurons with low firing rates. *Neural Computation*, 1999. **11**(7): 1621–1671.

46. Mattia, M., and P. Del Giudice, Attention and working memory: a dynamical model of neuronal activity in the prefrontal cortex. *Physical Review E*, 2002. **66**: 51917–51919.

47. Mattia, M., and P. Del Giudice, Finite-size dynamics of inhibitory and excitatory interacting spiking neurons. *Physical Review E, Statistical, Nonlinear, and Soft Matter Physics*, 2004. **70**(5 Pt 1): 052903.

48. Deco, G., and E.T. Rolls, Decision-making and Weber's Law: a neurophysiological model. *European Journal of Neuroscience*, 2006. **24**: 901–916.

49. Faisal, A.A., L.P. Selen, and D.M. Wolpert, Noise in the nervous system. *Nature Reviews Neuroscience*, 2008. **9**(4): 292–303.

50. Lisman, J.E., J.M. Fellous, and X.J. Wang, A role for NMDA-receptor channels in working memory. *Nature Neuroscience*, 1998. **1**(4): 273–275.

51. Wang, X.-J., Synaptic basis of cortical persistent activity: the importance of NMDA receptors to working memory. *Journal of Neuroscience*, 1999. **19**(21): 9587–9603.

52. Compte, A., et al., Synaptic mechanisms and network dynamics underlying spatial working memory in a cortical network model. *Cereb Cortex*, 2000. **10**(9): 910–923.

53. Wang, X.J., Synaptic reverberation underlying mnemonic persistent activity. *Trends in Neurosciences*, 2001. **24**(8): 455–463.

54. Tegner, J., A. Compte, and X.J. Wang, The dynamical stability of reverberatory neural circuits. *Biological Cybernetics*, 2002. **87** (5–6): 471–481.

55. Rolls, E.T., *Emotion Explained*. Oxford: Oxford University Press, 2005.

56. Coyle, J.T., G. Tsai, and D. Goff, Converging evidence of NMDA receptor hypofunction in the pathophysiology of schizophrenia. *Annals of the New York Academy of Sciences*, 2003. **1003**: 318–327.

57. Coyle, J.T., Glutamate and schizophrenia: beyond the dopamine hypothesis. *Cellular and Molecular Neurobiology*, 2006. **26**(4–6): 365–384.

58. Seamans, J.K., and C.R. Yang, The principal features and mechanisms of dopamine modulation in the prefrontal cortex. *Progress in Neurobiology*, 2004. **74**(1): 1–58.

59. Durstewitz, D., A few important points about dopamine's role in neural network dynamics. *Pharmacopsychiatry*, 2006. **39** (Suppl 1): S72–S75.

60. Durstewitz, D., *Dopaminergic modulation of prefrontal cortex network dynamics*, in *Monoaminergic Modulation of Cortical Excitability*, K.-Y. Tseng and M. Atzori, editors. New York: Springer, 2007, pp. 217–234.

61. Winterer, G., and D.R. Weinberger, Genes, dopamine and cortical signal-to-noise ratio in schizophrenia. *Trends in Neurosciences*, 2004. **27**(11): 683–690.

62. Rolls, E.T., *The Brain, Emotion, and Depression*. Oxford: Oxford University Press, 2018.

63. Rolls, E.T., The orbitofrontal cortex and emotion in health and disease, including depression. Neuropsychologia, 2019. **128**:14–43 doi: 10.1016/j. neuropsychologia.2017.09.021.

64. Rolls, E.T., The roles of the orbitofrontal cortex via the habenula in non-reward and depression, and in the responses of serotonin and dopamine neurons. *Neuroscience and Biobehavioral Reviews*, 2017. **75**: 331–334.

65. Rolls, E.T., A non-reward attractor theory of depression.

Neuroscience and Biobehavioral Reviews, 2016. **68**: 47–58.

66. Cheng, W., et al., Medial reward and lateral non-reward orbitofrontal cortex circuits change in opposite directions in depression. *Brain*, 2016. **139**(Pt 12): 3296–3309.

67. Wang, X.J., Probabilistic decision making by slow reverberation in cortical circuits. *Neuron*, 2002. **36**: 955–968.

68. Brody, C.D., R. Romo, and A. Kepecs, Basic mechanisms for graded persistent activity: discrete attractors, continuous attractors, and dynamic representations. *Current Opinion in Neurobiology*, 2003. **13**: 204–211.

69. Machens, C.K., R. Romo, and C.D. Brody, Flexible control of mutual inhibition: a neural model of two-interval discrimination. *Science*, 2005. **307**: 1121–1124.

70. Wong, K.F., and X.J. Wang, A recurrent network mechanism of time integration in perceptual decisions. *Journal of Neuroscience*, 2006. **26**(4): 1314–1328.

71. Rolls, E.T., *Emotion and Decision-Making Explained*. Oxford: Oxford University Press, 2014.

72. O'Kane, D., and A. Treves, Why the simplest notion of neocortex as an autoassociative memory would not work. *Network*, 1992. **3**: 379–384.

73. Rolls, E.T., *Memory, Attention, and Decision-making: A Unifying Computational Neuroscience Approach*. Oxford: Oxford University Press, 2008.

74. Rolls, E.T., *Information representation, processing and storage in the brain: analysis at the single neuron level*, in *The Neural and Molecular Bases of Learning*, J.-P. Changeux and M. Konishi, editors. Chichester: Wiley, 1987, pp. 503–540.

75. Rolls, E.T., *Functions of neuronal networks in the hippocampus and neocortex in memory*, in *Neural

Models of Plasticity: Experimental and Theoretical Approaches*, J.H. Byrne and W.O. Berry, editors. San Diego: Academic Press, 1989, pp. 240–265.

76. Rolls, E.T., *The representation and storage of information in neuronal networks in the primate cerebral cortex and hippocampus*, in *The Computing Neuron*, R. Durbin, C. Miall, and G. Mitchison, editors. Wokingham: Addison-Wesley, 1989, pp. 125–159.

77. Rolls, E.T., *Functions of neuronal networks in the hippocampus and cerebral cortex in memory*, in *Models of Brain Function*, R.M.J. Cotterill, editor. Cambridge: Cambridge University Press, 1989, pp. 15–33.

78. Rolls, E.T., Theoretical and neurophysiological analysis of the functions of the primate hippocampus in memory. *Cold Spring Harbor Symposia in Quantitative Biology*, 1990. **55**: 995–1006.

79. Rolls, E.T., *Functions of the primate hippocampus in spatial processing and memory*, in *Neurobiology of Comparative Cognition*, D.S. Olton and R.P. Kesner, editors. Hillsdale, NJ: Lawrence Erlbaum, 1990, pp. 339–362.

80. Rolls, E.T., Functions of the primate hippocampus in spatial and non-spatial memory. *Hippocampus*, 1991. **1**: 258–261.

81. Rolls, E.T., and R.P. Kesner, A computational theory of hippocampal function, and empirical tests of the theory. *Progress in Neurobiology*, 2006. **79**: 1–48.

82. Rolls, E.T., An attractor network in the hippocampus: theory and neurophysiology. *Learning and Memory*, 2007. **14**: 714–731.

83. Rolls, E.T., The storage and recall of memories in the hippocampo-cortical system. *Cell and Tissue Research*, 2018. **373**:577–604. doi: 10.1007/s00441-017-2744-3.

84. Marr, D., Simple memory: a theory for archicortex. *Philosophical Transactions of the* Royal Society *of London Series* B, *Biological Sciences*, 1971. **262**: 23–81.

85. McNaughton, B.L., and R.G.M. Morris, Hippocampal synaptic enhancement and information storage within a distributed memory system. *Trends in Neurosciences*, 1987. **10**(10): 408–415.

86. Levy, W.B., *A computational approach to hippocampal function*, in *Computational Models of Learning in Simple Neural Systems*, R.D. Hawkins and G.H. Bower, editors. San Diego: Academic Press, 1989, pp. 243–305.

87. McNaughton, B.L., Associative pattern completion in hippocampal circuits: new evidence and new questions. *Brain Research Reviews*, 1991. **16**: 193–220.

88. McClelland, J.L., B.L. McNaughton, and R.C. O'Reilly, Why there are complementary learning systems in the hippocampus and neocortex: insights from the successes and failures of connectionist models of learning and memory. *Psychological Review*, 1995. **102**: 419–457.

89. Ishizuka, N., J. Weber, and D.G. Amaral, Organization of intrahippocampal projections originating from CA3 pyramidal cells in the rat. *Journal of Comparative Neurology*, 1990. **295**: 580–623.

90. Kondo, H., P. Lavenex, and D.G. Amaral, Intrinsic connections of the macaque monkey hippocampal formation: II. CA3 connections. *Journal of Comparative Neurology*, 2009. **515**(3): 349–377.

91. Rolls, E.T., *The primate hippocampus and episodic memory*, in *Handbook of Episodic Memory*, E. Dere et al., editors. Amsterdam: Elsevier, 2008, pp. 417–438.

92. Rolls, E.T., and J.-Z. Xiang, Spatial view cells in the primate hippocampus, and memory recall. *Reviews in the Neurosciences*, 2006. **17**(1–2): 175–200.

93. Grady, C.L., Cognitive neuroscience of aging. *Annals of the New York Academy of Science*, 2008. **1124**: 127–144.

94. Miller, E.K., The "working" of working memory. *Dialogues in Clinical Neuroscience*, 2013. **15**(4): 411–418.

95. Wang, M., et al., NMDA receptors subserve persistent neuronal firing during working memory in dorsolateral prefrontal cortex. *Neuron*, 2013. **77**(4): 736–749.

96. Samson, R.D., and C.A. Barnes, Impact of aging brain circuits on cognition. *European Journal of Neuroscience*, 2013. **37**(12): 1903–1915.

97. Schliebs, R., and T. Arendt, The cholinergic system in aging and neuronal degeneration. *Behavioural Brain Research*, 2011. **221**(2): 555–563.

98. Kelly, K.M., et al., The neurobiology of aging. *Epilepsy Research*, 2006. **68**(Suppl 1): S5–S20.

99. Arnsten, A.F., and L.E. Jin, Molecular influences on working memory circuits in dorsolateral prefrontal cortex. *Progress in Molecular Biology and Translational Science*, 2014. **122**: 211–231.

100. Goldman-Rakic, P.S., E.C. Muly, 3rd, and G.V. Williams, D(1) receptors in prefrontal cells and circuits. *Brain Research Reviews*, 2000. **31**(2–3): 295–301.

101. Castner, S.A., G.V. Williams, and P.S. Goldman-Rakic, Reversal of antipsychotic-induced working memory deficits by short-term dopamine D1 receptor stimulation. *Science*, 2000. **287**(5460): 2020–2022.

102. Sikstrom, S., Computational perspectives on neuromodulation of aging. *Acta Neurochirurgica Suppl*, 2007. **97**(Pt 2): 513–518.

103. Diamond, A., Evidence for the importance of dopamine for prefrontal cortex functions early in life. *Philosophical Transactions of the Royal Society of London Series B, Biological Sciences*, 1996. **351**(1346): 1483–1493; discussion 1494.

104. Diamond, A., Consequences of variations in genes that affect dopamine in prefrontal cortex. *Cerebral Cortex*, 2007. **17**(Suppl 1): i161–i170.

105. Wang, M., et al., Alpha2A-adrenoceptors strengthen working memory networks by inhibiting cAMP-HCN channel signaling in prefrontal cortex. *Cell*, 2007. **129**(2): 397–410.

106. He, C., et al., Neurophysiology of HCN channels: from cellular functions to multiple regulations. *Progress in Neurobiology*, 2014. **112**: 1–23.

107. Grudzien, A., et al., Locus coeruleus neurofibrillary degeneration in aging, mild cognitive impairment and early Alzheimer's disease. *Neurobiology of Aging*, 2007. **28**(3): 327–335.

108. Moore, T.L., et al., Cognitive impairment in aged rhesus monkeys associated with monoamine receptors in the prefrontal cortex. *Behavioural Brain Research*, 2005. **160**(2): 208–221.

109. Downs, J.L., et al., Orexin neuronal changes in the locus coeruleus of the aging rhesus macaque. *Neurobiology of Aging*, 2007. **28**(8): 1286–1295.

110. Wang, M., et al., Neuronal basis of age-related working memory decline. *Nature*, 2011. **476**(7359): 210–213.

111. Carlyle, B.C., et al., cAMP-PKA phosphorylation of tau confers risk for degeneration in aging association cortex. *Proceedings of the National Academy of Sciences*

of the United States of America, 2014. **111**(13): 5036–5041.

112. Kesner, R.P., and E.T. Rolls, Role of long term synaptic modification in short term memory. *Hippocampus*, 2001. **11**: 240–250.

113. Lauterborn, J.C., et al., Chronic ampakine treatments stimulate dendritic growth and promote learning in middle-aged rats. *Journal of Neuroscience*, 2016. **36**(5): 1636–1646.

114. Burke, S.N. and C.A. Barnes, Neural plasticity in the ageing brain. *Nature Reviews Neuroscience*, 2006. **7**(1): 30–40.

115. Mesulam, N.-M., Human brain cholinergic pathways. *Progress in Brain Research*, 1990. **84**: 231–241.

116. Baxter, M.G., and D.J. Bucci, Selective immunotoxic lesions of basal forebrain cholinergic neurons: twenty years of research and new directions. *Behavioral Neuroscience*, 2013. **127**(5): 611–618.

117. Hasselmo, M.E., and M. Sarter, Modes and models of forebrain cholinergic neuromodulation of cognition. *Neuropsychopharmacology*, 2011. **36**(1): 52–73.

118. Bear, M.F., and W. Singer, Modulation of visual cortical plasticity by acetylcholine and noradrenaline. *Nature*, 1986. **320**: 172–176.

119. Fuhrmann, G., H. Markram, and M. Tsodyks, Spike frequency adaptation and neocortical rhythms. *Journal of Neurophysiology*, 2002. **88**(2): 761–770.

120. Abbott, L.F., et al., Synaptic depression and cortical gain control. *Science*, 1997. **275**(5297): 220–224.

121. Rolls, E.T., M.J. Burton, and F. Mora, Hypothalamic neuronal responses associated with the sight of food. *Brain Research*, 1976. **111**(1): 53–66.

122. Mora, F., E.T. Rolls, and M.J. Burton, Modulation during learning of the responses of neurones in the lateral hypothalamus to the sight of food. *Experimental Neurology*, 1976. **53**: 508–519.

123. Burton, M.J., E.T. Rolls, and F. Mora, Effects of hunger on the responses of neurones in the lateral hypothalamus to the sight and taste of food. *Experimental Neurology*, 1976. **51**: 668–677.

124. Wilson, F.A.W., and E.T. Rolls, Learning and memory are reflected in the responses of reinforcement-related neurons in the primate basal forebrain. *Journal of Neuroscience*, 1990. **10**: 1254–1267.

125. Wilson, F.A.W., and E.T. Rolls, Neuronal responses related to reinforcement in the primate basal forebrain. *Brain Research*, 1990. **509**: 213–231.

126. Rolls, E.T., et al., Activity of neurones in different forebrain structures during visual discrimination learning in the monkey. *Experimental Brain Research*, 1979. **32**: R39–R40.

127. Wilson, F.A.W., and E.T. Rolls, Neuronal responses related to the novelty and familiarity of visual stimuli in the substantia innominata, diagonal band of Broca and periventricular region of the primate. *Experimental Brain Research*, 1990. **80**: 104–120.

128. Rolls, E.T., et al., Neuronal responses related to visual recognition. *Brain*, 1982. **105**: 611–646.

129. Amaral, D.G., et al., *Anatomical organization of the primate amygdaloid complex*, in *The Amygdala*, J.P. Aggleton, editor. New York: Wiley-Liss, 1992, pp. 1–66.

130. Giocomo, L.M., and M.E. Hasselmo, Neuromodulation by glutamate and acetylcholine can change circuit dynamics by regulating the relative influence of afferent input and excitatory feedback. *Molecular Neurobiology*, 2007. **36**(2): 184–200.

131. Gil, Z., B.W. Connors, and Y. Amitai, Differential regulation of neocortical synapses by neuromodulators and activity. *Neuron*, 1997. **19**(3): 679–686.

132. Disney, A.A., K.V. Domakonda, and C. Aoki, Differential expression of muscarinic acetylcholine receptors across excitatory and inhibitory cells in visual cortical areas V1 and V2 of the macaque monkey. *Journal of Comparative Neurology*, 2006. **499**(1): 49–63.

133. Deco, G., and A. Thiele, Cholinergic control of cortical network interactions enables feedback-mediated attentional modulation. *European Journal of Neuroscience*, 2011. **34**(1): 146–157.

134. Power, J.M., and P. Sah, Competition between calcium-activated K^+ channels determines cholinergic action on firing properties of basolateral amygdala projection neurons. *Journal of Neuroscience*, 2008. **28**(12): 3209–3220.

135. Adelman, J.P., J. Maylie, and P. Sah, Small-conductance Ca^{2+}-activated K^+ channels: form and function. *Annual Review of Physiology*, 2012. **74**: 245–269.

136. Sah, P., and E.S. Faber, Channels underlying neuronal calcium-activated potassium currents. *Progress in Neurobiology*, 2002. **66**(5): 345–353.

137. Tovee, M.J., et al., Information encoding and the responses of single neurons in the primate temporal visual cortex. *Journal of Neurophysiology*, 1993. **70**(2): 640–654.

138. Liu, Y.H., and X.J. Wang, Spike-frequency adaptation of a generalized leaky integrate-and-fire model neuron. *Journal of Computational Neuroscience*, 2001. **10**(1): 25–45.

139. Lin, C.H., H.Y. Lane, and G.E. Tsai, Glutamate signaling in the pathophysiology and therapy of schizophrenia. *Pharmacology Biochemistry and Behavior*, 2012. **100**(4): 665–677.

140. Levin, E.D., Complex relationships of nicotinic receptor actions and cognitive functions. *Biochemical Pharmacology*, 2013. **86**(8): 1145–1152.

141. Zurkovsky, L., W.D. Taylor, and P.A. Newhouse, Cognition as a therapeutic target in late-life depression: potential for nicotinic therapeutics. *Biochemical Pharmacology*, 2013. **86**(8): 1133–1144.

142. Hu, N.W., T. Ondrejcak, and M.J. Rowan, Glutamate receptors in preclinical research on Alzheimer's disease: update on recent advances. *Pharmacology Biochemistry Behavior*, 2012. **100**(4): 855–862.

Mechanisms of Aging-Related Cognitive Decline

Stephen E. Nadeau

1 Introduction

Degenerative disorders that cause cognitive dysfunction have been revealed to be the final common result of an expanding number of mechanisms, with frontotemporal lobar degenerations and Parkinson's disease being outstanding examples. On the other hand, we still tend to view aging effects as a simple result of just plain getting old. As it turns out, mechanisms underlying aging-related alterations in cognitive function are proving to be far more varied and at least as complicated as those underlying dementing disorders. In the foregoing chapters, a host of processes have been identified that could account for these changes. They include processes related to a person's physical and mental condition (e.g., drugs taken, depression, and sleep disorders), changes in the mechanisms underlying various cognitive functions (detailed below), and the development of senescent physiology (Chapter 3) or pathology (Chapter 2). Some of these processes, particularly those related to personal conditions but also aging-related mechanistic changes and alterations in physiology, might be amenable to pharmacological or behavioral interventions. Some mechanistic changes are likely to reflect intrinsic limitations of the human brain. The mechanisms underlying senescent pathology remain obscure; however, given the magnitude of the probable contribution of some of this pathology, for example, myelin degradation, to cognitive dysfunction, at least some of these mechanisms could usefully be targeted for development of neurobiological interventions. It is becoming increasingly clear that, even though the growth of neurons is limited to the dentate gyrus of the hippocampus and the subependymal zones, the brain is a hyperdynamic machine that is kept on its course through the life span by the genome, which is susceptible to damage and the expression of which is susceptible to epigenetic changes (Chapter 3).

In any given elderly person with some impairment in cognitive function, it is not possible to determine with absolute confidence at any given time whether this impairment reflects aging-related changes in cognition or incipient dementia. Particularly in those aged greater than 80, such newly defined degenerative entities as primary age-related tauopathy (PART), hippocampal sclerosis of aging/cerebral age-related TDP-43 with sclerosis (CARTS) [1, 2], and cerebral arteriolosclerosis [3] become progressively more common (Chapter 2). Nevertheless, Alzheimer's disease remains the most common underlying cause of cognitive impairment up to age 100 and beyond. Cognitive hallmarks of Alzheimer's disease, such as impairment in episodic memory and anomia, are also major features of aging-related cognitive impairment, in which case they are most likely caused by senescent neurophysiology in the hippocampus and epigenetic (Chapter 3) and genetic changes [4] across the life span, as well as ontogenic changes in the brain (increasing neighborhood density and age of acquisition effects – see Chapter 8). A nearly certain diagnosis of Alzheimer's disease is now possible using biomarkers (positron emission tomographic imaging of tau and Aβ-amyloid and cerebrospinal fluid studies for tau and amyloid). However, because these studies are expensive and invasive, the best practical way of ruling out Alzheimer's disease as the cause of cognitive impairment is to demonstrate stability of function over the ensuing year.

In this chapter, I will systematically review non-degenerative processes associated with aging-related alterations in cognition, summarizing their potential impact on specific cognitive functions, as reviewed in earlier chapters, and seeking to bring order to this very complex subject.

2 Physical and Mental Condition

Cognitive impairment can be caused by a number of factors related to a person's condition that degrade cognitive function without necessarily causing brain damage. Many of these factors become more prevalent with advancing age. These include fatigue, the use of medications that affect central nervous system function, the presence of pain or situational stress, depression, and alterations in sleep. These factors, particularly drugs and pain, could directly degrade performance on neuropsychological tests. They also could be associated with progressive degradation of the neural substrate for cognitive function.

2.1 Pharmacologic Agents

It is beyond the scope of this chapter to review the many medications that may adversely impact brain function, particularly in late life. However, anticholinergic drugs, because of their importance, warrant some discussion. The substantial replacement of tricyclic antidepressants by serotonin selective reuptake inhibitors (SSRIs) or serotonin/norepinephrine reuptake inhibitors (SNRIs) has tremendously reduced the use of anticholinergic medications. However, the use of "bladder-specific" anticholinergic drugs, particularly in the elderly, in the treatment of urinary incontinence in women and urinary frequency and urgency caused by benign prostatic hyperplasia in men, poses a new source of concern. Newer anticholinergic drugs that do not cross the blood–brain barrier are actively pumped out of the central nervous system (CNS), or are purer agonists of the M3 muscarinic receptor (receptors in the CNS are M1), and therefore do not have CNS effects [5]. These include trospium, darifenacin, and fesoterodine. Unfortunately, old and inexpensive standbys, such as oxybutynin, with well-demonstrated adverse effects on cognition, continue to be widely used. The prescription of such drugs has been associated with an increased odds ratio for dementia [6]. Widespread concerns about the possible risks of benzodiazepines, particularly in combination with opioids, though based on methodologically flawed studies, are leading to a major shift to far less desirable alternatives, such as diphenhydramine (Benadryl) and quetiapine as hypnotics. Diphenydramine is a potent antihistaminergic (hence its sedative effect) but is also strongly anticholinergic.

2.2 Depression and Reduced Activity

The impact of depression on cognitive function has been the focus of almost innumerable studies. Conventional wisdom is that depression does impair cognition, even as the data are far from conclusive. Our own study of changes in cognitive function in patients with refractory depression treated with repetitive transcranial magnetic stimulation (rTMS) revealed that improvement in Hamilton Depression Rating Scale score bore no statistical relationship to changes in multiple domains of cognitive function [7]. However, chronic depression may have a degradative effect on cognitive function through a neuroplastic mechanism. The results of an elegant experiment by Langer and colleagues [8] show why this might be so. They obtained structural MRI scans in patients at the time of initial evaluation for a broken forearm and then 6 weeks later when the cast was removed. During this period, they observed measurable reduction in the thickness of cerebral cortex in the arm–hand region of the motor and somatosensory cortices contralateral to the casted arm, suggesting thinning of the neuropil (axons and dendrites, the anatomic substrates for synapses, which instantiate stored information). Before the age of GPS navigation, London taxi drivers had to have archival episodic memories of the streets in the sprawling city in which they operated. Gray matter volume of the mid- and posterior hippocampi is increased in these taxi drivers compared with controls (bus drivers) with equal travel experience but prespecified routes [9]. Presumably, this reflects increases in hippocampal neuropil – the volume of axons, dendrites, and glial processes. The results of these two studies were anticipated by a much earlier study by Merzenich and his collaborators [10]. Macaques were trained on a sensorimotor task (tracking an uneven rotating wheel with the second and third fingers). Cortical somatosensory area 3b was carefully mapped before and after training. The development of skill in performing the task was associated with a major expansion of the distal digit representations for the second and third fingers in association with reduction in the corresponding areas of representation for the other fingers and in the areas corresponding to more proximal portions of the second and third digits. These studies suggest that the brain is highly plastic, adjusting the amount of cortex invested in a task according to how heavily that particular cortex is engaged. The glutamate receptor α-amino-3-hydroxy-5-methyl-4-isoxazolepropionic acid (AMPA), the foundation of synaptic connection strengths, hence knowledge representation, has a half-life of 30 hours [11]. Thus, the stability of knowledge actually depends on the stability of an ongoing neuroplastic process.

Returning now to depression: daily physical and mental activity is often chronically reduced in patients with depression. One might, therefore, expect "use it or lose it" "atrophy" of cerebral structures whose activity is a marker of cognitive activity. Such "atrophy" has been observed in dorsolateral frontal [12] and anterior supragenual cingulate cortex [13] in patients with depression. Epidemiologic studies have found that the prevalence of depression in people over the age of 65 is 15.9% [14]. General practitioners detect, on average, 47% of cases of depression, and the specificity of diagnosis is 81%. Thus, half of patients with depression are going untreated. There does not appear to be an age effect on diagnostic accuracy.

These findings suggest that neural connectivity within the cortical gray matter, reflected indirectly in the quantity of neuropil, hence cortical thickness, is likely to be highly dynamic and related to the extent and intensity of engagement of particular regions of the cortex. These findings also suggest that imaging studies of cortical thickness need to take into account the possibility that alterations are not necessarily caused by degenerative disease and may be related to intensity and duration of cortical engagement. Emerging MRI techniques, such as neurite orientation dispersion and density imaging (NODDI, Chapter 4) might enable disentanglement of disuse atrophy from pathologic atrophy.

2.3 Sleep

It has long been recognized that sleep quality declines with advancing age [15]. Changes include shorter duration, more fragmented sleep, and reduced amount of slow wave sleep (SWS). These changes are likely to interfere with long-term memory formation and preservation. Two major mechanisms can be defined.

First, sleep has emerged as a crucial period for consolidation of memories [16]. Rapid eye movement (REM) sleep is implicated in the consolidation of nondeclarative memories (e.g., procedural memory). SWS is particularly implicated in the consolidation of episodic memories, via at least two broad mechanisms. Episodic memory retention is enhanced after SWS, suggesting that SWS inhibits the loss of the short-term hippocampal trace. However, there is also abundant evidence that SWS plays a role in memory consolidation as more typically conceived: the gradual transfer of information encoded by synaptic change confined to the hippocampus into changes in connectivity in

cerebral cortex (to the extent that these memories, by virtue of features shared with existing cortical knowledge, can be transferred to cortex [17–20]).

Second, aging-related changes in sleep are likely to interfere with processes underlying synaptic homeostasis [21]. Learning during wakefulness corresponds to increases or decreases in synaptic strengths within neural systems implicated in learning experiences. Eventually, this will lead to saturation of neural connectivity as, over time, synaptic strengths are driven to maximal or minimal values (Chapter 8). Not only does this steadily reduce learning capacity, but it also decreases the ability to selectively encode more important memories. The synaptic homeostasis hypothesis is that during wakefulness, there is, in aggregate, an overall strengthening of synaptic connectivity, while during SWS, there occurs a normalization of synaptic connectivity defined by comprehensive downgrading of synaptic connections strengths. This is constrained by a "survival of the fittest" process in which neural connectivity that is most implicated in the day's knowledge acquisition *and* implicated in existing long-term memory will be least weakened, or even strengthened, while neural connectivity that does not share these attributes will be differentially weakened. Thus, there is preservation of both the capacity for further learning (neuroplasticity) and the capacity for prioritization of knowledge to be retained.

Qualitative disorders of sleep such as obstructive sleep apnea and periodic limb movements of sleep (usually associated with restless limb syndrome) also become more prevalent with advancing age [22, 23]. Not only do these disorders disrupt sleep architecture, but they also cause daytime hypersomnolence, fatigue, and cognitive impairment. Obstructive sleep apnea and periodic limb movements of sleep are both treatable.

3 Mechanistic Changes in Network Processing with Aging

In this section, I will review changes that appear to reflect either the ontogenesis of brain structure and function over the life span or the intrinsic limitations of the brain.

3.1 Endogenous Neural Network Noise

A certain level of neural network noise is functionally indispensable as it helps to assure that a neural network will settle into the optimal attractor basin and not become trapped in a neighboring basin (Chapter 14). However, aging is accompanied by an increase in baseline neural activity – neural noise [24]. Excessive noise can interfere with network settling into any attractor basin, leading to nonresponses. It can also increase the chances of settling into a near-miss basin, something that could, for example, account for near-miss phonological and semantic errors in spoken language (Chapter 8). Increases in neural noise can also contribute to the slowing of processing observed in nearly all studies of aging effects by virtue of resultant slowing of the process of settling into stable representations (attractor states – see below). Neural noise is influenced by dopamine. Dopaminergic stimulation of D1 receptors elicits an inverted U-shaped curve response pattern (a recurring theme with catecholamines – one of the best examples being the Yerkes–Dodson law characterizing noradrenergic response patterns [25–27]). Dopaminergic stimulation of D2 receptors may have the opposite effect on response patterns [28, 29]. Low levels of D1 receptor stimulation are associated with elevated levels of background noise. Intermediate levels improve working memory primarily by suppressing task-irrelevant representations related to excessive background noise. High levels of D1 receptor stimulation impair working memory by suppressing delay-related firing for both irrelevant and relevant representations [29]. Dopamine (potentially augmented by administration of levo-dihydroxyphenylalanine, L-DOPA) stimulates both D1 and D2 receptors. Aging effects on dopamine systems will be discussed further below.

3.2 Neighborhood Density

In Chapter 8, it was noted that, in the course of a lifetime, a large amount of knowledge is accumulated. For example, an older person, when asked about members of the cat family, might respond not just with house cats, lions, tigers, leopards, and cheetahs, but also with ocelots, jaguars, panthers, bobcats, lynxes, snow leopards, servals, caracals, and margays. In other words, the semantic cat neighborhood becomes considerably more crowded (in contrast to the sparse neighborhood featured in Figure 8.1 of Chapter 8). Semantic neighborhood density is greater in the elderly [30]. An older person might also know of more features shared between semantic neighbors. The more features shared between a given exemplar and its neighbors, the broader its attractor basin (the

extreme breath of the mammal attractor basin reflects the astounding number of features that mammals hold in common). Given increased neighborhood density and broader attractor basins, there will tend to be greater overlap between neighboring basins. The latency to descend into the particular attractor basin specified by perceptual input, rather than a near neighbor basin that shares many features, will tend to increase. There will also tend to be more nonresponses that occur when the threshold for one discrete phonological representation is not met, and an increase in the propensity for semantic and phonological slips of the tongue.

Aging-related neighborhood density effects might be seen in any domain in which there is massive accumulation of knowledge or skills over the lifetime. In addition to semantic knowledge and phonologic sequence knowledge, this might include perceptual knowledge and motor skills. Perceptual knowledge is not limited to knowledge of objects as we commonly conceive them. As I have discussed elsewhere, many of the findings in the literature on magnitude estimation can be explained on the basis of limits in the spectrum of experience any one of us has with any particular stimulus modality [31]. For example, a person has extensive experience with line lengths (actual lines but also linear edges), but this experience is limited to a range of lengths, which defines their knowledge of lines. Thus, very long lines and very short lines are statistically likely to fall outside this experience and, therefore, to be underestimated or overestimated, respectively. This tendency to underestimate high magnitudes and overestimate small magnitudes is a recurring theme in the magnitude estimation literature. I make these points only to illustrate that we have vast knowledge of what might generally be regarded as merely featural. However, it is knowledge nonetheless and, therefore, potentially susceptible to aging-related neighborhood effects that might be construed as perceptual inaccuracy or enhanced variability of response rather than near misses. Such featural knowledge may have been of greater evolutionary advantage to our hominoid and Australopithecine ancestors than semantic knowledge. Aging-related neighborhood effects may contribute to the general difficulties in visual perception and the specific difficulties in facial recognition and the facial false-recognition biases noted in Chapter 5.

Emotional perception might also be affected by neighborhood density effects as we store more and more rich and finely textured emotional experiences with their associated visual, auditory, and limbically represented memories.

Skill knowledge is no less scalable than perceptual knowledge. There is a vast literature on ideomotor and limb kinetic praxis, in good part because these skills can be tested anywhere. However, many of the hundreds, if not thousands, of simple movements we execute every day are ballistic movements triggered by specific perceptual inputs deriving from specific contexts. For example, driving our cars involves an enormous repertoire of movements, and yet we do not have to think about putting the key in the ignition, opening the driver's side window, or adjusting the radio, even without looking at it. This domain of skills has scarcely been studied.

3.3 Age of Acquisition

As also discussed in Chapter 8, the acquisition of each new bit of knowledge through the lifetime likely corresponds to ever smaller adjustments in synaptic connection strengths as these strengths asymptotically approach maximum or minimum values. The net result is that early-acquired knowledge is more robust in the face of noise or brain damage, and late-acquired knowledge is more fragile. This gradual saturation of synaptic connectivity may be at least partly ameliorated by processes of synaptic homeostasis [21]. To the extent that synaptic homeostasis fails, the brain may be more likely to fail to generate a response involving late-acquired items. A good example is the tip of the tongue phenomenon that plagues all of us as we advance into late life. There is nothing that says that age of acquisition effects are limited to language (see Chapter 11, on motor programming). More generally, age of acquisition effects reflect the limitations of the cerebral neurobiologic machine: it eventually gets full. Furthermore, while preventing saturation of synaptic connectivity is a good thing, it might come at cost to a domain of knowledge that is not rehearsed for extended periods of time. For example, second language learners typically lose much of their facility if they do not speak the language for years.

Preclinical research has added another dimension to the age of acquisition story. In area 46 (dorsolateral prefrontal cortex) of aging macaques, there is a reduction in the density and an increase in the size of a particular dendritic spine, the so-called thin spine, which is characterized by a high density of N-methyl-D-aspartate (NMDA) glutamate channels (the major molecular mechanism for learning) [32]. In contrast, the density of so-called mushroom spines, which tend to have predominantly AMPA channels (the major substrate for established knowledge), remains stable. In this study, the correlation between the head volume of thin spines and rate of learning on a delayed non-match to sample test was -0.97. The findings of this study suggest that age of acquisition effects may be related in part to an aging-related decline in slender, NMDA channel-loaded, dendritic spines, which steadily, through the life span, reduce the neurobiologic potential for encoding new knowledge in the cortex.

3.4 Selective Engagement

Selective engagement is the bringing online of selected representations in selected neural networks [33], by eliciting alterations in the pattern of neural activity, alterations in the likelihood of neural firing, or selection of inputs that will produce neural firing [34, 35]. Selective engagement is a general term that encompasses the many mechanisms by which the brain allocates resources. In neurodynamical terms, the result of selective engagement is deepening of attractor basins [36]. Mechanisms of selective engagement underlie working memory and attention [33], both of which decline with age (Chapters 7, 8, 10, and 12). Working memory is not attention because it does not involve the focusing of sensory resources on a particular stimulus. However, it may rely on the same or similar underlying neural mechanisms, the physiology of which is altered in the aging process, as discussed in Chapter 14. Working memory capacity does decline with aging (Chapters 8 and 12). To the extent that this decline results in shallower postcentral attractor basins ([36] and Chapter 14), it could worsen neighborhood density effects, thereby contributing to such aging-related symptoms as anomia and impairment of syntax (Chapter 8). Potential mechanistically inspired treatment approaches are discussed below.

3.5 Balance of Volitional and Reactive Intention

The execution of any plan involves a balance between reactive intention and volitional or intentional intention. Reactive intention corresponds to the generation of a plan defined by a distributed representation in frontal cortex that is elicited by activity in postcentral cortex via anterior–posterior connectivity [37]. This connectivity was first defined by Chavis and Pandya [38] (see also [39, 40]). Reciprocal frontal-postcentral projections may also provide the substrate for working memory. Reactive intentional plans reflect well-learned strategies for dealing with everyday contingencies and are invaluable in enabling us to deal with the routine demands of life. For example, little or no planning is needed for routine driving until decisions have to be made (e.g., a turn at a particular intersection that is not part of one's daily route) or unexpected events occur. Little or no planning is needed to name familiar objects or produce verbal responses to simple questions. Volitional intention derives more exclusively from frontal cortical activity and involves the generation of plans that are tailor-made to deal with novel events or situations, future needs, and long-term goals. Aging may be associated with a general shift that favors reactive over volitional intention, leading to what are often characterized as failures of disengagement. The posterior to anterior shift in fMRI activation (PASA) seen in elderly individuals performing cognitively demanding tasks (Chapter 4) might be viewed as evidence against this hypothesis. However, this increased activation is best viewed as evidence of either aging-related loss of specificity of frontal engagement or the greater magnitude and extent of activation that commonly occurs with increased task difficulty.

The cause of the shift favoring reactive intention is uncertain. There are three possibilities. The lifelong accumulation of knowledge and experience may increase the power of postcentral representations deriving from semantic knowledge to drive intention. Aging-related pathology differentially affecting frontal cortex or deep white matter could disadvantage volitional intentional mechanisms (see Chapter 2). Aging-related changes in neurotransmitter function, most particularly norepinephrine, could produce the shift (see below). Attention-deficit hyperactivity disorder (ADHD) can usefully be viewed as an experiment of nature in which reactive intentional (and attentional) mechanisms are pathologically favored. Treatment of patients with ADHD with noradrenergic agents apparently shifts the balance in the direction of frontally mediated volitional mechanisms.

Many of the aging-related cognitive changes described in this book can be ascribed to this pathological shift between substrates for volitional (frontal) and reactive (postcentral) mechanisms. These include aging-related declines in volitional attention (Chapter 10) and related declines in perception stemming from inadequate attention to detail and context, for example, impaired visual perception in general and a specific bias toward false recognition of faces and insensitivity to environmental context in face learning (Chapter 5). This pathological shift could also account for aging-related impairment in working memory (Chapters 8 and 12), narrative discourse (Chapter 8), executive function (Chapter 12), and action-intention (Chapter 11), and the aging-related emotional positivity effect (Chapter 9). In particular, this shift can account for a number of phenomena relatable to aging-related decrements in executive functions, including increasing reliance on automatic responses/prepotent responses, greater reliance on crystallized knowledge, difficulty with self-initiation, cognitive rigidity, deterioration of cognitive control, defective response inhibition, pathological approach and utilization behavior, increased susceptibility to interference and distraction, tendencies to get stuck in set, increased dependency on the environment and greater benefit from perceptual cues (Chapter 12), diminished error awareness (which may be related in part to senescent attenuation of noradrenergic function (Chapter 10 and below)), impairment on tests that require disengagement and divergent thinking, such as the Wisconsin Card Sorting and Stroop color–word interference tests (Chapters 11 and 12), and loss of creativity (Chapter 13).

3.6 Neurotransmitters

Aging-related changes in neurotransmitter function are particularly important, both because of the impact these changes may have on cognitive functions and because deficits are maximally susceptible to pharmacological treatment. We already have many drugs that can potentiate the effects of modulating neurotransmitters such as acetylcholine, norepinephrine, dopamine, and serotonin. We also have drugs that can potentiate the activity of neurotransmitters, such as glutamate, that are the common currency of neural network processing.

3.6.1 Glutamate

Glutamatergic neurons comprise approximately 80% of all neurons in the cerebral cortex and thus constitute the primary engines of neural network processing (Chapter 14). The NMDA channel gates sodium, calcium, and potassium. The passage of sodium and potassium ions through these channels provides the major basis for neural electrophysiology. The passage of calcium is instrumental to the changes in synaptic strengths that constitute learning. Because the channel opens only in the context of simultaneous depolarization of its cell membrane and the presence of glutamate produced by an afferent synapse, it is a coincidence detector, thereby providing the basis for Hebbian learning. Presumably, there is slight loss of glutamatergic neurons with aging and it is unknown to what extent there is aging-associated attrition of synapses. However, animal studies have shown aging-related declines in NMDA receptor-gated glutamate channels, the extent to which varies from region to region [41]. The NMDA glutamate channel is a hetero-tetramer composed of two of four different proteins that cluster like staves of a barrel to form the ion channel. The combination of the proteins in these tetramers evolves through the life span. There is evidence of aging-related decline in NMDA glutamate channel function, and this has been correlated with declines in cognitive function in animals [41]. Unfortunately, because the populations of animals studied were small, it is not possible to tell how much unique variance in cognitive function was explained by NMDA channel dysfunction, above and beyond age per se. The consequence of a decline in NMDA glutamate channel function, as Edmund Rolls has pointed out (Chapter 14), would be to reduce the depths of attractor basins, thereby rendering cortical representations more susceptible to the effects of stochastic noise and less stable.

The other major glutamate-gated channel is the AMPA channel (also a hetero-tetramer), which is generally permeable only to sodium and potassium. Because AMPA channels open and close very quickly, relative to NMDA channels, they are responsible for most of the fast excitatory synaptic transmission in the central nervous system. Aging-related changes in AMPA channels have been less well studied [11].

Because the composition and function of NMDA and AMPA channels is related to their protein composition, the ultimate clues to their aging-related alterations will undoubtedly lie in a better understanding of the underlying molecular genetics. This is especially likely to be true for AMPA channels, which turnover very rapidly (half-life 30 hours) [11].

There is preclinical experimental evidence that the function of NMDA channels can be augmented by d-cycloserine, an old tuberculosis drug that is still available. D-cycloserine is a competitive agonist at the glycine site of the NMDA glutamate receptor. Treatment with the drug has been shown to improve cognitive function [41]. Treatment of young adults with d-cycloserine has been shown to enhance episodic memory acquisition [42], sleep-associated consolidation of declarative memory [43], training of working memory [44], and procedural memory acquisition [45]. There is also evidence that degradation in NMDA glutamate function over the life span may be related to augmentation of oxidative stress with aging ([41]; see also Chapter 3) and that oxidative inhibitors, such as N-acetylcysteine, a precursor to glutathione, can mitigate receptor dysfunction with beneficial effects on cognition. A number of clinical studies have been reported, predominantly in impaired populations (e.g., those with Alzheimer's disease, traumatic brain injury, and psychiatric disease), but the results have been inconclusive [46]. Finally, the drug piracetam, which potentiates AMPA receptor function, was tested in extensive clinical trials in the 1990s, predominantly as a potential adjuvant to reactive neuroplasticity immediately following stroke. An AMPAkine has been shown to mitigate reduction of dendritic branching, augment LTP, and improve long-term memory acquisition in middle-aged rats [47].

3.6.2 Acetylcholine

Rolls (Chapter 14) has described several mechanisms by which acetylcholine promotes cognitive function. Acetylcholine can usefully be viewed as the neurotransmitter of memory formation, both declarative and procedural – that is, as a neurotransmitter that promotes neural plasticity. Cholinergic neurons in the medial septal nuclei and the nucleus of the diagonal band of Broca project to the hippocampal formation, and cholinergic neurons in the nucleus basalis of Meynert project to the entire cerebral cortex. While Hebbian learning ("neurons that fire together wire together") is generally accepted as the driving mechanism for most of the synaptic modification that constitutes learning, neurons fire together extensively without wiring together because they need, in effect, to be told what is important to learn. This instruction is provided by a burst of acetylcholine. The basal forebrain nuclei are informed of what is important by projections to them from limbic structures and the orbitofrontal cortex – the arbiters of subjective value [48] (see also Chapter 14). Potentiation of nucleus basalis activity through micro-stimulation, precisely synchronized with auditory stimuli, has been shown to be capable of inducing complete rewiring of the primary auditory cortex of rats [49]. Saporotoxin-induced destruction of the nucleus basalis profoundly inhibits motor skill learning in rats [50]. Long ago, treatment with a scopolamine, a potent muscarinic acetylcholine receptor blocker, was shown to strongly inhibit episodic memory formation in human volunteers [51].

Nearly 40 years ago, profound loss of neurons in the basal forebrain was noted in Alzheimer's disease (AD). Tacrine, donepezil, rivastigmine, and galantamine, all inhibitors of acetylcholinesterase, have been shown to slow cognitive decline in patients with AD [52]. It has generally been assumed that the benefits of these acetylcholinesterase inhibitors were mediated through normalization of cortical and hippocampal acetylcholine in these patients. However, the studies reviewed above, as well as clinical trial data [53], suggest that the beneficial effects of cholinergic agents might be mediated through enhancement of neural plasticity, thereby exerting a palliative effect acting, as in Alzheimer's disease, to potentiate learning/relearning on an ongoing basis, thereby inhibiting the loss of knowledge and skills. Thus, patients with AD treated with acetylcholinesterase inhibitors may experience slower cognitive decline because they are able to take better advantage of the cognitive rehabilitation implicit in active participation in daily life.

It was also noted in Chapter 14 that acetylcholine elicits cortical activation, producing arousal, thus facilitating concentration and attention and deepening cortical attractor basins. It can decrease transmission in recurrent collateral excitatory connections, thereby reducing the effects of memories already stored in the recurrent collaterals so that they do not excessively influence the neuronal firing when new memories must be stored. Acetylcholine can act via a nicotinic receptor to enhance thalamocortical transmission. It can also inhibit adaptation to sustained high firing rates of cortical neurons.

The size of the cholinergic nuclei in the basal forebrain declines linearly across much of the life span, the decline accelerating somewhat after the age of 65 [54]. Corresponding changes in cortical choline acetyltransferase or acetyl cholinesterase have not, to our knowledge, been reported but can be assumed to drop in parallel with atrophy of the basal forebrain nuclei. There have been studies of acetylcholinesterase inhibitors as "neuro-enhancers" in normal participants [55] (see also Chapter 17). However, trials have been very small and, with few exceptions, limited to younger subjects. Thus, there has not been an adequate test of Rolls's neurodynamically motivated hypothesis on the potentially beneficial effects of cholinomimetic drugs on working memory, attention, and episodic memory (Chapter 14). Both short- and long-term trials might be considered: short-term trials to test the adjuvant effect on these cognitive functions, long-term trials to test the effects of enhanced neuroplasticity on learning and relearning, as reflected in greater retention of knowledge and skills.

3.6.3 Norepinephrine

Potentiation of noradrenergic function could provide a means for treatment of aging-related cognitive decline related to a pathologic imbalance between frontal (volitional) and postcentral (reactive) mechanisms of intention and attention, as it does in ADHD. More specifically, it could correct aging-related deficits in working memory function, and, as Robertson and Dockree surmise (Chapter 10), it could, via its effect on the mechanisms underlying working memory, increase frontal-postcentral connectivity in a way that would support error awareness. As noted in Chapter 14, norepinephrine, by reducing shunting inhibition of synaptic inputs, strengthens attractor networks, maintaining their stability for more prolonged periods. Shunting inhibition occurs when an excitatory postsynaptic potential (EPSP) traveling down a dendrite passes through a region in which an inhibitory postsynaptic potential has just been generated. The amplitude of the EPSP is thereby reduced.

The locus coeruleus is the source of all noradrenergic projections to the cerebrum. There is a 50% loss of locus coeruleus neurons between ages 1 and 104 [56]. Cell loss is not synonymous with loss of noradrenergic terminals as compensatory branching of axons can occur. Ligands for the norepinephrine transporter have been developed [57, 58]. Ding et al. [57] demonstrated a 65% decrease in transporter density in the pulvinar and hypothalamus between ages 25 and 54. As noted by Conrad and Chatterjee (Chapter 17), amphetamine, methylphenidate, and atomoxetine (which act on both noradrenergic and dopaminergic systems) have been shown to enhance attention, reaction time, short-term memory, and language learning. A study of macaque monkeys showed an aging-related decline in the firing rate of neurons in prefrontal cortex that normally support working memory by persistently firing during the delay period after stimulus presentation. Iontophoretic application of the alpha-2 agonist guanfacine significantly increased firing of these neurons [59]. Wilson et al. [60] reported a study of 165 normal human elderly participants in which cognitive functions were assessed serially for 5.8 years premortem, and cell densities of neurons in the locus coeruleus (norepinephrine), dorsal raphe (serotonin), substantia nigra (dopamine), and ventral tegmental area (dopamine) were determined postmortem. They found that cell density in the locus coeruleus uniquely accounted for rate of cognitive decline. Rate of decline in participants in the lowest quartile was approximately three times that of those in the upper 50th percentile.

Unfortunately, a phase II human study of guanfacine failed to show a treatment effect [61]. To our knowledge, studies have not been conducted employing alpha-1 or beta agonists or nonspecific adjuvants to noradrenergic function.

3.6.4 Dopamine

Augmentation of dopaminergic function could also provide a potential means for treatment of aging-related cognitive decline related to a pathologic imbalance between frontal, volitional, and postcentral reactive mechanisms of intention and attention. Robertson and Dockree (Chapter 10) pointed out that most of the aging-related variance in executive function (as operationally defined by performance on a spatial working memory test) can be accounted for by D1 receptor density [62] (see also Chapter 12). Aging-related decline in dopaminergic function could account for the more frequent manifestation of depression in the aged as anhedonia (Chapter 9). As Rolls has noted (Chapter 14), dopamine D1 receptor blockade can decrease the conductance of NMDA receptor–activated ion channels, thereby reducing

the depth of cortical attractor basins, particularly in prefrontal regions. In a recent meta-analysis of 95 studies involving a total of 2,611 individuals, the correlation of age with measures of D1 receptors, D2 receptors, and the dopamine transporter (a measure of density of dopaminergic synapses) was 0.68–0.77 [63]. Dopamine synthesis capacity in the striatum did not change with age, whereas there is some evidence that it declines in frontal cortex (synthesis is by aromatic amino acid decarboxylase located in axonal boutons). D1 receptors declined an average of 14% per decade after age 20; D2 receptors 8.2%; the dopamine transporter (striatum) 9.9%; and dopamine synthesis in the frontal cortex 10.8% and in the striatum 1.4%. The aging-related reduction in the dopamine transporter could have a compensatory effect as it would serve to reduce dopamine reuptake (the primary means by which dopamine is cleared from the synaptic cleft).

There have been more than 30 published trials of dopaminergic treatment (usually a single dose of L-DOPA 100–150 mg + benserazide 37.5 mg) in young adults. These studies have demonstrated positive drug effects on measures of executive function and, thus, provide proof of principle. The closest we come to studies of aged subjects is research on patients with Parkinson's disease on and off L-DOPA. Off L-DOPA, these patients exhibit impairments on the Tower of London task, spatial working memory tests, and task-switching paradigms. On the latter, they exhibit enhanced switching costs but reduced distractability relative to age-matched controls [29]. Both effects are reversed with resumption of L-DOPA treatment.

As noted in our discussion of the potential adverse effects of excessive background neural noise, the augmentation of working memory function and cognitive control by stimulation of D1 dopaminergic receptors is characterized by an inverted U-shaped dose–response curve. Optimal doses maximize suppression of neural activity associated with irrelevant responses without significantly compromising signal-related neural activity. Suboptimal doses fail to suppress background noise and super-optimal doses reduce both signal and background [29, 64]. Given the reduced levels of dopaminergic receptors and terminals in the aged, they are the most likely to benefit from L-DOPA, which stimulates both D1 and D2 receptors. The several available dopamine receptor agonists predominantly stimulate D2 receptors.

3.6.5 Serotonin

The entire cerebrum receives serotonergic afferents deriving from neurons in the dorsal raphe nucleus, which is located in the dorsal midline tegmentum at the junction between the midbrain and the pons. Seven serotonergic receptors have been identified, six of them metabotrophic (the action of serotonin (5-hydroxytriptamine, 5-HT) is mediated by G-protein coupled receptors (5-HT$_{1, 2, 4-7}$)) and one involving a ligand-gated cation channel (5-HT$_3$) [65]. 5-HT$_2$ receptors are implicated in depression. Serotonin action at some 5-HT receptors is excitatory and at others inhibitory. Serotonergic receptors are located variously on cholinergic, GABA-ergic, and glutaminergic neurons, some immediately adjacent to NMDA glutamate or GABA receptors. Data on aging-related changes affecting the serotonergic system are incomplete. The population of neurons in the dorsal raphe nucleus appears to be stable. The 5-HT transporter (the mechanism for reuptake of synaptic serotonin) appears to be stable, although as much as 50% loss over the lifetime has been noted in the cingulate gyrus. Aging-related reductions in 5-HT$_{1A}$, 5-HT$_{2A}$, and 5-HT$_4$ of 7–10% per decade have been documented.

The complexity of serotonergic systems has defied attempts to develop a unifying account of serotonin effects on cognitive function. However, experience using drugs that potentiate serotonergic activity to treat depression may be instructive. I have proposed that serotonergic input to the prefrontal cortex may, among other things, influence the balance of engagement between dorsolateral prefrontal cortex and orbitofrontal-limbic cortex and their relative contributions to the development of action plans [66] – in neurodynamical terms, altering the relative depths of attractor basins in the two domains. The dorsolateral prefrontal cortex provides the major basis for shaping of plans on the basis of objective input deriving from perception and semantic memory. In contrast, the orbitofrontal-limbic cortex plays a critical role in shaping plans on the basis of subjective value. Emotional valuation is subjective. In the 1940s and 1950s, undercutting of the orbitofrontal cortex (orbitofrontal leucotomy) was used extensively in the treatment of refractory depression [67]. Because of its effectiveness, it is the only psychosurgical procedure that lives on to this day in the form of ablative lesions or deep brain stimulation of the ventral anterior limb of the

internal capsule or the nucleus accumbens (both investigational). Orbitofrontal leucotomy serves to reduce the impact of limbic activity on plan development for thoughts and actions, freeing patients from the slavery imposed by the dysfunctional orbitofrontal-limbic system and allowing them to resume constructive thoughts and actions. Antidepressants, whether tricyclics, SSRIs, or SNRIs, appear to achieve the same end, albeit by chemical means. Furthermore, both orbitofrontal leucotomy and its modern variants and treatment with SSRIs is occasionally complicated by the development of a profound apathy syndrome. If our hypothesis on the mechanism for serotonergic effects on cognition is correct, then treatment with serotonergic drugs could augment dorsolateral prefrontal activity, attenuate orbitofrontal-limbic activity, or both. As predicted, administration of fluvoxamine, an SSRI, leads to advantageous performance on the Iowa Gambling Test, that is, a tendency to use a less risky strategy [68]. Furthermore, the short allelic variant of the serotonin transporter gene, which is associated with reduced expression of the gene and reduction of the serotonin transporter at the synapse, hence increased synaptic serotonin, is also associated with advantageous behavior on the Iowa Gambling Test [69].

To our knowledge, there have been no studies of the impact of SSRIs or SNRIs on cognitive function per se. However, a recent phase III trial of an atypical antidepressant, vortioxetine, involving 598 patients with depression, tested the impact of drug treatment on a number of executive functions, including the digit symbol substitution test, the Rey Auditory Verbal Learning Test, the Trail Making Test (parts A and B), the congruent and incongruent forms of the Stroop test, and simple and complex reaction times [70]. Vortioxetine inhibits serotonin reuptake and is a 5-HT$_{1D, 3 \& 7}$ receptor antagonist and a 5-HT$_{1A, B}$ agonist. Treatment with vortioxetine enhanced performance on all the tests listed with effect sizes in the 0.3–0.5 range. Improvement in depression accounted for only part of the variance in cognitive change, and substantial cognitive improvement was noted even in patients who exhibited no antidepressant effect.

3.7 Brain Ontogenesis

In Chapter 8, I reviewed the substantial evidence that, with increasing age, there is an increase in the relative incidence of Wernicke's aphasia in the context of brain injury (stroke or neoplasm). There is abundant evidence that the brain encodes knowledge of sequences, best exemplified in language (phonology, morphology, phrase structure, and syntax), praxis, and music. The hypothesis proposed to account for the increasing incidence of Wernicke's aphasia was that, over the course of the life span, such sequence knowledge expands to provide the basis for ever-longer sequences, perhaps, in the domain of language, including simple sentences and clauses, even as frontal cortex continues to provide the major substrate for sequential organization and modification of concept representations. On this basis, language sequence might be relatively preserved even with large frontal lesions that, in younger patients, produce Broca's aphasia. In this setting, serious disruptions of sequence would tend to occur mainly with posterior lesions that severely damage the major substrate for multi-morphemic sequence knowledge and its connectivity to the substrate for concept representations, yielding Wernicke's aphasia, because of either loss of this knowledge in the dominant hemisphere or inadequately developed knowledge in the nondominant hemisphere.

Can this expanding repertoire of phonological and morphological sequence knowledge account in any way for aging-related degradation of language function? Possibly so. If, with aging, there is a shift in the balance of volitional and reactive intention, as discussed earlier, this could lead to overreliance on postcentral systems. The consequence for language would be overreliance on the repertoire of sequences reinforced through a lifetime of speaking with associated loss of flexibility in adapting sentence structure to the unique demands of the conversational moment. Of course, such flexibility could also be lost because of degradation in prefrontal function. Unfortunately, we lack empirical evidence of aging-related impairment in syntactic function beyond that relatable to impairment in working memory.

Analogous reasoning should apply to praxis. Unfortunately for our argument, studies of praxis typically involve the ability to perform well-learned sequences involving tool use. The true test of prefrontally mediated praxis would be a test of praxis syntax: the creative development of new extended motor sequences to meet the particular demands of a novel situation. Perhaps it was an aging-related deficit in praxis syntax, due to either excessive influence by already learned sequences or diminished ability to

acquire new sequences, that accounted for Kenneth Heilman's difficulty in acquiring skill at golf in mid-life (Chapter 11).

4 Senescent Physiology

4.1 Hippocampal Physiology

Earlier in this chapter, I introduced the concept that the brain is highly plastic, adapting the extent of cortical investment in particular knowledge and skills according to how much these are routinely utilized, constrained, and promoted by the processes of synaptic homeostasis. Thinking about the brain in this way highlights the importance of lifelong ability to modify synaptic strengths, that is, to learn. Unfortunately, as detailed in Chapter 3, with advancing age, there is increased or more prolonged activation of redox signaling cascades, sometimes referred to as redox stress, which induce changes in Ca^{2+} regulation. By well-established mechanisms, this gradually shifts the balance between long-term potentiation (LTP) and long-term depression (LTD) in the direction of LTD. Changes in redox state and in Ca^{2+}-mediated effects on LTP and LDP are referred to as senescent physiology. The effects of senescent physiology have most clearly been shown in the hippocampus, accounting for the decline in episodic memory formation seen with aging (Chapter 7) and aging-related decline in capacity for recollection, which is hippocampally dependent, with relative sparing of familiarity, which is not (Chapter 12). The effects of senescent physiology have also been shown in prefrontal cortex (Chapter 3), accounting, at least in part, for degradation in executive functions observed with aging (Chapter 12). However, senescent physiology might also affect postcentral cortices.

LTP includes both short-term (early LTP) and long-term (late LTP) components. The glutamate-activated NMDA voltage-sensitive sodium/calcium ion channel–mediated calcium fluxes that underlie early LTP culminate in the insertion of additional, already available, AMPA glutamate channels in the postsynaptic membrane, thereby strengthening the synapse. We are unaware of any treatment studies directed at the senescent decline in early LTP described in Chapter 3. Gene transcription and protein synthesis – the basis for late LTP – are required for the transient synaptic strengthening achieved by early LTP to be sustained over the long run. There do exist treatment studies directed at late LTP, which is potentiated by dopamine [71]. Chowdhury et al. [72] tested the effect of L-DOPA 150 mg plus benserazide 37.5 mg in 32 healthy older adults (mean age 70.31 ± 3.22) on a recognition memory task involving indoor and outdoor scenes, some of which were linked with a monetary reward. L-DOPA treatment significantly increased "remember" hits 6 hours but not 2 hours after dosing, and the effect was observed only for unrewarded scenes. There was an inverted-U dose–response curve, such that the effect was maximal at a dose of 2 mg/kg and declined quite precipitously at lower or higher doses (dose variation deriving from variation in body weights of the participants). The fact that the effect was observed only for unrewarded stimuli suggested that it was achieved by dopaminergic potentiation of reward mechanisms. The fact that it was observed at 6 hours and not 2 hours suggested that it reflected hippocampal memory consolidation, a process that requires protein synthesis, and not hippocampal encoding. Comparable augmentation of verbal episodic memory has been demonstrated in a younger population [73]. In summary, aging-related deficits in hippocampal functions in general, including episodic memory formation and recollection, could be related to senescent pathology (Chapter 2), senescent physiology (Chapter 3), or decrements in acetylcholinergic or dopaminergic function.

Procedural memory acquisition does not depend on hippocampal mechanisms. Nevertheless, augmentation of procedural memory acquisition by L-DOPA treatment has been reported in older adults [74], involves the D1 receptor, and exhibits the expected inverted-U shaped dose–response curve [75].

4.2 Hippocampal Neurogenesis

Neuronal proliferation occurs throughout the lifetime in only two loci, the subependymal regions and the dentate gyrus of the hippocampus. Only the latter appears to be of functional importance. In fact, the continued proliferation of dentate neurons appears to play an essential role in episodic memory formation.

In the hippocampus, the approximately 20 million dentate granule cells receive extensive projections from the entorhinal cortex via the perforant pathway [19]. This input reflects the extensively overlapping representations supported by the cerebral cortex, almost the entirety of which projects to the entorhinal cortex via the perirhinal and parahippocampal

cortices. Very rapid competitive learning within the dentate serves to markedly reduce overlap between the input representations [19]. The cerebral cortex, with its extensive autoassociator networks and high degree of interconnectivity within networks (providing the basis for what are termed *dense* representations), is a highly effective instrument for detecting commonalities between representations. In contrast, processing by the dentate achieves the *sparse* (non-overlapping, non-orthogonal) representations needed for pattern separation. This sparseness is further enhanced by the very limited but powerful projections (via the mossy fibers) from any given granule cell to CA3 pyramidal neurons, and by the fact that CA3 pyramidal neurons respond only to the strongest inputs from the dentate. This ingenious system serves a foundational purpose. In the cortex, overlap between representations is essential to our capacity for building up general (semantic) knowledge from a series of individual experiences, our implicit understanding of the hierarchical organization of semantic domains (e.g., Labradors are dogs, which are canines, which are mammals, which are animals, which are vertebrates . . .), and for content-addressable memory (perceiving a single feature of a representation elicits the full representation). However, for learning to be specific to particular semantic exemplars or characteristics of exemplars, the overlaps between representations supported by cortical knowledge must be minimalized so that what is learned does not apply to entire semantic domains. Furthermore, the overlap must be minimalized so that new knowledge can be acquired without replacing old knowledge [18]. The dentate-CA3 system effectively eliminates the overlaps and achieves pattern separation [19, 76]. It enables the coding of small differences between cortical representations (e.g., those generated by perception of very similar objects) as episodic memories.

Dentate neurogenesis declines by about 75% across the life span [77]. The reasons for this decline are not known. The decline in dentate turnover has particular importance because it is young dentate neurons that achieve maximal pattern separation [76]. It could account for the aging-related increase in false facial recognition and reductions in visual discrimination ability on episodic memory tasks observed in older people (Chapter 5). More generally, it could lead to memory formation that is progressively more oblivious to the fact that "the devil is in the details."

5 Senescent Pathology

In Chapter 2, Anthony Yachnis described a host of gross and histological changes in the brain associated with aging.

5.1 General Changes

There is reduction is both gray and white matter volume. This could occur because of reduction in interstitial fluid in the brain, shrinkage of neurons and glia, reduction of myelin thickness, or axonal loss [78]. Whether it has implications for cognitive function is unknown. Aging is associated with a 5–10% loss of cortical neurons that is most marked in the hippocampus and the frontal cortex (Chapter 2). This may or may not have adverse consequences. Axons are the "business end" of neurons (they may have up to 10,000 times the volume of the cell body). Axons give rise to nearly all synapses, wherein the knowledge is stored as connection strengths, and they are capable of sprouting. A 10% loss of neurons could be more than compensated by an increase in axonal branches or synaptic density.

Aging is associated with the accumulation of a number of histologic markers, including lipofuschin, neurofibrillary tangles (polymerized phorphorylated tau), Hirano and Marinesco bodies, and corpora amylacea. Granulovacuolar degeneration, increases in glial fibrillary acid protein, and microvascular changes are also observed. We can only assume that these abnormalities reflect accumulating imperfections in genetic ("geniosenium" [4]), epigenetic (Chapter 3), molecular genetic, and molecular biological processes that result in the slow accumulation of nonfunctional end products – the senescent proteinopathy to which Yachnis alludes. Whether or not these end products impair the cellular machinery involved in cognitive function is unknown.

Astrocytes provide essential trophic support for neurons, mediate uptake and recycling of neurotransmitters (particularly important for glutamate, which can be neurotoxic), and are involved in maintenance of the blood–brain barrier. Aging is associated with transcriptional changes in astrocytes, likely mediated by epigenetic mechanisms, that favor the expansion of an inflammatory astrocytic phenotype that is characterized by reduced ability to support neural function and a propensity for production of complement and neurotoxic substances [79].

5.2 Myelin Changes

It was noted in Chapter 8 that transcallosal conduction velocities in elderly participants are 77–81% of those in younger participants [80], and central motor conduction velocities in the elderly are 81% of those in young participants [81]. These electrophysiologic changes strongly suggest alterations in myelin as myelin investment of axons enables saltatory conduction, increasing speed of conduction by a factor of 30–50. As described in Chapter 2, a number of aging-associated white matter changes have been noted. These include the macroscopic finding of myelin pallor (corresponding to leukoaraiosis on imaging studies) and electron microscopic findings of local demyelination, localized splitting of the major dense line of myelin, ballooning and reduplication of myelin sheaths, and separation of myelin from the axon [82]. As Liu et al. [82] note, there may be loss of integrity of the paranode, which anchors the myelin to the axolemma at nodes of Ranvier. To the extent that this occurs, nodes of Ranvier are lengthened, thereby inserting extended regions along the axon over which conduction velocity is reduced from 50 m/s to 1–2 m/s. The distance between nodes of Ranvier decreases with aging, thereby requiring more saltatory "hops" for the action potential to travel from the axon hillock near the cell body to axon terminals. With loss or disruption of myelin, there is an aging-related increase in radial diffusivity, an imaging measure of the tendency of water molecules to diffuse in directions transverse to axons [83].

Imaging studies have provided additional insights into the evolution of white matter changes through the life span (Chapter 4). Yeatman and colleagues [84] used an imaging sequence, R1 (1/T1), that is primarily driven by changes in myelin content. They found an inverse parabolic pattern of myelin density such that density increased steadily up to age 40–50 and then declined steadily thereafter, reaching levels at age 80 that were similar to those at age 8. Whereas all fiber tracts exhibited the same pattern, changes were most marked in ventral tracts, for example, temporal and orbitofrontal white matter. Magnitude of change was intermediate in more dorsal frontal white matter and the anterior third of the corpus callosum and least in motor pathways, the optic radiations, and the posterior two-thirds of the corpus callosum. There were no right–left hemispheric asymmetries.

Reduction of white matter conduction velocity of whatever cause could have substantial consequences for cognitive function. Aging-related impairment in processing speed accounts for 70–80% of the variance in other cognitive variables (Chapter 12). Cognitive processes in general depend on repeated back and forth, top-down/bottom-up transmission along white matter tracts as the brain settles into attractor states. Consider that a cognitive function with a 1-second latency would allow over 150 back-and-forth transmissions between fronto-polar and occipito-polar cortex, assuming an axonal conduction velocity of 50 meters per second and a brain length of 15 centimeters. Thus, aging-associated myelin changes could substantially account for reductions in processing speed and increases in reaction times (Chapter 11). Such reductions could have further ramifications. Cognitive processes that are particularly dependent on prefrontal function (Chapter 12), including creativity (Chapter 13), could be differentially slowed because of the length of the white matter tracts between prefrontal cortex and both postcentral cortices and subcortical structures. In partial support for this hypothesis, Serbruyns et al. [85] found that an imaging measure of myelin density, magnetization transfer ratio, accounted for 29% of the non-aging-associated variance in switching cost on a Navon-like figure task. Processes involving anterior callosal transmission might be similarly affected (Chapter 11). Aging-related myelin changes could degrade as well as slow processes like executive function and creativity that are dependent on the integrity of long intra- and interhemispheric connections. Working memory actually involves a combination of sustained cortical engagement and hippocampal encoding as episodic memory [86]. The longer that working memory must be sustained, the greater the reliance on the hippocampal system. Hippocampal function declines with aging (Chapter 7), substantially because of senescent physiology (Chapter 3). Some of the aging-related decrement in working memory could be due to this combination of slowed conduction and hippocampal dysfunction.

Whereas reduced central conduction velocities may provide an explanation for aging-related decrements in executive functions subserved by the lateral prefrontal cortex (Chapter 12), it is notable that executive functions particularly dependent on orbitofrontal cortex (processes requiring subjective judgment) are relatively spared [87], despite the greater aging-related pathology in ventral myelin [84]. This may mean that aging-related reduction in central conduction velocities is not so important, or that the influence of orbitofrontal-limbic function is intrinsically more sustained over time – in neurodynamical terms, that attractor states in this region tend to be more enduring (Chapter 14).

As noted in Chapter 8, reduction of conduction velocities could also differentially impact right hemisphere function (Chapters 9–11 and 13). There is reason to believe that one of the fundamental properties that distinguishes right and left hemisphere function is a greater extent of left hemisphere cortex dedicated to networks supporting categorical sequence knowledge (e.g., phonology, grammar, arithmetic, musical rhythm, and praxis) [88]. Such sequence knowledge is less likely to be important for the sorts of Gestalt processing long associated with the right hemisphere, for example, global attention, visuospatial function, affective prosody, emotional function (including recognition of facial emotions, the aging-related positivity effect, and alexithymia (Chapter 9)), musical melody, and personality. Much sequence knowledge may be adequately supported by networks characterized by relatively short white matter connections, for example, the phonologic and grammatic morphologic sequence knowledge that is supported predominantly by left perisylvian cortex. On the other hand, egocentric visuospatial function, for example, may depend on a representation of the entire spatial world, thus requiring engagement of the entire parietal and linked frontal association cortices and requiring use of many long white matter pathways.

Finally, axons in the cortical mantle are myelinated as well. Changes in cortical myelin, which mirror the aging-related changes in deep myelin [89], could alter the neurodynamical processes discussed by Rolls (Chapter 14).

6 Conclusion

In 1928, the brilliant scientist, extraordinary mentor, and Nobel laureate Santiago Ramon y Cajal stated that "once formed in youth, [synapses] cannot be newly formed after puberty and become immutable" [90]. In the modern era, this concept of CNS immutability has been qualified, as evidence of neuroplasticity, the mechanistic foundation for neurorehabilitation, has become manifest. However, as we have seen in this

Table 15.1 Dimensions of brain dynamics

Dimension	Approximate time scale
Internetwork and top-down/bottom-up intranetwork transmission during process of settling into attractor states that complete an action, e.g., word naming	0.025 seconds (gamma frequency)[a]
Achievement of early LTP instantiating episodic memory in hippocampus	1 second
Late LTP: interrogation of genome and protein synthesis	Hours
Synaptic turnover (AMPA receptor replacement)	Half-life 30 hours
Synaptic modification in process of memory consolidation	Sleep: daily
Synaptic modification in processes of synaptic homeostasis	Sleep: daily
Regional structural adaptation of neuropil (axodendritic architecture) to altered patterns of use	Weeks to months
Cerebral ontogenesis	Years
Evolution of aging-related changes in redox state	Years
Epigenetic evolution	Years
Time required for brain to fill with knowledge	100 years

[a] The exact role of gamma frequency oscillations remains uncertain. However, the frequency range (25–100 Hz) corresponds roughly to the time required for neural transmission from one brain region to another at 50 m/s.

book and in the mechanistic précis I have attempted in this chapter, it is now clear that even this modified version of the Ramon y Cajal concept has become outmoded. Perhaps nothing says this more emphatically than the discovery that the AMPA receptor, the very linchpin of synaptic strength and the foundation for our seemingly stable knowledge, has a half-life of 30 hours [11]. The brain is a hyper-dynamic machine. At one extreme, scores or even hundreds of back-and-forth neural transmissions occur between the various regions of the brain in less than a second as it settles into constellations of attractor states defining cerebral representations. Complete turnover of AMPA receptors occurs every 2 weeks. Regional changes in neuropil related to the activity of the organism and detectable with structural imaging can apparently take place in as little as a month. Changes involving epigenetics, evolution of the redox cycle, and alterations in white matter and neurotransmitters, as well as ontogenesis of the cerebrum, occur over decades (Table 15.1). As we have seen, ontogenesis over the life span involves important changes in the cerebral representation of language, a shift in the balance of frontal and postcentral processing favoring the latter, attenuation of right hemisphere functions, and deterioration of episodic memory.

It is now more accurate to characterize the brain as a slowly evolving steady-state machine. We must no longer confine our scientific inquiry to what influences change. We must turn the question around and ask, What mechanisms sustain the steady state despite its intrinsic mutability? We must consider the possibility that aberrant human behavior reflects inherent instability in the operation of a machine that is governed by nonlinear neurodynamics, hence chaotic properties. The evolution of cognitive function and its mechanistic underpinnings through the life span, detailed in this volume, appears, thankfully, to be more gradual, although not entirely linear.

There has long been a popular concept that the average person uses only 10% of their brain. We now know that we use 100% of our brains 100% of the time, even as the distribution of activity varies enormously depending on the constellation of environmental stimuli, stored knowledge, plans for thought or action, and waking/sleeping state. We also now have some evidence, presented in this book, that over the course of a full life span, we routinely plumb the limits of cerebral capabilities. Neighborhood effects empower generalization, inference, and synonymy early in life, but as neighborhoods become more crowded and working memory degrades, they apparently can become deleterious. The loss of flexibility of the synapse over the lifetime, with its limiting effect on learning and memory consolidation, has evidently been of sufficient importance to the survival of the species that mechanisms of synaptic homeostasis have evolved.

The remaining chapters in this book summarize our knowledge of how to bend the curve of evolution of the cerebral steady state over the life span in ways that enhance cognitive function and may provide some protection against the incursions of dementing processes. These chapters detail the near-term options. Looking beyond, one might address the

challenge of bending this curve in a different way. There are many varieties of brilliance. Some (e.g., Einstein, Bach, and savants) are inscrutable. However, we could agree that one characteristic of many "highly intelligent" people is that their brains are capable of storing an extraordinary quantity of knowledge and accessing it readily. This suggests that certain brains are better at handling some of the aging-related problems I have discussed. These include neighborhood density effects, age of acquisition effects, suboptimal synaptic homeostasis, reduced pattern separation, and degraded learning. The properties and processes involved may be susceptible to modification.

References

1. Nelson PT, Trojanowski JQ, Abner EL, Al-Janabi OM, Jicha GA, Schmitt FA, et al. "New old pathologies": AD, PART, and cerebral age-related TDP-43 with sclerosis [CARTS]. *Journal of Neuropathology and Experimental Neurology.* 2016;75:482–98.

2. Neltner JH, Abner EL, Jicha GA, Schmitt FA, Patel E, Poon LW, et al. Brain pathologies in extreme old age. *Neurobiology of Aging.* 2016;37:1–11.

3. Kryscio RJ, Abner EL, Nelson PT, Benbnett D, Schneider Js, Yu L, et al. The effect of vascular neuropathology on late-life cognition: results from the SMART Project. *Journal of Prevention of Alzheimer's Disease.* 2016;3:85–91.

4. Lodato MA, Rodin RE, Bohrson CL, Coulter ME, Barton AR, Kwon M, et al. Aging and neurodegeneration are associated with increased mutations in single human neurons. *Science.* 2018;359:555–9.

5. Chancellor MB, Staskin DR, Kay GG, Sandage BW, Oefelein MG, Tsao JW. Blood–brain barrier permeation and efflux exclusion of anticholinergics used in the treatment of overactive bladder. *Drugs Aging.* 2012;29:259–73.

6. Richardson K, Fox C, Maidment I, Steel N, Loke YK, Arthur A, et al. Anticholinergic drugs and risk of dementia: a case-control study. *British Medical Journal.* 2018;360: k1315.

7. Nadeau SE, Bowers D, Jones TL, Wu SS, Triggs WJ, Heilman KM. Cognitive effects of treatment of depression with repetitive transcranial magnetic stimulation. *Cognitive and Behavioral Neurology.* 2014;27:77–87.

8. Langer N, Hänggi J, Müller NA, Simmen HP, Jäncke L. Effects of limb immobilization on brain plasticity. *Neurology.* 2012;78:182–8.

9. Maguire EA, Woollett K, Spiers HJ. London taxi drivers and bus drivers: a structural MRI and neuropsychological analysis. *Hippocampus.* 2006;16:1091–101.

10. Jenkins WM, Merzenich MM, Recanzone G. Neocortical representational dynamics in adult primates: implications for neuropsychology. *Neuropsychologia.* 1990;28:573–84.

11. Henley JM, Wilkinson KA. AMPA receptor trafficking and the mechanisms underlying synaptic plasticity and cognitive aging. *Dialogues in the Clinical Neurosciences.* 2013;15:11–27.

12. Vasic N, Wolf ND, Sosic-Vasic Z, Connemann BJ, Sambataro F, von Strombeck A, et al. Baseline brain perfusion and brain structure in patients with major depression: a multimodal magnetic resonance imaging study. *Journal of Psychiatry and Neuroscience.* 2015;40:412–21.

13. Goodkind M, Eickhoff SB, Oathes DJ, Jiang Y, Chang A, Jones-Hagata LB, et al. Identification of a common neurobiological substrate for mental illness. *JAMA Psychiatry.* 2015;72:305–15.

14. Mitchell AJ, Vaze A, Rao S. Clinical diagnosis of depression in primary care: a meta-analysis. *Lancet.* 2009;374:609–19.

15. Mander BA, Winer JR, Walker MP. Sleep and human aging. *Neuron.* 2017;94:19–36.

16. Leger D, Debellemaniere E, Rabat A, Bayon V, Benchenane K, Chennaoui M. Slow-wave sleep: from the cell to the clinic. *Sleep Medicine Reviews.* 2018.

17. Alvarez P, Squire LR. Memory consolidation and the medial temporal lobe: a simple network model. *Proceedings of the National Academy of Sciences.* 1994;91:7041–5.

18. McClelland JL, McNaughton BL, O'Reilly RC. Why there are complementary learning systems in the hippocampus and neocortex: insights from the successes and failures of connectionist models of learning

and memory. *Psych Rev.* 1995;102:419–57.

19. Rolls ET. *Cerebral Cortex: Principles of Operation.* Oxford: Oxford University Press; 2016.

20. Squire LR, Zola-Morgan S. The medial temporal lobe memory system. *Science.* 1991;253:1380–6.

21. Tononi G, Cirelli C. Sleep and the price of plasticity; from synaptic and cellular homeostasis to memory consolidation and integration. *Neuron.* 2014;81:12–34.

22. Allen RP, Walters AS, Montplaisir J, Hening W, Myers A, Bell TJ, et al. Restless legs syndrome prevalence and impact. *Archives of Internal Medicine.* 2005;165:1286–92.

23. Lin CM, Davidson TM, Ancoli-Israel S. Gender differences in obstructive sleep apnea and treatment implications. *Sleep Med Rev.* 2008;12:481–96.

24. Voytek B, Kramer MA, Case J, Lepage KQ, Tempesta ZR, Knight RT, et al. Age-related changes in 1/f neural electrophysiological noise. *Journal of Neuroscience.* 2015;23:13257–65.

25. Yerkes RM, Dodson JD. The relation of strength of stimulus to rapidity of habit formation. *Journal of Comparative Neurology and Psychology.* 1908;18:459–82.

26. Devilbiss DM, Waterhouse BD. Norepinephrine exhibits two distinct profiles of action on sensory cortical neuron responses to excitatory synaptic stimuli. *Synapse.* 2004;37:273–82.

27. Devilbiss DM, Berridge CW. Cognition-enhancing doses of methylphenidate preferentially increase prefrontal cortex neuronal responsiveness. *Biological Psychiatry.* 2008;64:626–35.

28. Durstewitz D, Seamans J. The dual-state theory of prefrontal cortex dopamine function with relevance to catechol-o-

methyltransferase genotypes and schizophrenia. *Biological Psychiatry.* 2008;64:739–49.

29. Cools R, D'Esposito M. Inverted-U-shaped dopamine actions on human working memory and cognitive control. *Biological Psychiatry.* 2011;2011:e113–e125.

30. Conley P, Burgess C. Age effects on a computational model of memory. *Brain and Cognition.* 2000;43:104–8.

31. Nadeau SE. Attractor basins: a neural basis for the conformation of knowledge. In: Chatterjee A, Coslett HB, editors. *The Roots of Cognitive Neuroscience.* Oxford: Oxford University Press; 2014, pp. 305–33.

32. Dumutriu D, Hao J, Hara Y, Kaufmann J, Janssen WGM, Lou W, et al. Selective changes in thin spine density and morphology in monkey prefrontal cortex correlate with aging-relating cognitive impairment. *Journal of Neuroscience.* 2010;30:7507–15.

33. Nadeau SE, Crosson B. Subcortical aphasia. *Brain and Language.* 1997;58:355–402, 436–58.

34. Desimone R, Duncan D. Neural mechanisms of selective visual attention. *Annual Reviews of Neuroscience.* 1995;18:193–222.

35. Moran J, Desimone R. Selective attention gates visual processing in extrastriate cortex. *Science.* 1985;229:782–4.

36. Rolls ET, Deco G. Stochastic cortical neurodynamics underlying the memory and cognitive changes in aging. *Neurobiology of Learning and Memory.* 2015;118:150–61.

37. Nadeau SE, Heilman KM. Frontal mysteries revealed. *Neurology.* 2007;68:1450–3.

38. Chavis DA, Pandya DN. Further observations on corticofrontal connections in the rhesus monkey. *Brain Research.* 1976;117:369–86.

39. Goldman-Rakic PS. Cellular and circuit basis of working memory in prefrontal cortex of nonhuman primates. *Prog Brain Res.* 1990;85:325–36.

40. Ongür D, Price JL. The organization of networks within the orbital and medial prefrontal cortex of rats, monkeys and humans. *Cerebral Cortex.* 2000;10:206–19.

41. Kumar A. NMDA receptor function during senescence: implication on cognitive performance. *Front Neurosci.* 2015;9:473.

42. Onur OA, Schlaepfer TE, Kukolja J, Bauer A, Jeung H, Patin A, et al. The N-methyl-D aspartate receptor co-agonist d-cycloserine facilitates declarative learning and hippocampal activity in humans. *Biological Psychiatry.* 2010;67:1205–11.

43. Feld GB, Lange T, Gais S, Born J. Sleep-dependent declarative memory consolidation – unaffected after blocking NMDA or AMPA receptors but enhanced by NMDA coagonist D-cycloserine. *Neuropsychopharmacology.* 2013;38:2688–97.

44. Kuriyama K, Honma M, Shimazaki M, Horie M, Yoshiike T, Koyama S, et al. An N-methyl-D-aspartate receptor agonist facilitates sleep-independent synaptic plasticity associated with working memory capacity enhancement. *Scientific Reports.* 2011:1–7.

45. Kuriyama K, Honma M, Koyama S, Kim Y. D-cycloserine facilitates procedural learning but not declarative learning in healthy humans: a randomized controlled trial of the effect of D-cycloserine and valproic acid on overnight properties in the performance of non-emotional memory tasks. *Neurobiology of Learning and Memory.* 2011;95:505–9.

46. Skvarc DR, Dean OM, Byrne LK, Gray L, Lane S, Lewis M, et al. The

effect of N-acetylcysteine on human cognition – a systematic review. *Neuroscience and Biobehavioral Reviews.* 2017;78:44–56.

47. Lauterborn JC, Palmer LC, Jia Y, Pham DT, Hou B, Wang W, et al. Chronic ampakine treatments stimulate dendritic growth and promote learning in middle-aged rats. *Journal of Neuroscience.* 2016;36:1636–46.

48. Sarter M, Bruno JP. Cognitive functions of cortical acetylcholine: toward a unifying hypothesis. *Brain Research Reviews.* 1997;23:28–46.

49. Kilgard MP, Merzenich MM. Cortical map reorganization enabled by nucleus basalis activity. *Science.* 1998;279:1714–18.

50. Conner JM, Culberson A, Packowski C, Chiba AA, Tuszynski MH. Lesions of the basal forebrain cholinergic system impair task acquisition and abolish cortical plasticity associated with motor skill learning. *Neuron.* 2003;38:819–29.

51. Drachman DA, Leavitt J. Human memory and the cholinergic system. *Archives of Neurology.* 1974;30:113–21.

52. Schneider LS. Treatment of Alzheimer's disease with cholinesterase inhibitors. *Clin Geriatr Med.* 2001;17:337–58.

53. Doody RS, Geldmacher DS, Gordon B, Perdomo CA, Pratt RD, Donepezil Study Group. Open-label, multicenter, phase 3 extension study of the safety and efficacy of donepezil in patients with Alzheimer disease. *Archives of Neurology.* 2001;58:427–33.

54. Grothe M, Heinsen H, Teipel SJ. Atrophy of the cholinergic basal forebrain over the adult age range and in early stages of Alzheimer's disease. *Biological Psychiatry.* 2012;71:805–13.

55. Repantis D, Laisney O, Heuser I. Acetylcholinesterase inhibitors and memantine for neuroenhancement in healthy individuals: a systematic review. *Pharmacological Research.* 2010;61:473–81.

56. Manye Kf, McIntire DD, Mann DM, German DC. Locus coeruleus cell loss in the aging human brain: a nonrandom process. *Journal of Comparative Neurology.* 1995;358:79–87.

57. Ding Y-S, Singhal T, Planeta-Wilson B, Gallezot J-D, Nabulsi N, Labaree D, et al. PET imaging of the effects of age and cocaine on the norepinephrine transporter in the human brain using (S,S)-[(11)C]O-methylreboxetine and HRRT. *Synapse.* 2010;64:30–8.

58. Adhikarla V, Zeng F, Votaw JR, Goodman MM, Nye JA. Compartmental modeling of [^{11}C]MENET binding to the norepinephrine transporter in the healthy human brain. *Nuclear Medicine and Biology.* 2016;43:318–23.

59. Wang M, Gamo NJ, Yang Y, Jin LE, Wang X-J, Laubach M, et al. Neuronal basis of age-related working memory decline. *Nature.* 2011;476:210–13.

60. Wilson RS, Nag S, Boyle PA, Hizel LP, Yu L, Buchman AS, et al. Neural reserve, neural density in the locus ceruleus, and cognitive decline. *Neurology.* 2013;80:1202–8.

61. Barcelos NM, Van Ness PH, Wagner AF, MacAvoy MG, Mecca AP, Anderson GM, et al. Guanfacine treatment for prefrontal cognitive dysfunction in older participants: a randomized clinical trial. *Neurobiology of Aging.* 2018;70:117–24.

62. Bäckman L, Karlsson S, Fischer H, Karlsson P, Brehmer Y, Rieckmann A, et al. Dopamine D1 receptors and age differences in brain activation during working memory. *Neurobiology of Aging.* 2011;32:1849–56.

63. Karrer TM, Josef AK, Mata R, Morris ED, Samanez-Larkin GR. Reduced dopamine receptors and transporters but not synthesis capacity in normal aging adults: a meta-analysis. *Neurobiology of Aging.* 2017;57:36–46.

64. Vihayraghavan S, Wang M, Birnbaum SG, Williams GV, Arnsten AFT. Inverted-U dopamine D1 receptor actions on prefrontal neurons engaged in working memory. *Nature Neuroscience.* 2007;10:376–84.

65. Rodríguez JJ, Noristani HN, Verkhratsky A. The serotonergic system in ageing and Alzheimer's disease. *Progress in Neurobiology.* 2012;99:15–41.

66. Nadeau SE. Intentional disorders. In: Noseworthy JH, editor. *Neurological Therapeutics Principles and Practice*, 2nd ed, vol. 3. Oxon: Informa Healthcare; 2006, pp. 3108–23.

67. Elithorn A, Partridge M, McKissock W, Knight GC. Discussion on psychosurgery. *Proceedings of the Royal Society of Medicine.* 1959;52:203–10.

68. Bechara A, Damasio H, Damasio AR. Manipulation of dopamine and serotonin causes different effects on covert and overt decision-making. *Society for Neuroscience Abstracts.* 2001;27:126.

69. Miu AC, Crisan LG, Chis A, Ungureanu L, Druga B, Vulturar R. Somatic markers mediate the effect of serotonin transporter gene polymorphisms on Iowa Gambling Task. *Genes, Brain and Behavior.* 2012;11:398–403.

70. McIntyre RS, Lophaven S, Olsen CK. A randomized, double-blind, placebo-controlled study of vortioxetine on cognitive function in depressed adults. *International Journal of Neuropsychopharmacology.* 2014;17:1557–67.

71. Lisman J, Grace AA, Duzel E. A neoHebbian framework for

episodic memory: role of dopamine-dependent late LTP. *Trends in Neuroscience.* 2011;34:536–47.

72. Chowdhury R, Guitart-Masip M, Bunzeck N, Dolan RJ, Düzel E. Dopamine modulates episodic memory persistence in old age. *Journal of Neuroscience.* 2012;32:14193–204.

73. Knecht S, Breitenstein C, Bushuven S, Wailke S, Kamping S, Flöel A, et al. Levodopa: faster and better word learning in normal humans. *Annals of Neurology.* 2004;56:20–6.

74. Flöel A, Breitenstein C, Hummel F, Celnik P, Gingert C, Sawaki L, et al. Dopaminergic influences on formation of a motor memory. *Annals of Neurology.* 2005;58:121–30.

75. Fresnoza S, Paulus W, Mitsche MA, Kuo M-F. Nonlinear dose-dependent impact of D1 receptor activation on motor cortex plasticity in humans. *Journal of Neuroscience.* 2014;34:2744–53.

76. Brickman AM, Khan UA, Provenzano FA, Yeung L-K, Suzuki W, Schroeter H, et al. Enhancing dentate gyrus function with dietary flavanols improves cognition in older adults. *Nature Neuroscience.* 2014;12:1798–803.

77. Spalding KL, Bergmann O, Alkass K, Bernard S, Salehpour M, Huttner HB, et al. Dynamics of hippocampal neurogenesis in adult humans. *Cell.* 2013;153:1219–27.

78. Salvadores N, Sanhueza M, Manque P, Court FA. Axonal degeneration during aging and its functional role in neurodegenerative disorders. *Frontiers in Neuroscience.* 2017;11:1–21.

79. Clarke LE, Liddelow SA, Chakraborty C, Münch AE, Heiman M, Barres BA. Normal aging induces A1-like astrocyte reactivity. *Proceedings of the National Academy of Sciences USA.* 2018;115(8):e1896–e1905.

80. Davidson T, Tremblay F. Age and hemispheric differences in trancallosal inhibition between motor cortices: an ipsilateral silent period study. *BMC Neuroscience.* 2013;14:62.

81. Shibuya K, Park SB, Geevasinga N, Huynh W, Simon NG, Menon P, et al. Threshold tracking transcranial magnetic stimulation: Effects of age and gender on motor cortical function. *Clinical Neurophysiology.* 2016;127:2355–61.

82. Liu H, Yang Y, Xia Y, Zhu W, Leak RK, Wei Z, et al. Aging of cerebral white matter. *Ageing Research Reviews.* 2017;34:64–76.

83. Bennett IJ, Madden DJ, Vaidya CJ, Howard DV, Howard JH. Age-related differences in multiple measures of white matter integrity: a diffusion tensor imaging study of healthy aging. *Human Brain Mapping.* 2010;31:378–90.

84. Yeatman JD, Wandell BA, Mezer AA. Lifespan maturation and degeneration of human brain white matter. *Nature Communications.* 2014 Sep 17;5:4932.

85. Serbruyns L, Leunissen I, van Ruitenbeek P, Pauwels L, Caeyenberghs K, Solesio-Jofre E, et al. Alterations in brain white matter contributing to age-related slowing of task switching performance: the role of radial diffusivity and magnetization transfer ratio. *Human Brain Mapping.* 2016;37:4084–98.

86. Shrager Y, Levy DA, Hopkins RO, Squire LR. Working memory and the organization of brain systems. *J Neuroscience.* 2008;28:4818–22.

87. Macpherson SE, Philips LH, Della Sala S. Age, executive function and social decision making: a dorsolateral prefrontal theory of cognitive aging. *Psychology and Aging.* 2002;17:598–609.

88. Nadeau SE. Hemispheric asymmetry: what, why, and at what cost? *Journal of the International Neuropsychological Society.* 2010;27:1–3.

89. Mascalchi M, Toschi N, Ginestroni A, Giannelli M, Nicolai E, Aiello M, et al. Gender, age-related, and regional differences of the magnetization transfer ratio of the cortical and subcortical brain gray matter. *Journal of Magnetic Resonance Imaging.* 2014;40:360–6.

90. Ramon y Cajal S. *Degeneration and Regeneration of the Nervous System.* London: Oxford University Press; 1928.

Chapter 16

The Influence of Physical Exercise on Cognitive Aging

Jamie C. Peven, Chelsea M. Stillman, and Kirk I. Erickson

1 Introduction

Cognitive decline is a normal and widespread consequence of aging. Without promising drug interventions for reducing cognitive deficits, the field of cognitive aging has turned to nonpharmacologic treatments. Although there are several nonpharmacologic treatments (e.g., sleep, diet, cognitive training), in this chapter we discuss the effects of physical activity (PA) on cognitive and brain function in late adulthood. PA has well-known, robust benefits to many different parameters of physical, metabolic, and cardiovascular health, and there is now substantial evidence that PA benefits neurocognitive function as well. These effects of PA on neurocognitive health are the focus of the present chapter. Specifically, we present evidence that PA is a widely available and low-cost activity that might be effective at mitigating the public health burdens associated with aging-related cognitive changes. We seek to answer several questions, including whether there is strong evidence that PA influences cognition, and, if so, *why* would PA have these beneficial effects on cognition and the brain. In this chapter, we summarize the existing literature on the associations and effects of PA on cognitive and brain function in late adulthood.

1.1 Key Definitions

Before discussing research examining associations between physical activity and cognitive changes associated with brain aging, several terms must be defined. Although most individuals have a general understanding of the term "physical activity" and its many related terms (e.g., fitness), the ways in which these terms are used and operationalized in the context of scientific research is important for understanding the studies discussed in this chapter.

1.1.1 Physical Activity and Fitness

Physical activity (PA) is any movement that results in energy expenditure [1]. PA levels can be measured objectively (with actigraphy or other monitoring devices) or subjectively (with self-report questionnaires). Most current studies use wearable, objective monitoring devices to measure PA, though this is not always feasible in studies with large sample sizes. Due to higher costs for obtaining and using these devices, as well as the time to analyze the data, some studies elect to use self-report measures to collect information about PA habits. Objective and self-report metrics are often only modestly correlated, which suggests that there are some discrepancies between these measurement approaches. For example, people may overestimate the amount of time that they spend in moderate-intensity PA on self-report measures because of social desirability biases [2, 3].

There are multiple categories, or modes, of PA that people engage in that have different physiological effects: aerobic exercise (e.g., walking, jogging, swimming), muscle- and bone-strengthening (e.g., weight-lifting, jumping), balance training (e.g., walking backward), flexibility training (e.g., static or dynamic stretching), or activities that combine these effects (e.g., yoga, Tai Chi) [4]. Although it is likely that many modes of PA are beneficial, the majority of research on effects of PA on cognition has focused on aerobic exercise.

Different forms of activity result in varying amounts of energy being expended. Energy expenditure during PA is typically expressed in *metabolic equivalents* (METs), or the ratio of working metabolic rate to resting metabolic rate [5]. More METs are expended during "energy-expensive" activities. Energy expenditure during PA is related to the concept of "how much" PA is necessary to achieve optimal cognitive and brain effects. Aerobic exercise is among the most metabolically "expensive" forms of PA.

Identifying the appropriate *dose* of aerobic PA – perhaps the bare minimum dose – to improve specific health outcomes is critical for prescriptive purposes [4]. In the context of PA, dose can be characterized by intensity, frequency, and/or duration. The *intensity* of PA is the rate of energy expended and can be divided into four categories: sedentary, light, moderate, or vigorous. These categories are defined based on METs, although the intensity of PA can also be defined based on a person's maximal heart rate. The *frequency* of PA is how often, or the number of bouts, of moderate-vigorous PA (MVPA) a person engages in per day or per week. This is because MVPA is thought to be the intensity of PA necessary to obtain many of its salutary effects. The *duration* of PA is the length of time each PA bout lasts. The dose of PA necessary to achieve cognitive and brain benefits of activity is still an important and largely unanswered question as few studies to date have examined all three components of PA dose within the same study.

People who engage in high doses of PA are often interchangeably described as having a high level of "fitness." PA is distinct from fitness and it is important to understand how these terms differ in order to properly interpret studies using these various outcomes. Fitness can be conceptualized in multiple ways, including physical strength, environmental survival, ability to complete a task, or aerobic/cardiorespiratory functioning, only the latter of which is the focus of this chapter. *Cardiorespiratory fitness* (CRF) is the ability of the circulatory and respiratory systems to supply oxygen to the body during PA and is often expressed as a person's maximal oxygen uptake (VO_{2max}). CRF is closely related to the amount of PA a person engages in, but it is also influenced by a variety of other genetic and physiological factors. Thus, while PA and CRF often closely track together, they are not equivalent concepts. Further, these two variables may be differentially related to cognition, particularly in aging.

1.1.2 Research Designs

Given the various ways of quantifying PA discussed above, what are the most effective ways to measure its effects on cognition? A variety of research study designs can be used to examine the relationships between PA, CRF, and cognition. *Cross-sectional* studies utilize information taken from a single time point, effectively taking one "snapshot" of each person in a sample to infer relationships between variables. For example, to study the relationship between PA and aging in a cross-sectional design,

researchers would recruit individuals of various ages and assess their PA levels. They then correlate PA levels with participant age to test for an association. Cross-sectional studies can describe relationships between variables of interest, but, crucially, they *cannot* make claims about causality because PA is not directly manipulated. Cross-sectional designs, however, are often used when examining new relationships or when time and/or monetary resources are limited. An extension of the cross-sectional design is the *longitudinal observational* study. These studies involve taking multiple "snapshots" of a person at different time points, typically over the course of months or years. This study design is used in epidemiology to follow large cohorts and for assessing development of particular diseases. These studies have an advantage over the cross-sectional design in that they can make statements about temporal precedence, or changes over time in PA and any relevant outcomes because, although PA is still not manipulated, individuals are assessed at multiple time points. Yet, despite these strengths, the longitudinal design still has several limitations, including the nonrandomized nature of the sample. In other words, individuals who engage in greater PA earlier in life might also be behaving in many different ways from those engaging in lesser amounts of activity. This produces potential confounds, which inherently limit the causal claims that can be made.

The gold standard for testing causal relationships between variables is through a *randomized controlled trial* (RCT). RCTs are considered to be the "gold standard" of research designs because they allow investigators to make causal claims about the effects of a manipulated variable of interest by randomly assigning participants to different study conditions. These studies manipulate PA dose to understand changes in cognition and/or physical health after exercise interventions. To do this, participants are assigned to an active exercise group, which involves increased engagement in PA, or a control group, which involves a similarly social, but critically *non-aerobic*, activity (e.g., education, stretching). These studies also assume that the random assignment of participants to intervention groups will account for any nonshared environmental or genetic influences that could affect the results of the study. RCTs provide the strongest evidence for the influence of PA on cognitive aging because any observed changes in cognition can be attributed to the manipulated variable (i.e., PA) rather than to confounding variables due to the critical feature of random group assignment.

1.2 Learning Objectives

Several broad themes will be discussed throughout this chapter, including how PA affects brain and cognition in the context of aging. In order to assess the influence of PA on cognitive and brain aging, we will attempt to answer the following questions:

1. Are greater amounts of PA *associated with* better cognitive and brain health in older adults?

2. Is engaging in greater amounts of PA an effective approach for *improving* cognitive and brain health in older adults?

3. How do the above patterns translate to older adults with an existing pathology (e.g., those with cognitive impairment)?

2 How Cognition Relates to Physical Activity and Fitness

Learning, memory, processing speed, and executive functioning (EF) are the cognitive domains most susceptible to decline with aging. Many age-related neurodegenerative diseases initially show symptom patterns similar to those observed with healthy aging. However, as neurodegeneration progresses, the rate of decline often increases and may extend to other, typically "untouched" areas of cognition. In the following, we examine how PA may modulate the effects of normal and pathological aging processes on cognition.

2.1 Cross-Sectional Research

Some of the earliest work examining the effects of PA on cognition focused on the relationship between levels of PA and motor speed in aging [6, 7]. Spirduso and colleagues [6, 7] developed a research program centered around the observation that activity levels and general speed decrease in older adults. These researchers suspected that the biological basis for this phenomenon is related to the efficiency of neurotransmission within the brain's motor system. To test this idea, Spirduso and colleagues conducted some of the first cross-sectional studies of PA – initially using rodent models, then extending to older humans. They demonstrated that higher levels of PA (typically assessed via athletic or fitness status) were related to

faster reaction times in humans and better, more efficient dopamine transmission within motor brain circuits (e.g., more striatal dopamine receptors) in rodent models. This foundational work linked a physical behavior (i.e., PA) to a basic cognitive process (i.e., psychomotor speed), as well as a brain mechanism (i.e., dopamine transmission within the striatum). However, these early cross-sectional studies were limited by small sample sizes, and their narrow focus on one basic cognitive process made the results difficult to generalize to larger and more diverse populations or to other cognitive domains.

In larger cross-sectional studies of PA, cognition is often assessed with global measures (e.g., the Mini Mental State Examination (MMSE); [8]) that are quick to administer and easy to score. These global measurements can separate participants into "impaired" or "nonimpaired" categories. For example, Middleton and colleagues administered a modified MMSE to 9,344 older women and gave them a questionnaire to quantify the frequency and intensity of their PA at different times in their lives [9]. The authors found that, after controlling for relevant demographic variables such as age, education, and marital status, the women who were more active (i.e., who reported any regular PA) also had higher cognitive scores than those who were inactive at every age time point. While global metrics like the MMSE do not provide insight into which areas of cognition are more affected by being more physically active, they serve as evidence that living a healthier, more active lifestyle is temporally related to better cognitive functioning in late life. Further, the larger sample sizes in these studies support the conclusion that across age groups, higher PA is associated with better cognition.

In addition to cross-sectional measures of PA, measures of CRF are also associated with cognitive performance and some cognitive domains are more strongly associated with CRF than others. This is particularly true for EF. For example, Oberlin et al. examined the association between CRF and spatial working memory (a component of EF) in 154 low-active older adults [10]. CRF was measured with a graded maximum exercise test on a treadmill. Spatial working memory was assessed using a task that asked participants to remember the location of two, three, or four dots on a screen for several seconds and then respond to whether a red probe dot appeared in one of the same locations as the target dots or in a new location. Accuracy scores on each of the three conditions were averaged to create one mean score. After adjusting for age, gender, and education, the authors found that higher CRF was associated with greater accuracy on the task [10]. Similar patterns have been found for other components of EF. Higher CRF [11–13], as well as PA [14, 15], has been associated with better performance on tasks measuring set-shifting [11] and inhibitory control [12, 13].

The same general pattern is observed for memory performance. Older adults who are more fit and more active perform better on tests of episodic memory (e.g., [11, 13]). One study of older women examined the relationship between habitual PA and cognitive functioning in 16,370 registered nurses [14]. Participants completed a self-report questionnaire about leisure-time PA, which was assigned MET values according to a standardized list of activities [16]. The authors used the immediate and delayed recall portions of the East Boston Memory Test and a 10-word list from the Telephone Interview for Cognitive Status to create a composite verbal memory score. Weuve and colleagues found that older women engaging in the highest quintile of PA performed significantly better than their less-active counterparts on these verbal memory tests [14]. Their results held true for EF as well as global cognitive functioning. The domains of EF and memory are related to real-world behaviors, such as decision-making, impulsivity, and planning, and have functional relevance in the lives of healthy older adults. Thus, older adults with higher CRF and reporting more PA often perform better on these more complex tasks compared with their less fit and active counterparts.

In this type of research, it is important to keep in mind that associations between PA/CRF and cognitive function do not necessarily mean that being more active and/or fit leads to improved functioning. It is impossible to determine directionality with this type of research, as it is conceivable, for example, that those with better cognition tend to engage in higher levels of PA. This potential for bidirectional relationships between PA/CRF and cognitive functioning has spurred the field to design longitudinal and intervention studies that may help establish causality. Cross-sectional research is also limited by the ways in which PA is assessed. In larger studies, PA is often assessed via self-report questionnaires, most of which show poor correspondence to objectively measured PA levels [17]. Social desirability and social approval may influence the level of self-reported PA [2].

Although this bias may be reduced in the "oldest old" adults (i.e., those >85) [18], the poor correspondence between self-reported PA and objectively monitored PA makes it difficult to attribute variability in cognitive performance to PA levels alone, nor is it possible to determine dose–response effects. Exploring the evidence for and against whether higher CRF and/or more PA predict better, or preserved, cognitive performance in the same individuals over time is the next step in determining causality.

The cross-sectional research examining the relationships between PA/CRF and cognitive aging provides a critical foundation for understanding the relationships between physical activity and cognitive functioning. Studies using comprehensive neuropsychological assessments have shown that specific domains of cognition are differentially related to both age and PA/CRF. Despite the many differences in assessing PA and/or cognition across studies, a clear pattern has emerged: being more active and/or aerobically fit is associated with better cognitive function. Further exploring how these relationships persist or change across time can provide additional evidence that more PA and higher CRF are related to better cognition in late life.

2.2 Observational Longitudinal Research

There is mounting evidence from prospective observational studies that being more active and/or having higher CRF is associated with better cognition and reduced cognitive decline in populations with mild cognitive impairment (MCI) or dementia. In these studies, researchers examined the longitudinal trajectory of cognitive decline relative to CRF or PA over periods of 1-20 years after an initial cognitive assessment. Rather than examine changes in cognitive performance on specific tasks, most of the longitudinal research involving PA or CRF levels focuses on conversion from healthy cognitive status to cognitive impairment and/or dementia. One example of this comes from the Cooper Center Longitudinal Study, which followed 19,458 individuals from midlife into late life to examine the relationship between midlife CRF and incidence of dementia [19]. The authors found that participants in the highest age- and sex-adjusted quintile of CRF in midlife had 36% lower risk of developing dementia later in life. Compared with the quintile with the lowest CRF, participants in the second- and third-highest quintiles also had a reduced risk of developing dementia later in life by at least 22%. In healthy older adults, those who were more fit with regard to CRF tended to experience less cognitive decline over time compared with their peers who were not as fit.

Researchers can also use differences in PA levels to understand changes in cognitive functioning over time. For practical reasons, in longitudinal research, PA is often measured with self-report questionnaires. These questionnaires range from validated, detailed measures to simple "yes/no" items. Walking is the most common form of PA included in most studies and most self-reports, although some questionnaires, like the CHAMPS, also evaluate the frequency, duration, and intensity of self-reported exercise (e.g., asking if a participant worked hard enough to sweat). The frequency, duration, and intensity of PA is then converted into minutes of activity or energy expenditure and used in statistical analyses to determine the relationship between PA energy expenditure and cognitive functioning.

Just as higher CRF is associated with reduced risk of cognitive decline, being more active in late life is associated with lower risk of developing cognitive impairment and/or dementia [14, 20–25]. Particularly in the domains of EF and processing speed, older adults engaging in more habitual PA are less likely to experience the typical age-related declines in functioning [20, 26]. One of the first longitudinal studies followed 4,615 older adults (i.e., 65 years or older) for five years to determine the incidence of cognitive impairment over time [20]. Participants completed a comprehensive neuropsychological battery to assess cognitive functioning and were asked about the frequency and intensity of their physical exercise. Participant responses to the PA questions were categorized into low, moderate, or high levels of habitual PA. At follow-up, 721 (15.6%) were diagnosed with cognitive impairment or dementia. The authors controlled for age, sex, and education to eliminate potential confounds. The risk for developing cognitive impairment was reduced in participants engaging in high PA by 42%; the risk for developing any dementia was reduced in participants engaging in high PA by at least 37% and in participants engaging in moderate PA by at least 31%. Laurin and colleagues [20] further examined these relationships within each gender group and showed that only women had a 40% reduced risk of developing cognitive impairment when engaging in high levels of PA.

Meta-analyses examining the effects of PA on nondemented older adults show that engaging in higher levels of PA is associated with reduced risk of cognitive impairment [22, 24] and neurodegenerative disease [27]. One meta-analysis included 15 prospective studies of 33,816 nondemented adults and found that 3,210 of those participants (i.e., 9.5%) were cognitively impaired at follow-up between 1 and 12 years later [22]. Of the included study participants, those engaging in the highest level of PA had a 38% lower risk of developing cognitive impairment during the follow-up period. When low-to-moderate levels of PA were included in the analyses, the authors found that more activity overall was associated with a 35% lower risk of future cognitive impairment. Another meta-analysis specifically examined the risk for developing incident dementia, Alzheimer's disease (AD), or Parkinson's disease (PD) and included 16 prospective studies of 163,797 nondemented older adults who were followed from 3 to 30 years after the initial cognitive assessment [27]. Of the 163,797 participants, 3,219 (2%) were diagnosed with dementia, AD, or PD at follow-up. All the included studies controlled for age, with many of them also controlling for sex and/or body mass index. Five of the 16 studies controlled for apolipoprotein (APOE) genotype, as the ε4 variant is known to be associated with increased risk for developing AD. Additional covariates included other physical health (e.g., diabetes status, cholesterol) and/or mood (e.g., depressive symptoms) variables. All the included studies gauged PA engagement with self-report questionnaires and found that there was a reduced risk of developing a neurodegenerative disease for individuals engaging in the most PA (i.e., 28% lower risk of developing dementia overall, 45% lower risk of developing AD, and 18% lower risk of developing PD). Although these observational studies and their meta-analyses could not determine the type or dose of PA needed to maintain cognitive status, their results provide evidence that being more active is associated with maintenance of cognitive function later in life.

Despite the use of self-report questionnaires rather than objective metrics as the measure of PA, the results of these longitudinal studies are important in helping to understand the influence of PA on cognitive aging. Adults with MCI who are more physically active have a lower risk of conversion to dementia compared with those who are less active or inactive. Being physically active and fit in late life is associated with reduced risk of developing neurodegenerative diseases even if some cognitive impairment is already present [25]. A study by Grande and colleagues followed 176 older adults with MCI for approximately 3 years and measured their PA levels with a questionnaire about the type and frequency of their activities. At follow-up, the individuals in the highest tertile of PA had a 64% lower risk of converting from MCI to dementia relative to individuals in the lowest tertile of PA [25]. No other observational research has been done to evaluate the effects of PA or CRF in populations already suffering from some degree of cognitive impairment; however, some randomized clinical trials have examined how PA could alter the trajectory of cognitive decline and will be discussed in the next section.

Notably, "leisure time physical activity," or PA that occurred outside the workplace or commute, was the most effective in preventing cognitive impairment or further decline in longitudinal studies [28]. This is an important distinction because it means that older adults engaging in PA may have an advantage as it pertains to cognitive aging, although without corroborating evidence from randomized studies, this relationship cannot be causally attributed to PA. As the observational literature shows, engaging in greater amounts of PA is associated with maintenance of cognitive function.

However, there are some caveats to this type of research. Many longitudinal studies treat cognition as a dichotomous variable (i.e., impaired or not impaired). Although this may be the most feasible way to assess cognition in large samples, cognitive functioning can and should be examined on a continuous scale. As has been shown, cognitive domains do not decline at the same rate throughout the aging process, but this cannot be discerned with global metrics of cognition. Most importantly, these longitudinal studies did not manipulate PA and therefore were not able to determine causal relationships between increasing PA/CRF levels and improvements in cognitive function.

2.3 Randomized Controlled Trials

Studies of the relationships between cognitive performance and PA/CRF in cross-sectional and prospective longitudinal designs have hinted that that there might be a beneficial causal effect of engaging

in more PA on cognitive function in late life. However, the critical test for a causal relationship between these variables is to manipulate PA in the context of a randomized intervention. Overall, the evidence from RCTs suggests that increasing PA improves cognitive functioning in both cognitively normal individuals and patients with cognitive impairment. One of the first studies to examine these effects in healthy older adults recruited 43 community-dwelling, sedentary individuals to engage in aerobic exercise, strength and flexibility training, or to serve as no-contact controls [29]. A comprehensive neuropsychological battery was administered to all participants to evaluate attention, memory, and inhibitory control. Individuals in the exercise and toning/stretching groups participated in a 4-month intervention during which time they engaged in three supervised hours of their respective activity each week. The no-contact control group was tested before and after a 4-month period, which allowed researchers to control for practice effects (i.e., participants in both groups improving simply because they had done the tests before). After the intervention, the aerobic exercise group had a significantly increased VO_{2max} and their performance on the cognitive tests had improved relative to the strength training group and non-exercise controls. This was one of the earliest experiments showing that aerobic exercise training could improve cognitive functioning in healthy older adults. These findings are important because they highlight the benefits of aerobic over anaerobic exercise, as increases in CRF were observed only in the aerobic exercise group and were associated with improvements in cognitive task performance.

Meta-analyses of RCTs in healthy older adults have shown mixed evidence for the success of increasing PA/CRF in influencing cognitive functioning [30–32]. One of the first meta-analyses conducted included 18 exercise interventions [30]. The authors found that exercise interventions had the largest effect on EF, such that individuals randomized to the PA groups performed better on tests of EF than did the control groups (i.e., EF effect size was moderate to large at Hedges' g = 0.68, spatial and controlled test effect sizes were moderate at Hedges' g = 0.43–0.46, and speed test effect size was small at Hedges' g = 0.27). Further, the effects of PA were stronger with interventions that consisted of aerobic activity lasting at least 6 months, as well as in studies that contained more females. These studies identified duration, type of exercise, and sex as potentially important moderators of the effects of PA and provided preliminary evidence that there is a causal link between aerobic PA and cognitive functioning within healthy aging populations.

In one of the first demonstrations of how increasing PA improves cognition in impaired individuals, Lautenschlager and colleagues recruited 170 older adults who were either cognitively normal or diagnosed with MCI [33]. Participants completed the Community Healthy Activities Model Program for Seniors (CHAMPS) questionnaire [34] and wore a pedometer for seven days at baseline to measure habitual PA; participants were categorized into "active" (i.e., at least 70,000 steps per week) or "inactive" (i.e., fewer than 70,000 steps per week). They were then randomized to usual care/educational control or a PA intervention that consisted of at least three 50-minute, unsupervised home exercise sessions per week for 24 weeks. Participants were encouraged to choose enjoyable activities to improve adherence to the intervention. Cognitive function was assessed using the cognitive subscale of the Alzheimer's Dementia Assessment Scale (ADAS-Cog; [35]) and supplemental tests of EF and verbal fluency. The ADAS-Cog spans a variety of cognitive domains, including brief tests of memory and language processing. Participants' cognitive functioning was assessed again 6, 12, and 18 months after beginning the intervention. The authors controlled for age, sex, premorbid IQ, marital status, and cognitive scores from earlier time points to eliminate any confounding differences between their participant groups. After the 6-month intervention, participants randomized to the PA intervention had increased their steps per week by 9,000 – significantly more than the usual care group. This demonstrated the efficacy of the authors' PA intervention: their participants who had been trained to increase their PA were habitually more active than the educational control group. These participants also performed better on the ADAS-Cog overall. At the 18-month follow-up assessment, PA participants had increased their steps per week by 6,000, which was still significantly more than the usual care group. Additionally, the PA group had higher ADAS-Cog total and verbal memory scores, and lower Clinical Dementia Rating scores. This RCT demonstrated that increasing PA could reduce the rate of cognitive decline in individuals who were cognitively normal and reduce symptom progression in those already suffering from cognitive impairment.

In impaired populations, improving CRF and/or PA has beneficial effects on cognitive functioning [31, 32, 36]. A recent meta-analysis of 802 patients with dementia focused on the effects of aerobic, nonaerobic, and combined exercise interventions consisting of exercise and control groups [32]. The interventions ranged from 6 weeks to 1 year with the average intervention length being about 15 weeks. Participants in the exercise groups engaged in 40–840 minutes of activity per week, with an average of 183 minutes per week. Interventions that included a CRF component (i.e., aerobic and combined interventions) had positive effects on global measures of cognition (e.g., the MMSE, a clock drawing test), such that exercise groups showed a standardized mean difference 0.5 points higher on cognitive measures relative to control groups, regardless of dementia type. Importantly, the frequency of intervention, or number of minutes of PA per week the intervention attained, did not influence the positive effects of PA on cognitive functioning. This means that, in these populations of dementia patients, *any* PA is associated with better cognitive functioning relative to no PA. Thus, the threshold for the beneficial effects of PA may be lower in patient populations.

2.4 Disputing Evidence and Limitations in the Field

There have been many interventions that seek to increase CRF or habitual PA but no clear definition of the dose of PA required to preserve cognitive functioning has emerged. Rather, the methodologies used in each RCT differ with respect to PA intervention and cognitive assessments, making it difficult to discern the type and dose of PA that influences specific domains of cognition. It is also difficult to differentiate the effects of increasing CRF from increasing the amount of PA, as the two may be related in the context of an intervention. Some research indicates that increasing CRF is required to observe changes in cognition in the context of a PA intervention [37], though more research should examine whether CRF qualifies as an important mediator of the association.

Despite the wealth of evidence from RCTs demonstrating that PA benefits cognitive functioning, it is important to acknowledge that there are some studies, including meta-analyses, that have failed to find a significant effect of PA on cognition. These studies perpetuate skepticism about whether a simple and widely accessible activity, such as walking, is effective at promoting and preserving cognition in late life. For example, in a 12-week RCT of 126 older adults, both exercising and control groups showed equivalent improvements in cognition [38]. In addition, the largest and longest RCT of PA to date (the LIFE study) reported no significant improvements in cognition for the exercise compared with the control group [39]. However, an analysis of subgroups revealed a significant improvement in EF only in the oldest and most physically impaired participants. Finally, a recent meta-analysis argued that there is insufficient evidence that exercise is effective at improving cognitive performance in cognitively normal older adults [40]. These discrepant findings underscore the significant variability in results of PA studies.

The persistent disagreement about the effects of PA on cognitive outcomes highlights several limitations of the PA-cognition literature to date. First, most studies have had very small sample sizes (i.e., fewer than 50 participants per group), which can lead to spurious results that are either false positives or false negatives. Small samples also do not provide sufficient statistical power to closely examine the biological mediators or individual differences that could explain variability within and across studies. Second, most prior studies have used cognitive batteries that are insufficient for capturing the complexity and diversity of cognitive processes. Rather, they have used brief, global tests of cognition that cannot discriminate between specific cognitive domains. This makes combined analyses, such as those offered in some meta-analyses and reviews of the cognitive outcomes of PA, difficult to interpret. Third, there is considerable variability in quality control and intervention design across studies. In fact, many studies fail to report intervention adherence, compliance, or baseline fitness levels. Further, the duration of PA interventions ranges from less than 1 to more than 24 months, and few interventions closely monitor exercise intensity. This lack of dose reporting and monitoring (e.g., intensity and frequency characteristics of exercise) almost certainly contributes to heterogeneous findings across studies.

3 How the Brain Relates to Physical Activity and Fitness

PA influences cognition through several mechanisms and at several levels of brain structure and function

[41]. There are several ways to measure changes in brain structure and function with respect to PA. The majority of research on the neural effects of PA in humans has focused on structural brain changes using gray and white matter imaging techniques (see Chapter 4). Of note, it is not yet clear how structural changes relate to processes at the cellular and molecular level (e.g., new vasculature, new neurons, etc.). However, the cellular and molecular mechanisms through which PA influences the brain have been thoroughly studied in animal models and there is evidence to suggest that many of the same physiological changes occur in humans [42]. For example, increasing PA influences key growth factors that have downstream effects on energy maintenance and synaptic plasticity [43], both of which are altered with brain aging. Therefore, it is critical to understand how PA affects these two factors and thereby influences brain health later in life. However, cellular and molecular mechanisms in the human brain are difficult to measure. Therefore, research has centered on the more macro-level changes that can be linked to PA/CRF, for example, changes in brain structure and function.

Aging is broadly associated with reductions in gray and white matter volume and integrity. In general, however, there is a greater loss in white matter connectivity than a loss of neurons. In addition, some regions show more age-related losses than others [44]. Much of the literature examining reductions in brain volume or alterations in brain function focuses on the hippocampus and the prefrontal cortex – areas associated with memory (Chapter 7) and EF (Chapter 12), respectively (see also Chapter 3). These are the two domains of cognition that, with aging, tend to decline earliest. However, only relatively recently have studies begun to examine whether PA/CRF modifies the morphology of these brain areas in humans.

3.1 Cross-Sectional Research

The first studies examining how changes in the brain are related to CRF did not emerge until the early twenty-first century and focused on how CRF was associated with differences in brain volume across different areas of gray matter [45–47]. The majority of this cross-sectional research focused on the associations between the brain and CRF, rather than PA. One of the earliest studies in this area examined whether CRF was associated with gray matter volume in brain regions associated with EF [46]. In this study of 55 older adults, the authors used voxel-based morphometry (VBM) to measure the volume of gray and white matter on a point-by-point basis throughout the brain. The authors considered both age and CRF in their analyses, as age is associated with widespread reductions in brain volume. They found that highly fit older adults had experienced less tissue loss than their less-fit peers [46]. In the gray matter, these differences between more and less fit older adults were found in prefrontal, superior parietal, and temporal areas that are frequently associated with EF and memory. In white matter, these differences were primarily in the genu of the corpus callosum, the anterior portions of the white matter tracts that connect the left and right frontal hemispheres. These results provided some of the first evidence in humans that higher CRF was associated with reduced aging-related gray matter and white matter atrophy.

Just as higher CRF may be neuroprotective of gray matter, it may also be associated with preservation of the structural integrity of white matter [10, 48–50]. A previously discussed study by Oberlin and colleagues included two independent samples totaling 267 older adults and used diffusion tensor imaging (DTI) to evaluate the structural integrity of white matter microstructure [10]. In addition to finding that higher CRF was associated with better performance on a spatial working memory task, they also found that higher CRF was associated with higher fractional anisotropy (FA) – a quantification of white matter microstructural integrity. After controlling for age, gender, and education, the authors found that higher CRF levels were associated with higher FA in the anterior corona radiata, anterior internal capsule, fornix, cingulum, and corpus callosum across both samples [10]. Additionally, FA statistically mediated the relationship between CRF and spatial working memory, such that individuals with higher CRF had higher FA and better EF task performance (Figure 16.1). Maintaining CRF in late life is therefore associated with better structural integrity in both gray and white matter, specifically in areas that support EF and memory function. This cross-sectional work also suggests that associations with FA may be the path by which CRF is associated with better cognitive functioning. However, it is also possible that greater FA in deep white matter provides the basis for a more active lifestyle and better cognitive function, as the direction

of this relationship cannot be discerned from this study. Many studies have now replicated the associations seen with both gray [13, 45, 51, 52] and white matter [48–50] integrity and CRF in healthy older adults. As this field expands, more research is being conducted on populations with cognitive and neurologic impairments to better understand the variability of the relationship between CRF (and to some extent, habitual PA) in these samples.

Similar relationships between brain integrity and CRF [53, 54] have been established in older adults with MCI or dementia. One study of 22 amnestic MCI patients examined the relationship between CRF and both gray and white matter structural integrity by using VBM and a tract-based spatial statistics, respectively [53]. These authors found positive relationships between CRF and gray matter integrity in the left inferior parietal cortex, bilateral superior frontal cortices, and right superior orbitofrontal cortex, as measured with VBM. They also found positive associations between CRF and FA in the right inferior and superior longitudinal fasciculi, right inferior fronto-occipital fasciculus, and the genu of the corpus callosum. Although this study had a small sample size, it provided evidence that higher CRF, even in impaired populations, was associated with better brain structural integrity relative to individuals with lower CRF. Additional work in these populations is needed to determine whether CRF or PA is associated with brain function during later stages of cognitive impairment.

One limitation of the work linking CRF and/or PA to brain structure is that changes in structure are not a necessary precursor to changes in function. Put another way, "bigger isn't always better," and just because CRF is associated with larger gray matter volumes and higher white matter integrity does not necessarily mean that these outcomes are associated with better functioning. This limitation prompted researchers to examine PA/CRF in the context of brain function, which can be readily assessed in humans with modern fMRI paradigms.

Whereas higher CRF is associated with higher cortical and subcortical volumes in specific regions, fMRI studies reveal that higher CRF is also associated with more activity in these areas [55–58]. For example, one recent study examined blood-oxygen-level-dependent (BOLD) activity in an event-related dual-task fMRI paradigm and analyzed the associations between brain function and CRF [58] in

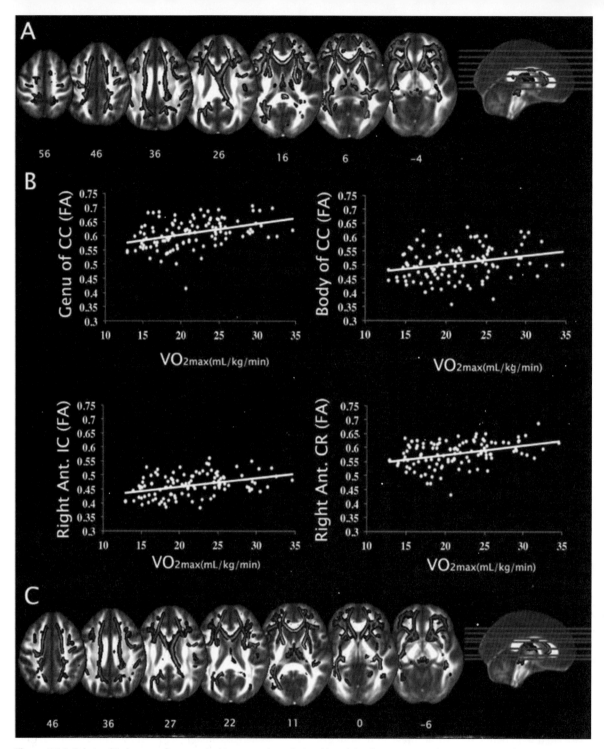

Figure 16.1 Relationship between fitness and white matter integrity in older adults. Shown are significant associations between cardiorespiratory fitness (CRF), fractional anisotropy (FA), and mean spatial working memory performance from Experiment 1 (of 2). (A) Clusters of voxels where fitness was significantly associated with FA. Warm-colored voxels show positive associations, cool-colored voxels demonstrate negative associations. Side panels indicate slice placements. Age, gender, and years of education were included as covariates. The z-plane coordinates of each slice, in MNI space, are presented at the bottom. For visualization purposes, tbss_fill was used to dilate statistical maps. (B) For illustration purposes, scatterplots and best-fit lines are shown for the relationship between CRF and FA in selected regions. (C) Spatial distribution of indirect path voxel clusters. Cyan-colored voxel clusters show a positive indirect effect, brown voxel clusters indicate a negative indirect effect. Ant, anterior; CC, corpus callosum; Ext, external; FA, fractional anisotropy; IC, internal capsule. From Oberlin et al. 2016 [10]. A black and white version of this figure will appear in some formats. For the color version, please refer to the plate section.

128 older adults. Participants completed VO_{2max} fitness testing and an EF paradigm that asked them to discriminate either numbers or letters in single- and dual-task conditions. The authors found that higher CRF was associated with better performance in the dual-task (i.e., more difficult) condition, but this result did not hold after controlling for age, sex, and education. In addition, comparison of patterns of brain activation between the single and dual tasks in relation to CRF revealed differential activity in the following specific areas: the anterior cingulate cortex/supplementary motor area (ACC/SMA), the thalamus/basal ganglia, the right motor/somatosensory cortex, the medial frontal gyrus, and the left somatosensory cortex. In these areas, heightened activation during the task was associated with higher CRF after controlling for age, sex, and education. Specifically, activity in the ACC/SMA mediated the relationship between CRF and dual-task performance, such that individuals with higher CRF had heightened activation in this area and better EF task performance. Results of studies such as this suggest that higher CRF in late life is related to better brain health despite age-related declines in neural integrity.

This brief overview illustrates the type of research being conducted to understand the associations between brain structure and function and PA/CRF. It appears that older adults who have higher CRF and/ or are more active are less likely to have reductions in brain tissue and loss of cognitive efficiency. These individuals have greater gray matter volume, more intact white matter microstructure, and greater BOLD signal changes in areas that support cognitive processing. However, these cross-sectional associations do not imply causality, and it is possible that older adults with better brain integrity self-select into healthier, more active lifestyles that are associated with greater CRF. Research using longitudinal and randomized controlled designs can provide more insight into the causality of this relationship.

3.2 Observational Longitudinal Research

While the majority of cross-sectional research has focused on CRF, longitudinal studies have historically focused on PA because of the ease of administering PA-related questionnaires to large samples. In these larger-scale studies, those who are more active tend to have better structural integrity in gray and white matter later in life [59–61]. For example, one study involved 299 older adults who completed a questionnaire that included a measurement of number of blocks walked per week at a baseline time point [59]. Nine years later, participants underwent structural neuroimaging to quantify gray matter volume. An additional 4 years later (i.e., 13 years after the baseline assessment), participants were clinically assessed for cognitive impairment. The authors found that walking at least 72 blocks per week at baseline was associated with increased gray matter volume in the frontal lobe, occipital lobe, entorhinal cortex, and hippocampus (Figure 16.2). In addition, increased gray matter volume was associated with a 50% lower risk of cognitive impairment on clinical adjudication. The results from this study suggest that higher PA is associated with reduced risk of cognitive impairment and greater gray matter volume.

Alterations in white matter integrity, assessed by quantification of FA or white matter lesions, can degrade the connectivity between different regions of the brain. As white matter integrity decreases, cognition can become impaired. In one study, 691 older adults completed a PA questionnaire at baseline and structural neuroimaging three years later to assess gray and white matter volume and integrity [60]. The participants in this study were part of the Lothian Birth Cohort and were assessed at baseline at age 70 and at follow-up at age 73. After controlling for age, social class, and health status, more PA at age 70 was associated with fewer white matter lesions at age 73. With fewer white matter lesions, cognition may be better preserved, even in healthy aging.

Greater levels of activity at baseline are associated with better follow-up brain integrity on both macro- and microstructural levels. This heightened structural integrity may be associated with both better maintenance of cognitive functions and better prevention of future cognitive decline, given the specific regions that seem to be affected by PA. Together, these observational longitudinal studies complement the results of the cross-sectional work summarized above, suggesting that greater PA may be protective against an age-related decline in structural integrity.

3.3 Randomized Controlled Trials

Cross-sectional and prospective studies are inherently limited in their ability to determine causal connections between PA and measures of brain health.

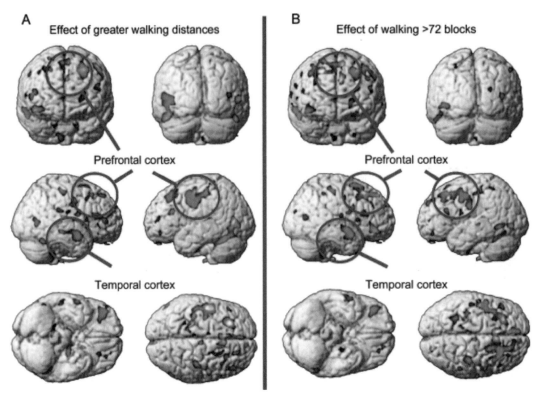

Figure 16.2 Brain regions associated with greater levels of walking. (A) Brain regions showing an association between greater amounts of physical activity (blocks walked) at baseline and greater gray matter volume. Statistical map is thresholded with a false discovery rate of p = 0.05 and a minimum cluster threshold of 100 contiguous voxels. (B) Brain regions showing greater volume in the highest activity quartile of the sample (>72 blocks walked in 2 weeks) compared with the bottom three quartiles. There were no reliable differences in brain volume among the bottom three quartiles. From Erickson et al., 2010 [57]. A black and white version of this figure will appear in some formats. For the color version, please refer to the plate section

Fortunately, evidence that PA *causes* brain changes comes from a growing number of RCTs, which have consistently demonstrated that moderate-intensity exercise for a period of at least 6 months is effective in altering both brain structure and function in a regionally specific manner, with the PFC and hippocampus most consistently affected [45]. For example, Erickson and colleagues recruited 120 cognitively normal older adults to participate in a moderate-intensity exercise RCT over the course of 1 year [62]. Participants were randomized to engage in PA (i.e., walking) 3 days per week, increasing the amount of time spent exercising each week until they reached 40 minutes per session, or were in a stretching and toning control group. After one year, the hippocampi, but not the caudate nuclei or thalamus, of the older adults in the exercise group had increased in size (Cohen's *d* = 0.315 (right) and 0.201 (left);

Figure 16.3). Here, only the participants engaging in frequent moderate-intensity exercise were able to mitigate the typical age-related tissue loss that is seen in the hippocampus. This RCT was the first of its kind to demonstrate that increasing PA could increase the size of this brain structure, which usually shows atrophy with older age.

More recent RCTs have demonstrated similar effects to those found by Erickson and colleagues, including one in healthy older adults [63] and one in older adults with MCI [64]. Colcombe and colleagues found in an RCT that a 6-month moderate-intensity exercise program increased the volume of the PFC and anterior cingulate cortex (ACC), but not the occipital cortex [65]. One recent meta-analysis combined the results from 14 aerobic exercise RCTs for a total of 737 participants to examine the effects of exercise on hippocampal volume [66]. The studies

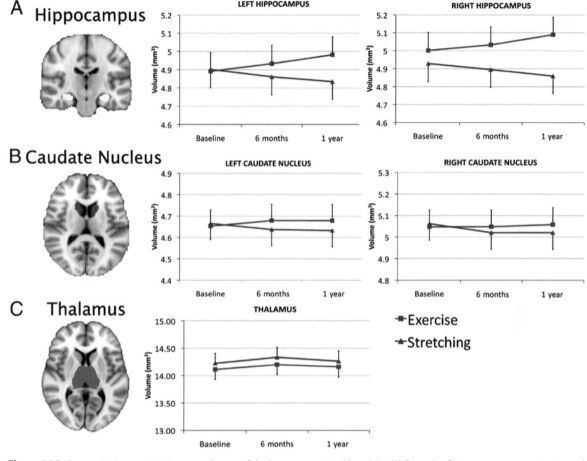

Figure 16.3 An exercise intervention increases the size of the hippocampus in older adults. (A) Example of hippocampus segmentation and graphs demonstrating a significant increase in hippocampus volume for the aerobic exercise group and a decrease in volume for the stretching control group. (B) Example of caudate nucleus segmentation and graphs demonstrating the change in volume for both groups. (C) Example of thalamus segmentation and graph demonstrating the change in volume for both groups. None of the changes was significant for the caudate or thalamus. From Erickson et al. 2011 [60]. A black and white version of this figure will appear in some formats. For the color version, please refer to the plate section.

varied in duration, ranging from three to 24 months and including two to five supervised exercise sessions per week. Six of the studies recruited healthy older adults while the remainder involved participants with depression, MCI, probable AD, and psychotic disorders, as well as healthy young adults. Firth and colleagues found that aerobic exercise did not have a significant effect on total hippocampal volume but did have a significant effect on left hippocampal volume. The authors posited that this effect was due to PA attenuating the typical age-related volume loss, rather than hippocampal volume increasing over time. Although this meta-analysis included a wide range of participants, it provides evidence that aerobic

PA is beneficial to specific brain regions. Thus, structural evidence from RCTs largely supports the findings from studies employing other research designs: that PA affects brain structure in both cortical and subcortical regions implicated in memory (i.e., hippocampus) and EF (i.e., PFC), but not in regions that perform more basic processing (i.e., thalamus, occipital cortex).

Similar specificity has emerged from fMRI studies assessing brain activation and functional connectivity – a measure of regional brain communication. For example, several research groups have shown that long-term moderate intensity PA increases brain activity in the PFC [67, 68] and functional connectivity between the PFC, the ACC, and the hippocampus [38, 55, 69] – regions involved in mediating episodic memory and EF. For example, Voss and colleagues conducted a 12-month RCT in which 65 older adults were randomly assigned to either an aerobic fitness or nonaerobic (i.e., stretching) intervention. Participants underwent resting state fMRI scans [70] at baseline, 6 months, and 12 months. From such studies, it is possible to infer which brain regions have correlated activation patterns over time. Voss and colleagues found that, compared with baseline, participants in the aerobic group had improved resting state functional connectivity. Specifically, the brains of participants in the aerobic exercise group exhibited greater functional connectivity in several large-scale brain networks including the default mode and central executive networks [55]. Changes in the functional connectivity of these networks were also associated with improved EF in the aerobic group, suggesting that fitness-related changes in functional brain communication were behaviorally relevant. Other groups have found similar results in brain areas and networks associated with memory and EFx [38, 67, 68]. These findings have important implications for maintaining cognitive function in late life as disruptions in the communication of these networks may be a key cause of cognitive dysfunction in aging.

To date, few interventions involving brain imaging studies have been conducted in older adults already suffering from MCI or dementia [36, 71]. Instead, RCTs have focused solely on improving or maintaining cognition by increasing CRF/habitual PA. One pilot study, however, included 76 older adults with probable AD who were randomized to a 6-month intervention involving either 150 minutes per week of activity or to a control treatment involving stretching and toning [36]. After the intervention, increases in CRF were associated with bilaterally increased hippocampal volume. This pilot study suggests that, despite diagnoses of MCI or probable AD, increasing aerobic exercise can reduce the burden of neurodegenerative diseases. Additional RCTs are underway investigating how PA interventions may alter CRF and brain outcomes in MCI and/or dementia patients [72, 73].

In sum, there is considerable evidence from cross-sectional studies, prospective longitudinal studies, and RCTs that moderate intensity aerobic exercise may be capable of improving brain structure and function in a domain and regionally specific manner. Randomized controlled trials that increase PA in older adults have demonstrated improvement in brain structural integrity and functional efficiency in key regions typically implicated in aging-related cognitive decline. Specifically, this increase in activity results in volumetric increases in areas critical for episodic memory and EF (e.g., the hippocampus and PFC) and in better functional connectivity between these areas and the rest of the brain. These interventions continue to provide evidence that increasing PA and CRF is a successful nonpharmacologic treatment that combats the neurodegeneration associated with healthy and pathological aging.

3.4 Contradictory Evidence and Limitations

A major limitation in research examining the relationships between PA/CRF and brain health is the sparsity of long-term RCTs, which are essential to making causal inferences about these relationships. Critical to this issue is the question of how long an intervention must be in order to maximize the likelihood of observing effects on brain outcomes. This question has yet to be answered and is a key limitation in the field of PA research. With the heterogeneity of RCT methodology, adherence rates, and PA compliance, it is difficult to discern the necessary dose of PA or to prescribe it as a nonpharmacologic treatment for prevention of age-related declines in cognition and brain health.

Although there are many associations between CRF and the brain, not as much is understood about *how* increasing PA alters brain structure and function. One proposed mechanism by which increasing PA improves neural integrity is through increasing levels of brain-derived neurotrophic factor (BDNF), a protein related to neuronal growth. Evidence for this mechanism comes almost exclusively from studies using animal models [74]. However, BDNF levels vary across the brain and cannot be directly measured in brain tissue in humans [75]. The protein can be measured in serum or plasma, but these assays may not accurately reflect how PA affects central BDNF. More advanced neuroimaging techniques may allow researchers to understand how increasing PA increases levels of BDNF, which then alter brain structure.

Just as no specific dose of PA has been clearly established to yield beneficial cognitive outcomes, the dose of PA required to achieve beneficial brain health outcomes, such as behaviorally relevant brain structure or function, has not yet been defined. Critically, this may be due to differences in the duration, frequency, and/or intensity of exercise utilized across RCTs. Instead, many interventions have been short (i.e., less than 6 months) or have utilized unsupervised exercise sessions, which results in uncertainty about participants' adherence or intensity. Future RCTs that manipulate PA (and seek to manipulate CRF) should consider these issues to make it possible to compare results across intervention without the concern that conclusions are limited due to methodological flaws or variability in study design.

4 Conclusions

PA is a promising nonpharmacologic intervention to prevent and treat typical aging-related declines in cognition and brain health. Both higher CRF and higher levels of PA have been shown to be associated with better cognitive task performance in healthy older adults, primarily for EF and memory. Higher CRF is associated with greater gray matter volume, better white matter microstructural integrity, and enhanced functional brain connectivity. Although it is not possible to determine from cross-sectional studies whether higher CRF leads to better brain health or if individuals with better brain integrity are leading lifestyles that result in higher CRF, the relationship between the two is unequivocal and likely bidirectional.

Longitudinal studies suggest that these associations between PA/CRF and cognition, as well as between PA/CRF and brain structure, are sustained over time. That is, those individuals who are more fit or more active at baseline tend to have better cognitive and brain health outcomes when evaluated at follow-up assessments many years later [14, 19–21, 23, 25, 59–61]. Older adults who have higher CRF and/or are more active may be protecting themselves against the cognitive and neural declines associated with aging. However, only RCTs can explicitly establish this causal relationship.

The apparent beneficial effects of higher CRF and PA for cognitive abilities in healthy older adults might extend to populations already suffering from cognitive decline. Longitudinal evidence shows that being more active may reduce the likelihood of converting from MCI to dementia by more than 60% and reduce the burden associated with neurodegenerative disease. The potential of PA to prevent or slow the progression of cognitive and neurologic decline translates to the potential for it to be used as a widely disseminated, readily accessible treatment for individuals at risk for neurodegenerative disease.

Increasing CRF and/or habitual PA may be neuroprotective. This has been shown in long-term RCTs (i.e., at least 6 months in duration) that report a reduction in decline in cognitive functioning and regionally specific brain volume in aerobic exercise groups relative to control groups [29, 31–33, 36, 38, 62, 64, 65]. The literature reviewed here suggests that cognitive functioning does not improve universally in all domains in older adults randomized to aerobic exercise groups. Rather, the effects associated with PA appear to be specific to EF and, somewhat less consistently, memory. The evidence also suggests that those in the aerobic exercise groups do not have the same rate of cognitive decline as their control group counterparts. Similarly, older adults in aerobic exercise groups do not experience as rapid age-related brain tissue loss as control participants. In spite of these overall favorable outcomes from exercise interventions, not all individuals increasing their PA experience the same degree of benefits. There is still considerable individual variability in the success of exercise interventions on brain health that may be mediated [41] or moderated [76] by a variety of central and peripheral factors. For example, cardiovascular variables, such as lower blood pressure or increased cerebral blood flow, are related to both PA and neurocognition and may mediate their relationship [77, 78]. Changes affecting the hypothalamic-pituitary axis, such as reduced stress, may also mediate this relationship through peripheral and central biological mechanisms. Individuals who actively improve their cardiovascular health or reduce stress through any number of modifiable lifestyle factors (e.g., diet, meditation) may be giving themselves a neurocognitive advantage later in life. Considering these relationships, future research should move the field toward a better understanding of which individuals can benefit most from increasing PA and the mechanisms by which PA exerts its effects. The studies reviewed here suggest that modifying one's lifestyle by increasing PA, even in late life, could prevent or delay cognitive impairment.

Despite the progress the field has made over the last two decades, there are several questions that still remain to be answered, for example: How long do the cognitive and neural benefits of an aerobic fitness program last? What dose of PA is optimal to maximize these neurocognitive benefits? and What factors contribute to the individual differences in the effects of PA training? As the field continues to progress and more RCTs are implemented, we can begin to answer these questions.

References

1. Caspersen CJ, Powell KE, Christenson GM. Physical activity, exercise, and physical fitness: definitions and distinctions for health-related research. *Public Health Rep.* 1985;100(2):126–31.

2. Adams SA, Matthews CE, Ebbeling CB, Moore CG, Cunningham JE, Fulton J, et al. The effect of social desirability and social approval on self-reports of physical activity. *Am J Epidemiol.* 2005;161 (4):389–98.

3. Prince SA, Adamo KB, Hamel ME, Hardt J, Connor Gorber S, Tremblay M. A comparison of direct versus self-report measures for assessing physical activity in adults: a systematic review. *Int J Behav Nutr Phys Act.* 2008;5 (56):56.

4. Committee PAGA. *2018 Physical Activity Guidelines Advisory Committee Scientific Report.* Washington, DC: US Department of Health and Human Services; 2018.

5. Pate RR, Pratt M, Blair SN, Haskell WL, Macera CA, Bouchard C, et al. Physical activity and public health. A recommendation from the Centers for Disease Control and Prevention and the American College of Sports Medicine. *JAMA.* 1995;273(5):402–7.

6. Spirduso W. Physical fitness, aging, and psychomotor speed: a review. *J Gerontol.* 1980;35 (6):850–65.

7. Spirduso W. Exercise and the aging brain. *Res Q Exerc Sport.* 1982;54(2):208–18.

8. Folstein M, Folstein S, McHugh P. "Mini-mental state": a practical method for grading the cognitive state of patients for the clinician. *J Psychiatr Res.* 1975;12 (3):189–98.

9. Middleton LE, Barnes DE, Lui LY, Yaffe K. Physical activity over the life course and its association with cognitive performance and impairment in old age. *J Am Geriatr Soc.* 2010;58 (7):1322–6.

10. Oberlin L, Verstynen T, Burzynska A, Voss M, Prakash R, Chaddock-Heyman L, et al. White matter microstructure mediates the relationship between cardiorespiratory fitness and spatial working memory in older adults. *NeuroImage.* 2016;131:91–101.

11. Freudenberger P, Petrovic K, Sen A, Toglhofer A, Fixa A, Hofer E, et al. Fitness and cognition in the elderly: the Australian Stroke Prevention Study. *Neurology.* 2016;86(5):418–24.

12. Dupuy O, Gauthier CJ, Fraser SA, Desjardins-Crepeau L, Desjardins M, Mekary S, et al. Higher levels of cardiovascular fitness are associated with better executive function and prefrontal oxygenation in younger and older women. *Front Hum Neurosci.* 2015;9:66.

13. Hayes SM, Hayes JP, Cadden M, Verfaellie M. A review of cardiorespiratory fitness-related neuroplasticity in the aging brain. *Front Aging Neurosci.* 2013;5:31.

14. Weuve J, Kang JH, Manson JE, Breteler MM, Ware JH, Grodstein F. Physical activity, including walking, and cognitive function in older women. *JAMA.* 2004;292 (12):1454–61.

15. Hillman CH, Motl RW, Pontifex MB, Posthuma D, Stubbe JH, Boomsma DI, et al. Physical activity and cognitive function in a cross-section of younger and older community-dwelling individuals. *Health Psychol.* 2006;25(6):678–87.

16. Ainsworth BE, Haskell WL, Leon AS, Jacobs DR, Jr., Montoye HJ, Sallis JF, et al. Compendium of physical activities: classification of energy costs of human physical activities. *Med Sci Sports Exerc.* 1993;25 (1):71–80.

17. Shephard R, Vuillemin A. Limits to the measurements of habitual physical activity by questionnaires. *Br J Sports Med.* 2003;37(3):197–206.

18. Innerd P, Catt M, Collerton J, Davies K, Trenell M, Kirkwood T, et al. A comparison of subjective and objective measures of physical activity from the Newcastle 85+ study. *Age and Ageing.* 2015;44 (4):691–4.

19. DeFina L, Willis B, Radford N, Gao A, Leonard D, Haskell W, et al. The association between midlife cardiorespiratory fitness levels and later-life dementia: a cohort study. *Ann Intern Med.* 2013;158(3):162–8.

20. Laurin D, Verreault R, Lindsay J, MacPherson K, Rockwood K. Physical activity and risk of cognitive impairment and dementia in elderly persons. *Arch Neurol.* 2001;58(3):498–504.

21. Etgen T, Sander D, Huntgeburth U, Poppert H, Forstl H, Bickel H. Physical activity and incident cognitive impairment in elderly persons: the INVADE study. *Arch Intern Med.* 2010;170(2):186–93.

22. Sofi F, Valecchi D, Bacci D, Abbate R, Gensini GF, Casini A, et al. Physical activity and risk of cognitive decline: a meta-analysis of prospective studies. *J Intern Med.* 2011;269(1):107–17.

23. Hamer M, Lavoie KL, Bacon SL. Taking up physical activity in later life and healthy ageing: the English longitudinal study of ageing. *Br J Sports Med.* 2014;48 (3):239–43.

24. Blondell S, Hammersley-Mather R, Veerman J. Does physical activity prevent cognitive decline and dementia? A systematic review and meta-analysis of longitudinal studies. *BMC Public Health.* 2014;14(1).

25. Grande G, Vanacore N, Maggiore L, Cucumo V, Ghiretti R, Galimberti D, et al. Physical activity reduces the risk of dementia in mild cognitive impairment subjects: a cohort study. *J Alzheimers Dis.* 2014;39 (4):833–9.

26. Bherer L, Erickson KI, Liu-Ambrose T. A review of the effects of physical activity and exercise on cognitive and brain functions in older adults. *J Aging Res.* 2013;2013:657508.

27. Hamer M, Chida Y. Physical activity and risk of neurodegenerative disease: a systematic review of prospective evidence. *Psychol Med.* 2009;39 (1):3–11.

28. Stephen R, Hongisto K, Solomon A, Lonnroos E. Physical activity and Alzheimer's disease: a systematic review. *J Gerontol A Biol Sci Med Sci.* 2017;72 (6):733–9.

29. Dustman R, Ruhling R, Russell E, Shearer D, Bonekat H, Shigeoka J, et al. Aerobic exercise training and improved neuropsychological function of older adults. *Neurobiol Aging.* 1984;5:35–42.

30. Colcombe S, Kramer AF. Fitness effects on the cognitive function of older adults: a meta-analytic study. *Psychol Sci.* 2003;14 (2):125–30.

31. Heyn P, Abreu BC, Ottenbacher KJ. The effects of exercise training on elderly persons with cognitive impairment and dementia: a meta-analysis. *Arch Phys Med Rehabil.* 2004;85(10):1694–704.

32. Groot C, Hooghiemstra A, Raijmakers P, van Berckel B, Scheltens P, Scherder E, et al. The effect of physical activity on cognitive function in patients with dementia: a meta-analysis of randomized control trials. *Ageing Res Rev.* 2016;25:13–23.

33. Lautenschlager N, Cox K, Flicker L, Foster J, van Bockxmeer F, Xiao J, et al. Effect of physical activity on cognitive function in older adults at risk for Alzheimer disease: a randomized trial. *JAMA.* 2008;300(9):1027–37.

34. Stewart AL, Mills KM, King AC, Haskell WL, Gillis D, Ritter PL. CHAMPS physical activity questionnaire for older adults: outcomes for interventions. *Med Sci Sports Exerc.* 2001;33 (7):1126–41.

35. Rosen WG, Mohs RC, Davis KL. A new rating scale for Alzheimer's disease. *Am J Psychiatry.* 1984;141 (11):1356–64.

36. Morris J, Vidoni E, Johnson D, Van Sciver A, Mahnken J, Honea R, et al. Aerobic exercise for Alzheimer's disease: a randomized controlled pilot trial. *PLoS ONE.* 2017;12(2).

37. Angevaren M, Aufdemkampe G, Verhaar HJ, Aleman A, Vanhees L. Physical activity and enhanced fitness to improve cognitive function in older people without known cognitive impairment. *Cochrane Database Syst Rev.* 2008;3(3).

38. Barnes DE, Santos-Modesitt W, Poelke G, Kramer AF, Castro C, Middleton LE, et al. The Mental Activity and eXercise (MAX) trial: a randomized controlled trial to enhance cognitive function in older adults. *JAMA Intern Med.* 2013;173 (9):797–804.

39. Sink KM, Espeland MA, Castro CM, Church T, Cohen R, Dodson JA, et al. Effect of a 24-month physical activity intervention vs health education on cognitive outcomes in sedentary older adults: the LIFE randomized trial. *JAMA.* 2015;314(8):781–90.

40. Young J, Angevaren M, Rusted J, Tabet N. Aerobic exercise to improve cognitive function in older adults without known cognitive impairment. *Cochrane Database Syst Rev.* 2015 Apr 22; (4):CD005381.

41. Stillman C, Cohen J, Lehman M, Erickson K. Mediators of physical activity on neurocognitive function: a review at multiple levels of analysis. *Frontiers in Human Neuroscience.* 2016 Dec 8;10:626.

42. Hamilton G, Rhodes J. Exercise regulation of cognitive function and neuroplasticity in the healthy and diseased brain. *Prog Mol Biol Transl Sci.* 2015;135:381–406.

43. Cotman C, Berchtold N, Christie L. Exercise builds brain health: key roles of growth factor cascades and inflammation. *Trends Neurosci.* 2007;30 (9):464–72.

44. Raz N, Lindenberger U, Rodrigue K, Kennedy K, Head D,

Williamson A, et al. Regional brain changes in aging healthy adults: general trends, individual differences and modifiers. *Cereb Cortex.* 2005;15(11):1676–89.

45. Erickson KI, Leckie R, Weinstein A. Physical activity, fitness, and gray matter volume. *Neurobiol Aging.* 2014;35(Suppl 2):S20–S28.

46. Colcombe S, Erickson KI, Raz N, Webb AG, Cohen NJ, McAuley E, et al. Aerobic fitness reduces brain tissue loss in aging humans. *J Gerontol A Biol Sci Med Scie.* 2003;58(2):M176–M180.

47. Erickson KI, Prakash R, Voss M, Chaddock-Heyman L, Hu L, Morris K, et al. Aerobic fitness is associated with hippocampal volume in elderly humans. *Hippocampus.* 2009;19 (10):1030–9.

48. Sen A, Gider P, Cavalieri M, Freudenberge P, Farzi A, Schallert M, et al. Association of cardiorespiratory fitness and morphological brain changes in the elderly: results of the Australian Stroke Prevention Study. *Neurodegener Dis.* 2012;10:135–7.

49. Burzynska A, Chaddock-Heyman L, Voss M, Wong C, Gothe N, Olson E, et al. Physical activity and cardiorespiratory fitness are beneficial for white matter in low-fit older adults. *PLoS ONE.* 2014;9 (9).

50. Tian Q, Simonsick E, Erickson KI, Aizenstein H, Glynn N, Boudreau R, et al. Cardiorespiratory fitness and brain diffusion tensor imaging in adults over 80 years of age. *Brain Research.* 2014;1588:63–72.

51. Schwarb H, Johnson C, Daugherty A, Hillman CH, Kramer AF, Cohen NJ, et al. Aerobic fitness, hippocampal viscoelasticity, and relational memory performance. *NeuroImage.* 2017;153:179–88.

52. Fletcher M, Low K, Boyd R, Zimmerman B, Gordon B, Tan C, et al. Comparing aging and fitness effects on brain anatomy. *Front Hum Neurosci.* 2016;10.

53. Teixeira C, Rezende T, Weiler M, Nogueira M, Campos B, Pegoraro L, et al. Relation between aerobic fitness and brain structures in amnestic mild cognitive impairment elderly. *Age (Dordr).* 2016 Jun;38(3):51.

54. Perea R, Vidoni E, Morris J, Graves R, Burns J, Honea R. Cardiorespiratory fitness and white matter integrity in Alzheimer's disease. *Brain Imaging Behav.* 2016;10(3):660–8.

55. Voss M, Prakash R, Erickson K, Basak C, Chaddock L, Kim J, et al. Plasticity of brain networks in a randomized intervention trial of exercise training in older adults. *Front Aging Neurosci.* 2010; 2.

56. Voss M, Weng T, Burzynska A, Wong C, Cooke G, Clark R, et al. Fitness, but not physical activity, is related to functional integrity of brain networks associated with aging. *NeuroImage.* 2016;131:113–25.

57. Albinet C, Mandrick K, Bernard P, Perrey S, Blain H. Improved cerebral oxygenation response and executive performance as a function of cardiorespiratory fitness in older women: a fNIRS study. *Front Aging Neurosci.* 2014;6.

58. Wong C, Chaddock-Heyman L, Voss M, Burzynska A, Basak C, Erickson KI, et al. Brain activation during dual-task processing is associated with cardiorespiratory fitness and performance in older adults. *Front Aging Neurosci.* 2015 Aug 12;7:154.

59. Erickson KI, Raji C, Lopez O, Becker J, Rosano C, Newman A, et al. Physical activity predicts gray matter volume in late adulthood: the Cardiovascular Health Study. *Neurology.* 2010;75 (16):1415–22.

60. Gow A, Bastin M, Maniega S, Valdes Hernandez M, Morris Z, Murray C, et al. Neuroprotective lifestyles and the aging brain: activity, atrophy, and white matter integrity. *Neurology.* 2012;79 (17):1802–8.

61. Best J, Rosano C, Aizenstein H, Tian Q, Boudreau R, Ayonayon H, et al. Long-term changes in time spent walking and subsequent cognitive and structural brain changes in older adults. *Neurobiol Aging.* 2017;57:153–61.

62. Erickson KI, Voss MW, Prakash RS, Basak C, Szabo A, Chaddock L, et al. Exercise training increases size of hippocampus and improves memory. *Proc Natl Acad Sci U S A.* 2011;108(7):3017–22.

63. Niemann C, Godde B, Voelcker-Rehage C. Not only cardiovascular, but also coordinative exercise increases hippocampal volume in older adults. *Front Aging Neurosci.* 2014;6.

64. Ten Brinke L, Bolandzadeh N, Nagamatsu L, Hsu C, Davis J, Miran-Khan K, et al. Aerobic exercise increases hippocampal volume in older women with probably mild cognitive impairment: a 6-month randomised controlled trial. *Br J Sports Med.* 2014;49(4):248–54.

65. Colcombe S, Erickson KI, Scalf P, Kim J, Prakash R, McAuley E, et al. Aerobic exercise training increases brain volume in aging humans. *J Gerontol A Biol Sci Med Sci.* 2006;61(11):1166–70.

66. Firth J, Stubbs B, Vancampfort D, Schuch F, Lagopoulos J, Rosenbaum S, et al. Effect of aerobic exercise on hippocampal volume in humans: a systematic review and meta-analysis. *NeuroImage.* 2018;166:230–8.

67. Smith J, Nielson K, Antuono P, Lyons J, Hanson R, Butts A, et al. Semantic memory functional MRI and cognitive function after exercise intervention in mild cognitive impairment.

J Alzheimer's Dis. 2013;37 (1):197–215.

68. Suzuki T, Shimada H, Makizako H, Doi T, Yoshida D, Ito K, et al. A randomized controlled trial of multicomponent exercise in older adults with mild cognitive impairment. *PLoS ONE.* 2013;8 (4):e61483.

69. Burdette J, Laurienti P, Espeland M, Morgan A, Telesford Q, Vechlekar C, et al. Using network science to evaluate exercise-associated brain changes in older adults. *Front Aging Neurosci.* 2010;2.

70. Biswal B, Kylen J, Hyde J. Simultaneous assessment of flow and BOLD signals in resting-state functional connectivity maps. *NMR in Biomedicine.* 1997;10 (4–5):165–70.

71. Reiter K, Nielson K, Smith T, Weiss L, Alfini A, Smith J. Improved cardiorespiratory fitness is associated with increased cortical thickness in mild cognitive impairment. *J Int Neuropsychol Soc.* 2015;21 (10):757–67.

72. Devenney K, Sanders M, Lawlor B, Olde Rikkert M, Schneider S, Group NS. The effects of an extensive exercise programme on the progression of mild cognitive impairment (MCI): study protocol for a randomised controlled trial. *BMC Geriatrics.* 2017;17(1).

73. Leeuwis A, Hooghiemstra A, Amier R, Ferro D, Franken L, Nijveldt R, et al. Design of the ECersion-VCI study: the effect of aerobic exercise on cerebral perfusion in patients with vascular cognitive impairment. *ALzheimer's & Dementia.* 2017;3 (2):157–65.

74. Cotman C, Berchtold N. Exercise: a behavioral intervention to enhance brain health and plasticity. *Trends Neurosci.* 2002;25(6):295–301.

75. Erickson KI, Miller D, Roecklein K. The aging hippocampus: interactions between exercise, depression, and BDNF. *Neuroscientist.* 2012;18 (1):82–97.

76. Leckie R, Weinstein A, Hodzic J, Erickson KI. Potential moderators of physical activity on brain health. *J Aging Res.* 2012;2012:948981.

77. Rosendorff C, Beeri M, Silverman J. Cardiovascular risk factors for Alzheimer's disease. *Am J Geriatr Cardiol.* 2007;16(3):143–9.

78. O'Donovan C, Lithander F, Raftery T, Gormley J, Mahmud A, Hussey J. Inverse relationship between physical activity and arterial stiffness in adults with hypertension. *J Phys Act Health.* 2014;11:272–7.

Pharmacological Cosmetic Neurology

Erin C. Conrad and Anjan Chatterjee

1 Introduction

"Cosmetic neurology," also referred to as "cognitive enhancement," is the practice of enhancing cognition and behavior in healthy people [1]. Although cosmetic neurology often refers to the enhancement of cognition, it can also refer to the enhancement of mood, movement, creativity, social finesse, and other psychological attributes. Cosmetic neurology carries the promise of an improved quality of life and productivity well into old age, as well as potential medical and social perils [2]. In this chapter, we review current drugs that can be used for enhancement, their potential efficacy, current cultural norms, and the ethical issues that arise from this practice.

2 Drugs Used for Cosmetic Neurology

Like its namesake, cosmetic surgery, which was first developed to treat disfiguring injuries resulting from World War I trench warfare, cosmetic neurology has roots in wartime applications [3]. Treatments for facial disfigurements from injuries in the field began to be applied to healthy people. This practice was in part driven by financial incentives and eventually cultural acceptance. Analogously, methamphetamine, one of the earliest cosmetic neurology drugs, was widely used in Germany during World War II to stimulate battle-weary soldiers [4, 5]. A medical officer reported early use of this drug during a 1942 battle involving German soldiers encircled by Russian troops at the Eastern Front. The exhausted soldiers were each given two tablets of methamphetamine and subsequently managed to break out of the encirclement, many becoming "euphoric" during the fight [6]. Cosmetic neurology, also driven by financial and social forces, has since evolved to include other drugs and has expanded beyond the military to the classroom, the workplace, and the home.

2.1 Stimulants

Stimulants include amphetamines, methylphenidate, atomoxetine, and modafinil. Multiple stimulants are currently approved to treat ADHD in the United States. Stimulants increase noradrenergic and dopaminergic transmission in frontoparietal attentional systems and the striatum [7]. They are the best-studied class of cognitive enhancers. Studies report evidence for improved attention [8], shorter reaction time [9–11], more accurate short-term memory [10, 12, 13], and improved language learning [14]. Stimulants have a greater effect during sleep deprivation [15]. Chess players on stimulants take longer to consider each move, improving their performance in untimed games, but display worse performance in more traditional games in which there is a time limit for each move [16]. The performance-enhancing effect of stimulants may not be mediated by directly increasing intelligence per se, but rather as a secondary effect of increased wakefulness, vigilance, or motivation [17]. Some argue that these drugs are better conceived as drive drugs than cognitive enhancers.

2.2 Cholinergic Medications

Cholinergic medications, including acetylcholinesterase inhibitors, acetylcholine precursors, and the direct nicotine agonist, increase normal cholinergic stimulation of the cerebral cortex via the nucleus basalis and cholinergic stimulation of the hippocampus via the medial septal nuclei and the nuclei of the diagonal bands of Broca [7, 18]. Acetylcholine acts on nicotinic and muscarinic receptors in the brain, and both receptors are thought to be important in cognition. Acetylcholinesterase inhibitors improve cognitive performance across multiple domains in patients with Alzheimer's disease and other forms of dementia, in part by guiding the development and maintenance of neuronal synaptic connections, a process that is disrupted in Alzheimer's disease [19–22]. They may improve episodic and verbal memory among healthy adults [23, 24]. In one preliminary study with commercial pilots, low doses of cholinesterase inhibitors improved performance during emergencies in flight simulations [25]. Like stimulants, the effect of these drugs may be mediated through increased levels of arousal (by potentiating the action of cholinergic nuclei in the midbrain reticular formation), as they also are more effective when the user is sleep deprived [23, 26, 27].

2.3 Others

Glutamatergic medications such as memantine, used to treat Alzheimer's disease, may improve visual memory in healthy adults [28, 29]. Calcium channel blockers improve memory acquisition, possibly by affecting cerebral circulation [30, 31]. Insulin resistance in diabetics is correlated with age-associated cognitive decline. There is conflicting evidence that the antihyperglycemic medication metformin may protect against this decline in patients with diabetes and pre-diabetes [32, 33]. Over-the-counter drugs used for enhancement include caffeine, an adenosine receptor antagonist that increases vigilance and working memory [9]; *Ginkgo biloba*, which has been proposed to improve cognition through its antioxidant properties, though there is no evidence of efficacy [34, 35]; *Bacopa monnieri*, which may improve delayed word recall in older adults [36]; piracetam, which has cholinergic and glutamatergic effects and has mixed evidence for efficacy in cosmetic neurology [37]; and curry (presumably through curcumin), which may improve Mini Mental Status Exam scores among the elderly [38]. Lysergic acid diethylamide (LSD) and psilocybin mushrooms, which are illegal in the United States and most of Europe, are increasingly used among young professionals in doses smaller than those used to achieve a high in order to augment mood, creativity, concentration, and problem-solving. This practice, known as "microdosing," is particularly popular in Silicon Valley [39, 40].

3 Prevalence of Cosmetic Neurology

The reported prevalence of cosmetic neurology varies widely across surveys depending on the nature of the survey, the cosmetic neurology drug being used, and the survey participants [41]. With this caveat, the practice of cosmetic neurology appears common.

Among students, reported lifetime use rates range from 5% to 40% and 18% for medical students specifically [42–48]. Among professionals, 9% of surgeons, 28% of poker players, and 19% of professionals in economics report using illicit or prescription drugs for enhancement [49–51]. Adults also use these pills outside school and work to improve their cognitive performance in daily life. Most of these data are from American populations. However, 15% of German elderly adults reported using ginkgo for cosmetic neurology [52].

4 Potential Advantages of Cosmetic Neurology

4.1 The Current Benefits of Cosmetic Neurology Are Unclear, and Probably Small

The enhancing effect of cosmetic neurology drugs on cognitive testing is inconsistent across trials, with little to no effect demonstrated in meta-analyses [15, 23]. Effects on more practical measures of intellectual success are equally underwhelming. Stimulants, the most commonly used cosmetic neurology drugs among students, do not actually improve grade point average [53]. Some studies find that people taking these drugs are more confident of their improved performance, even when such improvement is not evident in objective measures [54, 55].

These modest results should ground discussion on the potential individual and social effects of cosmetic neurology. However, many scientists, ethicists, and physicians are optimistic about their potential future benefits. Our improving understanding of cognitive neuroscience, the increasing prevalence of dementia in the aging population, and the need for treatments for conditions like depression, addiction, and attention deficit disorder will accelerate the development of new and more efficacious cosmetic neurology drugs [56, 57].

4.2 Benefits to the Individual

Cosmetic neurology offers the promise of improved cognitive performance, enhanced learning potential, increased motivation, facilitated social interactions, better mood, and improved ability to recover from stress [58, 59]. Both methylphenidate and lorazepam lessen the effect of emotional material on memory [60], and beta blockers prevent post-traumatic symptoms in car-crash victims [61]. Perhaps these drugs can be used to dull other painful – albeit less clinically significant – memories as well.

Cosmetic neurology may also enhance our autonomy [62, 63]. Our capacity for self-determination depends on our ability to act as rational agents. Improved verbal processing strengthens our ability to critically analyze others' claims and viewpoints, protecting us from deception. Enhanced memory gives us a more complete picture of ourselves and our world, aiding in self-reflection. And improved logical reasoning facilitates our free choice.

Cosmetic neurology may have particular utility among older adults. Aging begets an expected non-pathological cognitive decline, as distinct from dementia. Vocabulary and general knowledge tend to improve as we get older, but almost all other measures of cognition, including processing speed, attention, memory, visuospatial ability, and executive function, start declining as early as the third decade of life [64], as detailed in other chapters of this book. Although this decline is considered a normal part of healthy aging, it can greatly impact people's lives. Many are embarrassed by increasingly frequent tip-of-the-tongue episodes when trying to remember the names of acquaintances. Difficulty performing more complex executive tasks may lead to serious errors in managing finances. And as people live longer and the retirement age increases, cognitive changes may impact the ability of older adults to flourish and keep up with their younger colleagues.

4.3 Benefits to Society

Professionals such as pilots, physicians, and firefighters whose attention, reaction time, and problem-solving ability are critical for protecting the public may be able to perform their duties more safely with cosmetic neurology drugs, particularly under conditions of stress or sleep deprivation [65–68]. Sleep deprivation in people who work in these professions can be deadly. The case of Libby Zion, who died under the care of overworked medical residents, spurred advocacy for the regulation of resident work hours [69, 70]. But even today, residents routinely work 24 or more continuous hours without sleep, and the current physician shortage, combined with the aging population, makes it unlikely that we will have an abundance of well-rested physicians in the near future. Given the lack of available social

solutions to the physician shortage, should we turn to pharmacologic ones? If you had to receive care from either a sleep-deprived physician or a sleep-deprived physician on stimulants, which would you choose?

Enhancing the decision-making capacity of judges, whose decisions are less time critical but of equal consequence to those of physicians, may improve justice [71]. Retrials prompted by judges falling asleep mid-case show us that judges are subject to fatigue no less than physicians and pilots [72]. Also, judges make more lenient parole decisions at the beginning of the day and immediately after lunch [73], although the non-random order of prisoners without attorney representation may explain this effect [74]. The use of cosmetic neurology by judges might mitigate these unconscious biases [75].

More intelligent and creative thinking may also enhance economic productivity and accelerate new discoveries and inventions [76]. Paul Erdős, the author of more than 1,000 mathematics papers, is one of the most prolific mathematicians in history. He frequently used stimulants to enhance his mathematical prowess. In 1970 a friend concerned for his health bet him $500 that he couldn't stop amphetamines for a month. Erdős accepted the bet and won. However, he was frustrated by his lack of academic progress while off amphetamines, and told his friend at the end of the bet, "You've set mathematics back a month" [77].

We may also use cosmetic neurology to promote moral behavior, a concept referred to as moral enhancement. Some psychiatric disorders (most notably antisocial personality disorder) are characterized in part by a disregard for the rights of others. Therapy aimed at improving moral behavior in individuals with these disorders could be considered medical treatment [78]. We could also apply such therapies to less pathological moral deficiencies. One method would be to alter the underlying impulses that provoke immoral behavior. Just as naltrexone is used clinically to curb cravings for alcohol, drugs might be used to mitigate violent impulses or feelings of racism [79]. Conversely, we might take a pill that promotes empathy, trust, or altruism (oxytocin and SSRIs have this effect to some degree) [76, 80, 81]. Stimulants, cholinergic agents, and other cognitive enhancers discussed above could improve our ability to reason toward morally correct choices, assuming we start with good motives [80, 82].

5 Limits to Our Knowledge

Any discussion of the advantages and disadvantages of cosmetic neurology relies on adequate information about drug efficacy and adverse effects. Unfortunately, our knowledge is limited and may remain so for the foreseeable future.

5.1 Placebo Effects

A pervasive issue in trying to understand the specific effects of enhancing drugs is determining the extent of placebo effects [83, 84]. The belief that drugs are helpful often contributes to their demonstrable beneficial effects [85]. For example, people often feel better about their performance on stimulants even when there is no measurable improvement [86]. At a societal level, the greater the general belief that enhancements work, regardless of whether that belief is generated by the media or what peers say, the more likely people will experience positive effects of these medications. Such beliefs, if widespread, are likely to influence public policy regardless of limited scientific support.

5.2 Bias

There are several impediments to research on the effects of enhancing medications in healthy people. Most funding agencies do not support such research, making systematic progress difficult. The lack of funding and regulatory burdens prevents large multicenter randomized controlled trials. Accumulated data are often biased in fields with few researchers and small true effect sizes that might not be meaningful [87]. Inadequate statistical power, hence insufficient evidence of generalizability, is an endemic problem in studies of enhancements. These studies typically enroll small numbers of participants. Often the drugs are given once and, if repeated, only for relatively short durations. Because studies that show significant effects are more likely to be published, well-designed negative studies are not accounted for in any systematic manner. This publication bias is common in neuroscience [88]. As such, reviews of this literature and various meta-analyses may overestimate the effects of currently available enhancement medications.

6 Ethical Concerns of Cosmetic Neurology

6.1 Safety

Many physicians, scientists, and regulators worry that the medical risks and side effects outweigh the modest benefits of cosmetic neurology drugs. Stimulants have been subject to particular scrutiny. The established effect of stimulants on heart rate and blood pressure has caused concern over potential cardiovascular risks, leading the FDA to issue a black box warning in 2006 for all amphetamines and methylphenidate [89, 90]. However, since this warning, large retrospective cohort studies have demonstrated no increased risk of cardiovascular events with the use of any ADHD drugs by young adults or children [91, 92]. The relative cardiovascular safety of these drugs in young adults may not apply to older people with underlying atherosclerotic disease.

Other potentially concerning side effects of stimulants include decreased appetite, insomnia, and irritability [93]. Given the action of stimulants on the dopaminergic reward pathways, and given their similarity to drugs of abuse such as methamphetamine and cocaine, dependence and addiction are also concerns. However, prospective cohort studies have not found an increased risk of substance use disorders among people prescribed stimulants for ADHD [94, 95].

These are the risks of cosmetic neurology drugs when used to treat disease. We do not know the long-term effects of these drugs in *healthy* people. New, less-studied drugs present additional safety concerns [17, 96]. Physicians have argued that safety requirements for drugs should be more stringent when they are used for enhancement than when used to treat disease, as healthy individuals have less to gain and more to lose [97].

There are additional considerations when prescribing cosmetic neurology in older patients. Cosmetic neurology may produce greater gains in the elderly by restoring prior function. On this framing of the issue, the treatment-enhancement distinction is blurred and one might regard the use of enhancements as treatment. However, the higher incidence of hypertension, chronic obstructive pulmonary disease, and other risk factors, especially for cardiovascular disease in the elderly, is likely to also increase the risk of serious adverse effects of stimulant medications.

Some have pointed out a discrepancy between the actual and perceived benefits of cosmetic neurology [13, 98]. For instance, despite the lack of evidence for stimulants affecting academic performance, improving grades remains the primary reason students take stimulants [53]. If the hype surrounding cosmetic neurology outstrips the science, then users may be unknowingly putting themselves at risk for little benefit.

6.2 Inadvertent Cognitive Changes and Trade-offs

In addition to medical risk, cosmetic neurology pills may produce unintended psychological changes [99]. For instance, although stimulants show some benefit for cognitive function among sleep-deprived individuals, over longer periods of sleep deprivation, stimulants increase wakefulness but *not* cognitive performance, potentially instilling overconfidence in their users [54, 55]. In 2003, American pilots in Afghanistan spotted ground fire that was part of a Canadian military training exercise. Misinterpreting the exercise as hostile, the pilots – who were on amphetamines at the time to combat sleep deprivation – ignored an order to hold their fire, shooting and ultimately killing four of the Canadian soldiers. The pilots claimed that the drugs clouded their judgment [100].

Gaining function in one cognitive domain may also limit other abilities [101, 102]. By activating the noradrenergic system, stimulants may aggravate test anxiety. Also, enhancing concentration might harm the unfocused thought necessary for creativity [103]. There is some evidence that stimulants might impede performance on tasks that require cognitive flexibility, such as solving anagrams [104]. Amphetamines had no effect on overall performance on a battery of creativity tests; however, there was a small negative effect among the most creative individuals [105]. There are other potential trade-offs; for example, enhancing consolidation of long-term memories could reduce the adaptability of memory to changes in the environment [101].

6.3 Social Danger

Even when cosmetic neurology works as intended, an individual's enhanced intelligence, creativity, and productivity may carry some risk to others. History

gives us many examples (atomic bombs, biological weapons, cell phones, etc.) in which scientific progress can contribute to dangerous social results. Cosmetic neurology could potentially accelerate the development of harmful inventions. Of course, this risk exists with *any* intervention that improves intelligence, including basic education, but we consider the benefits of these cultural forms of enhancement to outweigh the risks. Some philosophers suggest that the solution to the dangers of cosmetic neurology – both cultural and pharmaceutical – is the development of moral enhancement as discussed above, and caution against cosmetic neurology that does not go hand in hand with moral enhancement [76].

6.4 Enhancement versus Treatment

Cosmetic neurology, like cosmetic surgery, deviates from medicine's stated goal of treating disease [106]. One can question the importance of the treatment/enhancement distinction with a thought experiment. Imagine two equally short boys – one afflicted with growth hormone deficiency and the other with short parents – who both want access to growth hormone pills. Although growth hormone would be treatment in the first boy and enhancement in the second, the practical effects of the pills would be identical in the two boys. By extension, why differentiate between cognitive treatment and cognitive enhancement [107]?

The treatment/enhancement distinction is particularly murky in age-associated cognitive changes. Although age-related cognitive decline is not considered pathological, its mechanisms, and more importantly its results, are similar to those of disease-related cognitive decline. Whereas cosmetic neurology is generally aimed at enhancing a person's baseline, in the elderly cosmetic neurology seeks to restore function to a prior baseline. Some have argued that the enhancement/restoration distinction is morally relevant and makes cosmetic neurology more permissible in the elderly than in young people [108]. However, as mentioned earlier, the potential risk of adverse effects is also likely to increase among the elderly, complicating an individual's decision to avail themselves of current available enhancement medications.

6.5 Inauthentic Pills

A major criticism of cosmetic neurology pills in surveys of public opinion is that drugs are unnatural.

The complaint depends on the form of the pill: the public is generally more accepting of vitamins, caffeine, and other natural supplements than they are of pharmaceuticals [109]. Even when the same enhancing substance is considered, people find it more morally acceptable if it is delivered by pill than by injection [110]. Pills are also considered less acceptable than nonpharmacological cosmetic neurology (such as exercise or computer training) [111]. Safety explains some of the difference, as people perceive pharmacological cosmetic neurology to be less safe than natural supplements [112]. The bias against pharmaceuticals may depend on familiarity with pharmaceuticals. A survey of medical students found no difference in acceptability between the use of pharmaceuticals and natural supplements for enhancement [113].

6.6 Inauthentic Achievements

Achievements with the aid of cosmetic neurology may also be interpreted as inauthentic, even amounting to cheating in competitive contexts such as standardized tests [114]. As with the use of calculators in school and specialized gear in athletics, "cheating" is defined by the pre-established rules of the game. So cosmetic neurology is cheating only if schools and other regulators say so. Regardless of how we define cheating, if a student, aided by a pill, does well on a test, then the pill arguably cheapens the success. But what if the pill is taken one month prior to the test, and the pill allows the student to study harder and retain more information? What if they take the pill years before the test, and the pill heightens their intelligence in a lasting way, making the test accurately reflect their newfound intelligence? Some argue that this intelligence is itself inauthentic, as it is the result of neither inborn potential nor hard work, discussed further below [115].

6.7 Inauthentic Selves

Will cosmetic neurology drugs erode our character by enabling intelligence through easier means ("gain without pain") [116]? Every new development that improves quality of life, from anesthesia to air conditioning, could also be argued to reduce character-building suffering. Yet we generally accept these convenient technologies [59]. But perhaps altering our intelligence rather than just our room temperature poses a greater risk to the human essence [106]. The President's Council on Bioethics wrote in 2003 that using unnatural means to change our thinking risks "flattening our souls" [117]. This discussion encroaches on concepts that vary widely across different individuals, cultures, and religions, making it challenging to definitively argue that the human soul is or is not harmed by cosmetic neurology [115]. The notion of changing ourselves through education, religion, travel, or even pills is not new or necessarily bad. Some have described experiences with psychedelic drugs that produced positive changes in their sense of self [118]. If it is acceptable to alter personhood with these external agents, then why not with cosmetic neurology?

6.8 Coercion

The potential use of cosmetic neurology for competition raises the question of whether the decision to use cosmetic neurology can be undertaken freely. If a student's peers are taking cosmetic neurology drugs, then the student may feel compelled to take drugs to level the playing field. As people age, they might feel pressure to enhance their cognition to keep up with or compete with younger workers, especially in a technologically changing and challenging workplace. On the other hand, any method of self-improvement – including learning to read – risks social coercion for similar reasons [115]. Social pressure to enhance oneself is not a harm in itself. But if cosmetic neurology is bad for *other* reasons, then the potential for coercion makes it even worse.

In addition to implicit pressures to keep pace with others, employers could explicitly demand that employees take pills to improve their workplace performance. This is not a remote concern: in the case of friendly fire on Canadian soldiers in Afghanistan, the American pilots claimed that they felt compelled by their superiors to use amphetamines or be dismissed from the mission [100]. This explicit coercion could be legislated against, although such legislation may have limited practical effect. It would be hard to prove that an employer gave unequal treatment because of an employee's unwillingness to use cosmetic neurology [119]. Explicit pressure might also arise in situations where benefits to the group might outweigh the rights of an individual. For example, might post-call medical residents be required to take drugs that counter errors made more likely by fatigue and sleep deprivation? Some even suggest that physicians have a moral responsibility to use enhancements [120].

6.9 Unequal Access

Cosmetic neurology may produce injustice through unequal access. Inequality is not inevitable: if cosmetic neurology were freely available to the public, it might mitigate rather than exacerbate inequalities by creating cognitive opportunities for the socially disadvantaged [121]. This optimistic possibility contrasts with the current social reality in which opportunities are disproportionately available to the wealthy. Where cosmetic neurology is available for pay, economic advantages become cognitive advantages [115]. Cosmetic neurology's potential for inequality is a reason for concern but likely not a reason for prohibition. The popularity of SAT prep classes reminds us that paying to promote your and your children's success is nothing new or currently framed as unacceptable. Cosmetic neurology is arguably more acceptable than the example of SAT prep classes: whereas only obtaining a higher score on the SAT alone might help a person gain entrance to a more prestigious college, enhancing a person's intelligence provides benefits to society that extend beyond the individual.

6.10 Children and Adolescents

Children and adolescents are a special case. On the one hand, their developing brains stand to benefit more from the effects of enhancing pills on neuroplasticity. However, this also puts them at greater risk. It is also unclear who should decide which children receive cosmetic neurology. Should a particular parent's wishes determine if a child is exposed to the potential risks and benefits of cosmetic neurology drugs? On the other hand, leaving the decision to the state would overrule parents' autonomy over raising their children. Citing these special concerns, the American Academy of Neurology issued guidance opposing cosmetic neurology for children [122].

7 Social Considerations

7.1 Inevitability

Regardless of the debate in the literature, cosmetic neurology is to some degree inevitable [31, 123]. A recent Netflix documentary released in March 2018 recounts the current widespread use of cosmetic neurology among students and workers in some sectors [124]. The use of stimulants for cosmetic neurology is essentially prohibited in the United States, as very few physicians prescribe stimulants in the absence of ADHD or other disease and sharing prescription medications with other people is illegal. The widespread use of prescription stimulants on college campuses despite this prohibition suggests that banning cosmetic neurology is practically impossible. It would be even more challenging to ban the use of over-the-counter medications for cosmetic neurology, as these are readily available to anyone. And if we did try to prohibit the use of over-the-counter medications for cosmetic neurology, where would we draw the line? If we ban ginkgo biloba, why not coffee?

Given that banning cosmetic neurology would be very difficult (and not clearly desirable), sociologists have instead turned their attention toward public policy that might foster responsible use. Universities that oppose cosmetic neurology could establish a social norm against it by defining cosmetic neurology in their honor codes as cheating [125]. We may be able to regulate cosmetic neurology drugs similarly to other legal nonprescription psychoactive drugs, such as nicotine and alcohol, with taxes, limited distribution, and age restrictions. However, as with alcohol and nicotine, this would not preclude abuses within or outside the legal system [126]. We could even license cosmetic neurology, requiring users to demonstrate an understanding of the risks before being allowed to purchase drugs. But, counterproductively, this would discourage those who have less cognitive capacity and thus could benefit the most from cosmetic neurology from pursuing it [115].

7.2 Public Opinion

Cultural norms about the use of enhancements have not coalesced into a consensus. Attitudes about enhancement are influenced by cultural contexts that vary [127]. Physicians, who would do the prescribing, may need to think beyond traditional disease models of care [1, 128–130]. Physicians are typically pragmatic about prescribing enhancements, but also ambivalent, viewing the practice as alleviating suffering while being wary of exaggerating social inequities [131, 132]. Approaching enhancement as a public health issue may advance the discussion [133].

Clinical neuroscientists and ethicists can lay the groundwork for broader public discussions. As of now, there is little agreement among academics [134]. Some regard the ethical concerns as exaggerated or ill-conceived [98, 135]. The attitude among the public also varies. Most of our information comes from surveys of young people, who show a divide between those who use enhancers and those who do not [136]. Nonusers more than users are concerned about medical safety and questions of fairness. Generally, both users and nonusers think that the decision to use enhancements is a matter of personal choice and oppose formal coercive policies, such as requiring use of enhancements in high-performance jobs (e.g., physicians, pilots).

Involving the public in the debate on cosmetic neurology is essential. First, it advances the ethical discussion: the public offers a diverse array of moral viewpoints and may anticipate future ethical considerations. Involving the public also prevents physicians, scientists, and ethicists from operating in isolation from the population they serve. Understanding which elements of cosmetic neurology the public finds acceptable and which they find morally concerning can help guide the development of cosmetic neurology drugs and shape socially conscious public policy. Many surveys, interviews, and focus groups have gathered opinion regarding cosmetic neurology, demonstrating large variability in respondents' opinions but largely reflecting the concerns raised by ethicists [136–147]. One limitation of these studies is that they largely surveyed students and primarily asked about the use of cosmetic neurology by students. Involving the larger public and addressing use

in and out of the workplace will reveal a broader range of opinions toward this growing application of cosmetic neurology.

8 Conclusion

Cosmetic neurology offers the potential for enhanced individual and social productivity across all ages, expanded human autonomy, and strengthened interpersonal relationships. At the same time, it carries the risk of medical and psychological harms as well as social perils. The growing excitement in the media and online toward "smart drugs" would suggest that the public holds an overwhelmingly optimistic view toward cosmetic neurology. However, surveys and focus groups reveal that the public is sensitive to the ethical concerns and is overall moderate in its opinion toward cosmetic neurology. The ambivalence among ethicists, healthcare workers, and the public toward cosmetic neurology is in part because the technology remains in its infancy. As we creep away from the modest scope of cosmetic neurology as it currently exists and toward one of its more robust potential incarnations, our discussions will shift from abstract promises and perils toward concrete benefits and harms. Anticipating the risks and engaging the public and professionals early helps guide the development of technology and policy to promote a socially responsible manifestation of cosmetic neurology.

References

1. Chatterjee A. Cosmetic neurology: the controversy over enhancing movement, mentation, and mood. *Neurology.* 2004;63(6):968–74.

2. Chatterjee A. Cosmetic neurology and cosmetic surgery: parallels, predictions, and challenges. *Camb Q Healthc Ethics.* 2007;16(2):129–37.

3. Haiken E. *Venus Envy: A History of Cosmetic Surgery.* Baltimore: Johns Hopkins University Press; 1997.

4. Snelders S, Pieters T. Speed in the Third Reich: metamphetamine (Pervitin) use and a drug history from below. *Soc Hist Med.* 2011;24(3):686–99.

5. Vearrier D, Greenberg MI, Miller SN, Okaneku JT, Haggerty DA. Methamphetamine: history, pathophysiology, adverse health effects, current trends, and hazards associated with the clandestine manufacture of methamphetamine. *Disease-a-Month.* 2012 Feb;58(2):38–89.

6. Steinkamp P. Pervitin (methamphetamine) tests, use and misuse in the German Wehrmacht. In: Eckart WU, editor. *Man, Medicine, and the State: The Human Body as an Object of Government Sponsored Medical Research in the 20th Century.* Stuttgart: Steiner; 2006, pp. 61–71.

7. Husain M, Mehta MA. Cognitive enhancement by drugs in health and disease. *Trends Cogn Sci.* 2011 Jan;15(1):28–36.

8. Sostek AJ, Buchsbaum MS, Rapoport JL. Effects of amphetamine on vigilance performance in normal and hyperactive children. *J Abnorm Child Psychol.* 1980 Dec;8(4):491–500.

9. Koelega HS. Stimulant drugs and vigilance performance: a review. *Psychopharmacology.* 1993;111(1):1–16.

10. Pigeau R, Naitoh P, Buguet A, McCann C, Baranski J, Taylor M, et al. Modafinil, d-amphetamine and placebo during 64 hours of

sustained mental work. I. Effects on mood, fatigue, cognitive performance and body temperature. *J Sleep Res.* 1995;4 (4):212–28.

11. Baranski JV, Pigeau R, Dinich P, Jacobs I. Effects of modafinil on cognitive and meta-cognitive performance. *Hum Psychopharm Clin.* 2004 Jul;19(5):323–32.

12. Elliott R, Sahakian BJ, Matthews K, Bannerjea A, Rimmer J, Robbins TW. Effects of methylphenidate on spatial working memory and planning in healthy young adults. *Psychopharmacology.* 1997 May;131(2):196–206.

13. Bagot KS, Kaminer Y. Efficacy of stimulants for cognitive enhancement in non-attention deficit hyperactivity disorder youth: a systematic review. *Addiction.* 2014 Apr;109 (4):547–57.

14. Breitenstein C, Wailke S, Bushuven S, Kamping S, Zwitserlood P, Ringelstein EB, et al. D-amphetamine boosts language learning independent of its cardiovascular and motor arousing effects. *Neuropsychopharmacology.* 2004 Sep;29(9):1704–14.

15. Repantis D, Schlattmann P, Laisney O, Heuser I. Modafinil and methylphenidate for neuroenhancement in healthy individuals: a systematic review. *Pharmacol Res.* 2010 Sep;62 (3):187–206.

16. Franke AG, Gränsmark P, Agricola A, Schühle K, Rommel T, Sebastian A, et al. Methylphenidate, modafinil, and caffeine for cognitive enhancement in chess: a double-blind, randomised controlled trial. *Eur Neuropsychopharmacol.* 2017 Mar;27(3):248–60.

17. Franke AG, Lieb K. Pharmacological neuroenhancement: substances and epidemiology. In: Hildt E,

Franke AG, editors. *Cognitive Enhancement: An Interdisciplinary Perspective.* Dordrecht: Springer Netherlands; 2013, pp. 17–27.

18. Fond G, Micoulaud-Franchi J-A, Brunel L, Macgregor A, Miot S, Lopez R, et al. Innovative mechanisms of action for pharmaceutical cognitive enhancement: a systematic review. *Psychiatry Res.* 2015;229(1):12–20.

19. Winblad B, Engedal K, Soininen H, Verhey F, Waldemar G, Wimo A, et al. A 1-year, randomized, placebo-controlled study of donepezil in patients with mild to moderate AD. *Neurology.* 2001 Aug 14;57(3):489–95.

20. Wesnes KA, McKeith IG, Ferrara R, Emre M, Del Ser T, Spano PF, et al. Effects of rivastigmine on cognitive function in dementia with Lewy bodies: a randomised placebo-controlled international study using the cognitive drug research computerised assessment system. *Dement Geriatr Cogn Disord.* 2002;13(3):183–92.

21. Rowan E, McKeith IG, Saxby BK, O'Brien JT, Burn D, Mosimann U, et al. Effects of donepezil on central processing speed and attentional measures in Parkinson's disease with dementia and dementia with Lewy bodies. *Dement Geriatr Cogn Disord.* 2007;23(3):161–7.

22. Ferreira-Vieira TH, Guimaraes IM, Silva FR, Ribeiro FM. Alzheimer's disease: targeting the cholinergic system. *Curr Neuropharmacol.* 2016;14 (1):101–15.

23. Repantis D, Laisney O, Heuser I. Acetylcholinesterase inhibitors and memantine for neuroenhancement in healthy individuals: a systematic review. *Pharmacol Res.* 2010 Jun;61 (6):473–81.

24. FitzGerald DB, Crucian GP, Mielke JB, Shenal BV, Burks D, Womack KB, et al. Effects of donepezil on verbal memory after

semantic processing in healthy older adults. *Cogn Behav Neurol.* 2008 Jun;21(2):57–64.

25. Yesavage JA, Mumenthaler MS, Taylor JL, Friedman L, O'Hara R, Sheikh J, et al. Donepezil and flight simulator performance: effects on retention of complex skills. *Neurology.* 2002 Jul 9;59 (1):123–5.

26. Chuah LYM, Chee MWL. Cholinergic augmentation modulates visual task performance in sleep-deprived young adults. *J Neurosci.* 2008 Oct 29;28(44):11369–77.

27. Chuah LYM, Chong DL, Chen AK, Rekshan WR 3rd, Tan J-C, Zheng H, et al. Donepezil improves episodic memory in young individuals vulnerable to the effects of sleep deprivation. *Sleep.* 2009 Aug;32 (8):999–1010.

28. Reisberg B, Doody R, Stöffler A, Schmitt F, Ferris S, Möbius HJ. Memantine in moderate-to-severe Alzheimer's disease. *N Engl J Med.* 2003 Apr 3;348(14):1333–41.

29. Rammsayer TH. Effects of pharmacologically induced changes in NMDA-receptor activity on long-term memory in humans. *Learn Mem.* 2001;8 (1):20–5.

30. Watfa G, Rossignol P, Kearney-Schwartz A, Fay R, Bracard S, Felblinger J, et al. Use of calcium channel blockers is associated with better cognitive performance in older hypertensive patients with subjective memory complaints. *J Hypertens.* 2010 Dec;28 (12):2485–93.

31. Rose SPR. "Smart drugs": do they work? Are they ethical? Will they be legal? *Nat Rev Neurosci.* 2002 Dec;3(12):975–9.

32. Ng TP, Feng L, Yap KB, Lee TS, Tan CH, Winblad B. Long-term metformin usage and cognitive function among older adults with diabetes. *J Alzheimers Dis.* 2014;41 (1):61–8.

33. Luchsinger JA, Ma Y, Christophi CA, Florez H, Golden SH, Hazuda H, et al. Metformin, lifestyle intervention, and cognition in the Diabetes Prevention Program Outcomes Study. *Diabetes Care.* 2017 Jul;40(7):958–65.

34. Solomon PR, Adams F, Silver A, Zimmer J, DeVeaux R. Ginkgo for memory enhancement: a randomized controlled trial. *JAMA.* 2002 Aug 21;288 (7):835–40.

35. Birks J, Grimley Evans J. Ginkgo biloba for cognitive impairment and dementia. *Cochrane Database Syst Rev.* 2007;2:CD003120.

36. Calabrese C, Gregory WL, Leo M, Kraemer D, Bone K, Oken B. Effects of a standardized *Bacopa monnieri* extract on cognitive performance, anxiety, and depression in the elderly: a randomized, double-blind, placebo-controlled trial. *J Altern Complement Med.* 2008 Jul;14 (6):707–13.

37. Flicker L, Evans JG. Piracetam for dementia or cognitive impairment. *Cochrane Database Syst Rev.* 2001;2:CD001011.

38. Ng T-P, Chiam P-C, Lee T, Chua H-C, Lim L, Kua E-H. Curry consumption and cognitive function in the elderly. *Am J Epidemiol.* 2006 Nov 1;164 (9):898–906.

39. Solon O. Meet the Silicon Valley-ites taking tiny hits of LSD to boost performance. *Wired.* 2016 Aug 24.

40. Johnstad PG. Powerful substances in tiny amounts: an interview study of psychedelic microdosing. *Nordic Studies on Alcohol and Drugs.* 2018;35(1):39–51.

41. Franke AG, Bagusat C, Rust S, Engel A, Lieb K. Substances used and prevalence rates of pharmacological cognitive enhancement among healthy subjects. *Eur Arch Psychiatry Clin Neurosci.* 2014 Nov;264(Suppl 1): S83–S90.

42. Singh I, Bard I, Jackson J. Robust resilience and substantial interest: a survey of pharmacological cognitive enhancement among university students in the UK and Ireland. *PLoS ONE.* 2014 Oct 30;9 (10):e105969.

43. Dietz P, Striegel H, Franke AG, Lieb K, Simon P, Ulrich R. Randomized response estimates for the 12-month prevalence of cognitive-enhancing drug use in university students. *Pharmacotherapy.* 2013 Jan;33 (1):44–50.

44. Babcock Q, Byrne T. Student perceptions of methylphenidate abuse at a public liberal arts college. *J Am Coll Health.* 2000 Nov;49(3):143–5.

45. McCabe SE, Knight JR, Teter CJ, Wechsler H. Non-medical use of prescription stimulants among US college students: prevalence and correlates from a national survey. *Addiction.* 2005 Jan;100 (1):96–106.

46. Arria AM, O'Grady KE, Caldeira KM, Vincent KB, Wish ED. Nonmedical use of prescription stimulants and analgesics: associations with social and academic behaviors among college students. *J Drug Issues.* 2008;38 (4):1045–60.

47. Arria AM, Wilcox HC, Caldeira KM, Vincent KB, Garnier-Dykstra LM, O'Grady KE. Dispelling the myth of "smart drugs": cannabis and alcohol use problems predict nonmedical use of prescription stimulants for studying. *Addict Behav.* 2013 Mar;38(3):1643–50.

48. Emanuel RM, Frellsen SL, Kashima KJ, Sanguino SM, Sierles FS, Lazarus CJ. Cognitive enhancement drug use among future physicians: findings from a multi-institutional census of medical students. *J Gen Intern Med.* 2013 Aug;28(8):1028–34.

49. Franke AG, Bagusat C, Dietz P, Hoffmann I, Simon P, Ulrich R, et al. Use of illicit and prescription

drugs for cognitive or mood enhancement among surgeons. *BMC Med.* 2013 Apr 9;11(1):102.

50. Caballero J, Ownby RL, Rey JA, Clauson KA. Cognitive and performance enhancing medication use to improve performance in poker. *J Gambl Stud.* 2016 Sep;32(3):835–45.

51. Dietz P, Soyka M, Franke AG. Pharmacological neuroenhancement in the field of economics – poll results from an online survey. *Front Psychol.* 2016 Apr 19;7:520.

52. Franke AG, Heinrich I, Lieb K, Fellgiebel A. The use of *Ginkgo biloba* in healthy elderly. *Age.* 2014;36(1):435–44.

53. Arria AM, Caldeira KM, Vincent KB, O'Grady KE, Cimini MD, Geisner IM, et al. Do college students improve their grades by using prescription stimulants nonmedically? *Addict Behav.* 2017 Feb;65:245–9.

54. Baranski JV, Pigeau RA. Self-monitoring cognitive performance during sleep deprivation: effects of modafinil, d-amphetamine and placebo. *J Sleep Res.* 1997 Jun;6 (2):84–91.

55. Sharp C. Cognitive enhancers – performance or problem? *Occup Med.* 2016 Mar;66(2):88–9.

56. Dekkers W, Rikkert MO. Memory enhancing drugs and Alzheimer's disease: enhancing the self or preventing the loss of it? *Med Health Care Philos.* 2007;10 (2):141–51.

57. Arce E, Ehlers MD. The mind bending quest for cognitive enhancers. *Clinical Pharmacology & Therapeutics.* 2017;101 (2):179–81.

58. Brand R, Wolff W, Ziegler M. Drugs as instruments: describing and testing a behavioral approach to the study of neuroenhancement. *Front Psychol.* 2016 Aug 17;7:1226.

59. Chatterjee A. Framing pains, pills, and professors. *Expositions*. 2008;2(2):139–46.

60. Brignell CM, Rosenthal J, Curran HV. Pharmacological manipulations of arousal and memory for emotional material: effects of a single dose of methylphenidate or lorazepam. *J Psychopharmacol*. 2007 Sep;21 (7):673–83.

61. Pitman RK, Sanders KM, Zusman RM, Healy AR, Cheema F, Lasko NB, et al. Pilot study of secondary prevention of posttraumatic stress disorder with propranolol. *Biol Psychiatry*. 2002 Jan 15;51 (2):189–92.

62. Clewis RR. Does Kantian ethics condone mood and cognitive enhancement? *Neuroethics*. 2017;10(3):349–61.

63. Schaefer GO, Kahane G, Savulescu J. Autonomy and enhancement. *Neuroethics*. 2014;7 (2):123–36.

64. Harada CN, Love MCN, Triebel KL. Normal cognitive aging. *Clin Geriatr Med*. 2013 Nov;29 (4):737–52.

65. English V, Sommerville A. *Boosting Your Brainpower, Ethical Aspects of Cognitive Enhancements: A Discussion Paper*. London: British Medical Association; 2007.

66. Lucke J, Partridge B. Towards a smart population: a public health framework for cognitive enhancement. *Neuroethics*. 2013;6 (2):419–27.

67. Maslen H, Santoni de Sio F, Faber N. With cognitive enhancement comes great responsibility? In: Koops B-J, Oosterlaken I, Romijn H, Swierstra T, van den Hoven J, editors. *Responsible Innovation 2*. Cham: Switzerland: Springer International Publishing; 2015, pp. 121–38.

68. Batéjat DM, Lagarde DP. Naps and modafinil as countermeasures for the effects of sleep deprivation on cognitive performance. *Aviat Space Environ Med*. 1999 May;70 (5):493–8.

69. Lerner BH. A case that shook medicine. *Washington Post*. 2006 Nov 28.

70. Lerner BH. A life-changing case for doctors in training. *New York Times*. 2009 Mar 3.

71. Chandler JA, Dodek AM. Cognitive enhancement in the courtroom. In: Jotterand F, Dubljevic V, editors. *Cognitive Enhancement: Ethical and Policy Implications in International Perspectives*. New York: Oxford University Press; 2016, pp. 329–45.

72. Grunstein RR, Banerjee D. The case of "Judge Nodd" and other sleeping judges – media, society, and judicial sleepiness. *Sleep*. 2007;30(5):625–32.

73. Danziger S, Levav J, Avnaim-Pesso L. Extraneous factors in judicial decisions. *Proc Natl Acad Sci*. 2011 Apr 26;108 (17):6889–92.

74. Weinshall-Margel K, Shapard J. Overlooked factors in the analysis of parole decisions. *Proc Natl Acad Sci U S A*. 2011 Oct 18;108 (42):E833.

75. Rachlinski JJ, Johnson SL, Wistrich AJ, Guthrie C. Does unconscious bias affect trial judges? *Notre Dame Law Review*. 2009;84(3):1195–246.

76. Persson I, Savulescu J. The perils of cognitive enhancement and the urgent imperative to enhance the moral character of humanity. *J Appl Philos*. 2008;25 (3):162–77.

77. Hoffman P. *The Man Who Loved Only Numbers: The Story of Paul Erdos and the Search for Mathematical Truth*. New York: Hyperion; 1998.

78. Carter S. Could moral enhancement interventions be medically indicated? *Health Care Anal*. 2017 Dec;25(4):338–53.

79. Douglas T. Moral enhancement. *J Appl Philos*. 2008 Aug;25 (3):228–45.

80. Shook JR. Neuroethics and the possible types of moral enhancement. *AJOB Neurosci*. 2012;3(4):3–14.

81. Ahlskog R. Moral enhancement should target self-interest and cognitive capacity. *Neuroethics*. 2017 Apr 26;10(3):363–73.

82. Harris J. Moral enhancement and freedom. *Bioethics*. 2010;25 (2):102–11.

83. Kirsch I. *The Emperor's New Drugs: Exploding the Antidepressant Myth*. New York: Basic Books; 2009.

84. Rutherford BR, Mori S, Sneed JR, Pimontel MA, Roose SP. Contribution of spontaneous improvement to placebo response in depression: a meta-analytic review. *J Psychiatr Res*. 2012 Jun;46(6):697–702.

85. Benedetti F. Mechanisms of placebo and placebo-related effects across diseases and treatments. *Annu Rev Pharmacol Toxicol*. 2008;48:33–60.

86. Ilieva I, Boland J, Farah MJ. Objective and subjective cognitive enhancing effects of mixed amphetamine salts in healthy people. *Neuropharmacology*. 2013 Jan;64:496–505.

87. Ioannidis JPA. Why most published research findings are false. *PLoS Med*. 2005 Aug;2(8): e124.

88. Button KS, Ioannidis JPA, Mokrysz C, Nosek BA, Flint J, Robinson ESJ, et al. Power failure: why small sample size undermines the reliability of neuroscience. *Nat Rev Neurosci*. 2013 May;14 (5):365–76.

89. Wilens TE, Hammerness PG, Biederman J, Kwon A, Spencer TJ, Clark S, et al. Blood pressure changes associated with medication treatment of adults with attention-deficit/

hyperactivity disorder. *J Clin Psychiatry*. 2005 Feb;66(2):253–9.

90. Nissen SE. ADHD drugs and cardiovascular risk. *N Engl J Med*. 2006;354(14):1445–8.

91. Habel LA, Cooper WO, Sox CM, Arnold Chan K, Fireman BH, Arbogast PG, et al. ADHD medications and risk of serious cardiovascular events in young and middle-aged adults. *JAMA*. 2011;306 (24):2673–83.

92. Cooper WO, Habel LA, Sox CM, Arnold Chan K, Arbogast PG, Craig Cheetham T, et al. ADHD drugs and serious cardiovascular events in children and young adults. *N Engl J Med*. 2011;365 (20):1896–904.

93. Busardò FP, Kyriakou C, Cipolloni L, Zaami S, Frati P. From clinical application to cognitive enhancement: the example of methylphenidate. *Curr Neuropharmacol*. 2016;14 (1):17–27.

94. Biederman J, Monuteaux MC, Spencer T, Wilens TE, Macpherson HA, Faraone SV. Stimulant therapy and risk for subsequent substance use disorders in male adults with ADHD: a naturalistic controlled 10-year follow-up study. *Am J Psychiatry*. 2008 May;165 (5):597–603.

95. Barkley RA, Fischer M, Smallish L, Fletcher K. Does the treatment of attention-deficit/hyperactivity disorder with stimulants contribute to drug use/abuse? A 13-year prospective study. *Pediatrics*. 2003 Jan;111 (1):97–109.

96. Brühl AB, Sahakian BJ. Drugs, games, and devices for enhancing cognition: implications for work and society. *Ann N Y Acad Sci*. 2016 Apr;1369(1):195–217.

97. Banjo OC, Nadler R, Reiner PB. Physician attitudes towards pharmacological cognitive enhancement: safety concerns are

paramount. *PLoS ONE*. 2010 Dec 14;5(12):e14322.

98. Partridge BJ, Bell SK, Lucke JC, Yeates S, Hall WD. Smart drugs "as common as coffee": media hype about neuroenhancement. *PLoS ONE*. 2011 Nov 30;6(11): e28416.

99. Schermer M. Changes in the self: the need for conceptual research next to empirical research. *Am J Bioeth*. 2009 May;9(5):45–7.

100. Shanker T, Duenwald M. Threats and responses: military; bombing error puts a spotlight on pilots' pills. *New York Times*. 2003 Jan 19.

101. Schermer M, Bolt I, de Jongh R, Olivier B. The future of psychopharmacological enhancements: expectations and policies. *Neuroethics*. 2009;2 (2):75–87.

102. Davis NJ. A taxonomy of harms inherent in cognitive enhancement. *Front Hum Neurosci*. 2017 Feb 14;11. ArtID: 63.

103. Heilman KM, Nadeau SE, Beversdorf DO. Creative innovation: possible brain mechanisms. *Neurocase*. 2003 Oct;9(5):369–79.

104. Beversdorf DQ, Hughes JD, Steinberg BA, Lewis LD, Heilman KM. Noradrenergic modulation of cognitive flexibility in problem solving. *Neuroreport*. 1999 Sep 9;10(13):2763–7.

105. Farah MJ, Haimm C, Sankoorikal G, Smith ME, Chatterjee A. When we enhance cognition with Adderall, do we sacrifice creativity? A preliminary study. *Psychopharmacology*. 2009 Jan;202 (1–3):541–7.

106. Fukuyama F. *Our Posthuman Future: Consequences of the Biotechnology Revolution*. New York: Farrar, Straus and Giroux; 2002.

107. Daniels N. Normal functioning and the treatment-enhancement

distinction. *Camb Q Healthc Ethics*. 2000 Summer;9(3):309–22.

108. Reiner PB. Distinguishing between restoration and enhancement in neuropharmacology. *Virtual Mentor*. 2010 Nov 1;12(11):885–8.

109. Caviola L, Faber NS. Pills or push-ups? Effectiveness and public perception of pharmacological and non-pharmacological cognitive enhancement. *Front Psychol*. 2015;6:1852.

110. Scheske C, Schnall S. The ethics of "smart drugs": moral judgments about healthy people's use of cognitive-enhancing drugs. *Basic Appl Soc Psych*. 2012;34 (6):508–15.

111. Specker J, Schermer MHN, Reiner PB. Public attitudes towards moral enhancement. Evidence that means matter morally. *Neuroethics*. 2017 Jul 27;10 (3):405–17.

112. Bergström LS, Lynöe N. Enhancing concentration, mood and memory in healthy individuals: an empirical study of attitudes among general practitioners and the general population. *Scand J Public Health*. 2008 Jul;36(5):532–7.

113. Kudlow PA, Naylor KT, Xie B, McIntyre RS. Cognitive enhancement in Canadian medical students. *J Psychoactive Drugs*. 2013 Sep;45(4):360–5.

114. Greely H, Sahakian B, Harris J, Kessler RC, Gazzaniga M, Campbell P, et al. Towards responsible use of cognitive-enhancing drugs by the healthy. *Nature*. 2008;456(7223):702–5.

115. Bostrom N, Sandberg A. Cognitive enhancement: methods, ethics, regulatory challenges. *Sci Eng Ethics*. 2009 Sep;15 (3):311–41.

116. Kass LR. Ageless bodies, happy souls: biotechnology and the pursuit of perfection. *The New Atlantis*. 2003 Spring;1(1):9–28.

117. President's Council on Bioethics (U.S.), Kass L. *Beyond Therapy: Biotechnology and the Pursuit of Happiness.* New York: Harper Perennial; 2003.

118. Elliot C. American bioscience meets the American dream. *Am Prospect.* 2003;14(6):38.

119. Appel JM. When the boss turns pusher: a proposal for employee protections in the age of cosmetic neurology. *J Med Ethics.* 2008 Aug;34(8):616–18.

120. Enck GG. Pharmaceutical enhancement and medical professionals. *Med Health Care Philos.* 2014 Feb;17(1):23–8.

121. Ray KS. Not just "study drugs" for the rich: stimulants as moral tools for creating opportunities for socially disadvantaged students. *Am J Bioeth.* 2016;16(6):29–38.

122. Graf WD, Nagel SK, Epstein LG, Miller G, Nass R, Larriviere D. Pediatric neuroenhancement: ethical, legal, social, and neurodevelopmental implications. *Neurology.* 2013 Mar 26;80 (13):1251–60.

123. Cakic V. Smart drugs for cognitive enhancement: ethical and pragmatic considerations in the era of cosmetic neurology. *J Med Ethics.* 2009 Oct;35 (10):611–15.

124. Klayman A. *Take Your Pills.* Netflix; 2018.

125. Sattler S, Sauer C, Mehlkop G, Graeff P. The rationale for consuming cognitive enhancement drugs in university students and teachers. *PLoS ONE.* 2013 Jul 17;8(7):e68821.

126. Lucke J, Partridge B, Forlini C, Racine E. Using neuropharmaceuticals for cognitive enhancement: policy and regulatory issues. In: Clausen J, Levy N, editors. *Handbook of Neuroethics.* Dordrecht: Springer Netherlands; 2014, pp. 1085–100.

127. Shook JR, Galvagni L, Giordano J. Cognitive enhancement kept within contexts: neuroethics and informed public policy. *Front Syst Neurosci.* 2014 Dec 5;8:228.

128. Synofzik M. Ethically justified, clinically applicable criteria for physician decision-making in psychopharmacological enhancement. *Neuroethics.* 2009;2 (2):89–102.

129. Bostrom N. Drugs can be used to treat more than disease. *Nature.* 2008;451(7178):520.

130. Ravelingien A, Braeckman J, Crevits L, De Ridder D, Mortier E. "Cosmetic neurology" and the moral complicity argument. *Neuroethics.* 2009;2(3):151–62.

131. Ott R, Lenk C, Miller N, Neuhaus Bühler R, Biller-Andorno N. Neuroenhancement – perspectives of Swiss psychiatrists and general practitioners. *Swiss Med Wkly.* 2012 Nov 27;142:w13707.

132. Hotze TD, Shah K, Anderson EE, Wynia MK. "Doctor, would you prescribe a pill to help me . . . ?" a national survey of physicians on using medicine for human enhancement. *Am J Bioeth.* 2011 Jan;11(1):3–13.

133. Outram SM, Racine E. Developing public health approaches to cognitive enhancement: an analysis of current reports. *Public Health Ethics.* 2011;4(1):93–105.

134. Heinz A, Kipke R, Heimann H, Wiesing U. Cognitive neuroenhancement: false assumptions in the ethical debate. *J Med Ethics.* 2012 Jun;38 (6):372–5.

135. Zohny H. The myth of cognitive enhancement drugs. *Neuroethics.* 2015;8(3):257–69.

136. Schelle KJ, Faulmüller N, Caviola L, Hewstone M. Attitudes toward pharmacological cognitive enhancement – a review. *Front Syst Neurosci.* 2014 Apr 17;8:53.

137. Bell S, Partridge B, Lucke J, Hall W. Australian university students' attitudes towards the acceptability and regulation of pharmaceuticals to improve academic performance. *Neuroethics.* 2013;6 (1):197–205.

138. Aikins RD. Academic performance enhancement: a qualitative study of the perceptions and habits of prescription stimulant–using college students. *J Coll Stud Dev.* 2011;52(5):560–76.

139. Desantis AD, Hane AC. "Adderall is definitely not a drug": justifications for the illegal use of ADHD stimulants. *Subst Use Misuse.* 2010;45(1–2):31–46.

140. Dodge T, Williams KJ, Marzell M, Turrisi R. Judging cheaters: is substance misuse viewed similarly in the athletic and academic domains? *Psychol Addict Behav.* 2012 Sep;26 (3):678–82.

141. Fitz NS, Nadler R, Manogaran P, Chong EWJ, Reiner PB. Public attitudes toward cognitive enhancement. *Neuroethics.* 2014;7 (2):173–88.

142. Franke AG, Bonertz C, Christmann M, Engeser S, Lieb K. Attitudes toward cognitive enhancement in users and nonusers of stimulants for cognitive enhancement: a pilot study. *AJOB Prim Res.* 2012;3 (1):48–57.

143. Franke AG, Lieb K, Hildt E. What users think about the differences between caffeine and illicit/ prescription stimulants for cognitive enhancement. *PLoS ONE.* 2012;7(6):e40047.

144. Partridge B, Bell S, Lucke J, Hall W. Australian university students' attitudes towards the use of prescription stimulants as cognitive enhancers: perceived patterns of use, efficacy and safety. *Drug Alcohol Rev.* 2013;32 (3):295–302.

145. Partridge B, Lucke J, Hall W. A comparison of attitudes toward cognitive enhancement and legalized doping in sport in a community sample of Australian

adults. *AJOB Prim Res*. 2012;3
(4):81–6.

146. Sabini J, Monterosso J. Judgments
of the fairness of using

performance enhancing drugs.
Ethics Behav. 2005;15(1):81–94.

147. Sattler S, Forlini C, Racine É,
Sauer C. Impact of contextual

factors and substance
characteristics on perspectives
toward cognitive enhancement.
PLoS ONE. 2013;8(8):e71452.

Chapter 18

Cognitive Rehabilitation in Healthy Aging

Nicole D. Anderson and Gordon Winocur

1 Introduction

Cognitive aging is associated with decline in a broad range of functions including episodic learning and memory, working memory [1], processing speed [2], and executive functioning [3]. Compared with their younger counterparts, older adults have difficulty encoding new information, retrieving events from the past [1], and remembering to do things in the future (prospective memory) [4]. They perform poorly on tasks requiring one to hold and manipulate information in mind and experience difficulty multitasking and executing complex plans. Significant research has focused on improving these cognitive abilities in older adults. The outcomes of this research are essential for clinicians trying to improve the everyday functioning of their patients, as well as for advancing our theoretical understanding of the malleability of cognitive aging.

Successful cognitive rehabilitation should meet three criteria: efficacy, transfer, and maintenance. First, rehabilitation is successful if it is efficacious, that is, leads to improved performance in areas targeted by the intervention. Second, a successful intervention should transfer beyond the specific materials or task parameters trained. Transfer can be near, intermediate, or far. For example, in the context of memory rehabilitation, near transfer refers to improvements to untrained memoranda in otherwise similar task formats; intermediate transfer refers to improvements in other areas of function within the trained cognitive domain (e.g., spatial memory and event memory); and far transfer refers to gains in other cognitive domains or in different aspects of everyday life. Third, a successful intervention should result in improvements that maintain (i.e., persist) after completion of the intervention. Developing a rehabilitation intervention that is efficacious, transfers well, and has long-lasting benefits for older adults remains a major challenge for clinicians and researchers concerned with normal cognitive aging.

There have been two traditional approaches toward cognitive rehabilitation. The goal of restorative approaches is to repair the affected cognitive processes by directly retraining them, usually in an adaptive manner whereby the task becomes progressively more difficult as the learner meets specified performance criteria. For example, in working memory training, participants may start with a 1-back task, in which individual stimuli are presented in successive trials, and participants are instructed to press one button if the current stimulus matches the one that immediately preceded it, or to press another button if it does not match the prior stimulus. When a performance criterion is met in a given session (e.g., 90% accuracy), the difficulty is increased to 2-back (where now participants are detecting stimuli that match the ones presented two trials prior), and then to 3-back, and so on. Restorative approaches are based on the notion that by improving the targeted cognitive processes, training should transfer to other cognitive functions and tasks that rely on these processes. In the working memory example, this could include another n-back task with different stimuli (near transfer), other working memory tasks (intermediate transfer), or other cognitive domains such as fluid intellectual abilities or even real-life everyday functioning (far transfer).

The second traditional approach to cognitive rehabilitation is compensatory, which aims to offset cognitive decrements by bypassing the impairment or by identifying alternate means to achieve good performance. A key compensatory approach is strategy training – teaching individuals mnemonic strategies to bolster memory performance, or problem-solving strategies to improve management of daily life. Compensatory cognitive interventions are often "multimodal," addressing other factors that could be affecting performance, such as self-efficacy, stress, or lifestyle.

This review describes restorative approaches and compensatory approaches to cognitive rehabilitation in healthy older adults, in that order. Other interventions that have had cognitive outcome measures, such as physical exercise, diet, meditation, leisure-based approaches, neurostimulation, or pharmacotherapy, are outside the scope of this review, as are the effects of cognitive rehabilitation on neural outcomes (e.g., brain structure or activity).

2 Restorative Approaches to Cognitive Rehabilitation

Restorative approaches to cognitive rehabilitation in healthy older adults have primarily targeted episodic memory, working memory, and various aspects of attention and executive functioning that are particularly vulnerable to the effects of aging.

2.1 Episodic Memory Training

Episodic memory is learning and retrieval of personally experienced events (e.g., what happened at a birthday party last month); the "items" (e.g., the birthday cake) are remembered along with their context (e.g., what type of cake it was and that cousin Mary spilled it down her dress) to create a rich mnemonic trace that allows one to engage in what Endel Tulving called "mental time travel" to reexperience past events or imagine future events [5]. The goal of episodic memory training is to restore the mnemonic processes that are most affected by normal aging. Repetition lag training [6] is a classic example. This approach was inspired by evidence for a dissociation in the effects of aging on two memory processes: recollection, the ability to remember information bound to its original context (such as remembering who told you a recent fact that you learned, or precisely where you placed a specific object), undergoes significant age-related declines, while familiarity for a prior event, lacking any accompanying memory for the context, is relatively spared with aging (see [7] for a meta-analysis). The original repetition lag procedure has a study phase involving learning a list of words. In a following test phase, the studied words are intermixed with new words in a recognition test, but every new word is presented a second time with a variable number of other studied and other new words intervening between the two presentations of each new word. Participants are to respond "yes" only to the studied words, and to respond "no" to new words, both times that they are presented. The first presentation of new words will amplify their familiarity, leading to erroneous endorsements of their repetition unless that familiarity is offset by recollection that these words are familiar because they are from the test phase and not the study phase. Jennings and Jacoby [6] used this paradigm in healthy older adults, gradually increasing the number of intervening words between the two presentations of the new words (the "lag") as participants achieved a specified performance criterion. Training lasted 7 days (~1 hour of training per day). Control participants were individually yoked to a trained participant and received the same lags over the seven days, but in a random order. As an abbreviated example, if a trained participant advanced through the lags in the following order: 2, 2, 4, 4, 4, 8, 12, 12, then a control participant may have received the same lags, but in this random order: 4, 12, 2, 8, 4, 12, 2, 4. Training success was established by comparing basal (lag at which performance criterion was met on the first day) and ceiling (lag at which this criterion was met on the last day) performance. Basal performance was a lag of two for both groups, but the ceiling level of the trained group far exceeded that of the control group.. These results suggested that older adults can benefit from repeated practice in deploying recollection to offset the misleading influences of familiarity.

The efficacy of repetition lag training for older adults has been replicated in numerous studies [8–13]. The first objective evidence that repetition lag training eliminates aging-related decrements in recollection on the trained task, and is maintained 3 months after training, was provided by Anderson et al. [8]. Whether or not repetition lag training promotes transfer is less clear. Some studies have found intermediate transfer to other memory tasks thought to rely on recollection (e.g., n-back, digit span, and spatial span), and far transfer to the AX-CPT test of inhibitory attention [9, 11]. In this latter test, a series of cue–probe letters is presented (e.g., B and then Y), and participants are to press a target response key only to the probe X when it is preceded by the cue A; the probe X is presented on the majority of A-cue trials, leading to a high rate of false alarms to non-X probes that follow an A cue. However, other studies showed no transfer to tasks such as reading span, word list learning, visuospatial learning, and working memory measures such as n-back and self-ordered pointing [8, 11, 13].

Bellander et al. [14] proposed that repetition lag training helps to improve working memory and not episodic memory, which is why it fails to transfer to other episodic memory tests. This account, however, does not align with the failure of repetition lag training to transfer to working memory measures such as *n*-back, self-ordered pointing, and a Sternberg task (see [8] for an example). Anderson et al. [8] offered an alternative explanation for the limited transfer of repetition lag training. Their explanation was based on evidence that different regions of the medial temporal lobes mediate episodic memory encoding for different types of information, providing support for the representational models of medial temporal lobe contributions to perception and episodic memory (e.g., [15, 16]). Anderson et al. [8] suggested that there is no monolithic recollection, but rather that recollection can be fractionated by type (e.g., for recency or temporal context, for modality, or for voice), such that training one type of recollection (e.g., recency or temporal context in the classic repetition lag paradigm) does not necessarily transfer to other types of recollection.

Motivated by concerns about the repetition lag paradigm, Bellander et al. [14] chose to train associative memory processes in healthy older adults. Associative memory relies on recollection (e.g., [17]), but the training methods Bellander et al. used did not entail recollection training per se. In 24 sessions over six weeks, older adults learned object–word pairs, knowing that either associative memory (experimental group) or item memory would be tested (control group). The list length increased or decreased from session to session in an adaptive manner in the experimental group as participants met or failed the performance criterion, but stayed at a fixed shorter length throughout training for the control group. Outcome measures included near transfer tests of associative and item memory, intermediate transfer tests of visuospatial memory, and far transfer tests of reasoning. Both groups improved on all outcome domains from pre-test to post-test, but the experimental group improved more than the control group only on the item memory test. Thus, this study failed to demonstrate efficacy of associative memory training and did not find evidence for intermediate or far transfer. These results are reminiscent of the relative failure of repetition lag training to show intermediate or far transfer. Given that repetition lag training strengthens episodic *retrieval* processes,

whereas associative memory training (as implemented by Bellander et al.) targets episodic associative *encoding*, these results may dampen enthusiasm for these restorative approaches toward episodic memory rehabilitation in healthy aging.

Zimmermann et al. [18] randomized older adult participants to object-location associative memory training using three distinct tasks, or to an active control procedure, carried out in 30 sessions over 6 weeks. Training was adaptive, imposing greater difficulty as participants met the performance criterion. Outcome measures – including other spatial memory tests (near transfer), verbal memory tasks (intermediate transfer), and visuospatial reasoning tasks (far transfer) – were administered at baseline, midway through training, immediately post-training, and 4 months post-training. Object-location memory training resulted in significant near and far (but not intermediate) transfer, and gains were maintained four months post-training. The authors concluded that the object-location memory training used in their study was both domain and process specific in that both the near and far transfer tasks required self-generated associations with visuospatial information, whereas the near transfer tasks required appreciation of semantic (verbal) associations. This interpretation aligns with that of Anderson et al. [8] in emphasizing the specificity of restorative episodic memory training, but offers more hope for transfer – near or far – provided that the transfer tasks rely on the same types of representations and processes.

2.2 Working Memory Training

Working memory refers to simultaneous short-term storage and manipulation of information held in conscious awareness. For example, when adding two three-digit numbers, a person has to remain consciously aware of these numbers, using auditory repetition or visual imagery when carrying a tens value from one column to the next column, as well as remembering the sum of the ones values in the preceding column. The study by Dahlin et al. [19] sparked interest in working memory training in healthy older adults. They examined working memory performance before and after 5 weeks of working memory training involving five different tasks, relative to a no-contact control group. In four of these tasks, the participants viewed a variable-length series of stimuli (letters, numbers, colors, or spatial locations), and when the list ended, reported the four most recently presented stimuli. The list lengths became more difficult when participants met a training criterion of 80% in the letter memory task. In the fifth working memory task, a "keep track" task, 15 words were presented serially, and for each word, participants indicated which of a set of provided categories the word belonged to. When the trial ended, participants had to remember the most recent word in each category. As training progressed, the number of possible categories increased. The outcome measures included one of the trained tasks, as well as an untrained n-back task. Performance gains were greater in the training group compared with the control group on the trained tasks, but not on the n-back task. These early results suggested that working memory training is efficacious but does not transfer. However, the small sample size of this study should be heeded ($n = 11$ trained and $n = 8$ control). On the other hand, many other studies of working memory training in healthy older adults have been published since that original report and most of them report gains in the criterion (trained) task ([20–35; but see [36] for an exception). The finding that participants improve on a well-practiced task is not surprising. The results of studies examining the transfer of working memory training are more mixed, with some studies reporting a lack of transfer [27, 32–34], and others reporting near and sometimes far transfer [20–26, 28–31, 35, 36].

Even among those studies reporting transfer of training, transfer typically is not successful to all measures hypothesized to improve as a result of training. Of the studies that included follow-up assessments to ascertain maintenance of working memory training effects, nearly all found that the participants maintained their post-treatment performance (i.e., performance on a trained working task remains improved relative to baseline after a delay; [20–24, 26, 35, 36], but see [25], who found no maintenance after a year delay in participants with a mean age of 80). Furthermore, maintenance of transfer effects appears more fleeting than maintenance of training effects ([20–23]; but see [24] and [35] for evidence of sustained transfer effects).

Karbach and Verhaeghen [37] conducted a meta-analysis combining working memory *and* executive functioning training studies. They reported significant efficacy of working memory and executive training on the criterion (trained) measures.

Moreover, the two types of training were similarly efficacious and younger and older adults showed comparable training gains on the criterion measures. Finally, their meta-analysis showed greater near than far transfer, although both were significant. Their general conclusion was that executive function and working memory training are effective at improving cognition broadly in younger and older adults. They argued that the fact that working memory and executive functioning both transfer to measures of fluid intelligence might have important implications for daily functioning. Melby-Lervåg and Hulme [38] critiqued this later conclusion, however, and reanalyzed the working memory training data after accounting for baseline differences in the studies and whether the control groups were active or passive. They found no evidence that such training transfers to fluid intelligence (after removing one outlier study). In general, it appears that working memory training improves older adults' performance on the trained task, that gains are maintained after training is completed, and that benefits can transfer, at least to other working memory tasks.

2.3 Attention/Executive Functioning Training

Much of attention training research among healthy older adults has focused on improving divided attention, which is the ability to carry out two tasks simultaneously (for an early example, see [39]). A dominant approach in this vein has been variable-priority training, in which participants are trained to vary the relative priority they give to the two tasks across blocks of trials. For example, in one block, participants might be instructed to emphasize both tasks equally (50:50), in another block to focus primarily on one task (80:20), and in yet another to focus on the other task (20:80). The degree of improvement on both tasks and transfer to other tasks is then compared between participants receiving variable-priority training and participants receiving fixed-priority training (i.e., 50:50 throughout). The initial application of this approach in a cognitive aging study had younger and older adults perform two executive functioning tasks simultaneously over four sessions [40]. One of these tasks was a monitoring task in which participants had to monitor six continuously changing gauges and reset them as soon as they reached the critical regions; participants could not see the level of the gauges without sampling one at a time. At the same time, participants performed an alpha-numeric task in which expressions such as K – 3 (letters in the alphabet) were presented to the participants (answer: H), and they had to indicate whether the current answer was greater or lesser than the previous answer (e.g., if the previous alpha-numeric answer was F, then H is greater than F). The two age groups had similarly greater improvements on the trained tasks. Transfer to a new dual task involving executive functioning and working memory was greater in those who received variable priority training than in those who received fixed priority training, regardless of age. Subsequent work has replicated these training [41–43] and near transfer effects [41, 43]. Other studies, however, have found comparable training [44] and transfer [42] effects in fixed and variable priority training.

Another well-studied attention training paradigm is processing speed training [45]. Processing speed training is an adaptive computerized training paradigm in which participants discriminate targets from distractors, initially only in central locations, then in mixed central and peripheral locations, both at progressively faster presentation speeds when participants perform accurately. As will be discussed in a later section of this chapter, in an early, large, randomized, controlled trial, processing speed training led to significant improvements in older adults' perceptual discrimination abilities, and these gains were maintained for 1 and 2 years [46]. While processing speed training did not transfer to measures of everyday functioning at these time points, subsequent work has demonstrated improvements on far transfer measures such as timed instrumental activities of daily living [47, 48], on-road driving performance [49] and an increased number of days people drove their vehicle per week [50], as well as decreased dementia risk [51].

Other attention training paradigms have focused on specific aspects of attention that are particularly affected by healthy aging. For example, Mishra et al. [52] trained 16 older adults to inhibit distracting information (and, interestingly, 10 older rats, using the same paradigm, but with a food reward rather than a points reward). In each trial of 36 blocks of training, divided into 12 sessions spanning 4–6 weeks, the older adults heard a target tone and then three trial tones. The participants had to decide if the trial tones included the target tone. The target tone was

present in 20% of the trials. In the adaptive training paradigm, the nontarget distractor tones were initially fairly distinct in frequency from the target tone, but as participants improved on the task, the distractor tones became more similar to the target. Compared with an untrained control group, the trained older adults (and rats) improved their tone discrimination to a level that surpassed that of an untrained young adult group. This was driven by a reduction in false alarms to nontarget distracting tones. Training also transferred to an untrained working memory span task but not to a sustained attention task or to a working memory task that involved interference. The authors suggest that this training fine-tuned the older adults' perceptual inputs, effectively leading to less "noisy" signals.

Rolle et al. [53] trained spatial attention using a Posner-like cuing paradigm. In their version of the Posner task, all cues were valid but training was adaptive, with progressively less spatial cue information provided as participants improved over 5 hours of training over 2 weeks. Compared with an active control group, trained younger and older adults improved their spatial attention. Training also transferred to an unrelated test of spatial working memory, a change detection task in which participants were presented with an array of 2, 4, 6, or 8 colored squares, followed by a 900-ms retention interval, and then a probe that appeared in one of the locations of the previously presented array. Participants were to indicate whether the probe color matched the color of the square that had appeared in that location. Together, these efforts to train divided attention, processing speed, inhibitory processes, and spatial attention suggest that adaptive attention training is effective for healthy older adults, often transfers to other cognitive tasks, and, in the case of processing speed training, appears to influence measures of everyday life such as instrumental activities of daily living and driving performance.

While the above-mentioned studies focused on training attention toward external stimuli, another study trained older adults to self-regulate their attentional and executive skills in the service of goal-directed plans. Van Hooren et al. [54] studied a group of 69 adults who were 55 years of age or older and had complaints about their cognitive functioning. Participants were randomized to receive either goal management training in 12 sessions over 6 weeks or to a wait-list control condition. Goal management training (cf. [55]) involves breaking a larger goal (e.g., planning a vacation) into a series of prioritized smaller sub-goals and in performing the tasks necessary to achieve these sub-goals. One learns to periodically stop ongoing activity and evaluate whether one's current activity is moving one closer to attainment of the current sub-goal. Goal management training includes training in relaxation/mindfulness to support staying present in the moment and involves homework requiring people to practice goal management in their everyday lives [54]. Van Hooren et al. hypothesized that goal management training would have stronger effects on subjective cognitive failures (as measured by the Cognitive Failures Questionnaire, CFQ) than on executive functioning (as measured by a standardized Stroop test), given its focus on everyday life problems. Outcome assessments occurred twice prior to the intervention (or commencement of the wait period), to account for practice effects; immediately after the intervention or control period; and again 7 weeks post-intervention or control. Compared with the waitlist control group, goal management training resulted in reduced complaints about executive functioning and annoyance with cognitive failures, both immediately post-intervention and 7 weeks later. However, it had no effect on the total CFQ score. Reduced anxiety was also evident in the trained group in the long-term follow-up assessment, but not immediately post-training. By contrast, goal management training had no effect on depression or on performance on the Stroop interference task. These results suggest that a fairly brief, albeit intensive course of training can reduce the frequency of cognitive slips in older adults' everyday lives, as well as the annoyance that such slips engender.

2.4 Individual Differences in Restorative Cognitive Rehabilitation Efficacy and Transfer

Who benefits from restorative approaches to cognitive rehabilitation? Among older adults, gains achieved with repetition lag training [10] and transfer effects deriving from working memory training [20, 35] decline with advancing age. Nevertheless, it is encouraging that older seniors (e.g., 80+ years of age) have demonstrated significant training effects [22, 25]. Older adults' repetition lag training gains have also been linked to crystallized intelligence and individual differences in the deployment of effective encoding strategies [10], while working memory

transfer effects have been linked to the magnitude of gains on the trained task [35]. More work is needed to identify the personal characteristics that determine who benefits from restorative approaches to cognitive rehabilitation among healthy older adults.

3 Compensatory Approaches to Cognitive Rehabilitation in Healthy Older Adults

3.1 Memory Strategy Approaches

Although *knowledge* about effective memory strategies is largely unaffected by healthy aging [56, 57], one hallmark feature of cognitive aging is the reduced ability to *self-initiate* effective encoding strategies such as semantic elaboration and visual imagery [58, 59]. Fortunately, older adults can be trained to use self-initiated effective encoding strategies, in word list learning, face–name learning, and working memory tasks (e.g., [60–65]). For example, Kirchhoff et al. [66] engaged a small group ($n = 16$) of seniors in two 60- to 90-minute sessions of strategy training. Participants were taught to think about the pleasantness and personal relevance of a list of words and to make a sentence for each of the presented words. Post-training, when learning a new list of words, participants were less likely to report not using any strategy and were more likely to report using both the pleasantness and personal relevance strategies. Recognition performance for the words also improved. These authors later reported that the memory gains were driven by increases in recollection and decreases in familiarity [67]. Most studies of these types of mnemonic strategies have not assessed maintenance of their use post-training. One encouraging result reported by Gross and Rebok [68] was that the use of a trained semantic clustering strategy mediated performance both on a word list learning task and on a measure of everyday functioning 5 years post-training. Whether these results can be replicated and extended to other strategies such as semantic elaboration and visual imagery should be the focus of future research.

The method of loci is another self-initiated encoding strategy. In this strategy, one learns a list of words or objects by imagining placing them in a series of familiar places, for example, places in one's home while imagining walking through rooms. Older adults can learn how to use this strategy successfully

[69–71]. However, the majority of older adults do not continue to use the strategy on their own [72, 73], perhaps due to its complexity [74], which makes it impractical for application in many real-life scenarios.

Training using the "implementation intentions" strategy can be used to improve prospective memory [75, 76]. It involves use of specific if-then plans (e.g., "if [or when] I see Susan, I will give her my book"). When teaching the implementation intentions strategy to older adults, Chasteen, Park, and Schwarz [77] had them perform a computerized working memory task in which the background screen color was different on every trial. Participants were instructed to perform two prospective memory tasks: (1) pressing a key whenever a certain background color was presented and (2) writing the day of the week in the upper right corner of any piece of paper provided to them. To manipulate implementation intentions, before the task started, half of the participants were instructed to imagine pressing the designated key when the specified background color was presented. The other half of the participants were to imagine writing the day of the week on each piece of paper. Both groups stated out loud their respective intention. Implementation intentions significantly increased remembering to write the day of the week at the top of each sheet but did not increase remembering to press the key in response to the designated screen background color. The authors argued that implementation intentions were ineffective in the latter case because the background screen color was not salient enough to effectively trigger retrieval of the intention. Although the results of individual studies on implementation intentions in older adults are mixed, a meta-analysis identified a medium to large effect size of 0.59 SD [78], suggesting that this strategy is generally efficacious in bolstering older adults' prospective memory.

A meta-analysis of the efficacy of memory strategy training (of all types) in older adults yielded an overall training gain of 0.73 SD compared with 0.37 in the sham or active control groups and 0.36 in the no-contact control groups [79]. A later meta-analysis revealed a similar 0.31 SD training gain relative to control groups when adjusting for practice effects [80]. Transfer effects explored in the earlier meta-analysis [79], however, were limited, suggesting that older adults struggle when trying to apply learned strategies to novel situations. One intriguing exception to this trend is the study of Brom and Kliegel [81].

They reported improved blood pressure monitoring adherence in older adults in the week following a single session of implementation intention training. It should be noted, however, that participants in that study had not monitored their blood pressure regularly prior to this study, presumably because they did not need to. It remains to be determined if the success of this strategy generalizes to individuals who need to conduct regular health monitoring.

Not only are older adults less likely to use mnemonic strategies until trained to use them, but memory strategy training is often less efficacious: if younger and older adults are trained to deploy a given strategy, both groups improve, but the younger adults show greater gains in memory performance (e.g., [63, 70]). These strategy production and utilization deficits have been attributed to aging-related decrements in attentional, executive, and working memory resources, and indeed older adults are more likely to use and benefit from memory strategies if given more time or other forms of support for their utilization (see [63] for a comprehensive discussion of these findings).

The vast majority of studies that have examined the effects of mnemonic strategy training on memory performance in older adults have involved only one or two sessions and have taught only a single strategy or two, often combined. One notable exception is the ACTIVE trial [46], in which 711 older adults were taught a variety of mnemonic strategies (e.g., semantic organization, visual imagery, semantic association, method of loci) and practiced them using laboratory tasks and everyday tasks (e.g., remembering a shopping list). This memory training group was compared with a reasoning training group ($n = 705$), a speed of process training group ($n = 712$), and a no-contact control group ($n = 704$). The three training groups received 10 sessions of training over a 5- to 6-week interval. Memory, reasoning, and processing speed, as well as daily functioning (activities of daily living and driving measures) were assessed at baseline, immediately post-training, and at 1 and 2 years follow-up, with multiple booster sessions offered to a random 60% of participants in the three training groups after initial training was completed. Those assigned to memory training improved on the memory measures immediately and 1, 2 [46], and 5 years later [82], but not 10 years post-training [83]. Notwithstanding the absence of improvement at 10-year follow-up, 5 years is impressive for long-term maintenance of mnemonic strategy training.

The primary discovery of the ACTIVE trial, however, was the specificity of training effects: at the immediate post-training and 1- and 2-year follow-up assessments, each training type induced gains only on the outcomes targeted by the training received and not on the other cognitive or daily functioning measures [46]. The ACTIVE trial results recapitulate a running theme in memory rehabilitation research: gains are often limited to the domain trained. However, gains following memory training were identified in instrumental activities of daily living [83] and health-related quality of life [84] 5 years post-training. The ACTIVE trial results suggest that the efficacy, maintenance, and transfer of mnemonic strategy training for older adults can be enhanced if training is extended over multiple sessions and if multiple mnemonic strategies are taught. Perhaps this type of intervention would show earlier transfer to everyday functioning if it were combined with other interventions (e.g., relaxation, self-efficacy). These are the features that characterize multimodal approaches to compensatory memory rehabilitation, which are discussed next.

3.2 Multimodal Approaches

Multimodal approaches to cognitive rehabilitation teach participants cognitive strategies and aim to address other psychological factors that affect cognitive performance, such as attention and relaxation. Multimodal cognitive rehabilitation programs often also contain an educational component that involves discussing lifestyle factors affecting cognition, such as exercise, diet, cognitive activities, and social engagement. Many multimodal cognitive rehabilitation studies have focused on memory. In an early study, Stigsdotter and Bäckman [85] compared memory performance on three tasks before and after 2 months of a weekly training involving one of three treatments: (1) a multimodal mnemonic (imagery, organization, method of loci), attention, and relaxation training program ($n = 9$); (2) an active control cognitive activation program including problem-solving, logical thinking, and visuospatial skills training ($n = 9$), and (3) a no-contact control ($n = 10$). Performance on one of the three outcome measures (the Buschke Selective Reminding test) was improved immediately after training and these gains were maintained 6 months later, but only in the multimodal memory intervention group. No group improved on the other two outcome

measures (digit span and Benton visual retention), both of which can be viewed as transfer measures to which the trained mnemonics would be less applicable. This early study served as a proof of principle that multimodal memory rehabilitation programs effectively improve performance on the tasks targeted by training, but it does not address whether the non-mnemonic features of the program contribute to its efficacy. Importantly, these authors later compared the multimodal program with memory training alone and reported greater efficacy with the multimodal program [86]. They reassessed both groups 3.5 years later and found long-term maintenance of multifactorial memory training effects [87].

A number of other studies have followed that initial study, describing group-based multimodal memory programs, typically four to nine sessions in length, covering memory strategies and addressing expectations for healthy aging-related memory changes and memory self-efficacy. Many of these programs teach people both internal memory strategies and the effective use of external memory strategies, such as using calendars and writing things down. Most programs engage participants in applying the memory strategies in lifelike scenarios, for example, remembering the names of people, and remembering grocery lists. The conclusion to be drawn from most of these studies is that such programs improve objective memory performance ([88–97], but see [98–100] for null effects on memory performance). Gains in memory performance have also been reported among older adults with extremely low levels of education [95]. Participants in most programs have shown increased knowledge about mnemonic strategies and have reported their increased use in everyday life ([92, 94, 96, 99], but see [98, 100] for exceptions). Decreased memory complaints and/or increased memory self-efficacy are other important outcomes of multimodal memory programs ([92, 93, 95–97, 99], with the exception of [89]). Some of these studies have also reported maintenance of gains for 1–6 months ([94, 100]; see also [96] for subjective, but not objective gains). Vandermorris et al. [101] conducted a qualitative study of 11 participants in one of these programs [100] and found that participants learned to be more accepting of and less worried about their aging-related memory impairment and had an increased motivation to make lifestyle changes. Wiegand et al. [100] also reported a significant increase in participants' likelihood of making positive lifestyle changes (e.g., engaging in more relaxation strategies and in more cognitively engaging activities) and a decreased intention to seek medical care for their memory issues.

One unique multimodal cognitive rehabilitation program combined memory strategy training with goal management training and psychosocial training, provided over 3 months in three 4-week modules (for the methodology of this study, see [102]). This study recruited seniors who had subjective memory or cognitive concerns but who performed normally on a series of neuropsychological tests. Half of the participants received the program soon after recruitment (the early training group), and half received it after a wait-list delay (the late training group). Executive functioning (e.g., planning), memory, and psychosocial functioning were assessed at baseline and after the three modules, and at two 3-month intervals after the completion of the intervention. Memory training taught participants about memory, factors that affect memory (e.g., fatigue, stress, medical conditions), and its relation to brain function. The use of various external and internal memory strategies was also taught and practiced with homework. A modified version of the Goal Management Training program of Levine et al. [55] was used to teach participants to use a "stop-state-split" strategy when confronted with complex tasks in order to avoid absentminded action slips. This strategy included (1) stopping ongoing activities to assess goal attainment, (2) stating or defining the main features of the task, and (3) splitting larger goals into sub-goals [103]. Finally, psychosocial training focused on self-efficacy, locus of control, realistic goal setting, and combating ageist stereotypes. Participants worked on an individually selected goal at home in their spare time.

The outcomes of this trial were reported in multiple papers [103–105]. In terms of memory gains, improvements were noted in secondary memory (i.e., memory after a short delay) and long-term memory, and in the application of strategies to boost memory performance. Furthermore, these gains were maintained up to 6 months later [104]. To assess the effects of the intervention on executive functioning, simulated complex real-life tasks were developed, such as planning an efficient carpool schedule, taking into account who was or was not a driver, how many passengers each car could accommodate, and the passengers' pickup locations. Improved simulated real-life task performance was found, and participants

engaged in more stopping and checking behavior as the task was carried out. These effects were maintained 6 months (early training group) and 3 months (late training group) later [103]. Finally, to assess psychosocial gains, measures of happiness, quality of life, self-efficacy, depression, optimism, and locus of control were combined into a single outcome. Gains were observed immediately post-intervention and were maintained 6 months later [105].

One interesting result from this study was that gains were greater in the early than late training group. Specifically, gains in memory performance and strategy use in the early training group outstripped those of the late training group [104]; gains were numerically, albeit not significantly, greater on the simulated complex real-life tasks for the early compared with late training group [103]; and gains and maintenance in the psychosocial outcomes were greater in the early training group [105]. The authors attributed these findings to the late training groups' failure to fully understand that their intervention would be delayed and the disappointment that came along with this.

Together, these various results suggest that group-based multimodal cognitive rehabilitation programs are effective in teaching mnemonic strategies to seniors, that these strategies are retained in both the short and the long term, that they may have significant benefits for seniors' ability to cope with the cognitive changes that occur with healthy aging, and that they might yield healthcare savings. Future research should focus on devising objective measures of everyday life strategy implementation and the influence of strategy implementation on everyday functioning and healthcare utilization.

4 Conclusions and Future Directions

The evidence is overwhelming that cognitive rehabilitation for older adults is efficacious, in the sense that they can learn to perform better on a trained task, acquire appropriate strategies, and learn how to implement them. Moreover, cognitive gains achieved with both restorative and compensatory approaches appear to persist weeks or months after the interventions are completed. The problem for many forms of cognitive rehabilitation for older adults lies in transfer of training: there is little evidence of transfer of restorative memory process training beyond the domains and processes trained, and evidence of the effects of compensatory memory and multimodal approaches on "real world" functioning has to date been predominately subjective. Still, the fact that older adults who participate in such efforts have increased self-efficacy is important, as this may have repercussions for critical outcomes such as healthcare utilization. Attention and executive function training appear to hold more promise in affecting real-world outcomes, and in the case of processing speed training, even dementia risk. Future work should focus on identifying the personal characteristics that predict who will benefit most from training and on development and more widespread use of objective measures of the impact of cognitive rehabilitation on older adults' everyday functioning.

Acknowledgments

This work was supported by a Discovery grant from the Natural Sciences and Engineering Research Council of Canada (#238861) awarded to NDA, and by a grant from the Canadian Institutes for Health Research (#MGP 6694) to GW. We thank the editors of this volume and Mariam Sidrak for editorial assistance. Portions of this chapter were adapted from N. D. Anderson, "Memory rehabilitation in healthy aging," in B. G. Knight, S. D. Neupert, N. D. Anderson, H.-W. Wahl, and N. A. Pachana (eds.), *The Oxford Encyclopedia of Psychology and Aging* (Oxford University Press, 2019).

References

1. Nyberg L, Lövden M, Riklund K, et al. Memory aging and brain maintenance. *Trends Cogn Sci* 2012; **16**: 292–305.

2. Rabbitt P. Speed of visual search in old age: 1950 to 2016. *J Gerontol Psychol Sci* 2017; **72**: 51–60.

3. West RL. An application of prefrontal cortex function theory to cognitive aging. *Psychol Bull* 1996; **120**: 272–92.

4. Kliegel M, Ballhausen N, Hering A, et al. Prospective memory in older adults: Where are we now and what is next. *Gerontology* 2016; **62**: 459–66.

5. Tulving E. Memory and consciousness. *Can Psychol* 1985; **26**: 1–12.

6. Jennings JM, Jacoby LL. Improving memory in older adults: Training recollection. *Neuropsychol Rehabil* 2003; **13**: 417–40.

7. Koen JD, Yonelinas AP. The effects of healthy aging, amnestic mild cognitive impairment, and Alzheimer's disease on recollection and familiarity: A meta-analytic review. *Neuropsychol Rev* 2014; **24**: 332–54.

8. Anderson ND, Ebert PL, Grady CL, et al. Repetition lag training

eliminates age-related recollection deficits (and gains are maintained after three months) but does not transfer: Implications for the fractionation of recollection. *Psychol Aging* 2018; **33**: 93–108.

9. Bailey H, Dagenbach D, Jennings JM. The locus of the benefits of repetition-lag memory training. *Aging Neuropsychol Cogn* 2011; **18**: 577–93.

10. Bissig D, Lustig C. Who benefits from memory training? *Psychol Sci* 2007; **18**: 720–6.

11. Jennings JM, Webster LM, Kleykamp BA, et al. Recollection training and transfer effects in older adults: Successful use of a repetition-lag procedure. *Aging Neuropsychol Cogn* 2005; **12**: 278–98.

12. Lustig C, Flegal KE. Targeting latent function: Encouraging effective encoding for successful memory training and transfer. *Psychol Aging* 2008; **23**: 754–64.

13. Stamenova V, Jennings JM, Cook SP, et al. Training recollection in healthy older adults: Clear improvements on the training task, but little evidence of transfer. *Front Hum Neurosci* 2014; **8**: 898.

14. Bellander M, Eschen A, Lövdén M, et al. No evidence for improved associative memory performance following process-

based associative memory training in older adults. *Front Aging Neurosci* 2017; **8**: 326.

15. Saksida LM, Bussey TJ. The representational-hierarchical view of amnesia: Translation from animal to human. *Neuropsychologia* 2010; **48**: 2370–84.

16. Ranganath C. A unified framework for the functional organization of the medial temporal lobes and the phenomenology of episodic memory. *Hippocampus* 2010; **20**: 1263–90.

17. Troyer AK, Murphy KJ, Anderson ND, et al. Associative recognition in mild cognitive impairment: Relationship to hippocampal volume and apolipoprotein E. *Neuropsychologia* 2012; **50**: 3721–8.

18. Zimmermann K, von Bastian CC, Röcke C, et al. Transfer after process-based object-location memory training in healthy older adults. *Psychol Aging* 2016; **31**: 798–814.

19. Dahlin E, Neely AS, Larsson A, et al. Transfer of learning after updating training mediated by the striatum. *Science* 2008; **320**, 1510–12.

20. Borella E, Carretti B, Cantarella A, et al. Benefits of training

visuospatial working memory in young-old and old-old. *Dev Psychol* 2014; **50**: 714–27.

21. Borella E, Carretti B, Riboldi F, et al. Working memory training in older adults: Evidence of transfer and maintenance effects. *Psychol Aging* 2010; **25**: 767–78.

22. Borella E, Carretti B, Zanoni G, et al. Working memory training in old age: An examination of transfer and maintenance effects. *Arch Clin Neuropsychol* 2013; **28**: 331–47.

23. Borella E, Carretti B, Sciore R, et al. Training working memory in older adults: Is there an advantage of using strategies? *Psychol Aging* 2017; **32**: 178–91.

24. Brehmer Y, Westerberg H, Bäckman L. Working-memory training in younger and older adults: Training gains, transfer, and maintenance. *Front Hum Neurosci* 2012; **6**: 63.

25. Buschkuehl M, Jaeggi SM, Hutchison S, et al. Impact of working memory training on memory performance in old-old adults. *Psychol Aging* 2008; **23**: 743–53.

26. Dahlin E, Nyberg L, Bäckman L, et al. Plasticity of executive functioning in young and older adults: Immediate training gains, transfer, and long-term maintenance. *Psychol Aging* 2008; **23**: 720–30.

27. Goghari VM, Lawlor-Savage L. Comparison of cognitive change after working memory training and logic and planning training in healthy older adults. *Front Aging Neurosci* 2017; **9**: 39.

28. Heinzel S, Schulte S, Onken J, et al. Working memory training improvements and gains in non-trained cognitive tasks in young and older adults. *Aging Neuropsychol Cogn* 2014; **21**: 146–73.

29. Heinzel S, Lorenz RC, Pelz P, et al. Neural correlates of training and transfer effects in working memory in older adults. *NeuroImage* 2016; **134**: 236–49.

30. Payne BR, Stine-Morrow EAL. The effects of home-based cognitive training on verbal working memory and language comprehension in older adulthood. *Front Aging Neurosci* 2017: **9**: 256.

31. Richmond LL, Morrison AB, Chein JM, et al. Working memory training and transfer in older adults. *Psychol Aging* 2011; **26**: 813–22.

32. Von Bastian CC, Langer N, Jäncke L, et al. Effects of working memory training in young and old adults. *Mem Cognit* 2013; **41**: 611–24.

33. Wayne RV, Hamilton C, Jones Huyck J, et al. Working memory training and speech in noise comprehension in older adults. *Front Aging Neurosci* 2016; **8**: 49.

34. Zinke K, Zeintl M, Eschen A, et al. Potentials and limits of plasticity induced by working memory training in old-old age. *Gerontology* 2012; **58**: 79–87.

35. Zinke K, Zeintl M, Rose NS, et al. Working memory training and transfer in older adults: Effects of age, baseline performance, and training gains. *Dev Psychol* 2014; **50**: 304–15.

36. McAvinue LP, Golemme M, Castorina M, et al. An evaluation of a working memory training scheme in older adults. *Front Aging Neurosci* 2013; **5**: 20.

37. Karbach J, Verhaeghen P. Making working memory work: A meta-analysis of executive-control and working memory training in older adults. *Psychol Sci* 2014; **25**: 2027–37.

38. Melby-Lervåg M, Hulme C. There is no convincing evidence that working memory training is effective: A reply to Au et al. (2014) and Karbach and Verhaeghen (2014). *Psychon Bull Rev* 2016; **23**: 324–30.

39. McDowd JM. The effects of age and extended practice on divided attention performance. *J Gerontol* 1986; **41**: 764–9.

40. Kramer AF, Larish JF, Strayer DL. Training for attentional control in dual task settings: A comparison of young and old adults. *J Exp Psychol: Applied* 1995; **1**: 50–76.

41. Belleville S, Mellah S, de Boysson C, et al. The pattern and loci of training-induced brain changes in healthy older adults are predicted by the nature of the intervention. *PLoS ONE* 2014; **9**: e102710.

42. Bier B, de Boysson C, Belleville S. Identifying training modalities to improve multitasking in older adults. *Age* 2014; **36**: 9688.

43. Lussier M, Bugaiska A, Bherer L. Specific transfer effects following variable priority dual-task training in older adults. *Restor Neurol Neurosci* 2017; **35**: 237–50.

44. Bherer L, Kramer AF, Peterson MS, et al. Training effects in dual-task performance: Are there age-related differences in plasticity of attentional control? *Psychol Aging* 2005; **20**: 695–709.

45. Ball K, Beard B, Roenker D, et al. Visual search: Age and practice. *Invest Ophthalmol Vis Sci* 1988; **29**: 448.

46. Ball K, Berch DB, Helmers KF, et al. Effects of cognitive training interventions with older adults. *JAMA* 2002; **288**: 2271.

47. Edwards JD, Wadley VG, Myers RS, et al. Transfer of a speed of processing intervention to near and far cognitive functions. *Gerontology* 2002; **48**: 329–40.

48. Edwards JD, Wadley VG, Vance DE et al. The impact of speed of processing training on cognitive and everyday performance. *Aging Ment Health* 2005; **9**: 262–71.

49. Roenker DL, Cissell GM, Ball KK, et al. Speed-of-processing and driving simulator training results in improved driving performance. *Hum Factors* 2003; **45**: 218–33.

50. Ross LA, Edwards JD, O'Conner ML, et al. The transfer of cognitive speed of processing training to older adults' driving mobility across 5 years. *J Gerontol Psychol Sci* 2016; **71**: 87–97.

51. Edwards JD, Xu H, Clark DO, et al. Speed of processing training results in lower risk of dementia. *Alzheimers Dement* 2017; **3**: 603–11.

52. Mishra J, de Villers-Sidani E, Merzenich M, et al. Adaptive training diminishes distractibility in aging across species. *Neuron* 2014; **84**: 1091–103.

53. Rolle CE, Anguera JA, Skinner SN, et al. Enhancing spatial attention and working memory in younger and older adults. *J Cogn Neurosci* 2017; **29**: 1483–97.

54. van Hooren SAH, Valentijn SAM, Bosma H, et al. Effect of a structured course involving goal management training in older adults: A randomised controlled trial. *Patient Educ Couns* 2007; **65**: 205–13.

55. Levine B, Robertson IH, Clare L, et al. Rehabilitation of executive functioning: An experimental-clinical validation of goal management training. *J Int Neuropsychol Soc* 2000; **6**: 299–312.

56. Hertzog C, Hultsch DF. Metacognition in adulthood and old age. In: Craik FIM, Salthouse TA, eds. *The handbook of aging and cognition* (2nd ed.). Mahwah, NJ: Erlbaum, 2000; 417–66.

57. Hultch DF, Hertzog C, Dixon RA. Age differences in metamemory: Resolving the inconsistencies. *Can J Psychol* 1987; **41**: 193–208.

58. Craik FIM. On the transfer of information from temporary to permanent memory. *Philos Trans R Soc Lond B Biol Sci* 1983; **302**: 341–59.

59. Craik FIM. A functional account of age differences in memory. In: Klix F, Hagendorf H, eds. *Human memory and cognitive capabilities, mechanisms, and performances.* Amsterdam: Elsevier, 1986; 409–22.

60. Bailey HR, Dunlosky J, Hertzog C. Does strategy training reduce age-related deficits in working memory? *Gerontology* 2014; **60**: 346–56.

61. Craik FIM, Byrd M. Aging and cognitive deficits: The role of attentional resources. In: Craik FIM, Trehub S. eds. *Aging and cognitive processes.* New York: Plenum, 1982; 191–211.

62. Troyer AK, Hafliger A, Cadieux MJ, et al. Name and face learning in older adults: Effects of level of processing, self-generation, and intention to learn. *J Gerontol: Psychol Sci* 2006; **61**: 67–74.

63. Kuhlmann BG, Touron DR. Aging and memory improvement through semantic clustering: The role of list-presentation format. *Psychol Aging* 2016; **31**: 771–85.

64. Yesavage JA. Imagery pretraining and memory training in the elderly. *Gerontology* 1983; **29**: 271–5.

65. Yesavage JA, Rose TL, Bower GH. Interactive imagery and affective judgments improve face–name learning in the elderly. *J Gerontol* 1983; **38**: 197–203.

66. Kirchhoff BA, Anderson BA, Barch DM, et al. Cognitive and neural effects of semantic encoding strategy training in older adults. *Cereb Cortex* 2012; **22**: 788–99.

67. Kirchhoff BA, Anderson BA, Smith SE, et al. Cognitive training-related changes in hippocampal activity associated with recollection in older adults. *NeuroImage* 2012; **62**: 1956–64.

68. Gross AL, Rebok GW. Memory training and strategy use in older adults: Results from the ACTIVE study. *Psychol Aging* 2011; **26**: 503–37.

69. Anschutz L, Camp CJ, Markley RP, et al. Maintenance and generalization of mnemonics for grocery shopping by older adults. *Exp Aging Res* 1985; **11**: 157–60.

70. Kliegl R, Smith J, Baltes PB. Testing-the-limits and the study of adult age differences in cognitive plasticity of a mnemonic skill. *Dev Psychol* 1989; **25**: 247–56.

71. Yesavage JA, Rose TL. Semantic elaboration and the method of loci: A new trip for older learners. *Exp Aging Res* 1984; **10**: 155–9.

72. Anschutz L, Camp CJ, Markley RP, et al. Remembering mnemonics: A three-year follow-up on the effects of mnemonics training in elderly adults. *Experimental Aging Research* 1987; **13**: 141–3.

73. Gross AL, Brandt J, Bandeen-Roche K, et al. Do older adults use the method of loci? Results from the ACTIVE study. *Exp Aging Res* 2014; **40**: 140–63.

74. Brooks JO 3rd, Friedman L, Yesavage JA. A study of the problems older adults encounter when using a mnemonic technique. *Int Psychogeriatrs* 1993; **5**: 57–65.

75. Gollwitzer PM. Implementation intentions. *Am Psychol* 1999; **54**: 493–503.

76. Gollwitzer PM, Sheeran P. Implementation intentions and goal achievement: A meta analysis of effects and processes. *Adv Exp Soc Psychol* 2006; **38**: 69–119.

77. Chasteen AL, Park DC, Schwarz N. Implementation intentions and facilitation of prospective memory. *Psychol Sci* 2001; **12**: 457–61.

78. Chen X-J, Wang Y, Liu L-L, et al. The effect of implementation intentions on prospective memory: A systematic and meta-analytic review. *Psychiatry Res* 2015; **226**: 14–22.

79. Verhaeghen P, Marcoen A, Goossens L. Improving memory performance in the aged through mnemonic training: A meta-analytic study. *Psychol Aging* 1992; **7**: 242–51.

80. Gross AL, Parisi JM, Spira AP, et al. Memory training interventions for older adults: A meta-analysis. *Aging Ment Health* 2012; **16**: 722–34.

81. Brom SS, Kliegel M. Improving everyday prospective memory performance in older adults: Comparing cognitive process and strategy training. *Psychol Aging* 2014; **29**: 744–55.

82. Rebok GW, Langbaum JB, Jones RN, et al. Memory training in the ACTIVE study: How much is needed and who benefits? *Aging Ment Health* 2013; **25**: 21S–42S.

83. Rebok GW, Ball K, Guey LT, et al. Ten-year effects of the advanced cognitive training for independent and vital elderly cognitive training trial on cognition and everyday functioning in older adults. *J Am Geriatr Soc* 2014; **62**: 16–24.

84. Wolinsky FD, Unverzagt FW, Smith DM, et al. The ACTIVE cognitive training trial and health-related quality of life: Protection that lasts 5 years. *J Gerontol: Med Sci* 2006; **61**: 1324–9.

85. Stigsdotter A, Bäckman L. Multifactorial memory training with older adults: How to foster maintenance of improved performance. *Gerontology* 1989; **35**: 260–7.

86. Stigsdotter Neely A, Bäckman L. Maintenance of gains following multifactorial and unifactorial memory training in late adulthood. *Educ Gerontol* 1993; **19**: 105–17.

87. Stigsdotter Neely A, Bäckman L. Long-term maintenance of gains from memory training in older adults: Two 3 1/2-year follow-up studies. *J Gerontol* 1993; **48**: P233–7.

88. Belleville S, Gilbert B, Fontaine F, et al. Improvement of episodic memory in persons with mild cognitive impairment and healthy older adults: Evidence from a cognitive intervention program. *Dement Geriatr Cogn Disord* 2006; **22**: 486–99.

89. Best DL, Hamlett KW, Davis SW. Memory complaint and memory performance in the elderly: The effects of memory-skills training and expectancy change. *Appl Cogn Psychol* 1992; **6**: 405–16.

90. Dellefield KS, McDougall GJ. Increasing metamemory in older adults. *Nurs Res* 1996; **45**: 284–90.

91. Fabre C, Massé-Biron J, Chamari K, et al. Evaluation of quality of life in elderly healthy subjects after aerobic and/or mental training. *Arch Gerontol Geriatr* 1999; **28**: 9–22.

92. Fairchild JK, Scogin FR. Training to enhance adult memory (TEAM): An investigation of the effectiveness of a memory training program with older adults. *Aging Mentl Health* 2010; **14**: 364–73.

93. Hastings EC, West RL. The relative success of a self-help and a group-based memory training program for older adults. *Psychol Aging* 2009; **24**: 586–94.

94. Kinsella GJ, Ames D, Storey E, et al. Strategies for improving memory: A randomized trial of memory groups for older people, including those with mild cognitive impairment. *J Alzheimer Dis* 2016; **49**: 31–43.

95. Lima-Silva TB, Ordonez TN, Santos GD, et al. Effects of cognitive training based on metamemory and mental images. *Dement Neuropsychol* 2010; **4**, 114–19.

96. Mohs RC, Ashman TA, Jantzen K, et al. A study of the efficacy of a comprehensive memory enhancement program in healthy elderly persons. *Psychiatry Res* 1998; **77**: 183–95.

97. West RL, Bagwell DK, Dark-Freudeman A. Self-efficacy and memory aging: The impact of a memory intervention based on self-efficacy. *Aging Neuropsychol Cogn* 2008; **15**: 302–29.

98. McDougall GJ, Becker H, Pituch K, et al. The SeniorWISE study: Improving everyday memory in older adults. *Arch Psychiatr Nurs* 2010; **24**: 291–306.

99. Troyer AK. Improving memory knowledge, satisfaction, and functioning via an education and intervention program for older adults. *Aging Neuropsychol Cogn* 2001; **8**: 256–68.

100. Wiegand MA, Troyer AK, Gojmerac C, et al. Facilitating change in health-related behaviors and intentions: A randomized controlled trial of a multidimensional memory program for older adults. *Aging Ment Health* 2013; **17**: 806–15.

101. Vandermorris S, Davidson S, Au A, et al. "Accepting where I'm at": A qualitative study of the mechanisms, benefits, and impact of a behavioral memory intervention for community-dwelling older adults. *Aging Ment Health* 2017; **21**: 895–901.

102. Stuss DT, Robertson IH, Craik FIM, et al. Cognitive rehabilitation in the elderly: A randomized trial to evaluate a new protocol. *J Int Neuropsychol Soc* 2007; **13**: 120–31.

103. Levine B, Stuss DT, Winocur G, et al. Cognitive rehabilitation in the elderly: Effects on strategic behavior in relation to goal management. *J Int Neuropsychol Soc* 2007; **13**: 143–52.

104. Craik FIM, Winocur G, Palmer H, et al. Cognitive rehabilitation in the elderly: Effects on memory. *J Int Neuropsychol Soc* 2007; **13**: 132–42.

105. Winocur G, Palmer H, Dawson DR, et al. Cognitive rehabilitation in the elderly: An evaluation of psychosocial factors. *J Int Neuropsychol Soc* 2007; **13**: 153–65.

Chapter 2

Preventing Cognitive Decline and Dementia

Yat-Fung Shea and Steven T. DeKosky

1 Introduction

"Dementia" is derived from Latin words *de*, meaning "out of" and *mens*, meaning "mind" [1]. Unfortunately, the word "dementia" is stigmatizing in many cultures as people believe that it is a curse or form of punishment. In addition, relatives or primary caregivers may misinterpret "dementia" as a normal aging process [1]. These mistaken beliefs lead to delay in diagnosis when symptoms manifest, and people may not believe that "dementia" can be treated. The latest edition of the Diagnostic and Statistical Manual of Mental Disorders (DSM-5) has replaced the word "dementia" with "major neurocognitive disorder" and the early, milder symptomatic phase is designated as "mild neurocognitive disorder" [2]. For this chapter, we will use the terms "dementia" and "Alzheimer's disease" (AD), as both have been the targets of most of the dementia research of the past 30 years. The most common dementia etiology is AD, followed by vascular dementia/vascular cognitive impairment (VaD/VCI) and dementia with Lewy bodies (DLB) [3].

Dementia occurs mainly in people over 65 years of age [3] and in the earliest mild states may be confused with normal aging. Beginning in the third to fourth decade of life, there are variable, usually slight, but universal declines in cognitive functions that extend across the life span, involving memory, attention, information processing, and executive function, as detailed in earlier chapters. Such changes occur at a rate of 0.2–0.8 standard deviations per decade, depending on the cognitive domain [4]. With the increase in longevity of the global population due to improvements in public health (e.g., better sanitation and ready access to clean water) and medical care, the global population is aging, and dementia is perhaps the greatest global challenge for health and social care. Forty-seven million people suffered from dementia in 2015, and the number is going to triple by 2050 as

some 131 million "Baby Boomers" age into their 70s, 80s, and beyond [5]. In the United States, the prevalence of dementia among persons older than 70 was estimated to be 14.7% in 2010 [6]. The financial costs are immense, and these diseases result in great burdens on the patient, caregivers, and society. The global cost of dementia was estimated to be $818 billion in 2015, and approximately 85% of this is related to burden on family and society [3]. In the United States, according to estimates by the Alzheimer's Association, direct medical expenditures related to dementia were $236 billion in 2016 and will rise to $1 trillion in 2050 [6]. Even this startling figure does not fully take into account some of the indirect costs, for example, lost productivity as caregivers quit their jobs to care for patients, providing nearly 18.1 billion hours of assistance at a cost of around $220 billion annually [6].

AD is the most well-studied dementia so far. With advances in neuroimaging, especially positron emission tomography (PET) employing tracers that bind to β-amyloid in the brain (Aβ-PET), in vivo detection of amyloid plaques is possible [7]. Among people with normal cognition, the prevalence of amyloid pathology identified on Aβ-PET increases from 10% at age 50 to 44% at age 90 [8]. Amyloid deposition develops in patients' brains 20–30 years before clinical manifestations emerge, predominantly after 65 years of age but sometimes earlier [8].

Over the past two decades, multiple clinical trials studying potential disease-modifying agents have failed to demonstrate clinical benefits among patients with mild to moderate AD [9–12]. However, the long asymptomatic period (when aging adults have positive amyloid markers but normal cognition) provides opportunities for implementation of interventions to prevent cognitive decline. Such an approach, if successful, will have immense financial, personal, and familial impact. It has been estimated that if any preventive strategy can delay the onset of dementia by 5 years, there would be a 50% decrease in dementia prevalence several decades later; this strategy could save up to $91 billion in 2027 and $164 billion by 2047 [13]. Therefore, the development of strategies to prevent or delay cognitive decline and dementia is important.

A number of risk factors for cognitive decline and dementia have been identified in retrospective studies, many of which could easily be modified with minimal side effects. We will discuss these opportunities in some detail, as well as the hypothesized mechanisms by which they might provide benefit. We shall also review ongoing clinical trials aiming at prevention or delay of dementia (with the recognition that these will be changing with some regularity) and review potential issues in designing future clinical trials.

2 Importance of Modifiable Risk Factors

Factors that are known to increase or decrease the risk of dementia may be modifiable. Neurodegenerative changes in the brain can begin to develop 20–30 years prior to onset of cognitive symptoms [8]. Thus far, clinical trials of potential disease-modifying agents have failed to demonstrate clinical usefulness in symptomatic patients. This suggests that modifiable risk factors for AD should be aggressively addressed during midlife, for example, between 40 and 60 years of age. Midlife appears to be the time, as with atherosclerotic cardiovascular disease, that such interventions might reduce late-life risk. The combination of poorer education (e.g., primary school level), hypertension, obesity, hearing impairment, depression, diabetes mellitus (DM), sedentary lifestyle, smoking, and lack of social engagement accounts in statistical models for 35% of the variance in dementia incidence. However, it accounts for only 7% of the variance among people who lack the apolipoprotein E $\varepsilon4$ allele (ApoE$\varepsilon4$), which increases the risk of AD significantly [3]. The mechanisms by which these modifiable risk factors act to increase the risk of dementia include elevated risk of atherosclerotic vascular disease; increases in insulin resistance, oxidative stress, and cortisol levels; and a reduction in brain-derived neurotrophic factor (BDNF) and possibly other trophic factors [14]. We shall review these modifiable risk factors and summarize the latest clinical evidence of the impact of treating them on the risk of dementia (Figure 19.1).

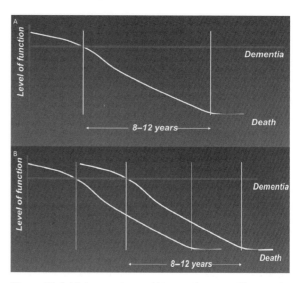

Figure 19.1 (A) Averaged natural history of cognitive/functional decline in Alzheimer's disease. The first vertical yellow line represents the onset of detectable symptoms; the second (white) line indicates approximate time of death. (B) Effect of a successful prevention or disease-modifying delay strategy. The curve of deterioration will be shifted to the right, delaying the onset of initial symptoms and subsequent decline to dementia. At the time when a person would have died if untreated, they would have only mild to moderate symptoms. If symptom onset is delayed by, e.g., 5 years, AD prevalence will be reduced 40% or more several decades later, and more people would die of a competing mortality with milder or no symptoms. If the delay in onset were extended to 10 years, the majority of cases of AD would be prevented, since the prevalence increases with age greater than 70 and thus most treated people would die of a competing mortality while cognitively normal or much less severely impaired. A black and white version of this figure will appear in some formats. For the color version, please refer to the plate section.

2.1 Education

Low education has been well reported as a risk factor for dementia, as demonstrated by differential prevalence of dementia as a function of education level in several populations [15, 16]. Recent epidemiological studies in several countries, including the United States, United Kingdom, Canada, Sweden, and the Netherlands, have reported declines in age-specific dementia incidence or prevalence[17–22], while dementia incidence in China and dementia prevalence in Japan has increased [23–25]. The decline in age-specific dementia incidence or prevalence has been attributed to increases in education in recent decades [3]. Education is believed to increase the brain's cognitive reserve through enhancement of neuronal branching, synaptic growth, and cognitive circuit efficiency [26, 27]. It is posited that, with enhanced cognitive reserve, cognitive deficits may not appear until neurodegenerative pathology is more advanced [26, 27]. Low education, currently defined as education that is limited to primary school or below [3], has been reported to increase the risk of dementia by 60% (RR 1.59, 95% CI 1.26–2.01) [3]. The consistent finding that greater education is associated with diminished risk in older subjects at risk for AD suggests that encouraging education and learning throughout life may diminish the risk of developing AD.

2.2 Intellectual Activities and Social Activities

Consistent with the theorized mechanism of cognitive reserve, day-to-day intellectual activities may help to delay the onset of dementia. The potential value of a number of intellectual activities, include reading newspapers and books, playing music, dancing, playing games (board games, card games, or mahjong), and gambling, has been studied [28–36] (see also Chapter 18). A recent meta-analysis included 19 studies on the effects of such cognitive activities. It revealed a 31% decrease in risk of cognitive impairment and a 42% decrease in risk of dementia in association with these activities [37]. These mentally stimulating activities were associated with better memory, speed of processing, and executive functioning. However, multiple confounding factors necessitate caution. People engaging in more intellectual activities are more likely to be aware of their health and to practice a healthier lifestyle, including avoiding smoking, exercising regularly, and maintaining a balanced diet, all of which are known to reduce the risk of dementia. These intellectual activities involve social and recreational components associated with positive experiences. People with mild cognitive impairment (MCI) may lack the capacity or motivation to engage in complicated leisure activities [30], in which case neurodegenerative disease may be responsible for diminished participation in mentally stimulating activities. Lee et al. [30] recently addressed some of these limitations in a Hong Kong study involving 15,582 community-living Chinese individuals ≥ 65 years of age without dementia who were followed for 6 years. They assessed the impact of intellectual activities while controlling for lifestyle factors (i.e., physical exercise, adequate fruit and vegetable intake, smoking, and recreational and social activities). Over a median follow-up

of 5 years, 9% of the subjects developed dementia. After exclusion of those individuals who developed dementia during the first 3 years of the study, the intellectual activities "group" had a 29% lower dementia incidence (OR 0.71, 95% CI 0.60–0.84, p < 0.001) [30]. Thus, intellectual activities appeared to be associated with reduction in risk, even after separating out the potential contribution of healthy lifestyle and higher social activity.

Enrichment of the social component of leisure activities has been shown to reduce the risk of dementia by 32% [29]. Improvement in social contacts correlates with a reduction in dementia risk [3]. Social isolation may increase dementia risk because of cognitive inactivity, leading to lower cognitive reserve, a higher risk of depression or physical inactivity, and a higher risk of hypertension [38] and coronary artery disease [39]. Although better estimation of the effect of intellectual activities on dementia risk can be achieved by controlling for the effect of social activities, as Lee et al. have done [30], the potential effect of social contact on intellectual or leisure activities cannot be discounted.

2.3 Speaking Multiple Languages

An individual who uses two languages or dialects in daily life is bilingual; a polyglot is one who speaks more than two languages [40]. During language production, language selection and inhibition of lexical competitors implicate both cortical (left prefrontal cortex, bilateral supramarginal, and anterior cingulate gyri) and subcortical structures (left caudate nucleus) [40]. To speak one language, one must suppress neural instantiation of the other language system [41]. Bilingualism is hypothesized to boost brain plasticity by increasing the quantity of neural substrate engaged by language production (gray and white matter) [41]. It is also associated with better performance on executive control, recall, and letter and category fluency tasks [41]. The number of spoken languages is inversely correlated with risk of dementia, and some studies have suggested that bilingualism can delay the onset of dementia by 4–5 years [41].

Craik et al. performed a retrospective review of 102 bilingual (BL) and 109 monolingual (ML) patients with probable AD who were evaluated in a memory clinic in Toronto between January 2007 and December 2009 [42]. The BL AD patients first experienced symptoms when they were 5.1 years older than the ML patients (p < 0.0001) [42]. The two groups had no prior differences in cognitive functions or occupational level, although the ML patients had received more formal education. There was no apparent effect of immigration status [42]. Alladi et al. reviewed the case records of 648 patients with dementia (391 BL, 257 ML) seen in a memory clinic between June 2006 and October 2012 and found that BL patients developed dementia of any type 4.5 years later than the ML patients (p < 0.0001). A significant difference in age of onset was found for AD (3.2 years later, p = 0.013), frontotemporal dementia (6 years, p = 0.001), and vascular dementia (3.7 years, p = 0.012) [43]. The effect of BL on age of dementia onset remained significant even after adjusting for potential confounding factors such as education, sex, occupation, and urban versus rural residence [43].

Functional imaging has also provided evidence of effects of bilingualism on brain reserve and metabolic connectivity in patients with AD. Perani et al. [44] studied 85 AD patients (45 BL, 40 ML) with ^{18}flurodeoxyglucose positron emission tomography (FDG PET). They found that the cortical area of cerebral hypometabolism was larger in the BL than in the ML AD patients. However, the BL group outperformed the ML group in cognitive testing (visuospatial short term memory, verbal short term, and long term memory, p-values < 0.001) [44]. These findings suggest that the BL patients had greater cognitive reserve. Bilingual patients, when compared with ML patients, exhibited increased metabolism in the orbitofrontal, inferior frontal, and cingulate cortices (i.e., executive control and default mode networks), suggesting engagement of compensatory circuitry to complete the tasks [44]. In another study, BL patients had less severe preclinical AD as defined by cerebrospinal fluid (CSF) biomarkers (abnormal amyloid with or without abnormal tau), and BL AD patients had lower levels of CSF total tau and less age-associated increases in total tau or phosphorylated tau. These findings suggest that bilingualism may not only enhance cognitive reserve; it may delay neurodegeneration in AD patients [45].

The effects of bilingualism extend to patients with MCI [46]. Among amnestic MCI patients, the BL patients exhibited a later age of onset than the ML patients [47].

Among aging Chinese BL people in Hong Kong, gray matter volume in the left and right inferior parietal lobules was significantly greater than in ML individuals [48]. Further, second language (L2) naming performance correlated with gray matter volume in the left inferior parietal lobule (R = 0.311, p = 0.047) while L2 exposure correlated with the right inferior parietal lobule volume [48]. Young normal BL individuals have greater gray matter volume in the anterior cingulate cortex and parietal lobes and highly proficient L2 learners have larger tissue volumes in the left superior temporal gyrus and right hippocampus [49], suggesting a physical basis for higher cognitive reserve. However, no study has demonstrated similar structural differences in patients suffering from MCI.

2.4 Physical Activity and Exercise

Prospective, randomized trials have shown that exercise or physical activity can prevent or slow cognitive decline in normal and cognitively impaired elderly participants (see Chapter 16). Observational studies also suggest that exercise may reduce the risk of cognitive impairment [50, 51]. Another major advantage of physical activity is its low cost and its beneficial effect on risk of cardiovascular and cerebrovascular events and diabetes mellitus (DM) [52, 53]. For elderly subjects, it may reduce the risk of falls and depression and improve overall function [54–56]. Exercise may reduce dementia risk by multiple mechanisms. Regular resistance training for at least 5 weeks increases blood levels of brain-derived neurotrophic factor (BDNF) [57]. Regular exercise stimulates release of fibronectin type III domain-containing protein 5 (FNDC5) from muscle and the subsequent cleaved product irisin induces expression of BDNF in the hippocampus [58]. Insulin resistance [59] and cerebral oxidative stress are reduced by exercise (see also Chapter 3). Exercise reduces oxidative stress by increasing the activity of antioxidant enzymes, including catalase and superoxide dismutase, thereby reducing the products of neuronal lipid peroxidation [60, 61].

A meta-analyses involving 163,797 nondemented participants in 16 prospective studies showed that the highest physical activity category was associated with a 28% reduction in the incidence of dementia (RR 0.72, 95% CI 0.60–0.86) and a 45% reduction in incidence of AD (RR 0.55, 95% CI 0.36–0.84) [50]. Leisure time physical activity (involving a wide variety of sports activities) also was associated with reduced risk of AD.

It is less clear whether occupational activity can reduce dementia risk. Higher occupation-related physical activity (i.e., manual work) could be related to lower social class or lower education levels, both risk factors for dementia [51]. Previous meta-analyses included retrospective studies that were limited by recall bias, and people of different countries and cultures might have different self-perceptions of physical activity.

Given that published studies have involved different types, durations, and intensities of physical activity, it is not yet possible to recommend any specific type, duration, or intensity of exercise as most beneficial to cognitive health.

2.5 Sleep and Sleep Disturbances

There is growing evidence of an association between insomnia and dementia, particularly AD [62]. In cognitively normal subjects, insomnia worsens memory, the ability to integrate visual and semantic information, and executive function [63]. There are multiple mechanisms by which sleep disturbances might increase the risk of dementia. Sleep is a vital period for amyloid-beta (Aβ) clearance from the CSF via the glymphatic system [62]. CSF Aβ levels are lowest in the morning and rise gradually through the day [64]. During sleep, there is a 60% increase in the interstitial space, which facilitates the convection exchange of CSF with interstitial fluid and facilitates removal of CSF Aβ [65]. Inflammation and oxidative stress increase Aβ deposition; deep sleep can mitigate both processes [66]. There has been less study of the relationship between sleep and tau pathology or tau hyperphosphorylation (p-tau), but poor sleep in cognitively normal subjects can increase CSF tau/Aβ42 and p-tau/Aβ42 ratios [67].

Recently Shokri-Kojori et al. reported a study of 20 cognitively normal young subjects (mean age 39.8 years) that assessed the effects of acute sleep deprivation on brain amyloid load (assessed by Aβ-PET) [68]. They found that acute sleep deprivation resulted in a higher amyloid load in the hippocampus, parahippocampal gyrus, thalamus (especially on the right side), putamen, and right precuneus [68]. It is not known whether treatment of insomnia can reduce the risk of dementia, although the role of the glymphatic system in Aβ clearance suggests that it may do so. Multiple studies have demonstrated an association between long-term exposure to benzodiazepines and increased risk of dementia [69, 70]. However, association does not prove causation, and studies employing propensity risk-matching are needed.

3 Traumatic Brain Injury

There has been increasing interest over the last decade in whether head injury increases risk of dementia or AD. Professional athletes in various sports, including football, boxing, soccer, wrestling, ice hockey, rugby, and baseball, as well as military personnel exposed to either deceleration or blast trauma, are well known to be at risk of repeated head injury [71]. The severity of traumatic brain injury (TBI) can be classified simply in terms of presence or absence of history of loss of consciousness (LOC) [72]. More complicated classification schemes incorporate duration of loss or alteration of consciousness and post-traumatic amnesia to grade injury as mild, moderate, or severe [73]. Mild TBI is defined as injury associated with normal structural imaging, LOC of 0–30 minutes, altered consciousness lasting from a moment up to 24 hours, and post-traumatic amnesia lasting up to 1 day [73]. Moderate TBI is defined by a Glasgow Coma Score (GCS) of 9–12 out of 15 and LOC from 20 minutes up to 6 hours; severe TBI is defined by LOC longer than 6 hours and GCS of 8 or less. The presence of pathologies related to TBI can lower the threshold for the development of additional pathologic processes, for example, those underlying AD, and accelerate the development of clinical symptoms [71, 72]. Mechanisms linking TBI with dementia or AD include diffuse axonal injury with subsequent cerebral atrophy, facilitation of formation of amyloid plaques and neurofibrillary tangles, white matter degeneration, and chronic neuroinflammation [74, 75].

A recent systematic review and meta-analysis that included data from 32 studies, involving more than two million individuals, showed that head injury increased the risk of dementia by 63% (RR 1.63, 95% CI 0.67–1.27) and AD by 51% (RR 1.51, 95% CI 1.26–1.80) [72]. A recent cohort study, including nearly 180,000 veterans with TBI, found that even mild TBI without LOC increased the risk of dementia by a factor of 2.4 (HR 2.36, 95% CI 2.10–2.66) [71], while moderate to severe TBI increased risk by a factor of 3.8 (HR 3.77, 95%CI 3.63–3.91) [71]. Not all studies have detected a relationship between TBI severity and dementia risk [72]. Other studies have suggested a higher risk of dementia in male subjects [76] or ApoEε4 carriers [77] who experience TBI.

4 Diet

Many different approaches, for example, altering dietary patterns, medical foods, nutraceutical supplementation, and dietary macro- and micronutrients, have been used to study the effects of diet in preventing or slowing cognitive decline. These strategies are predicted to have few side effects [78]. We shall focus on approaches supported by some scientific evidence.

The best-studied dietary pattern is the Mediterranean diet (Med-diet), the main components of which are fruits, vegetables, legumes, cereals, and olive oil, together with moderate consumption of red wine and low consumption of red meat and dairy products. The Med-diet has been associated with reduced risk of cognitive impairment, MCI, and AD, and reduced progression of MCI to AD [79–82]. A variant involving either mixed nuts or extra virgin olive oil (EVOO) has been compared with a standard diet, coupled with advice to limit fat, in a randomized controlled trial (RCT) [83]. The Med-diet with mixed nuts led to an improvement on a memory composite score, while the Med-diet with EVOO yielded better episodic memory and attention and improvement in frontal and global cognition composite scores [83]. The Dietary Approach to Stop Hypertension (DASH) and the Mediterranean-DASH diet Intervention for Neurodegenerative Delay (MIND) diets were associated with lower rates of cognitive decline and reduction in AD rates [81]. These diets were thought to work via a plant-based antioxidant effect [84]. EVOO and nuts contain phenolic compounds with antioxidant effects that prevent neurodegeneration in animal models [85], increase synthesis of neurotrophic factors, stimulate neurogenesis, and modulate neuronal signaling [86]. EVOO also contains n-3 fatty polyunsaturated fatty acids (PUFAs), the potential effects of which are described below [78].

PUFAs are one of the most well-studied macronutrients for prevention of cognitive decline. Long-chain (LC) PUFAs include docosahexaenoic acid (DHA), eicosapentaenoic acid (EPA), and arachidonic acid (ARA) [87]. Populations with high intake of fish, monounsaturated fatty acids, and LC PUFAs have a lower risk of cognitive decline [88]. Dietary supplementation with n-3 PUFAs has been shown in RCTs

to improved executive function, letter fluency, immediate and long-delay free recall, spatial and nonspatial working memory, white matter microstructural integrity, regional gray matter volume (including left hippocampus and precuneus), and electroencephalographic P300 latency [89–93]. PUFAs are important components of neural cell membrane phospholipids. PUFAs increase the effects of antioxidative enzymes, which protect against oxidative stress and reduce neuronal death and the formation and aggregation of Aβ [94] (see also Chapter 3). PUFAs also have anti-inflammatory effects [95].

Polyphenols, including flavonoids, found in berries, grapes, and red wine; curcumin from turmeric; and resveratrol from grapes and red wine [78] have been found to have beneficial effects on declarative and spatial memory, episodic memory, working memory, executive function, and immediate and delayed recall. They also have been found on functional MRI studies [92, 96–100] to increase functional connectivity between the hippocampus and frontal, parietal, and occipital areas, and to enhance cerebral blood volume (a surrogate measure of synaptic density) in the dentate gyrus [96]. The dentate gyrus is involved in pattern separation.

Multidomain approaches to prevention of cognitive decline include diet, exercise, vascular risk factor reduction, and cognitive training [78]. The Finnish Geriatric Intervention Study to Prevent Cognitive Impairment and Disability (FINGER) was a 2-year multidomain lifestyle intervention involving 631 participants in the intervention and 629 in the control group, all aged 60–77 years at baseline [101]. The intervention resulted after 2 years in a mean change in neuropsychological battery Z scores of 0.2 in the intervention group and 0.16 in the control group [101]. These intriguing findings suggested that a multidomain intervention could improve or maintain cognitive functioning in at-risk older people. Perhaps more importantly, this study raised the possibility that attending to these lifestyle factors earlier in life, especially in midlife, when AD pathology first emerges, could have an even greater benefit.

There have also been studies of dietary intervention to prevent cognitive decline with negative findings [78]. These studies are characterized by great heterogeneity in study samples, study duration, and type of intervention. Thus, it is not possible to draw simple conclusions on the efficacy of dietary approaches, in general, in preventing dementia, much less the best dietary approach. Further, in many places in the world (notably, in the countries surrounding the Mediterranean Sea), the effects of diet are conflated with the effects of regular exercise (walking to purchase food every day), social interactions, and physical exercise associated with work (e.g., fishing and farming).

5 Vascular Disease: Hypertension, Diabetes Mellitus, and Obesity

Midlife hypertension is a risk factor for dementia, including VaD/VCI and AD [102]. Hypertension is estimated to account for 2% of all dementias [3]. Potential mechanisms include disturbances of cerebral circulatory regulation, reduction of vascular reserve, and promotion of ischemic injury [103]. Such disturbances have also been proposed to contribute to accumulation of vascular amyloid, thereby potentiating the development of amyloid angiopathy [104]. Hypertension also causes white matter disease, micro-infarcts, and micro-hemorrhages, all of which contribute to cognitive impairment [105, 106]. In addition, vascular damage appears to be additive to the pathology of AD in causing clinical dementia. In the Religious Orders Study, over 50% of the autopsy-diagnosed cases of AD also had significant vascular pathology, whereas only 25% had exclusively AD pathology. It remains uncertain whether treatment with antihypertensive drugs can reduce the risk of dementia [102], although meta-analyses have demonstrated a strong trend toward reduction in the risk of dementia by 13% (HR 0.87, 95% CI 0.76–1.00) [107]. Another meta-analysis also demonstrated a reduction in cognitive decline in treated subjects by an adjusted mean difference of 0.42 (95% CI 0.30–0.53) [108].

Obesity is associated with insulin resistance, pre-diabetes, and diabetes mellitus (DM). DM is a risk factor for dementia and AD [3]. Insulin-degrading enzyme (IDE) metabolizes both insulin and Aβ. Thus, increased insulin associated with insulin resistance, by competing with Aβ at IDE sites, reduces the breakdown and clearance of Aβ [109]. Insulin resistance also increases the activity of glycogen synthase kinase-3 (GSK3), which in turn increases the phosphorylation of tau, thereby stimulating formation of neurofibrillary tangles (NFT) [109]. Chronic hyperglycemia reduces the expression of the blood–brain barrier glucose transporter, possibly resulting in reduced central nervous system glycolysis and ATP production

and affecting both neuronal and astrocytic function [109]. Obesity and diabetes both stimulate a pro-inflammatory environment within the body, which can activate microglial cells and promote oxidative stress [109]. It remains to be confirmed whether regular physical exercise, by reducing obesity, prediabetes, or DM itself, can reduce the risk of dementia. A number of ongoing clinical trials are seeking to determine whether some diabetic medications, including intranasal insulin, can reduce the risk of progression from MCI to dementia [110].

6 Issues Related to Ongoing and Future Clinical Trials

Apart from targeting modifiable risk factors, it is possible to target the underlying pathophysiological mechanisms of dementia in asymptomatic subjects (Figure 19.2). AD is the best-studied dementia in this regard. A number of potential medications have been tested in clinical trials or are in the planning phase. These therapeutic interventions include drugs targeting amyloid accumulation (e.g., antibodies such as solanezumab and gantenerumab) [111], reducing amyloid production (e.g., the beta secretase inhibitor atabecestat) [112], suppressing oxidative stress (e.g., nonsteroidal anti-inflammatory agents [113], selenium, and vitamin E [114]), and targeting insulin resistance (e.g., pioglitazone) [115]. Unfortunately, none of the agents so far tested has been found to be effective. These studies have, however, taught us important lessons for future clinical trials bearing on (1) choice of potential medications, (2) safety of potential medications, (3) patient groups that should be targeted, and (4) study design and sample size estimation.

It is now known that the amyloid plaques of AD begin to develop 20 or more years before the emergence of clinical symptoms, so it is logical to consider the use of potentially preventive medications or interventions in clinically asymptomatic subjects [8]. However, since only a relatively small proportion of cognitively normal individuals will eventually develop MCI or AD (Table 19.1), without the ability to select subjects at higher risk, a sample size of several thousand subjects would be needed for a prevention study in AD, together with a sufficiently long follow-up time to allow adequate numbers of AD cases to emerge (Table 19.2). The long follow-up required presents difficulties in adherence to the experimental

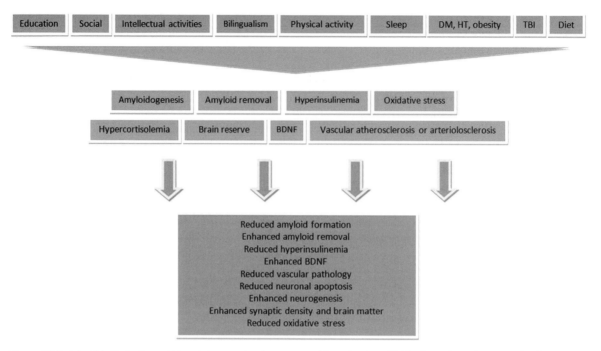

Figure 19.2 Potential effects of a multidomain interventional strategy on AD mechanisms. BDNF = brain-derived neurotrophic factor; DM = diabetes mellitus; HT = hypertension; TBI = traumatic brain injury.

medications, especially if the route of administration is anything but oral. Drop-out rates in such studies typically approach 30%. Because the medications will be administered to healthy subjects, they must have minimal side effects. This will be true even if the population is selected for higher risk of AD than the general population – for example, people with the APOEε4 allele. Unexpected risks in such trials may emerge. For example, the atabecestat trial had to be stopped because of a high incidence of hepatic injury [112], and the gamma-secretase inhibitors caused skin tumors.

Studies can be enriched by recruiting high-risk subjects, thereby reducing the sample size required. For AD clinical trials, such risks include older age, positive family history [113], heterozygosity or homozygosity for the APOEε4 allele [112], a positive Aβ-PET scan [116], and a CSF "AD profile" (low Aβ, high tau, and high phosphorylated-tau [112]). However, while studies restricted to higher risk participants can achieve greater efficiency and reduce the total time needed to determine whether an intervention works, response rates in subsequent studies of more broadly representative populations may be lower because of the greater heterogeneity of these

populations. Volunteer participants usually have broader knowledge of the disease and may have healthier lifestyles than the general population. Participants selected for higher risk or from specialty clinics may not be representative, and the results of a successful intervention in a large clinical trial involving such participants may not be translatable to the general population. Clinical trials are very costly, even when restricted to higher-risk populations. This has dampened the enthusiasm of the pharmaceutical industry, engendering the notion that neurodegenerative diseases pose insurmountable challenges. At least one major company has withdrawn from studies in AD and Parkinson's disease after a several-billion-dollar investment.

There must be strong preclinical data on both safety and efficacy to justify initiation of clinical trials. There must also be clear evidence of engagement with the expected molecular target and adequate information on appropriate dosing [117]. A double-blind, randomized controlled design is essential. Assessment instruments must be sensitive enough to detect changes in cognitive status, even among initially clinically normal subjects. Trials must be powered to enable robust statistical testing of a priori hypotheses

Table 19.1 Age-associated incidence of Alzheimer's disease according to natural history data

Age range	Bachman et al. (1993), Framingham (n = 2,117)	Incidence (%/year) Hebert et al. (1995), East Boston Study (n = 2,313)	Kawas et al. (2000), Baltimore Longitudinal Study of Aging (n = 1,236)	Average (%/year)
65–69	0.5	0.6	0.1	0.4
70–74	1.6	1.0	0.4	1.0
75–79	3.0	2.0	0.9	2.0
80–84	5.4	3.3	2.2	3.6
> 85	7.3	8.4	6.5	7.4

Table 19.2 Estimated sample size requirement using alpha value of 0.05, two-tailed $p < 0.05$ with 80% power of detecting difference in outcome

Treatment effect (% reduction from placebo)	Incidence in placebo group 5.0%	7.5%	10.0%
50%	2,000	1,300	950
40%	3,200	2,100	1,550
30%	6,000	4,000	3,000
20%	14,000	9,000	6,660

bearing on clinical outcomes and biomarkers. The statistical analyses must be adjusted for multiple outcomes if such are proposed [63]. Anticholinergic medications must be excluded as they can impair cognition [118]. Further, the experimental medication must not have significant anticholinergic effects [4]. Finally, from previous neuropathological studies, it is known that elderly patients, even if asymptomatic, are likely to have multiple pathologies that may contribute to future cognitive decline. These may include AD pathologies (amyloid plaques and NFT), as well as vascular pathology and synucleinopathy [119]. Among autopsied cases without cognitive impairment, there was evidence of mixed pathology in 9.4%; the corresponding figure among MCI subjects was 19.4% [119]. Current strategies for potential disease-modifying agents target one particular mechanism of neurodegeneration; that may render them less effective than desired. Combinations of various preventive medications, as used in cancer and heart disease, must be tested in future. Since it is difficult and time consuming to recruit an entirely new cohort

for a subsequent clinical trial testing another strategy (which would also take several more years to complete while the AD epidemic is continuing to expand), it will be important to consider using prespecified adaptive study designs that anticipate the advent of new data during the conduct of a study [116], or adding new treatment or endpoints to existing treatment trials [114].

In summary, future clinical trials face many obstacles. However, despite the financial costs and difficulties, such trials are vital to finding potentially useful preventive strategies for AD. Table 19.3 summarizes the current ongoing AD prevention trials.

7 Conclusions

At the moment, there are no clinically useful treatments available for AD that modify the long-term course of the disease. Research on potential ways to prevent dementia remains vital. Current evidence supports a number of nonspecific preventive strategies, including encouraging education, increasing

Table 19.3 Summary of current clinical prevention trials

Names of the trials (target number of subjects)	Target group	Medications/ interventions used	Primary outcome measures
DIAN-TU (n = 438) [111]	Individuals with known PSEN1, PSEN2, or APP mutation; age within 15 years before to 10 years after the affected parent's age of onset; cognitively normal or with MCI or mild dementia (CDR 0-1)	Gantenerumab, solaneuzumab, atabecestat[a]	DIAN-TU cognitive composite score (weeks 52, 104, 156, and 208)
Alzheimer Prevention Initiative (API) (n = 252) [120]	Individuals carrying the PSEN1 E280A mutation; MMSE ≥ 24 if < 9 years of education or ≥ 24 if with ≥ 9 years of education; without any evidence of cognitive impairment	Crenezumab	API Autosomal-Dominant Alzheimer's Disease composite cognitive test total score at week 260
Anti-Amyloid Treatment in Asymptomatic Alzheimer's Disease (A4) trial (n = 1,150) [116]	Subjects between 65 and 85 years old; MMSE 25–30; CDR = 0; Logical Memory II score 6–18; AV45 demonstrated amyloid positivity	Solanezumab	Change from baseline of the ADCS Pre-clinical Alzheimer Cognitive Composite
Aerobic Exercise for Older Adults at Increased Risk of Alzheimer's Disease and Related Dementias BIMII (n = 264) [121]	Inactive (defined by physical activity questionnaire), aged 50–80, subjective cognitive impairment and ≥ 1 vascular risk factor (HT, DM, obesity, hyperlipidemia, current smoking, and history of CAD without symptoms in past 5 years)	Supervised 6-month aerobic (walk/ jog) training 3 days per week; control group with stretching and toning without aerobic exercise	Change in cognition assessed by the neuropsychological test battery at 6 months and follow-up at 18 months
Exercise in Adults with Mild Memory Problems (EXERT) (n = 300)	65–89 years old, MMSE ≥ 24 (with ≥ 13 years of education) or ≥ 22 (< 13 years of education), CDR = 0.5, impaired delayed verbal recall, sedentary or underactive as determined by survey assessment	Moderate/high intensity aerobic exercise (training with up to 70–80% of heart rate reserve for 30 minutes) twice per week for 12 months; control intervention: stretching, or balance or range of motion program with exercise < 35% of heart rate reserve for 30 minutes	Cognitive function composite score at 12 months

ADCS = Alzheimer's Disease Cooperative Study; AV45 = florbetapir; BIMII = Aerobic Exercise for Older Adults at Increased Risk of Alzheimer's Disease and Related Dementias; CAD = coronary artery disease; CDR = Clinical Dementia Rating; DIAN-TU = Dominantly Inherited Alzheimer Network Trial: An opportunity to prevent dementia; DM = diabetes mellitus; HT = hypertension; MCI = mild cognitive impairment; MMSE = Mini-Mental State Examination; PSEN1 = Presenilin 1; PSEN2 = Presenilin 2
[a] Currently not in active recruitment because of risk of liver injury.

challenging leisure activities, learning more than one language, avoiding head injuries, maintaining good sleep habits, making healthy dietary choices, and aggressively treating cardiovascular risk factors.

Population health recommendations such as these, initiated in midlife, may aid in decreasing the burden of dementia in the future, until effective preventive as well as disease-modifying medications are developed.

References

1. Mukadam N LG. Reducing the stigma associated with dementia: approaches and goals. *Aging Health*. 2012;8:377–86.

2. Association AP. *Diagnostic and Statistical Manual of Mental Disorders* (DSM-5). Washington, DC: American Psychiatric Publishing; 2013.

3. Livingston G, Sommerlad A, Orgeta V, Costafreda SG, Huntley J, Ames D, et al. Dementia prevention, intervention, and care. *Lancet*. 2017;390 (10113):2673–734.

4. Salthouse T. *Major Issues in Cognitive Aging*. New York: Oxford University Press; 2010.

5. Alzheimer's Disease International. World Alzheimer Report 2016. Available from www.alz.co.uk/ research/world-report-2016.

6. Deb A, Thornton JD, Sambamoorthi U, Innes K. Direct and indirect cost of managing Alzheimer's disease and related dementias in the United States. *Expert Rev Pharmacoecon Outcomes Res*. 2017;17 (2):189–202.

7. Johnson KA, Minoshima S, Bohnen NI, Donohoe KJ, Foster NL, Herscovitch P, et al. Appropriate use criteria for amyloid PET: a report of the Amyloid Imaging Task Force, the Society of Nuclear Medicine and Molecular Imaging, and the Alzheimer's Association. *Alzheimers Dement*. 2013;9(1): e1–e16.

8. Jansen WJ, Ossenkoppele R, Knol DL, Tijms BM, Scheltens P, Verhey FR, et al. Prevalence of cerebral amyloid pathology in persons without dementia: a meta-analysis. *JAMA*. 2015;313 (19):1924–38.

9. Doody RS, Thomas RG, Farlow M, Iwatsubo T, Vellas B, Joffe S, et al. Phase 3 trials of solanezumab for mild-to-moderate Alzheimer's disease. *N Engl J Med*. 2014;370 (4):311–21.

10. Egan MF, Kost J, Tariot PN, Aisen PS, Cummings JL, Vellas B, et al. Randomized trial of verubecestat for mild-to-moderate Alzheimer's disease. *N Engl J Med*. 2018;378 (18):1691–703.

11. Honig LS, Vellas B, Woodward M, Boada M, Bullock R, Borrie M, et al. Trial of solanezumab for mild dementia due to Alzheimer's disease. *N Engl J Med*. 2018;378 (4):321–30.

12. Salloway S, Sperling R, Fox NC, Blennow K, Klunk W, Raskind M, et al. Two phase 3 trials of bapineuzumab in mild-to-moderate Alzheimer's disease. *N Engl J Med*. 2014;370(4):322–33.

13. Brookmeyer R, Gray S, Kawas C. Projections of Alzheimer's disease in the United States and the public health impact of delaying disease onset. *Am J Public Health*. 1998;88 (9):1337–42.

14. Schelke MW, Attia P, Palenchar DJ, Kaplan B, Mureb M, Ganzer CA, et al. Mechanisms of risk reduction in the clinical practice of Alzheimer's disease prevention. *Front Aging Neurosci*. 2018;10:96.

15. Ott A, van Rossum CT, van Harskamp F, van de Mheen H, Hofman A, Breteler MM. Education and the incidence of dementia in a large population-based study: the Rotterdam Study. *Neurology*. 1999;52(3):663–6.

16. Qiu C, Backman L, Winblad B, Aguero-Torres H, Fratiglioni L. The influence of education on clinically diagnosed dementia incidence and mortality data from the Kungsholmen Project. *Arch Neurol*. 2001;58(12):2034–9.

17. Langa KM, Larson EB, Crimmins EM, Faul JD, Levine DA, Kabeto MU, et al. A comparison of the prevalence of dementia in the United States in 2000 and 2012. *JAMA Intern Med*. 2017;177 (1):51–8.

18. Langa KM, Larson EB, Karlawish JH, Cutler DM, Kabeto MU, Kim SY, et al. Trends in the prevalence and mortality of cognitive impairment in the United States: is there evidence of a compression of cognitive morbidity? *Alzheimers Dement*. 2008;4 (2):134–44.

19. Manton KC, Gu XL, Ukraintseva SV. Declining prevalence of dementia in the U.S. elderly population. *Adv Gerontol*. 2005;16:30–7.

20. Qiu C, von Strauss E, Backman L, Winblad B, Fratiglioni L. Twenty-year changes in dementia occurrence suggest decreasing incidence in central Stockholm, Sweden. *Neurology*. 2013;80 (20):1888–94.

21. Satizabal CL, Beiser AS, Chouraki V, Chene G, Dufouil C, Seshadri S. Incidence of dementia over three decades in the Framingham Heart Study. *N Engl J Med*. 2016;374(6):523–32.

22. Schrijvers EM, Verhaaren BF, Koudstaal PJ, Hofman A, Ikram MA, Breteler MM. Is dementia incidence declining? Trends in dementia incidence since 1990 in the Rotterdam Study. *Neurology*. 2012;78(19):1456–63.

23. Chan KY, Wang W, Wu JJ, Liu L, Theodoratou E, Car J, et al.

Epidemiology of Alzheimer's disease and other forms of dementia in China, 1990–2010: a systematic review and analysis. *Lancet*. 2013;381(9882):2016–23.

24. Dodge HH, Buracchio TJ, Fisher GG, Kiyohara Y, Meguro K, Tanizaki Y, et al. Trends in the prevalence of dementia in Japan. *Int J Alzheimers Dis*. 2012;2012:956354.

25. Okamura H, Ishii S, Ishii T, Eboshida A. Prevalence of dementia in Japan: a systematic review. *Dement Geriatr Cogn Disord*. 2013;36(1–2):111–18.

26. Valenzuela MJ. Brain reserve and the prevention of dementia. *Curr Opin Psychiatry*. 2008;21 (3):296–302.

27. Meng X, D'Arcy C. Education and dementia in the context of the cognitive reserve hypothesis: a systematic review with meta-analyses and qualitative analyses. *PLoS ONE*. 2012;7(6):e38268.

28. Akbaraly TN, Portet F, Fustinoni S, Dartigues JF, Artero S, Rouaud O, et al. Leisure activities and the risk of dementia in the elderly: results from the Three-City Study. *Neurology*. 2009;73(11):854–61.

29. Karp A, Paillard-Borg S, Wang HX, Silverstein M, Winblad B, Fratiglioni L. Mental, physical and social components in leisure activities equally contribute to decrease dementia risk. *Dement Geriatr Cogn Disord*. 2006;21 (2):65–73.

30. Lee ATC, Richards M, Chan WC, Chiu HFK, Lee RSY, Lam LCW. Association of daily intellectual activities with lower risk of incident dementia among older Chinese adults. *JAMA Psychiatry*. 2018;75(7):697–703.

31. Paillard-Borg S, Fratiglioni L, Winblad B, Wang HX. Leisure activities in late life in relation to dementia risk: principal component analysis. *Dement Geriatr Cogn Disord*. 2009;28 (2):136–44.

32. Paillard-Borg S, Fratiglioni L, Xu W, Winblad B, Wang HX. An active lifestyle postpones dementia onset by more than one year in very old adults. *J Alzheimers Dis*. 2012;31(4):835–42.

33. Valenzuela M, Brayne C, Sachdev P, Wilcock G, Matthews F, Medical Research Council Cognitive Function and Ageing Study. Cognitive lifestyle and long-term risk of dementia and survival after diagnosis in a multicenter population-based cohort. *Am J Epidemiol*. 2011;173 (9):1004–12.

34. Verghese J, Lipton RB, Katz MJ, Hall CB, Derby CA, Kuslansky G, et al. Leisure activities and the risk of dementia in the elderly. *N Engl J Med*. 2003;348 (25):2508–16.

35. Wilson RS, Bennett DA, Bienias JL, Aggarwal NT, Mendes De Leon CF, Morris MC, et al. Cognitive activity and incident AD in a population-based sample of older persons. *Neurology*. 2002;59(12):1910–14.

36. Wilson RS, Mendes De Leon CF, Barnes LL, Schneider JA, Bienias JL, Evans DA, et al. Participation in cognitively stimulating activities and risk of incident Alzheimer disease. *JAMA*. 2002;287(6):742–8.

37. Yates LA, Ziser S, Spector A, Orrell M. Cognitive leisure activities and future risk of cognitive impairment and dementia: systematic review and meta-analysis. *Int Psychogeriatr*. 2016;28(11):1791–806.

38. Yang YC, Boen C, Gerken K, Li T, Schorpp K, Harris KM. Social relationships and physiological determinants of longevity across the human life span. *Proc Natl Acad Sci U S A*. 2016;113 (3):578–83.

39. Hemingway H, Marmot M. Evidence based cardiology: psychosocial factors in the aetiology and prognosis of coronary heart disease. Systematic review of prospective cohort studies. *BMJ*. 1999;318 (7196):1460–7.

40. Calvo N, Garcia AM, Manoiloff L, Ibanez A. Bilingualism and cognitive reserve: a critical overview and a plea for methodological innovations. *Front Aging Neurosci*. 2015;7:249.

41. Perani D, Abutalebi J. Bilingualism, dementia, cognitive and neural reserve. *Curr Opin Neurol*. 2015;28(6):618–25.

42. Craik FI, Bialystok E, Freedman M. Delaying the onset of Alzheimer disease: bilingualism as a form of cognitive reserve. *Neurology*. 2010;75(19):1726–9.

43. Alladi S, Bak TH, Duggirala V, Surampudi B, Shailaja M, Shukla AK, et al. Bilingualism delays age at onset of dementia, independent of education and immigration status. *Neurology*. 2013;81 (22):1938–44.

44. Perani D, Farsad M, Ballarini T, Lubian F, Malpetti M, Fracchetti A, et al. The impact of bilingualism on brain reserve and metabolic connectivity in Alzheimer's dementia. *Proc Natl Acad Sci U S A*. 2017;114 (7):1690–5.

45. Estanga A, Ecay-Torres M, Ibanez A, Izagirre A, Villanua J, Garcia-Sebastian M, et al. Beneficial effect of bilingualism on Alzheimer's disease CSF biomarkers and cognition. *Neurobiol Aging*. 2017;50:144–51.

46. Bialystok E, Craik FI, Binns MA, Ossher L, Freedman M. Effects of bilingualism on the age of onset and progression of MCI and AD: evidence from executive function tests. *Neuropsychology*. 2014;28 (2):290–304.

47. Ossher L, Bialystok E, Craik FI, Murphy KJ, Troyer AK. The effect of bilingualism on amnestic mild cognitive impairment. *J Gerontol B Psychol Sci Soc Sci*. 2013;68 (1):8–12.

48. Abutalebi J, Canini M, Della Rosa PA, Green DW, Weekes BS. The neuroprotective effects of bilingualism upon the inferior parietal lobule: a structural neuroimaging study in aging Chinese bilinguals. *J Neurolinguistics*. 2015;33:3–13.

49. Grundy JG, Anderson JAE, Bialystok E. Neural correlates of cognitive processing in monolinguals and bilinguals. *Ann N Y Acad Sci*. 2017;1396 (1):183–201.

50. Hamer M, Chida Y. Physical activity and risk of neurodegenerative disease: a systematic review of prospective evidence. *Psychol Med*. 2009;39 (1):3–11.

51. Stephen R, Hongisto K, Solomon A, Lonnroos E. Physical activity and Alzheimer's disease: a systematic review. *J Gerontol A Biol Sci Med Sci*. 2017;72 (6):733–9.

52. Mora S, Cook N, Buring JE, Ridker PM, Lee IM. Physical activity and reduced risk of cardiovascular events: potential mediating mechanisms. *Circulation*. 2007;116 (19):2110–18.

53. Aune D, Norat T, Leitzmann M, Tonstad S, Vatten LJ. Physical activity and the risk of type 2 diabetes: a systematic review and dose-response meta-analysis. *Eur J Epidemiol*. 2015;30(7):529–42.

54. Almeida OP, Khan KM, Hankey GJ, Yeap BB, Golledge J, Flicker L. 150 minutes of vigorous physical activity per week predicts survival and successful ageing: a population-based 11-year longitudinal study of 12 201 older Australian men. *Br J Sports Med*. 2014;48(3):220–5.

55. Blake H, Mo P, Malik S, Thomas S. How effective are physical activity interventions for alleviating depressive symptoms in older people? A systematic review. *Clin Rehabil*. 2009;23 (10):873–87.

56. de Labra C, Guimaraes-Pinheiro C, Maseda A, Lorenzo T, Millan-Calenti JC. Effects of physical exercise interventions in frail older adults: a systematic review of randomized controlled trials. *BMC Geriatr*. 2015;15:154.

57. Yarrow JF, White LJ, McCoy SC, Borst SE. Training augments resistance exercise induced elevation of circulating brain derived neurotrophic factor (BDNF). *Neurosci Lett*. 2010;479 (2):161–5.

58. Wrann CD, White JP, Salogiannnis J, Laznik-Bogoslavski D, Wu J, Ma D, et al. Exercise induces hippocampal BDNF through a PGC-1alpha/FNDC5 pathway. *Cell Metab*. 2013;18(5):649–59.

59. Watson GS, Craft S. The role of insulin resistance in the pathogenesis of Alzheimer's disease: implications for treatment. *CNS Drugs*. 2003;17 (1):27–45.

60. Devi SA, Kiran TR. Regional responses in antioxidant system to exercise training and dietary vitamin E in aging rat brain. *Neurobiol Aging*. 2004;25 (4):501–8.

61. Somani SM, Husain K. Exercise training alters kinetics of antioxidant enzymes in rat tissues. *Biochem Mol Biol Int*. 1996;38 (3):587–95.

62. Proserpio P, Arnaldi D, Nobili F, Nobili L. Integrating sleep and Alzheimer's disease pathophysiology: hints for sleep disorders management. *J Alzheimers Dis*. 2018;63 (3):871–86.

63. Dmitrienko A, D'Agostino RB, Sr. Multiplicity considerations in clinical trials. *N Engl J Med*. 2018;378(22):2115–22.

64. Lucey BP, Gonzales C, Das U, Li J, Siemers ER, Slemmon JR, et al. An integrated multi-study analysis of intra-subject variability in cerebrospinal fluid amyloid-beta concentrations collected by lumbar puncture and indwelling lumbar catheter. *Alzheimers Res Ther*. 2015;7(1):53.

65. Xie L, Kang H, Xu Q, Chen MJ, Liao Y, Thiyagarajan M, et al. Sleep drives metabolite clearance from the adult brain. *Science*. 2013;342(6156):373–7.

66. Mander BA, Winer JR, Jagust WJ, Walker MP. Sleep: a novel mechanistic pathway, biomarker, and treatment target in the pathology of Alzheimer's disease? *Trends Neurosci*. 2016;39 (8):552–66.

67. Sprecher KE, Koscik RL, Carlsson CM, Zetterberg H, Blennow K, Okonkwo OC, et al. Poor sleep is associated with CSF biomarkers of amyloid pathology in cognitively normal adults. *Neurology*. 2017;89 (5):445–53.

68. Shokri-Kojori E, Wang GJ, Wiers CE, Demiral SB, Guo M, Kim SW, et al. Beta-amyloid accumulation in the human brain after one night of sleep deprivation. *Proc Natl Acad Sci U S A*. 2018;115 (17):4483–8.

69. Chan TT, Leung WC, Li V, Wong KW, Chu WM, Leung KC, et al. Association between high cumulative dose of benzodiazepine in Chinese patients and risk of dementia: a preliminary retrospective case-control study. *Psychogeriatrics*. 2017;17(5):310–16.

70. Penninkilampi R, Eslick GD. A systematic review and meta-analysis of the risk of dementia associated with benzodiazepine use, after controlling for protopathic bias. *CNS Drugs*. 2018;32(6):485–97.

71. Barnes DE, Byers AL, Gardner RC, Seal KH, Boscardin WJ, Yaffe K. Association of mild traumatic brain injury with and without loss of consciousness with dementia in US military veterans. *JAMA Neurol*. 2018;75 (9):1055–61.

72. Li Y, Li Y, Li X, Zhang S, Zhao J, Zhu X, et al. Head injury as a risk factor for dementia and Alzheimer's disease: a systematic review and meta-analysis of 32 observational studies. *PLoS ONE*. 2017;12(1):e0169650.

73. Defense Centers of Excellence for Psychological Health and Traumatic Brain Injury. Department of Defense coding guidance for traumatic brain injury fact sheet. Updated September 2010. Available from https://health.mil/About-MHS/Defense-Heath-Agency/Research-and-Development.

74. Abrahamson EE, Ikonomovic MD, Ciallella JR, Hope CE, Paljug WR, Isanski BA, et al. Caspase inhibition therapy abolishes brain trauma-induced increases in Abeta peptide: implications for clinical outcome. *Exp Neurol*. 2006;197(2):437–50.

75. DeKosky ST, Abrahamson EE, Ciallella JR, Paljug WR, Wisniewski SR, Clark RS, et al. Association of increased cortical soluble abeta42 levels with diffuse plaques after severe brain injury in humans. *Arch Neurol*. 2007;64(4):541–4.

76. Fleminger S, Oliver DL, Lovestone S, Rabe-Hesketh S, Giora A. Head injury as a risk factor for Alzheimer's disease: the evidence 10 years on; a partial replication. *J Neurol Neurosurg Psychiatry*. 2003;74(7):857–62.

77. Sundstrom A, Nilsson LG, Cruts M, Adolfsson R, Van Broeckhoven C, Nyberg L. Increased risk of dementia following mild head injury for carriers but not for non-carriers of the APOE epsilon4 allele. *Int Psychogeriatr*. 2007;19(1):159–65.

78. Solfrizzi V, Agosti P, Lozupone M, Custodero C, Schilardi A, Valiani V, et al. Nutritional intervention as a preventive approach for cognitive-related outcomes in cognitively healthy older adults: a systematic review. *J Alzheimers Dis*. 2018;64(s1):S229–S254.

79. Psaltopoulou T, Sergentanis TN, Panagiotakos DB, Sergentanis IN, Kosti R, Scarmeas N. Mediterranean diet, stroke, cognitive impairment, and depression: a meta-analysis. *Ann Neurol*. 2013;74(4):580–91.

80. Singh B, Parsaik AK, Mielke MM, Erwin PJ, Knopman DS, Petersen RC, et al. Association of Mediterranean diet with mild cognitive impairment and Alzheimer's disease: a systematic review and meta-analysis. *J Alzheimers Dis*. 2014;39(2):271–82.

81. Solfrizzi V, Custodero C, Lozupone M, Imbimbo BP, Valiani V, Agosti P, et al. Relationships of dietary patterns, foods, and micro- and macronutrients with Alzheimer's disease and late-life cognitive disorders: a systematic review. *J Alzheimers Dis*. 2017;59(3):815–49.

82. Lourida I, Soni M, Thompson-Coon J, Purandare N, Lang IA, Ukoumunne OC, et al. Mediterranean diet, cognitive function, and dementia: a systematic review. *Epidemiology*. 2013;24(4):479–89.

83. Valls-Pedret C, Sala-Vila A, Serra-Mir M, Corella D, de la Torre R, Martinez-Gonzalez MA, et al. Mediterranean diet and age-related cognitive decline: a randomized clinical trial. *JAMA Intern Med*. 2015;175(7):1094–103.

84. Sofi F, Abbate R, Gensini GF, Casini A. Accruing evidence on benefits of adherence to the Mediterranean diet on health: an updated systematic review and meta-analysis. *Am J Clin Nutr*. 2010;92(5):1189–96.

85. Bullo M, Lamuela-Raventos R, Salas-Salvado J. Mediterranean diet and oxidation: nuts and olive oil as important sources of fat and antioxidants. *Curr Top Med Chem*. 2011;11(14):1797–810.

86. Del Rio D, Rodriguez-Mateos A, Spencer JP, Tognolini M, Borges G, Crozier A. Dietary (poly) phenolics in human health: structures, bioavailability, and evidence of protective effects against chronic diseases. *Antioxid Redox Signal*. 2013;18(14):1818–92.

87. Janssen CI, Kiliaan AJ. Long-chain polyunsaturated fatty acids (LCPUFA) from genesis to senescence: the influence of LCPUFA on neural development, aging, and neurodegeneration. *Prog Lipid Res*. 2014;53:1–17.

88. Solfrizzi V, Frisardi V, Capurso C, D'Introno A, Colacicco AM, Vendemiale G, et al. Dietary fatty acids in dementia and predementia syndromes: epidemiological evidence and possible underlying mechanisms. *Ageing Res Rev*. 2010;9(2):184–99.

89. Jaremka LM, Derry HM, Bornstein R, Prakash RS, Peng J, Belury MA, et al. Omega-3 supplementation and loneliness-related memory problems: secondary analyses of a randomized controlled trial. *Psychosom Med*. 2014;76(8):650–8.

90. Pase MP, Grima N, Cockerell R, Stough C, Scholey A, Sali A, et al. The effects of long-chain omega-3 fish oils and multivitamins on cognitive and cardiovascular function: a randomized, controlled clinical trial. *J Am Coll Nutr*. 2015;34(1):21–31.

91. Tokuda H, Sueyasu T, Kontani M, Kawashima H, Shibata H, Koga Y. Low doses of long-chain polyunsaturated fatty acids affect cognitive function in elderly Japanese men: a randomized controlled trial. *J Oleo Sci*. 2015;64(6):633–44.

92. Witte AV, Kerti L, Hermannstadter HM, Fiebach JB,

Schreiber SJ, Schuchardt JP, et al. Long-chain omega-3 fatty acids improve brain function and structure in older adults. *Cereb Cortex*. 2014;24(11):3059–68.

93. Boespflug EL, McNamara RK, Eliassen JC, Schidler MD, Krikorian R. Fish oil supplementation increases event-related posterior cingulate activation in older adults with subjective memory impairment. *J Nutr Health Aging*. 2016;20 (2):161–9.

94. Pietinen P, Ascherio A, Korhonen P, Hartman AM, Willett WC, Albanes D, et al. Intake of fatty acids and risk of coronary heart disease in a cohort of Finnish men. The Alpha-Tocopherol, Beta-Carotene Cancer Prevention Study. *Am J Epidemiol*. 1997;145 (10):876–87.

95. Schaefer EJ, Bongard V, Beiser AS, Lamon-Fava S, Robins SJ, Au R, et al. Plasma phosphatidylcholine docosahexaenoic acid content and risk of dementia and Alzheimer disease: the Framingham Heart Study. *Arch Neurol*. 2006;63 (11):1545–50.

96. Brickman AM, Khan UA, Provenzano FA, Yeung LK, Suzuki W, Schroeter H, et al. Enhancing dentate gyrus function with dietary flavanols improves cognition in older adults. *Nat Neurosci*. 2014;17 (12):1798–803.

97. Kean RJ, Lamport DJ, Dodd GF, Freeman JE, Williams CM, Ellis JA, et al. Chronic consumption of flavanone-rich orange juice is associated with cognitive benefits: an 8-wk, randomized, double-blind, placebo-controlled trial in healthy older adults. *Am J Clin Nutr*. 2015;101(3):506–14.

98. Mastroiacovo D, Kwik-Uribe C, Grassi D, Necozione S, Raffaele A, Pistacchio L, et al. Cocoa flavanol consumption improves cognitive function, blood pressure control, and metabolic profile in elderly subjects: the Cocoa, Cognition, and Aging (CoCoA) Study – a randomized controlled trial. *Am J Clin Nutr*. 2015;101(3):538–48.

99. Nilsson A, Salo I, Plaza M, Bjorck I. Effects of a mixed berry beverage on cognitive functions and cardiometabolic risk markers; a randomized cross-over study in healthy older adults. *PLoS ONE*. 2017;12(11):e0188173.

100. Sarubbo F, Esteban S, Miralles A, Moranta D. Effects of resveratrol and other polyphenols on sirt1: relevance to brain function during aging. *Curr Neuropharmacol*. 2018;16(2):126–36.

101. Ngandu T, Lehtisalo J, Solomon A, Levalahti E, Ahtiluoto S, Antikainen R, et al. A 2 year multidomain intervention of diet, exercise, cognitive training, and vascular risk monitoring versus control to prevent cognitive decline in at-risk elderly people (FINGER): a randomised controlled trial. *Lancet*. 2015;385 (9984):2255–63.

102. Iadecola C. Hypertension and dementia. *Hypertension*. 2014;64 (1):3–5.

103. Pires PW, Dams Ramos CM, Matin N, Dorrance AM. The effects of hypertension on the cerebral circulation. *Am J Physiol Heart Circ Physiol*. 2013;304(12): H1598–H1614.

104. Park L, Zhou J, Zhou P, Pistick R, El Jamal S, Younkin L, et al. Innate immunity receptor CD36 promotes cerebral amyloid angiopathy. *Proc Natl Acad Sci U S A*. 2013;110(8):3089–94.

105. Faraco G, Iadecola C. Hypertension: a harbinger of stroke and dementia. *Hypertension*. 2013;62(5):810–17.

106. Iadecola C. The pathobiology of vascular dementia. *Neuron*. 2013;80(4):844–66.

107. McGuinness B, Todd S, Passmore P, Bullock R. Blood pressure lowering in patients without prior cerebrovascular disease for prevention of cognitive impairment and dementia. *Cochrane Database Syst Rev*. 2009 (4):CD004034.

108. Forette F, Seux ML, Staessen JA, Thijs L, Babarskiene MR, Babeanu S, et al. The prevention of dementia with antihypertensive treatment: new evidence from the Systolic Hypertension in Europe (Syst-Eur) study. *Arch Intern Med*. 2002;162(18):2046–52.

109. Riederer P, Korczyn AD, Ali SS, Bajenaru O, Choi MS, Chopp M, et al. The diabetic brain and cognition. *J Neural Transm (Vienna)*. 2017;124(11):1431–54.

110. Femminella GD, Bencivenga L, Petraglia L, Visaggi L, Gioia L, Grieco FV, et al. Antidiabetic drugs in Alzheimer's disease: mechanisms of action and future perspectives. *J Diabetes Res*. 2017;2017:7420796.

111. Bateman RJ, Benzinger TL, Berry S, Clifford DB, Duggan C, Fagan AM, et al. The DIAN-TU Next Generation Alzheimer's prevention trial: adaptive design and disease progression model. *Alzheimers Dement*. 2017;13 (1):8–19.

112. ClinicalTrials.gov. An Efficacy and Safety Study of Atabecestat in Participants Who Are Asymptomatic at Risk for Developing Alzheimer's Dementia (EARLY). 2015. Updated June 13, 2018. Available from https://clinicaltrials.gov/ct2/show/NCT02569398?term=JNJ-54861911.

113. Alzheimer's Disease Anti-inflammatory Prevention Trial Research G. Results of a follow-up study to the randomized Alzheimer's Disease Anti-inflammatory Prevention Trial (ADAPT). *Alzheimers Dement*. 2013;9(6):714–23.

114. Kryscio RJ, Abner EL, Caban-Holt A, Lovell M, Goodman P, Darke

AK, et al. Association of antioxidant supplement use and dementia in the Prevention of Alzheimer's Disease by Vitamin E and Selenium Trial (PREADViSE). *JAMA Neurol.* 2017;74(5):567–73.

115. ALZFORUM. There's no tomorrow for TOMMORROW. 2018. Updated January 25, 2018. Available from www.alzforum.org/news/research-news/theres-no-tomorrow-tommorrow#comment-26186.

116. ClinicalTrials.gov. Clinical trial of solanezumab for older individuals who may be at risk for memory loss (A4). 2013. Updated December 22, 2017. Available from https://clinicaltrials.gov/ct2/show/NCT02008357?term=A4+study&rank=1.

117. DeKosky ST, Williamson JD, Fitzpatrick AL, Kronmal RA, Ives DG, Saxton JA, et al. Ginkgo biloba for prevention of dementia: a randomized controlled trial. *JAMA*. 2008;300 (19):2253–62.

118. Fox C, Smith T, Maidment I, Chan WY, Bua N, Myint PK, et al. Effect of medications with anti-cholinergic properties on cognitive function, delirium, physical function and mortality: a systematic review. *Age Ageing.* 2014;43(5):604–15.

119. Schneider JA, Arvanitakis Z, Leurgans SE, Bennett DA. The neuropathology of probable Alzheimer disease and mild cognitive impairment. *Ann Neurol.* 2009;66(2):200–8.

120. ClinicalTrails.gov. A study of crenezumab versus placebo in preclinical presenilin1 (PSEN1) E280A mutation carriers to evaluate efficacy and safety in the treatment of autosomal-dominant Alzheimer's disease (AD), including a placebo-treated non-carrier cohort. 2013. Updated April 13, 2018. Available from https://clinicaltrials.gov/ct2/show/NCT01998841.

121. ClinicalTrails.gov. Aerobic exercise for older adults at increased risk of Alzheimer's disease and related dementias (BIMII). 2017. Updated January 16, 2018. Available from https://clinicaltrials.gov/ct2/show/NCT03035851?term=Prevention&recrs=ad&type=Intr&cond=Alzheimer%27s+disease&draw=2&rank=16.

Index